Spumaretroviruses

Spumaretroviruses

Editors

Arifa S. Khan
Dirk Lindemann
Martin Löchelt

MDPI • Basel • Beijing • Wuhan • Barcelona • Belgrade • Manchester • Tokyo • Cluj • Tianjin

Editors
Arifa S. Khan
Center for Biologics Research and Evaluation
USA

Dirk Lindemann
Technische Universität Dresden
Germany

Martin Löchelt
German Cancer Research Center (DKFZ)
Germany

Editorial Office
MDPI
St. Alban-Anlage 66
4052 Basel, Switzerland

This is a reprint of articles from the Special Issue published online in the open access journal *Viruses* (ISSN 1999-4915) (available at: https://www.mdpi.com/journal/viruses/special_issues/spumaretroviruses).

For citation purposes, cite each article independently as indicated on the article page online and as indicated below:

LastName, A.A.; LastName, B.B.; LastName, C.C. Article Title. *Journal Name* **Year**, *Volume Number*, Page Range.

ISBN 978-3-0365-0594-7 (Hbk)
ISBN 978-3-0365-0595-4 (PDF)

Contents

About the Editors . . . . **ix**

Preface to "Spumaretroviruses" . . . . **xi**

Ottmar Herchenröder, Martin Löchelt, Florence Buseyne, Antoine Gessain, Marcelo A. Soares, Arifa S. Khan and Dirk Lindemann
Twelfth International Foamy Virus Conference—Meeting Report
Reprinted from: *Viruses* **2019**, *11*, 134, doi:10.3390/v11020134 . . . . **1**

André F. Santos, Liliane T. F. Cavalcante, Cláudia P. Muniz, William M. Switzer and Marcelo A. Soares
Simian Foamy Viruses in Central and South America: A New World of Discovery
Reprinted from: *Viruses* **2019**, *11*, 967, doi:10.3390/v11100967 . . . . **13**

Sandra M. Fuentes, Eunhae H. Bae, Subhiksha Nandakumar, Dhanya K. Williams and Arifa S. Khan
Genome Analysis and Replication Studies of the African Green Monkey Simian Foamy Virus Serotype 3 Strain FV2014
Reprinted from: *Viruses* **2020**, *12*, 403, doi:10.3390/v12040403 . . . . **29**

Anupama Shankar, Samuel D. Sibley, Tony L. Goldberg and William M. Switzer
Molecular Analysis of the Complete Genome of a Simian Foamy Virus Infecting *Hylobates pileatus* (pileated gibbon) Reveals Ancient Co-Evolution with Lesser Apes
Reprinted from: *Viruses* **2019**, *11*, 605, doi:10.3390/v11070605 . . . . **45**

Pakorn Aiewsakun, Peter Simmonds and Aris Katzourakis
The First Co-Opted Endogenous Foamy Viruses and the Evolutionary History of Reptilian Foamy Viruses
Reprinted from: *Viruses* **2019**, *11*, 641, doi:10.3390/v11070641 . . . . **67**

Shannon M. Murray and Maxine L. Linial
Simian Foamy Virus Co-Infections
Reprinted from: *Viruses* **2019**, *11*, 902, doi:10.3390/v11100902 . . . . **85**

Thamiris S. Miranda, Cláudia P. Muniz, Silvia B. Moreira, Marina G. Bueno, Maria Cecília M. Kierulff, Camila V. Molina, José L. Catão-Dias, Alcides Pissinatti, Marcelo A. Soares and André F. Santos
Eco-Epidemiological Profile and Molecular Characterization of Simian Foamy Virus in a Recently-Captured Invasive Population of *Leontopithecus chrysomelas* (Golden-Headed Lion Tamarin) in Rio de Janeiro, Brazil
Reprinted from: *Viruses* **2019**, *11*, 931, doi:10.3390/v11100931 . . . . **95**

Magdalena Materniak-Kornas, Martin Löchelt, Jerzy Rola and Jacek Kuźmak
Infection with Foamy Virus in Wild Ruminants—Evidence for a New Virus Reservoir?
Reprinted from: *Viruses* **2020**, *12*, 58, doi:10.3390/v12010058 . . . . **109**

Rikio Kirisawa, Yuko Toishi, Hiromitsu Hashimoto and Nobuo Tsunoda
Isolation of an Equine Foamy Virus and Sero-Epidemiology of the Viral Infection in Horses in Japan
Reprinted from: *Viruses* **2019**, *11*, 613, doi:10.3390/v11070613 . . . . **125**

Sarah R. Kechejian, Nick Dannemiller, Simona Kraberger, Carmen Ledesma-Feliciano, Jennifer Malmberg, Melody Roelke Parker, Mark Cunningham, Roy McBride, Seth P. D. Riley, Winston T. Vickers, Ken Logan, Mat Alldredge, Kevin Crooks, Martin Löchelt, Scott Carver and Sue VandeWoude
Feline Foamy Virus is Highly Prevalent in Free-Ranging *Puma concolor* from Colorado, Florida and Southern California
Reprinted from: *Viruses* **2019**, *11*, 359, doi:10.3390/v11040359 . . . . **137**

Liliane T. F. Cavalcante, Cláudia P. Muniz, Hongwei Jia, Anderson M. Augusto, Fernando Troccoli, Sheila de O. Medeiros, Carlos G. A. Dias, William M. Switzer, Marcelo A. Soares and André F. Santos
Clinical and Molecular Features of Feline Foamy Virus and Feline Leukemia Virus Co-Infection in Naturally-Infected Cats
Reprinted from: *Viruses* **2018**, *10*, 702, doi:10.3390/v10120702 . . . . **147**

Carmen Ledesma-Feliciano, Ryan M. Troyer, Xin Zheng, Craig Miller, Rachel Cianciolo, Matteo Bordicchia, Nicholas Dannemiller, Roderick Gagne, Julia Beatty, Jessica Quimby, Martin Löchelt and Sue VandeWoude
Feline Foamy Virus Infection: Characterization of Experimental Infection and Prevalence of Natural Infection in Domestic Cats with and without Chronic Kidney Disease
Reprinted from: *Viruses* **2019**, *11*, 662, doi:10.3390/v11070662 . . . . **169**

Maïwenn Bergez, Jakob Weber, Maximilian Riess, Alexander Erdbeer, Janna Seifried, Nicole Stanke, Clara Munz, Veit Hornung, Renate König and Dirk Lindemann
Insights into Innate Sensing of Prototype Foamy Viruses in Myeloid Cells
Reprinted from: *Viruses* **2019**, *11*, 1095, doi:10.3390/v11121095 . . . . **191**

Wenhu Cao, Erik Stricker, Agnes Hotz-Wagenblatt, Anke Heit-Mondrzyk, Georgios Pougialis, Annette Hugo, Jacek Kuźmak, Magdalena Materniak-Kornas and Martin Löchelt
Functional Analyses of Bovine Foamy Virus-Encoded miRNAs Reveal the Importance of a Defined miRNA for Virus Replication and Host–Virus Interaction
Reprinted from: *Viruses* **2020**, *12*, 1250, doi:10.3390/v12111250 . . . . **211**

Magdalena Materniak-Kornas, Juan Tan, Anke Heit-Mondrzyk, Agnes Hotz-Wagenblatt and Martin Löchelt
Bovine Foamy Virus: Shared and Unique Molecular Features In Vitro and In Vivo
Reprinted from: *Viruses* **2019**, *11*, 1084, doi:10.3390/v11121084 . . . . **231**

Birgitta M. Wöhrl
Structural and Functional Aspects of Foamy Virus Protease-Reverse Transcriptase
Reprinted from: *Viruses* **2019**, *11*, 598, doi:10.3390/v11070598 . . . . **257**

Ga-Eun Lee, Eric Mauro, Vincent Parissi, Cha-Gyun Shin and Paul Lesbats
Structural Insights on Retroviral DNA Integration: Learning from Foamy Viruses
Reprinted from: *Viruses* **2019**, *11*, 770, doi:10.3390/v11090770 . . . . **275**

Suzhen Zhang, Xiaojuan Liu, Zhibin Liang, Tiejun Bing, Wentao Qiao and Juan Tan
The Influence of Envelope C-Terminus Amino Acid Composition on the Ratio of Cell-Free to Cell-Cell Transmission for Bovine Foamy Virus
Reprinted from: *Viruses* **2019**, *11*, 130, doi:10.3390/v11020130 . . . . **291**

Yogendra Singh Rajawat, Olivier Humbert and Hans-Peter Kiem
In-Vivo Gene Therapy with Foamy Virus Vectors
Reprinted from: *Viruses* **2019**, *11*, 1091, doi:10.3390/v11121091 . . . . **307**

About the Editors

Arifa S. Khan, Ph.D. is a Supervisory Microbiologist and Head, Molecular Retrovirology Unit, Division of Viral Product, Office of Vaccines Research and Review, Center for Biologics Evaluation and Research, U.S. Food and Drug Administration. She has broad retrovirus experience including in vivo and in vitro infections of simian foamy viruses, human and simian immunodeficiency viruses, murine leukemia viruses, and feline leukemia viruses. Her primary regulatory responsibilities include a safety review of viral vaccines and cell substrates for known and novel viruses that could be unintentionally introduced, including exogenous and endogenous viruses. The research program is focused on the development and standardization of advanced, sensitive and broad virus detection assays for adventitious virus detection in biologics such as high-throughput sequencing and investigating factors involved in cross-species transmission of retroviruses and virus–virus and virus–host interactions that result in human infections including simian foamy virus and HIV-1.

Dirk Lindemann, Ph.D. is a Professor of Molecular Virology at the Institute of Virology, Medical Faculty of the Technische Universität Dresden, in Dresden, Germany. He teaches classes in Virology for medical and biology students. His lab has a longstanding interest in the molecular and cell biology of various retroviruses. Research has strong focus on the molecular and cellular aspects of foamy virus replication, the interaction of these viruses with the host cell, including the innate immune system and intracellular trafficking networks. Furthermore, his lab develops novel or improved gene transfer systems based on different types of retroviruses, which in several cases, exploit some of the unique features of foamy viruses.

Martin Löchelt, Ph.D. is Professor of Molecular Virology at the Research Program Infection, Inflammation and Cancer, Division Viral Transformation Mechanisms, German Cancer Research Center (DKFZ), Heidelberg, Germany. He teaches at the Faculties for Medicine and Biosciences at Heidelberg University. His interests and research activities cover retroviral/spumaviral gene expression, particle assembly and release, pathogenicity including animal experimentation, host–virus interaction and co-evolution using in vitro selection screening, cellular restriction mechanisms and viral counter-defense, and vaccine vector development including replication-competent engineered foamy viruses. In addition, he studies infection- and inflammation-induced oncogenesis via APOBEC3 cytidine deaminases.

Preface to "Spumaretroviruses"

As this is being written, we are in the midst of the coronavirus disease 2019 (COVID-19) pandemic, with millions of deaths occurring throughout the world [1]. This reminds us again of the great impact of zoonoses and the importance of research in this area for protecting the human population against zoonotic diseases. Many of the past pandemics, most notably influenza in 1918, and recent outbreaks in the 21st century, such as influenza and Ebola, have been due to the transmission of RNA viruses from domestic and wild animals. Another example is the human immunodeficiency virus type 1 (HIV-1) retrovirus, responsible for the ongoing global AIDS/HIV-1 epidemic. HIV-1 arose by cross-species transmission of a simian immunodeficiency virus (SIV) from nonhuman primates [2]. It should be noted that zoonotic transmission of simian foamy viruses (SFVs), which belong to the distinct retrovirus subfamily Spumaretrovirinae [3], is currently occurring from infected nonhuman primates to humans, although the number of cases reported is still low [4]. Fortunately, SFV infections are latent, and there is no evidence of human-to-human transmission [5, 6], although there seems to be high transmission between nonhuman primates (since SFVs are widely prevalent in all nonhuman primate species). At present, there is no clear evidence that FVs on their own are associated with disease in zoonotically infected humans or in their natural hosts, which includes simians, bovines, equines, caprines, and felines, or upon transmissions between related animal species [4, 7]. However, FVs may be co-factors in other retroviral infections [7, 8] and could exacerbate the pathogenesis of some viruses in case of co-infections [9]. Thus, diverse FVs can be good models to further our understanding of zoonotic transmission and to develop mitigation strategies against cross-species infections.

This Special Issue provides a collection of reviews and research articles presenting recent perspectives and progress in spumaretrovirus research to continue updating our understanding of the FV biology and virus–host interactions that could provide insights for addressing potential concerns related to human infections that may emerge. Additionally, the unique properties of FVs, that places them in the separate retrovirus subfamily of Spumaretrovirinae, have led researchers to develop them as gene therapy vectors and to use endogenous FV sequences for studies on host species evolution/co-evolution and virus–host co-adaptation. The content of this Special Issue includes reviews and research articles on SFVs of Old World and New World nonhuman primates and nonprimate FVs from bovine, caprine, equine, and feline hosts.

The contributions to this Special Issue on "Spumaretroviruses" start with the meeting report of the "Twelfth International Foamy Virus Conference" held in Dresden, Germany, in 2018. We then continue with papers related to genomes and evolution, which include a review on SFVs from the New World, two reports concerning whole genome characterization of SFV isolates from Old World monkeys, and description of ancient, endogenous FVs from reptiles and the importance of the env gene for potential host function. The next collection of papers describes naturally occurring and experimental FV infections and co-infections of their native hosts like simians, equines, and felines. In addition, the potential contribution of FVs to complex disease syndromes is discussed. The following two articles are related to host–virus interactions in innate immunity and host gene expression upon FV infection. The next set of papers includes three reviews and one research paper on the overall molecular biology of FVs as well as specialized topics including FV reverse transcription, integration, virus transmission, and particle release. Additionally, we refer you to a recent review on FV assembly and release [10]. The final two papers in this Special Issue are reviews related to general FV vector development in vivo and to new strategies targeting blood stem cells.

This Special Issue provides key areas of scientific development and technological advancements in spumaretroviruses, which we hope will be a knowledge base for further research to gain insights into understanding the virus–host balance controlling human infections.

Acknowledgements: We thank the authors for their contributions to the Special Issue "Spumaretroviruses". We acknowledge all of the Editorial Office team from Viruses for providing administrative support and all reviewers involved in the peer review process.

References

1. Morens, D.M.; Daszak, P.; Markel, H.; Taubenberger, J.K. Pandemic COVID-19 Joins History's Pandemic Legion. *mBio* **2020**, *11*.

2. Sharp, P.M.; Hahn, B.H., Origins of HIV and the AIDS pandemic. *Cold Spring Harb. Perspect. Med.* **2011**, *1*, a006841.

3. Khan, A.S.; Bodem, J.; Buseyne, F.; Gessain, A.; Johnson, W.; Kuhn, J.H.; Kuzmak, J.; Lindemann, D.; Linial, M.L.; Lochelt, M.; et al. Spumaretroviruses: Updated taxonomy and nomenclature. *Virology* **2018**, *516*, 158–164.

4. Pinto-Santini, D.M.; Stenbak, C.R.; Linial, M.L. Foamy virus zoonotic infections. *Retrovirology* **2017**, *14*, 55.

5. Rua, R.; Gessain, A. Origin, evolution and innate immune control of simian foamy viruses in humans. *Curr. Opin. Virol.* **2015**, *10*, 47–55.

6. Lambert, C.; Batalie, D.; Montange, T.; Betsem, E.; Mouinga-Ondeme, A.; Njouom, R.; Gessain, A.; Buseyne, F. An Immunodominant and Conserved B-Cell Epitope in the Envelope of Simian Foamy Virus Recognized by Humans Infected with Zoonotic Strains from Apes. *J .Virol.* **2019**, *93*.

7. Materniak-Kornas, M.; Tan, J.; Heit-Mondrzyk, A.; Hotz-Wagenblatt, A.; Lochelt, M. Bovine Foamy Virus: Shared and Unique Molecular Features In Vitro and In Vivo. *Viruses* **2019**, *11*.

8. Cavalcante, L.T.F.; Muniz, C.P.; Jia, H.; Augusto, A.M.; Troccoli, F.; Medeiros, S.O.; Dias, C.G.A.; Switzer, W.M.; Soares, M.A.; Santos, A.F. Clinical and Molecular Features of Feline Foamy Virus and Feline Leukemia Virus Co-Infection in Naturally-Infected Cats. *Viruses* **2018**, *10*.

9. Choudhary, A.; Galvin, T.A.; Williams, D.K.; Beren, J.; Bryant, M.A.; Khan, A. S. Influence of naturally occurring simian foamy viruses (SFVs) on SIV disease progression in the rhesus macaque (Macaca mulatta) model. *Viruses* **2013**, *5*, 1414–1430.

10. Lindemann, D.; Hutter, S.; Wei, G.; Lochelt, M. The Unique, the Known, and the Unknown of Spumaretrovirus Assembly. *Viruses* **2021**, *13*.

Arifa S. Khan, Dirk Lindemann , Martin Löchelt
Editors

viruses

MDPI

Meeting Report

Twelfth International Foamy Virus Conference—Meeting Report

Ottmar Herchenröder [1], Martin Löchelt [2], Florence Buseyne [3,4], Antoine Gessain [3,4], Marcelo A. Soares [5], Arifa S. Khan [6] and Dirk Lindemann [7,8,*]

1 Institut für Experimentelle Gentherapie und Tumorforschung, Universitätsmedizin Rostock, 18057 Rostock, Germany; ottmar.herchenroeder@med.uni-rostock.de
2 Department of Viral Transformation Mechanisms, Research Program Infection, Inflammation and Cancer, 69120 Heidelberg, Germany; m.loechelt@dkfz.de
3 Unité d'épidémiologie et physiopathologie des virus oncogènes, Institut Pasteur, 75015 Paris, France; florence.buseyne@pasteur.fr (F.B.); antoine.gessain@pasteur.fr (A.G.)
4 CNRS UMR 3569, Institut Pasteur, 75015 Paris, France
5 Departamento de Genética, Universidade Federal do Rio de Janeiro, Rio de Janeiro 21941-590, Brazil; masoares@inca.gov.br
6 Laboratory of Retroviruses, Division of Viral Products, Center for Biologics Evaluation and Research, U.S. Food and Drug Administration, Silver Spring, MD 20993, USA; arifa.khan@fda.hhs.gov
7 Institute of Virology, Medical Faculty "Carl Gustav Carus", Technische Universität Dresden, 01307 Dresden, Germany
8 Center for Regenerative Therapies Dresden, Technische Universität Dresden, 01307 Dresden, Germany
* Correspondence: dirk.lindemann@tu-dresden.de; Tel.: +49-351-458-6210

Received: 25 January 2019; Accepted: 29 January 2019; Published: 1 February 2019

Abstract: The 12th International Foamy Virus Conference took place on 30–31 August 2018 at the Technische Universität Dresden, Dresden, Germany. The meeting included presentations on current research on non-human primate and non-primate foamy viruses (FVs; also called spumaretroviruses) as well as keynote talks on related research areas in retroviruses. The taxonomy of foamy viruses was updated earlier this year to create five new genera in the subfamily, *Spumaretrovirinae*, based on their animal hosts. Research on viruses from different genera was presented on topics of potential relevance to human health, such as natural infections and cross-species transmission, replication, and viral-host interactions in particular with the immune system, dual retrovirus infections, virus structure and biology, and viral vectors for gene therapy. This article provides an overview of the current state-of-the-field, summarizes the meeting highlights, and presents some important questions that need to be addressed in the future.

Keywords: foamy virus; spumaretrovirus; cross-species virus transmission; zoonosis; restriction factors; immune responses; FV vectors; virus replication; latent infection

1. Introduction

The baroque city of Dresden, Germany and its modern biomedical research campus set the stage for the 12th International Foamy Virus Conference hosted and organized by Dirk Lindemann and his team. Based on a 24-year-old tradition since the first meeting, which was held in 1994 in London (Table 1), Dirk arranged an exciting scientific program on current aspects of foamy viruses (FVs), also known as spumaretroviruses.

Table 1. Foamy virus conference history.

Year	Location	Key Findings Reported
1994	London, UK	• Identification of "human foamy virus (HFV)" being the result of a zoonotic transmission of a chimpanzee FV • Involvement of a defective HFV genome in viral latency • Details of Tas-dependent HFV transcriptional control involving internal and LTR promoter
1997	Herzogenhorn, Germany	• Full-length sequence of a feline FV isolate • Reverse transcription during virus morphogenesis results in infectious FVs with a DNA genome • First generation replication-deficient PFV vectors
1999	Gif-sur-Yvette, France	• Characterization of an equine FV isolate • FV glycoprotein-mediated subviral particle formation • FV glycoprotein leader peptide-dependent viral particle release mechanism
2002	Atlanta, GA, USA	• Application of 2nd generation replication-deficient PFV vector for hematopoietic stem cell gene transfer • Viral genome-dependent FV Pol encapsidation mechanism
2004	Würzburg, Germany	• Identification of FV Bet as inhibitor of the APOBEC restriction factors • ESCRT-complex-dependent FV release • First generation replication-deficient feline FV vector systems
2006	Seattle, WA, USA	• Successful treatment of canine leukocyte adhesion deficiency by FV vector-mediated HSC gene transfer • Centrosomal latency of incoming FV capsids in resting cells • Identification of in vivo sites of FV replication in infected primates
2008	Heidelberg, Germany	• CRM1-mediated nuclear export of unspliced FV RNAs • PFV protease structure
2010	Argos, Greece	• Host cells DDX6 protein involvement in PFV genome encapsidation • Heparan sulfate as FV Env-dependent attachment factor
2012	Bethesda, MD, USA	• Structure of the PFV Gag N-terminus in complex with FV Env LP peptides • Innate sensing of FV by plasmacytoid dendritic cells • Pseudotyping of FV vectors by heterologous viral glycoproteins
2014	Puławy, Poland	• Discovery of BFV LTR encoded microRNAs • Host cell Polo-like kinase interaction with PFV Gag involved in proviral integration • Update of FV taxonomy and new nomenclature proposed
2016	Paris, France	• Structure of the central domain of PFV Gag • Genetic diversity of the *env* gene in zoonotic gorilla and chimpanzee FV strains
2018	Dresden, Germany	• Identification of ISG PHF11 as cellular restriction factor of FVs • Cross species dynamics of feline FV • A FV vector system for transient expression of CRISPR/Cas genome engineering tools

FVs are the only type of viruses in the subfamily of *Spumaretrovirinae*, while all other retroviruses belong to the *Orthoretrovirinae*. A biannual meeting brings together most of the FV researchers from different international institutions to present their progress and discuss new developments, and also provides a platform for collaborations. The presentations at the Dresden meeting reflected the dynamics of the field: New and evolving topics, "old" questions being addressed with new technologies, and identification of priority topics that need attention in the coming years. The scientific and generational changes in the field were noted by first-time participating scientists in the meeting. Meanwhile, some topics addressed at past gatherings have now apparently been solved, for instance, the acceptance of the uniqueness of the FV replication strategy, which has led to the establishment of *Spumaretrovirinae* as a separate subfamily of retroviruses, followed by an updated taxonomy and nomenclature [1]. As another milestone, it had been the integrase protein of the prototype FV (PFV; designated as SFVpsc_huHSRV.13), which led to the first successful crystallization of a complete retroviral intasome complex and subsequent ultrastructural analyses of the active intermediates [2]. Thus, the FV integrase serves as the template structure for all retroviral/retroid element integrases. Due to their unique molecular biology, FVs may be considered relevant models to study yet unidentified principles of (retro-)virology. Ultimately, the taxonomic "upgrade" could draw other virologists' attention to these viruses and eventually get more scientists involved in FV research.

In addition to presentations on many aspects of basic, applied, and translational biology of a constantly growing number of new and molecularly characterized FV isolates from diverse hosts, there were keynote presentations from related fields as well as opportunities that were provided for informal discussions and scientific exchange.

2. Summary of Scientific Sessions

The session chairs in consultation with the speakers developed the summaries below, which provide an overview of the current status and future directions for advancing the topic.

2.1. Epidemiology of Natural and Zoonotic Infections (Session Chair: Ottmar Herchenröder)

FVs are infectious agents that persistently infect primate, feline, bovine, and equine species as well as chiropterans (bats). Generally, FVs co-evolve with their host species. Having been an issue of debate in the early decades of FV research, we nowadays know that humans are not natural hosts of FVs. However, transmissions of simian FVs (SFV) to man are not uncommon in natural habitats shared by humans and non-human primates (NHPs), or in settings where the latter are held in captivity, such as in zoos or primate research centers. In contrast to the most prominent example of interspecies transmissions of retroviruses to man that initiated the worldwide AIDS epidemic caused by human immunodeficiency viruses (HIV), FVs are considered apathogenic in both their natural hosts and after interspecies transmissions.

In this session, researchers from the U.S., Brazil, and France gave further insights on the epidemiology of FVs and transmissions between species. Sue VandeWoude (Colorado State University, Fort Collins, CO, USA) reported on her group's comparative epidemiologic surveys amongst mountain lions and domestic cats that share, in part, habitats in the Rocky Mountains foothills. Feline FVs (FFVs) are highly prevalent in these wild animals and, interestingly, interspecies transmissions from domestic cats to mountain lions were frequent as documented by sequence comparisons. Vice versa, FV from mountain lion (*Puma concolor*), was not seen in domestic cats, presumably, as the interaction between individuals of both species necessary for virus transmission may usually not allow the pet to walk away unscathed [3]. Marcelo Soares' group (Universidade Federal do Rio de Janeiro, Rio de Janeiro, Brazil) had previously isolated and characterized FVs from a series of New World NHPs in Brazil. In Dresden, Marcelo's co-worker, Cláudia Muniz, added new data on interspecies transmissions of SFVs from the "invading species", Golden-headed lion tamarin (*Leontopithecus chrysomelas*), to the endangered local population of Golden lion tamarins *(Leontopithecus rosalia*) in the greater Rio de Janeiro area. This study also underlined the validity and robustness of oral swabs as a non-invasive method to achieve both species assignment and FV isolation and characterization [4]. Antoine Gessain (Institut Pasteur, Paris, France) presented a case-control study executed by French and Cameroonian scientists amongst hunters in Cameroon's south-eastern rain forests that gave pause for thought whether simian FV-infections after interspecies transmissions always remain benign over the lifetime of the human recipient. The cases presented with deviations in several blood parameters in comparison to controls matching in residence, age, and social status [5]. Since clinical assessments did not differ between the cases and the controls, the data are reassuring for infected people. However, this study and most previous reports suffer from a strong bias as only apparently healthy individuals were studied. The audience's attention was brought back to domestic animals by Magdalena Materniak-Kornas (National Veterinary Research Institute, Puławy, Poland), who analyzed co-infections with gammaherpesviruses and bovine FV (BFV) in cows suffering from post-partum metritis. By multiplex qPCR and Elisa techniques, the researchers found a good number of animals coinfected with both virus species [6]. Whether FVs have any influence on the clinical onset and burden of metritis in cattle remains speculative.

Altogether, some general beliefs hold true after this latest gathering of FV researchers. First, FV infections are common in numerous species, including livestock and many of those we humans conceive affection for, such as apes, monkeys, and of course cats. Second, FV infections remain in both the natural hosts or the foreign recipients after interspecies transmissions, apparently apathogenic as consented in the aftermath of the first FV conference (Table 1) [7]. More recent data, however, imply an association with hematologic abnormalities [5] and demand further research. Third, unlike many other retroviruses, FV distribution is a worldwide affair and those viruses appear phylogenetically more ancient than their pathogenic counterparts. As such, FVs may be considered as models to study in depth retrovirus biology and evolution.

The author of this section had a long time ago propagated FV isolates in Cf2Th, a cell line derived from canine thymus, which eventually resulted in the first complete sequence of a chimpanzee FV [8]. Cf2Th cells are very permissive for several FVs, although all canine species are considered free from non-endogenous retroviruses. With the surprises FV have entertained virologists over the last decades, he wonders, whether some day one will isolate a FV from man's best companion, the dog. Similarly, it may be worth to look again whether any rodents harbor FVs.

2.2. Interactions of Foamy Viruses with the Immune System (Session Chairs: Antoine Gessain, Marcelo A. Soares)

Immunological aspects of infection by FV are still poorly characterized, both in naturally infected animals and in human infections after cross-species transmission. This scarcity of data includes both innate and acquired immunity, and several issues are still to be addressed in these areas.

What do we know about the immune responses directed against FVs? Several findings suggest strongly an efficient control of SFVs by the immune system in NHPs. These include the apparent lack of pathogenicity of SFVs in vivo, restriction of SFV RNA expression mainly to the oral cavity, and seemingly the gastrointestinal tract in some NHP species, as well as the very limited genetic variability in vivo. Furthermore, recent data indicate that FVs are susceptible to several restriction factors (see virus-host interactions Section 2.4), demonstrating the role of innate immunity in SFV infection, as well as, in some instances, in humans infected by SFVs of zoonotic origin [9,10]. In contrast, the control of SFV replication by innate immunity (antiviral molecules and cells), as well as adaptive immune responses (virus-specific antibodies and T lymphocytes), remain poorly characterized in NHP and even less in humans infected by an SFV.

The following questions remain poorly answered: (i) Can an immunodepression or a viral co-infection alter the pathogenicity of FVs in animal models and in natural infections? (ii) What are the molecular mechanisms by which FVs are efficiently sensed by innate immune cells? This will allow us to better understand how SFVs trigger an innate immune response, especially interferon (IFN) production, which has been demonstrated in blood plasmacytoid dendritic cells, a quite relevant model [11]. (iii) What is the respective part of each arm of the immune system in the modulation of FV infection and the apparent lack of pathogenicity of these viruses, especially in the context of zoonotic infection? (iv) What is the efficacy of antiviral activity of antibodies, especially the role and importance of neutralizing antibodies in vivo?

Answers to some of these questions were given at this meeting. Concerning immunosuppression and FV infection, a previous study has demonstrated that SIV coinfection in a macaque model led to expanded tissue tropism of SFV [12]. Conversely, SFV infection accelerated clinical progression, immunodeficiency, and viral load after SIV infection [13]. Thus, Cláudia Muniz and colleagues (Universidade Federal do Rio de Janeiro, Rio de Janeiro, Brazil) performed experiments in order to study the kinetics of SFV viral loads during immunosuppressive therapy, i.e., with tacrolimus, a drug commonly used to prevent graft rejection after transplantation. SFV DNA load was stable without major variation during the immunosuppression period in the two studied groups. The authors concluded that the immune mechanisms affected by tacrolimus, mostly T lymphocytes, were unable to modulate SFV replication at least during the chronic phase of the infection. In a South American NHP (*Brachyteles arachnoides*) with symptoms indicative of clinical immunodepression, likely due to infection by a simian type-D retrovirus (SRV), the same team demonstrated the presence of very high SFV DNA levels in the saliva and identified a new isolate, SFVbar [14]. Furthermore, transcriptome analysis from blood yielded SRV-related transcripts, but failed to identify SFVbar RNA, suggesting that SFVbar remained latent in PBMCs despite the immunocompromised status of the host.

Concerning antibodies, Florence Buseyne and colleagues (Institut Pasteur, Paris, France) demonstrated the presence of potent neutralizing antibodies in humans infected by zoonotic gorilla and chimpanzee FVs. Furthermore, Florence showed that the antibodies are directed against conserved epitopes located in the dimorphic domain of the surface envelope protein. The neutralization patterns provided evidence for persistent expression of viral proteins and a high prevalence of viral co-infection by two different viruses diverging in the *env* SU gene [15].

Mathilde Couteaudier and colleagues (Institut Pasteur, Paris, France) investigated whether plasma antibodies can inhibit SFV cell-to-cell transmission. Indeed, SFV transmission is considered highly cell-to-cell associated. Interestingly, she demonstrated that plasma samples from humans infected by zoonotic SFV, selected for their potent ability to neutralize cell-free virus, were unable to inhibit virus cell-to-cell spread.

In a second session devoted to the interaction between FV and the immune system, Florence Buseyne and colleagues (Institut Pasteur, Paris, France) characterized an immunodominant epitope located in the leader region of the SFV envelope protein (SFVpsc_huHSRV.13, aa 96–110) and recognized by the plasma antibodies of most SFV-infected hunters from Central Africa, similar to what has been recently described in FFV infections [16]. Whereas plasma from subjects infected with SFV derived from gorillas strongly recognized peptides corresponding to that envelope region of SFV from apes and other Old World primates, recognition was poor or absent to the respective peptides from SFV infecting more distant New World primates or from a specific African green monkey strain, suggesting evolutionary constraints in the adaptive immune responses observed. Whether the magnitude of such antibody responses can serve as proxies of overall adaptive immunity against SFV still remains to be determined.

By using FFV, Cláudia Muniz and coworkers (Universidade Federal do Rio de Janeiro, Rio de Janeiro, Brazil) had determined the effect of coinfections between FV and other retroviruses, in this case, the feline leukemia virus (FeLV) in domestic cats. Since FeLV causes immunodeficiency in their natural hosts, the feline model can also be used to understand the kinetics of FFV infection in the context of immunosuppresion. The investigators found that among FeLV/FFV-coinfected cats, those displaying an FeLV regressive infection (that tends to spontaneous clearance of the virus in the infected host), FFV replication and potential transmissibility is also reduced in the oral cavity, suggesting a synergistic interaction of both retroviruses as recently confirmed by Powers et al. [17]. On the other hand, FFV proviral loads in the peripheral blood did not differ between cats with or without clinical signs after FeLV infection, again highlighting a lack of association between FV replication and the general immunosuppressive status of the host, as pointed out in the studies conducted in NHP described above.

The last two presentations of the session addressed the role of innate immunity on FV infection in a very complementary manner. Jakob Weber and coworkers (Technische Universität Dresden, Dresden, Germany) showed the utility of the Phorbol 12-myristate 13-acetate (PMA)-differentiated monocytic cell line, THP-1, as a model system to study innate sensing in macrophages and monocytes, the likely first immune cell types to contact FV particles in infected tissues. The researchers found that incubation of these cells with PFV resulted in the induction of interferon-stimulated genes (ISGs). Furthermore, they demonstrated that PFV sensing is independent of Tas expression and integration of the proviral genome, but rather occurs at cell entry and requires access to the cytoplasm of the infected cell, with reverse-transcribed DNA being a likely recognized molecule. Maïwenn Bergez and colleagues (Paul-Ehrlich-Institut, Langen, Germany) showed that transduction of PFV vector particles into both THP-1 cells and primary human monocyte-derived dendritic cells induces the expression of the interferon regulatory factor 3 (IRF3)-dependent ISGs. Such induction was highly attenuated when RT-deficient viruses were used or azidothymidine was added during transduction, confirming that the newly reverse-transcribed PFV DNA acts as a pathogen-associated molecular pattern that stimulates the host cell innate immune system. The cytosolic sensors involved in the innate immune response to FV infection are yet to be determined.

2.3. *Molecular and Cellular Biology of Foamy Viruses (Session Chair: Arifa S. Khan)*

The development of advanced molecular tools and new generation biochemical reagents have enabled us to re-visit important questions regarding the biology and replication of FVs. Our current knowledge regarding the FV life cycle is mainly based on studies with SFVpsc_huHSRV.13, since this was initially believed to be a human FV (until it was sequenced and identified as a chimpanzee FV, which had infected a human by cross-species transmission). The information has been expanded based on FV isolates from other NHP species and extended by studies on FFVs and BFVs. The majority of the early work is based on laboratory virus strains. Although a few efforts are currently directed at studying the biology of natural FV isolates, most are from NHPs and only recently have also included New World monkeys. This research gap is further being addressed by studies investigating natural infections of FVs in bovine and feline species. Moreover, the availability of new and more sensitive assays that can investigate the different steps of FV replication, from infection/entry through integration/expression, resulting in release/exit, are important for understanding natural virus transmission and cross-species infections in humans by NHP FVs. To aid these goals, there is a need to develop reagents and functional assays for studying the molecular and cellular biology of naturally-occurring FV isolates. This session highlighted applications of new molecular tools and assays for investigating critical steps in spumaretrovirus replication.

Stefanie Richter from the Lindemann laboratory (Technische Universität Dresden, Dresden, Germany) reported on the adaptation of the fluorescent-based β-lactamase (BlaM) fusion assay [18] for FVs to obtain new insights about the kinetics and temperature requirements of FV Env-mediated fusion. The study used BlaM-containing SFVpsc_huHSRV.13 single-round vector particles habouring either SFVpsc_huHSRV.13 or SFVmcy_FV21 Env proteins and the Pac2 zebrafish embryonic cell line, which was previously thought to be resistant to FV Env-mediated entry [19]. Using Pac2 cells loaded with the fluorescent BlaM substrate CCF4-AM, the researchers demonstrated that this cell line was permissive for FV Env-mediated fusion. These results highlighted the potential of this approach for providing insight into the differences seen in the susceptibility of cells to FV infection.

Ivo Glück from the Lamb laboratory (Ludwig-Maximilians-Universität, München, Germany) presented on the application of the TrIC method [20] to track steps involved in the fusion process of single FV particles in live HeLa cells. Virus particles used in the study contained the viral envelope protein (Env) tagged with mCherry and the capsid protein (Gag) tagged with eGFP. By tracking the eGFP signal and locally cross-correlating the eGFP and mCherry intensities, the individual viral fusion events could be visualized as the capsid separated from the envelope. The analysis revealed a previously undetected intermediate step in the FV fusion process, in which the capsid and envelope signals are separated by approximately 300 nm, but remain tethered for an average of 7.1 min before full separation. An important next step is to identify the linking component that tethers the viral capsid to the envelope.

Martin Löchelt (German Cancer Research Center, Heidelberg, Germany) extended the previous identification of the chromatin binding site (CBS) in PFV Gag by functionally characterizing a highly conserved motif of the CBS of the Gag protein of FFV. It was demonstrated that the RYG residues in the QPQRYG motif are, in addition, essential during the early stages of infection after entry into the cytosol since mutagenesis of RYG abrogated the accumulation of Gag and proviral DNA in the nucleus and, subsequently, DNA integration into the host genome, similar to mutations within the chromatin binding. The results confirmed that chromatin binding by foamy virus Gag is a shared feature among FVs belonging to diverse genera and mediated by a conserved protein region located at the C-terminus of Gag, which is of prime importance for the provirus integration site. This motif likely influences the incoming virus capsid or its disassembly intermediates, but not newly synthesized Gag or its assembly products. The study, which was recently published [21] provides a strategy for comparing different FVs for mechanism and host cell conditions that can influence the efficiency of integration.

FV research using new assays and methodologies can be further enhanced and extended by the development of advanced technologies, such as next generation or high-throughput sequencing

(NGS, HTS), which has emerged as a powerful tool that can help to investigate various aspects of virus biology and replication. In particular, transcriptomics and genomics studies using NGS could help determine the virus-host interactions that result in the seemingly general FV latency and limited expression seen in natural infections. The results from such studies may aid in predicting potential outcomes of FV infections in humans.

2.4. Mechanisms of Virus–Host Interactions: Cellular Antiviral Factors and Viral Antagonists (Session Chair: Florence Buseyne)

The interactions of FVs with their hosts were shaped by millions of years of coevolution [22]. FV have a ubiquitous tropism in vitro and numerous cross-species transmission events occurred in their evolutionary history. Thus, these viruses escape most constitutively expressed restriction factors. On the other hand, they are sensitive to the action of type I and type II IFN in vitro and are apparently apathogenic in vivo. Among the ISG products, TRIM5α, N-myc-interactor, IFP35, TRIM19, APOBEC, and tetherin were described to inhibit FV, while MxB and SAMHD1 had no action, and some discordant results are thus far unresolved. The currently open questions in the field, summarized after the former FV conference in 2016 [23], were about the role of restriction factors and IFN-induced genes in controlling FV gene expression in vivo in their natural hosts and in humans after cross-species transmission. Lack of knowledge on the induction and action of non-IFN antiviral actors (inflammasome, cytokines, and miRNA) were striking.

This conference provided new insights on four topics. Carsten Münk (Heinrich-Heine-Universität Düsseldorf, Düsseldorf, Germany) presented on APOBEC3s, which are potent inhibitors of FV. The viral Bet protein is the single antiviral factor antagonist described for FV. Its mechanism of action is unique: Bet prevents APOBEC3s incorporation into viral particles and thereby, provides protection of FVs, as well as lentiviruses, if Bet is expressed in trans, against APOBEC3s' antiviral activity. Conversely, Carmen Ledesma-Feliciano reported in the FV vector session (see 2.6) that the feline immunodeficiency virus (FIV) Vif protein can replace the FFV Bet protein in vitro, but the chimeric virus was attenuated in vivo [24]. These in vivo attenuated phenotypes of Bet-deficient FV highlighted that additional Bet functions impacting FVs interaction with their hosts are waiting to be described.

Wenhu Cao from the Löchelt laboratory (German Cancer Research Center, Heidelberg, Germany) presented new results on bovine FV (BFV) miRNAs. BFV encodes miRNAs with a noncanonical biogenesis involving RNA polymerase III, generation of a single pri-miRNA, and its processing into three functional miRNAs. Cellular proteins were identified whose expression were suppressed by BFV miRNA and this was shown to result in repression of IFN-β and NF-κB pathways. Importantly, deletion of miRNA led to in vivo attenuation of BFV, confirming the major role of miRNAs in virus-host interactions.

Melissa Kane from the Bieniasz laboratory (The Rockefeller University, New York, NY, USA) presented new data based on results from the screening of nearly 500 human and macaque antiviral genes against 11 retroviruses, including the PFV [25]. The screen identified the ISG PHD finger protein 11 (PHF11) as a PFV-specific inhibitor. In vitro, PFV was unable to escape PHF11 restriction. PHF11 is involved in DNA damage signaling and DNA repair, and inhibits an early step in FV replication.

Arifa Khan (U.S. Food and Drug Administration, Silver Spring, MD, USA) presented the careful characterization of SFV-infected human A549 cell clones with various viral expression patterns, defined by viral DNA and RNA expression and production of infectious virions. Clones with fully latent and actively replicating SFV were analyzed for gene expression using next generation sequencing. Cells infected with different macaque SFV strains with widely different kinetics were included in the screen. Data overview showed diversity across strains in their ability to modulate IFN-signaling and other immune activation pathways.

Important questions and future directions were highlighted at the meeting. Data pointed to the uniqueness of FV (Bet, miRNA, and the PHF11) with elegant studies starting with molecular understanding of the activity of an FV component to in vivo assessment of its action. Such specificities open new molecular medicine applications, such as expression of heterologous regulatory RNA by BFV miRNA. The interest of high-throughput assays associated with well-validated in vitro models was evident and indeed, the PHF11 will not be identified by a hypothesis-driven strategy as early as with the comprehensive approach used [25]. In the future, new input is expected from modern biology approaches to identify cellular factors regulating viral replication and latency.

2.5. Structural Studies of Foamy Virus Proteins (Session Chair: Martin Löchelt)

Structural biology provides challenging insights into the molecular and atomic organization and underlying functions of proteins and molecular assemblies of high complexity. In addition, structural biology is a major tool in drug discovery and optimization and has enormous implications for translational research, medical care, and disease prevention. Under these perspectives, the current state-of-the-art of FV structural biology, focused in particular on integrase (IN) and the Gag structural proteins, was summarized in excellent reviews by Paul Lesbats (CNRS UMR5234, Bordeaux, France) and Jonathan Stoye (The Francis Crick Institute, London, United Kingdom).

FV Pol proteins share most of the conserved sequence motifs with the other retroviruses. However, their expression mode via a spliced transcript, resulting in the lack of a Gag-Pol fusion protein, most probably determines the uniqueness of FV particle assembly, genome incorporation, protein processing, capsid maturation, and reverse transcription. Another unique feature is the lack of processing of FV Pol precursor molecules to release the protease [3,22,26].

After a lot of unsuccessful attempts using other retroviruses, PFV IN was the first retroviral IN to be crystallized in its active form and as a high-molecular mass complex together with its target DNA [2]. Based on this structure and subsequent new data, highly divergent degrees of IN oligomerization in intasomes has been described for different retroviruses [27]. Here, PFV IN tetramers contrast other retroviral octo- and hexadecameric arrangements that make up the active intasomes. It is possible that the comparably low degree of PFV IN oligomerisation favored or even allowed its crystallization and thus, its structural analysis. Based on his experience in retroviral IN interactions with chromatin, Paul Lesbats described the interaction of the PFV chromatin-binding site with histones confirming and extending knowledge on C-terminal Gag residues involved in this process that contributes to FV integration site selection [28].

FV Gag and that of other retroviruses largely perform equivalent functions. However, several features, including the absence of genome-binding Cys-His motifs and a major homology region, the limited Gag processing at a very C-terminal site, and the essential requirement of N-terminal Gag and Env LP domains for particle release, are fundamentally different from that of other retroviruses [29]. The N-terminal and central domains of the unique FV Gag proteins are the focus of Jonathan Stoye's past and current activities. Here, structural studies strongly target evolutionary issues related to retroviral capsid structures and their interaction with host-encoded restriction factors. Jonathan described structural analyses that identified two independent domains in a central part of FV Gag, which most probably derived from sequence duplications [30]. Surprisingly, these structures reveal a greater and unforeseen similarity to the Ty3 retrotransposon-derived mammalian protein ARC, than to conventional retroviral capsid proteins [31].

In summary, structural studies of FV Pol proteins have shown that they are highly related to those of other retroviruses and in the case of IN, even serve as model structures for the whole virus family. By contrast, although the amino-terminal and central domains of FV-Gag have been structurally characterized, the evolutionary origin and relationship with orthoretroviral Gag and exapted proteins found in mammalian genomes is the subject of current FV structural studies. Other FV proteins, most of them with unique features, have at large not been targets of high-resolution studies. Structural studies of FV Env are limited to a low-resolution (9 Å). Cryo-EM structure revealed the trimeric nature of the PFV Env $gp80^{SU}$ spike [32] and the crystal structure an Env $gp18^{LP}$ peptide bound to the N-terminal domain of PFV Gag [33]. Further high-resolution structural analyses of Env from two distinct serotypes of primate and feline FV SU could greatly foster the understanding of virus neutralization and the overlap with receptor binding, and may even support identification of the FV receptor(s). Finally, structural data on the non-canonical FV Tas transcriptional transactivator and the enigmatic Bet protein that counteracts APOBEC3-mediated restriction, but may also fulfil many additional functions, would fertilize further research on these essential and FV-specific proteins [34].

2.6. Development and Application of Foamy Virus Vector Systems (Session Chair: Dirk Lindemann)

Over the last 50 years human gene therapy has developed from fiction to become reality. After approval of the first gene therapy drugs several years ago, the last 24 months have seen a good number of new gene therapy drugs being approved and entering the market. The majority of them are based on viral gene ferries, which is also true for drugs currently being examined in gene therapy trials worldwide. This most likely reflects the fact that viruses may be considered as evolutionarily optimized nucleic acid delivery entities, although it took researchers decades to develop viral vector systems with optimized features of transduction efficiency, balanced expression control, and safety. Retroviral vectors are still the most frequent gene ferries used in gene therapy clinical trials and approved drugs. Gammaretroviral vectors based on murine leukemia virus were the first gene ferries being used in clinical trials. They were also employed in the SCID-X1 clinical trials around the turn of the century and were the first gene transfer tools with unequivocal therapeutic benefits for the patients. Lentiviral vectors based on HIV-1 were developed only later. Due to their ability to also efficiently transduce non-mitotic cells they have become more popular, which can be seen by the rising number of clinical trials using them as gene delivery tools.

The first vector systems based on FV were developed about 20 years ago [26,35]. FV have several natural features of a good candidate gene transfer vector, such as one of the largest retroviral genomes, an infectious DNA genome, a favorable integration site profile, and an extremely broad tropism. Most important is their apparent apathogenicity in both natural and zoonotic infections that renders them attractive for gene delivery. Furthermore, they have shown promising therapeutic results in preclinical studies using animal model systems [26,35]. However, so far, FV vectors or individual components of FV, such as the FV Env protein, have not been used in human gene therapy clinical trials.

Karol Budzik from the Russell laboratory (Mayo Clinic, Rochester, NY, USA) summarized his efforts to develop an FV platform for oncolytic virotherapy. SFVpve virus produced from a chimeric infectious molecular clone, which was derived from two chimpanzee FV strains (PAN1, PAN2), showed higher oncolytic activity in vitro than either parental strain or the PFV isolate in a variety of tumor cell lines. Furthermore, a U251 glioblastoma-derived reporter cell line was established and used to demonstrate in vivo replication of FV in a mouse model. This provides the basis for further examination of the tumoricidal potential of this new chimeric SFV strain or armed versions thereof in animal model systems.

Carmen Ledesma-Feliciano from the VandeWoude laboratory (Colorado State University, Fort Collins, CO, USA) presented a recently published study on the experimental infection in domestic cats with a replication-competent wild type and a novel FFV vaccine vector candidate expressing a truncated FFV-Bet/FIV-Vif fusion protein [24]. In vitro analysis in feline cells showed a requirement of FIV Vif expression without an FFV Bet N-terminal tag for efficient viral replication. In contrast, inoculation of immunocompetent domestic cats revealed a poor replication capacity of the vaccine vector in comparison to wild-type FFV. This suggests a yet uncharacterized role of FFV Bet for in vivo replication besides its anti-APOBEC activity.

Fabian Lindel from the Lindemann laboratory (Technische Universität Dresden, Dresden, Germany) reported on a novel PFV based vector system for largely transient expression of CRISPR/Cas9 genome editing tools in various target tissues. The system exploits the previously described natural feature of FV to encapsidate and efficiently transmit non-viral RNAs, which was exploited to express Cas9 fully transient in transduced cells. When combined with integration-deficient retroviral vectors harboring a U6 promoter-driven sgRNA, efficient gene inactivation was achieved in different target cell types. Additionally, the inclusion of a donor DNA template enabled efficient gene editing of reporter or cellular genes by homology directed repair mechanisms.

Finally, Jennifer Donau from the Valtink laboratory (Technische Universität Dresden, Dresden, Germany) summarized her work towards the establishment of a therapeutic proliferation stimulation strategy for primary human ocular tissues. She reported on the identification of viral and cellular proliferation promoting factors for immortalization of primary human corneal endothelial (CEC) or retinal pigment epithelial (RPE) cells upon stable transduction by lentiviral vectors pseudotyped by FV glycoproteins. Furthermore, she demonstrated that integration-deficient lentiviral vectors are not suited for transient growth stimulation in a therapeutic setting due to their residual non-viral mediated integration potential, which results in stable immortalization of primary tissues. At the end, she referred to her first attempts to achieve growth stimulation in these primary target tissues by transient expression of proliferation promoting factors using FV-mediated non-viral RNA gene transfer.

3. Keynote Lectures

The first keynote lecture was given by Welkin E. Johnson (Boston College, Chestnut Hill, MA, USA). Welkin presented an overview of a comparative study of ancient *env* genes of endogenous retroviral elements that provides insight into the co-evolution of retroviruses and their vertebrate hosts. He reviewed examples of potential cases of exaptations, whereby former endogenous retrovirus (ERV) *env* genes are preserved by purifying evolutionary selection and now provide cellular functions, for example, in the development (syncytins-mediated trophoblast fusion) or antiviral defense against extant viruses (ERV-mediated superinfection resistance). Furthermore, he summarized his and other people's work on the origins and exaptive evolution of the ERV-Fc locus in mammals.

Frank Buchholz (Technische Universität Dresden, Dresden, Germany) delivered the second keynote lecture reviewing his and other researchers' work on programmable nucleases and designer recombinases for genome surgery. He presented examples from his lab using CRISPR/Cas9 library screens to dissect driver mutations from passenger mutations in human cancer cell lines as an approach towards a personalized cancer therapy. Furthermore, he summarized the pioneering work of his and Joachim Hauber's laboratory (Heinrich-Pette-Institut, Hamburg, Germany) on the broad-range anti-HIV-1 recombinase Brec1 and presented the latest results from experiments using humanized mouse models.

4. Conclusions

Two major goals were achieved by the 12th International Foamy Virus Meeting. First, bringing together most of the senior and junior scientists in the field with expertise in different disciplines for a scientific exchange and providing the opportunity for discussing ongoing, and initiating new collaborations. Second, attracting new people to the field, which was reflected by several first-time attendees, whose presentations strongly underlined the interdisciplinary character of the meeting and demonstrated the continued interest in this unique type of retrovirus. We enjoyed lively discussions after the individual presentations and in the breaks. We hope that the session summaries and highlights provided in this report illustrate that there is so much to be discovered and learned from FVs and will encourage interested researchers to join us at the 13th International Spumaretrovirus Conference, which is being planned for 2020 in Rio de Janeiro, Brazil. More information can be obtained by the conference host: Marcelo Soares masoares@biologia.ufrj.br.

Author Contributions: All authors participated in the writing and editing of the manuscript. All meeting participants approved their presentation summaries and consented to mentioning of their names and affiliations.

Acknowledgments: The meeting was supported by grants from the Deutsche Forschungsgemeinschaft (DFG, German Research Foundation, Projektnummer 406942900); from the Boehringer Ingelheim Stiftung; and the TU Dresden's Institutional Strategy (F-003661-533-Ü5D-1250000), funded by the Excellence Initiative of the German Federal and State Governments. No funding was received for covering the costs to publish this meeting report in open access.

Conflicts of Interest: The authors declare no conflict of interest. The funding agencies had no role in the decision to publish this report.

References

1. Khan, A.S.; Bodem, J.; Buseyne, F.; Gessain, A.; Johnson, W.; Kuhn, J.H.; Kuzmak, J.; Lindemann, D.; Linial, M.L.; Lochelt, M.; et al. Spumaretroviruses: Updated taxonomy and nomenclature. *Virology* **2018**, *516*, 158–164. [CrossRef]
2. Hare, S.; Gupta, S.S.; Valkov, E.; Engelman, A.; Cherepanov, P. Retroviral intasome assembly and inhibition of DNA strand transfer. *Nature* **2010**, *464*, 232–236. [CrossRef] [PubMed]
3. Kehl, T.; Tan, J.; Materniak, M. Non-simian foamy viruses: Molecular virology, tropism and prevalence and zoonotic/interspecies transmission. *Viruses* **2013**, *5*, 2169–2209. [CrossRef]
4. Muniz, C.P.; Zheng, H.; Jia, H.; Cavalcante, L.T.F.; Augusto, A.M.; Fedullo, L.P.; Pissinatti, A.; Soares, M.A.; Switzer, W.M.; Santos, A.F. A non-invasive specimen collection method and a novel simian foamy virus (SFV) DNA quantification assay in New World primates reveal aspects of tissue tropism and improved SFV detection. *PLoS ONE* **2017**, *12*, e0184251. [CrossRef] [PubMed]
5. Buseyne, F.; Betsem, E.; Montange, T.; Njouom, R.; Bilounga Ndongo, C.; Hermine, O.; Gessain, A. Clinical Signs and Blood Test Results Among Humans Infected With Zoonotic Simian Foamy Virus: A Case-Control Study. *J. Infect. Dis.* **2018**, *218*, 144–151. [CrossRef]
6. Materniak-Kornas, M.; Osinski, Z.; Rudzki, M.; Kuzmak, J. Development of a Recombinant Protein-based ELISA for Detection of Antibodies Against Bovine Foamy Virus. *J. Vet. Res.* **2017**, *61*, 247–252. [CrossRef] [PubMed]
7. Weiss, R.A. Reverse transcription. Foamy viruses bubble on [news]. *Nature* **1996**, *380*, 201. [CrossRef]
8. Herchenröder, O.; Renne, R.; Loncar, D.; Cobb, E.K.; Murthy, K.K.; Schneider, J.; Mergia, A.; Luciw, P.A. Isolation, cloning, and sequencing of simian foamy viruses from chimpanzees (SFVcpz): High homology to human foamy virus (HFV). *Virology* **1994**, *201*, 187–199. [CrossRef]
9. Pinto-Santini, D.M.; Stenbak, C.R.; Linial, M.L. Foamy virus zoonotic infections. *Retrovirology* **2017**, *14*, 55. [CrossRef]
10. Rua, R.; Gessain, A. Origin, evolution and innate immune control of simian foamy viruses in humans. *Curr. Opin. Virol.* **2015**, *10*, 47–55. [CrossRef]
11. Rua, R.; Lepelley, A.; Gessain, A.; Schwartz, O. Innate sensing of foamy viruses by human hematopoietic cells. *J. Virol.* **2012**, *86*, 909–918. [CrossRef] [PubMed]
12. Murray, S.M.; Picker, L.J.; Axthelm, M.K.; Linial, M.L. Expanded tissue targets for foamy virus replication with simian immunodeficiency virus-induced immunosuppression. *J. Virol.* **2006**, *80*, 663–670. [CrossRef] [PubMed]
13. Choudhary, A.; Galvin, T.A.; Williams, D.K.; Beren, J.; Bryant, M.A.; Khan, A.S. Influence of naturally occurring simian foamy viruses (SFVs) on SIV disease progression in the rhesus macaque (Macaca mulatta) model. *Viruses* **2013**, *5*, 1414–1430. [CrossRef] [PubMed]
14. Muniz, C.P.; Cavalcante, L.T.F.; Dudley, D.M.; Fedullo, L.P.; Pissinatti, A.; O'Connor, D.H.; Santos, A.F.; Soares, M.A. First Complete Genome Sequence of a Simian Foamy Virus Infecting the Neotropical Primate Brachyteles arachnoides. *Microbiol. Resour. Announc.* **2018**, *2*, e00839-18. [CrossRef] [PubMed]
15. Lambert, C.; Couteaudier, M.; Gouzil, J.; Richard, L.; Montange, T.; Betsem, E.; Rua, R.; Tobaly-Tapiero, J.; Lindemann, D.; Njouom, R.; et al. Potent neutralizing antibodies in humans infected with zoonotic simian foamy viruses target conserved epitopes located in the dimorphic domain of the surface envelope protein. *PLoS Pathog.* **2018**, *14*, e1007293. [CrossRef] [PubMed]
16. Mühle, M.; Bleiholder, A.; Löchelt, M.; Denner, J. Epitope Mapping of the Antibody Response Against the Envelope Proteins of the Feline Foamy Virus. *Viral. Immunol.* **2017**, *30*, 388–395. [PubMed]
17. Powers, J.A.; Chiu, E.S.; Kraberger, S.J.; Roelke-Parker, M.; Lowery, I.; Erbeck, K.; Troyer, R.; Carver, S.; VandeWoude, S. Feline Leukemia Virus (FeLV) Disease Outcomes in a Domestic Cat Breeding Colony: Relationship to Endogenous FeLV and Other Chronic Viral Infections. *J. Virol.* **2018**, *92*, e00649-18. [CrossRef] [PubMed]
18. Jones, D.M.; Padilla-Parra, S. The beta-Lactamase Assay: Harnessing a FRET Biosensor to Analyse Viral Fusion Mechanisms. *Sensors* **2016**, *16*, 950. [CrossRef]
19. Stirnnagel, K.; Lüftenegger, D.; Stange, A.; Swiersy, A.; Müllers, E.; Reh, J.; Stanke, N.; Grosse, A.; Chiantia, S.; Keller, H.; et al. Analysis of prototype foamy virus particle-host cell interaction with autofluorescent retroviral particles. *Retrovirology* **2010**, *7*, 45. [CrossRef]

20. Dupont, A.; Stirnnagel, K.; Lindemann, D.; Lamb, D.C. Tracking image correlation: Combining single-particle tracking and image correlation. *Biophys. J.* **2013**, *104*, 2373–2382. [CrossRef]
21. Wei, G.; Kehl, T.; Bao, Q.; Benner, A.; Lei, J.; Lochelt, M. The chromatin binding domain, including the QPQRYG motif, of feline foamy virus Gag is required for viral DNA integration and nuclear accumulation of Gag and the viral genome. *Virology* **2018**, *524*, 56–68. [CrossRef] [PubMed]
22. Rethwilm, A.; Bodem, J. Evolution of foamy viruses: The most ancient of all retroviruses. *Viruses* **2013**, *5*, 2349–2374. [CrossRef] [PubMed]
23. Buseyne, F.; Gessain, A.; Soares, M.A.; Santos, A.F.; Materniak-Kornas, M.; Lesage, P.; Zamborlini, A.; Löchelt, M.; Qiao, W.; Lindemann, D.; et al. Eleventh International Foamy Virus Conference-Meeting Report. *Viruses* **2016**, *8*, 318. [CrossRef] [PubMed]
24. Ledesma-Feliciano, C.; Hagen, S.; Troyer, R.; Zheng, X.; Musselman, E.; Slavkovic Lukic, D.; Franke, A.M.; Maeda, D.; Zielonka, J.; Munk, C.; et al. Replacement of feline foamy virus bet by feline immunodeficiency virus vif yields replicative virus with novel vaccine candidate potential. *Retrovirology* **2018**, *15*, 38. [CrossRef] [PubMed]
25. Kane, M.; Zang, T.M.; Rihn, S.J.; Zhang, F.; Kueck, T.; Alim, M.; Schoggins, J.; Rice, C.M.; Wilson, S.J.; Bieniasz, P.D. Identification of Interferon-Stimulated Genes with Antiretroviral Activity. *Cell Host Microbe.* **2016**, *20*, 392–405. [CrossRef] [PubMed]
26. Lindemann, D.; Rethwilm, A. Foamy virus biology and its application for vector development. *Viruses* **2011**, *3*, 561–585. [CrossRef] [PubMed]
27. Engelman, A.N.; Cherepanov, P. Retroviral intasomes arising. *Curr. Opin. Struct. Biol.* **2017**, *47*, 23–29. [CrossRef] [PubMed]
28. Lesbats, P.; Serrao, E.; Maskell, D.P.; Pye, V.E.; O'Reilly, N.; Lindemann, D.; Engelman, A.N.; Cherepanov, P. Structural basis for spumavirus GAG tethering to chromatin. *Proc. Natl. Acad. Sci. USA* **2017**, *114*, 5509–5514. [CrossRef]
29. Müllers, E. The foamy virus Gag proteins: What makes them different? *Viruses* **2013**, *5*, 1023–1041. [CrossRef]
30. Ball, N.J.; Nicastro, G.; Dutta, M.; Pollard, D.J.; Goldstone, D.C.; Sanz-Ramos, M.; Ramos, A.; Müllers, E.; Stirnnagel, K.; Stanke, N.; et al. Structure of a Spumaretrovirus Gag Central Domain Reveals an Ancient Retroviral Capsid. *PLoS Pathog.* **2016**, *12*, e1005981. [CrossRef]
31. Taylor, W.R.; Stoye, J.P.; Taylor, I.A. A comparative analysis of the foamy and ortho virus capsid structures reveals an ancient domain duplication. *BMC Struct. Biol.* **2017**, *17*, 3. [CrossRef] [PubMed]
32. Effantin, G.; Estrozi, L.F.; Aschman, N.; Renesto, P.; Stanke, N.; Lindemann, D.; Schoehn, G.; Weissenhorn, W. Cryo-electron Microscopy Structure of the Native Prototype Foamy Virus Glycoprotein and Virus Architecture. *PLoS Pathog.* **2016**, *12*, e1005721. [CrossRef] [PubMed]
33. Goldstone, D.C.; Flower, T.G.; Ball, N.J.; Sanz-Ramos, M.; Yap, M.W.; Ogrodowicz, R.W.; Stanke, N.; Reh, J.; Lindemann, D.; Stoye, J.P.; et al. A Unique Spumavirus Gag N-terminal Domain with Functional Properties of Orthoretroviral Matrix and Capsid. *PLoS Pathog.* **2013**, *9*, e1003376. [CrossRef] [PubMed]
34. Lukic, D.S.; Hotz-Wagenblatt, A.; Lei, J.; Rathe, A.M.; Mühle, M.; Denner, J.; Münk, C.; Löchelt, M. Identification of the feline foamy virus Bet domain essential for APOBEC3 counteraction. *Retrovirology* **2013**, *10*, 76. [CrossRef] [PubMed]
35. Trobridge, G.D.; Horn, P.A.; Beard, B.C.; Kiem, H.P. Large animal models for foamy virus vector gene therapy. *Viruses* **2012**, *4*, 3572–3588. [CrossRef] [PubMed]

viruses

MDPI

Review

Simian Foamy Viruses in Central and South America: A New World of Discovery

André F. Santos [1], Liliane T. F. Cavalcante [1], Cláudia P. Muniz [1], William M. Switzer [2] and Marcelo A. Soares [1,3,*]

1 Departamento de Genética, Universidade Federal do Rio de Janeiro, Rio de Janeiro 21941-617, RJ, Brazil; andre20@globo.com (A.F.S.); liliane.tavaresdefaria@gmail.com (L.T.F.C.); claudia.muniz16@gmail.com (C.P.M.)
2 Laboratory Branch, Division of HIV/AIDS Prevention, National Center for HIV/AIDS, Hepatitis, STD, and TB Prevention, Centers for Disease Control and Prevention, Atlanta, GA 30329, USA; bis3@cdc.gov
3 Programa de Oncovirologia, Instituto Nacional de Câncer, Riod e Janeiro, RJ 20231-050, RJ, Brazil
* Correspondence: masaores@inca.gov.br; Tel.: +55-21-3207-6591

Received: 30 September 2019; Accepted: 18 October 2019; Published: 20 October 2019

Abstract: Foamy viruses (FVs) are the only exogenous retrovirus to date known to infect neotropical primates (NPs). In the last decade, an increasing number of strains have been completely or partially sequenced, and molecular evolution analyses have identified an ancient co-speciation with their hosts. In this review, the improvement of diagnostic techniques that allowed the determination of a more accurate prevalence of simian FVs (SFVs) in captive and free-living NPs is discussed. Determination of DNA viral load in American primates indicates that oral tissues are the viral replicative site and that buccal swab collection can be an alternative to diagnose SFV infection in NPs. Finally, the transmission potential of NP SFVs to primate workers in zoos and primate centers of the Americas is examined.

Keywords: spumaretrovirus; new world primates; simian retrovirus

1. Introduction

Spumaretroviruses are complex, exogenous retroviruses in the *Spumaretrovirinae* subfamily known to infect different mammalian orders, such as nonhuman primates (NHPs), felines, bovines and equines [1]. In NHPs, spumaretroviruses are also called simian foamy viruses (SFVs). Despite being the only reported exogenous retrovirus known to infect neotropical primates (NPs), as first reported in 1973 [2], little is known about this viral infection. Recently published studies using improved molecular and serologic techniques for SFV diagnosis in NPs have shed light on the prevalence, transmission routes and zoonotic potential of these NP viruses.

2. Neotropical Primates: Taxonomy and Evolution

The word "primate" is derived from Latin *primat* that means prime or first rank. The Primates order has the third most abundant number of species among mammals, only behind Chiroptera (bats) and Rodentia (rodents) [3]. Although the exact number of species is still in discussion with constant changes in taxonomic classification, there are between 261 and 504 species described to date divided into 16 families and 79 genera [3,4]. Primates are distributed across four global regions: Latin America, mainland Africa, Madagascar, and Asia, covering 90 countries (Figure 1) [3]. Common features of the Primates order include a large brain in relation to the body size, accurate binocular color vision, opposable thumbs and a sophisticated social system. The common ancestor of the Primates order is estimated to have originated about 60–80 million years ago (MYA) based on evidence of small mammals adapted to live in trees and with the oldest fossil found in Africa [5].

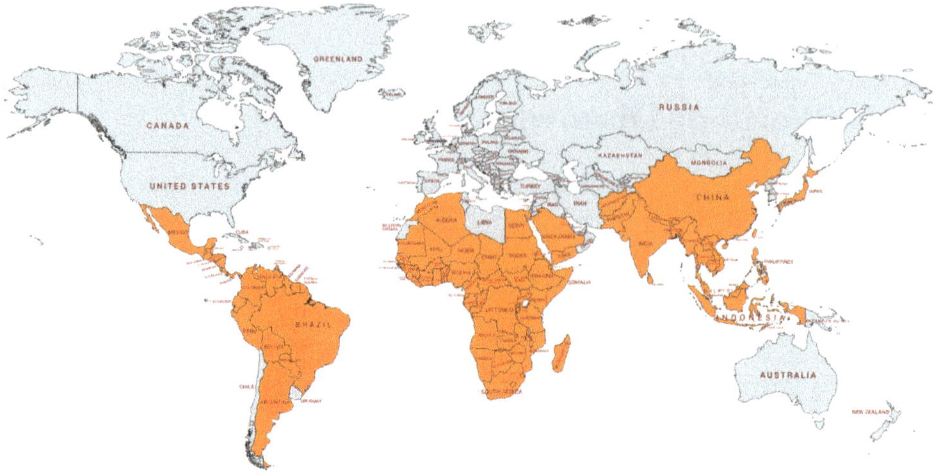

Figure 1. Global primate distribution. In orange, countries with native species of primates. Data were extracted from IUCN/SSC Primate Specialist group web site www.primate-sg.org/threat_primate_habitat_country/ on August 15th. Graph art was generated using mapchart.net.

Primates radiated to five infraorders, of which the infraorder Simiiformes emerged about 36–50 MYA and is divided in the parvorders Catarrhini (Old World monkeys, great apes, gibbons, and humans) and Platyrrhini (neotropical monkeys). The parvorder Catarrhini consists of three families: Cercopithecidae, Hominidae and Hylobatidae. The Cercopithecidae family, also known as Old World primates (OWPs), is the largest family, with 32 genera and 138 species described living in Africa and Asia [4]. Examples of OWPs include the *Macaca* (macaques), *Papio* (baboons), *Cercocebus* (mangabeys) and *Mandrillus* (mandrills) genera, all primates lacking prehensile tails. The Hylobatidae family harbors Asian primates known as gibbons, considered small apes [6]. The Hylobatidae is considered a sister clade of the Hominidae family, composed of the great apes (the largest primate species) and includes four genera: *Pongo* (orangutan), *Gorilla* (gorilla), *Pan* (bonobo and chimpanzee) and *Homo* (human) [4].

The parvorder Platyrrhini, also known as neotropical primates (NPs), is composed of Latin American primates descendent from African Cercopithecidae primates that reached South America about 40 MYA [4,7]. The spread of NPs in South and Central America resulted in a broad radiation that permitted the occupation of a large range of biomes from Mexico to the Argentinian Patagonia, leading to a great diversity of morphology and body size [8]. NPs are small to mid-sized animals, ranging from the world's smallest primate pigmy marmoset (*Cebuella pygmae*; 14–16 cm in length) to the Southern muriqui (*Brachyteles acrachnoides*; 55–70 cm in length). Other unique features of Platyrrhini include a flat nose compared to OWPs (originating the name of the parvorder) and a prehensile tail. NPs also lack trichromatic vision, which is characteristic of OWPs [9]. In contrast to OWPs, most NP species constitute monogamous pairs, and provide extensive paternal care of young [10]. With respect to diet, NPs eat fruits, nuts, flowers, insects, bird eggs, spiders, and small mammals [11].

Platyrrhini is divided into three families (Atelidae, Cebidae, and Pitheciidae), 21 genera and at least 170 species according to recent molecular analyses [4], of which 42% are threatened (www.primate-sg.org/primate_diversity_by_region/). Since the 2000s, 19 novel species and subspecies have been described in the region, with the most recent being a new titi monkey species (*Plecturocebus grovesi* sp. nov.), described in 2019 [12].

3. Diversity and Origin of SFVs in the Americas

SFVs have been shown to naturally infect most nonhuman primates (NHPs), including NPs, OWPs, and prosimians [13,14]. For over 60 years of spumavirus study, most research focused on SFVs in OWPs. In 1973, the presence of a syncytium-forming virus was first detected in a spider monkey (*Ateles* sp.) brain culture, classified then as SFV-8 [2] and currently named SFVaxx after the revision of foamy virus nomenclature in 2018 [15]. The original classification using numbers was based on serologic neutralizing activity, with consecutive numbers used for those isolates with undetectable or weak neutralizing activity to known SFVs indicative of infection with a divergent variant. The current SFV classification uses a three-letter code for the host species name with the first letter of the host genus and the next two letters derived from the first two letters of the species or subspecies. If the species or subspecies is unknown, the letters "xx" are used. Hence, SFVaxx refers to SFV from an *Ateles* monkey for which the species is not known. In 1975, an SFV infecting capuchin monkeys (*Cebus* sp.) was isolated and called SFV-9 [16]. In 1976, another strain of SFV was isolated from red uacari (*Cacajao rubicundus*) lymphocytes in a co-culture with kidney cells from a nocturnal monkey (*Aotus* sp.) [17]. Early in the 1980s, a fourth neotropical SFV was characterized in skin explants of 46 healthy white-tufted marmosets (*Callithrix jaccus*) [18]. Not until 2007 was the complete genome of SFVaxx obtained, 34 years after it was first isolated [19]. In 2010, complete SFVssc and SFVcja genomes, which infect squirrel monkeys (*Saimiri sciureus*) and white-tufted marmosets (*Callithrix jaccus*), respectively, were reported [20].

While phylogenetic analysis of short polymerase (*pol*) sequences demonstrated the co-evolution of SFVs with their NHP hosts [14], only one sequence from SFVaxx was available at the time to fully understand the evolutionary trajectory of SFVs in NPs. Phylogenetic analysis of the three complete SFV genomes from NPs with those from OWPs and a prosimian showed SFVs clustering into three major clades, reflecting the evolutionary split between NP (parvorder Platyrhini), OWP (parvorder Catarrhini), and prosimian (Strepsirrhini suborder) hosts [20]. More recently, complete SFV genomes were obtained from *Sapajus xanthosternos*, the yellow-breasted capuchin (SFVsxa), and *Brachyteles arachnoides*, the wooly spider monkey (SFVbar) [21,22]. Additionally, partial SFV *pol* and/or LTR/*gag* sequences (around 500-bp) were obtained from SFV strains infecting 20 different NP species from 10 genera, encompassing all three NP families (Table 1) [23–25]. Nonetheless, the complete or partial characterization of these few strains is still poor when compared to the wide diversity of NPs, with more than 150 species described. Furthermore, another 16 species from 11 NP genera had indirect evidence of foamy virus (FV) infection, characterized by diagnostic PCR, Western blot detection and/or detectable DNA viral load (VL) by quantitative PCR (qPCR) (Table 1). The size of the DNA fragments generated by these PCR techniques (192-bp) was, however, too small to enable robust phylogenetic inferences from those species, since this region is very conserved among the different strains and therefore has a low phylogenetic signal for resolution of related strains.

Table 1. Simian foamy virus (SFV) diversity in neotropical primates revealed by virus detection and complete or partial genome characterization.

Primate Family	Genus	Common Name	Complete Genome [1]	Partial Genome (LTR/*gag* and/or *pol*) [1]	Diagnostic-PCR and/or qPCR and/or WB Serology [1]
Cebidae	*Aotus*	owl monkey			SFVaaz, SFVatr, SFVani
	Callimico	marmoset			SFVcgo
	Callithrix	marmoset	SFVcja	SFVcge	SFVcau
	Cebus	capuchin		SFVcal	SFVcol
	Leontopithecus	tamarin		SFVlro, SFVlcm	SFVlcp
	Mico	marmoset			SFVmhu
	Saguinus	tamarin			SFVsbi, SFVsfu, SFVsmi, SFVsoe
	Saimiri	squirrel monkey	SFVssc	SFVsbo, SFVsus	
	Sapajus	capuchin	SFVsxa	SFVsap, SFVsfl, SFVsro	
Atelidae	*Alouatta*	howler monkey		SFVabe, SFVaca, SFVagu, SFVase	SFVapl
	Ateles	spider monkey	SFVaxx	SFVage, SFVahy, SFVach	SFVafu, SFVapn
	Brachyteles	wooly spider monkey	SFVbar		
	Lagothrix	wooly monkey		SFVlla	
Pitheciidae	*Cacajao*	uakari	—	SFVcca, SFVcme	
	Callicebus	titi	—	—	SFVcmo
	Pithecia	saki	—	SFVppi	

[1] Species definition for SFV by primate genera: *Aloutta*: SFVabe (*Alouatta belzebul*), SFVaca (*Alouatta caraya*), SFVagu (*Alouatta guariba*), SFVase (*Alouatta seniculus*); SFVapl (*Alouatta palliata*); *Aotus*: SFVaaz (*Aotus azarae*), SFVatr (*Aotus trivirgatus*), SFVani (*Aotus nigriceps*); *Ateles*: SFVage (*Ateles geoffroyi*), SFVahy (*Ateles hybridus*), SFVach (*Ateles chamek*), SFVafu (*Ateles fusciceps*), SFVapn (*Ateles paniscus*), SFVaxx (*Ateles* sp.); *Brachyteles*: SFVbar (*Brachyteles aracnoides*); *Cacajao*: SFVcca (*Cacajao calvus*), SFVcme (*Cacajao melanocephalus*); *Callicebus*: SFVcmo (*Callicebus moloch*); *Callimico*: SFVcgo (*Callimico goeldii*); *Callithrix*: SFVcau (*Callithrix aurita*), SFVcge (*Callithrix geoffroyi*), SFVcja (*Callithrix jaccus*); *Cebus*: SFVcal (*Cebus albifrons*), SFVcol (*Cebus olivaceus*); *Lagothrix*: SFVlia (*Lagothrix lagotricha*) *Leontopithecus*: SFVlcm (*Leontopithecus chrysomelas*), SFVlcp (*Leontopithecus chrysopygus*), SFVlro (*Leontopithecus rosalia*); *Mico*: SFVmhu (*Mico humeralifer*); *Pithecia*: SFVppi (*Pithecia pithecia*); *Saguinus*: SFVsbi (*Saguinus bicolor*), SFVsfu (*Saguinus fuscicollis*), SFVsmi (*Saguinus midas*), SFVsoe (*Saguinus oedipus*); *Saimiri*: SFVsbo (*Saimiri boliviensis*), SFVssc (*Saimiri sciureus*), SFVsbo (*Saimiri ustus*); *Sapajus*: SFVsap (*Sapajus apella*), SFVsfl (*Sapajus flavius*), SFVsro (*Sapajus robustus*), SFVsxa (*Sapajus xanthosternos*).

Phylogenetic analysis of the genetic sequences of NP SFV isolates has allowed for the determination of their evolutionary history, which shows distinct evolutionary lineages. Furthermore, genetic characterization of endogenous FVs integrated into mammals, reptiles, amphibians and fish [14,26–31] has permitted elucidation of the genetic relationships between exogenous and endogenous FVs, revealing strong evidence of an ancient co-speciation of FVs with their hosts since the origin of marine vertebrates around 500 MYA [27]. The co-speciation hypothesis of SFVs with their primate hosts has also been demonstrated in OWPs and NPs at the family, genus and species levels occurring around 43 MYA [24,25,32]. The phylogeny of NP SFVs also reflects the evolutionary relationships of their hosts, but with some exceptions. For example, SFVs from monkeys in the Pithecidae family (Pithecia, Cacajao, Chiropotes) are not monophyletic as expected with co-evolution and SFV *pol* sequences from Saimiri are paraphyletic to those from monkeys in the Cebidae family instead of being sister taxa in accordance with the co-evolutionary hypothesis (Figure 2). These unexpected phylogenetic relationships may result from only short sequences being analyzed or from cross-species infections, as further discussed below.

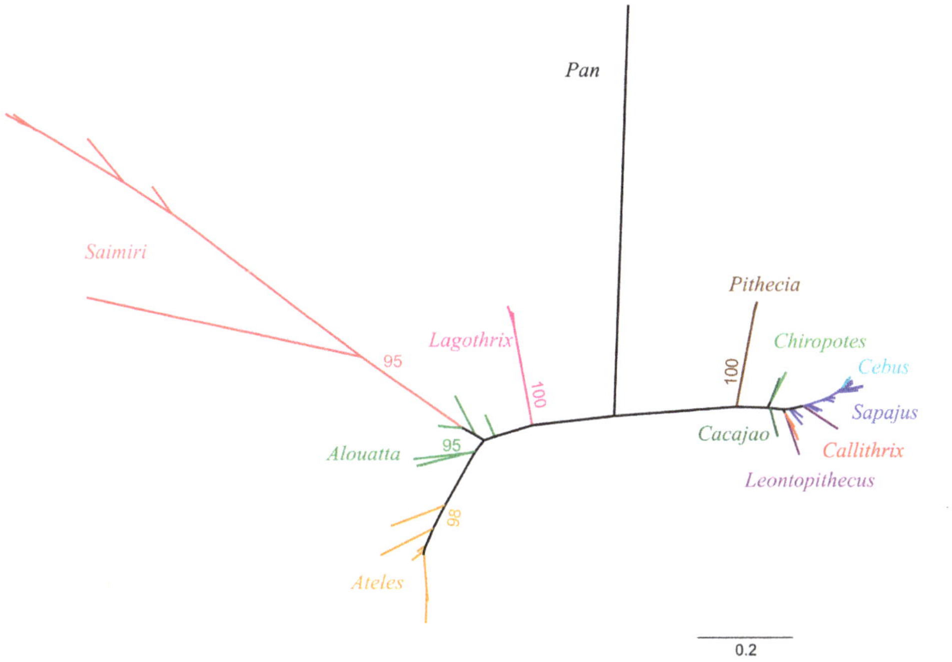

Figure 2. Phylogenetic relationships of simian foamy viruses from neotropical primates (NPs). Unrooted tree inferred by maximum likelihood analysis of an alignment of 411 nucleotides of partial polymerase sequences with 1000 bootstrap replicates. Different NP genera and bootstrap values are indicated by distinct colors. Distance bar is shown at the bottom.

Comparison of complete SFV genomes among primate hosts revealed some interesting features (Figure 3). For example, the mean size of the *pol* gene is highly conserved among SFVs infecting OWPs and NPs (average of 3435-bp and 3436-bp, respectively) [21]. Similarly, the envelope (*env*) gene lengths are also comparable with a mean size of 2949-bp in NP SFVs and 2962-bp in OWP SFVs. The length of these two genes also appears to be conserved in feline and equine FVs. The exception is the bovine FV *pol* gene, which is 3660-bp in length [21]. The size of the *gag* gene coding for the group specific antigen is conserved within both NP (range of 1817–2071-bp) and OWP SFVs (range of 1872–1974-bp) [21,22,33]. The exception is SFVssc, which has the shortest *gag* gene (1716-bp) of all

SFVs described to date. The long terminal repeat (LTR) region has a mean length of 1696-bp among OWP SFVs, with the longest LTR in SFVs infecting a pileated gibbon (SFVhpi), at 2074-bp [21,33], while an SFV infecting Cebidae has the shortest LTR among FVs (1061–1080-bp). SFVaxx has LTRs ranging from 1129-bp (SFVbar) to 1251-bp (SFVasp) in length [21,22]. Whether gene or LTR length differences among SFVs affect their biological functions remains to be elucidated.

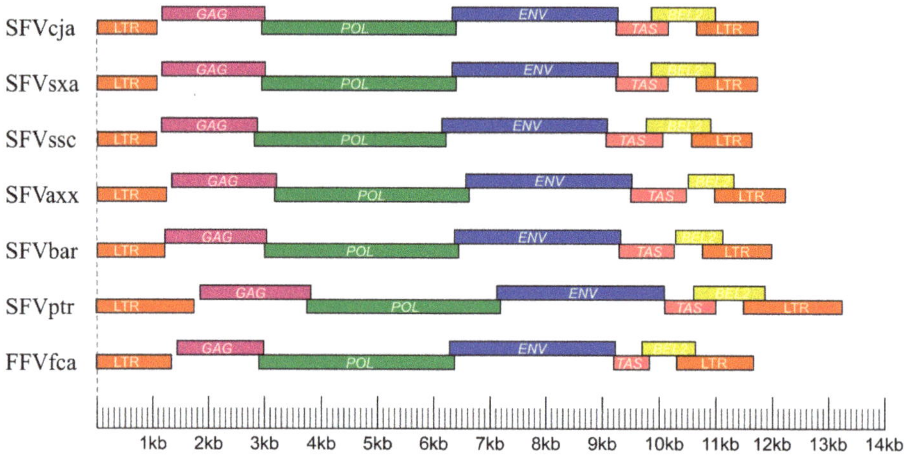

Figure 3. Structural organization of complete simian foamy virus (SFV) and feline foamy virus (FFV) genomes. SFVcja (*Callithrix jaccus*), SFVsxa (*Sapajus xanthosternos*), SFVssc (*Saimiri sciureus*), SFVaxx (*Ateles* sp.), SFVbar (*Brachyteles aracnoides*), SFVptr (*Pan troglodytes*), FFVfca (*Feline catus*). LTR, long terminal repeat; GAG, group specific antigen, POL, polymerase; ENV, envelope; TAS, transcriptional activator; BEL2, between the ENV and LTR.

4. NP SFV Prevalence and Viral Detection Methodologies

Very little is known about the prevalence of SFV in wild NP populations, while studies of captive animals are relatively common (Table 2). A seminal study in 1975 with *Ateles sp.* (spider monkeys) determined that 61% of specimens had antibodies against SFVaxx [16]. Another study conducted in the 1980s with 90 marmosets (*Callithrix jaccus* and *Saguinus* sp.) living in a colony in the United States (U.S.), found a 54% SFV seroprevalence only in *Callithrix* specimens [18]. However, these studies were performed using in-house serological assays that were not validated and standardized, and therefore the reported SFV serological prevalence may have been overestimated by the lack of specificity of the test and/or possible cross-reactivity.

Table 2. Simian foamy virus prevalence in neotropical primates.

Study	Methodology	Sites	Prevalence
Hooks, 1975 [2]	Serology	Colony	61%
Marczynska et al., 1981 [18]	Serology	Colony	54%
Muniz et al., 2013 [23]	Diag. PCR [1]	Brazilian zoo and primatology center Wild primates	23% 29%
Ghersi et al., 2015 [25]	Serology and Diag. PCR	Peruvian and US zoos Peruvian rescue center Illegal trade market	45–47% 19%
Muniz et al., 2015 [24]	Serology and Diag. PCR	Brazilian zoo and primatology center	51%

[1] Diagnostic PCR.

Decades later in 2013, a large study examined 332 NP samples from 15 genera using molecular testing to detect 192-bp *pol* NP SFV sequences in peripheral blood mononuclear cells (PBMCs), including—for the first time—samples collected from wild monkeys [23]. The PCR assay used in this study had a 100% sensitivity using PBMC specimens from Western blot (WB)-positive monkeys from seven NP genera (*Alouatta*, *Aotus*, *Ateles*, *Cacajao*, *Callithrix*, *Cebus*, and *Pithecia*), except for *Saimiri* specimens, with four PCR-positive specimens being WB-negative [34]. The WB used combined antigens from extracts of CfTh2 cells infected with two NP SFV isolates from *Callithrix jaccus* (SFVcja) and *Ateles* sp. (SFVaxx), representing two out of the three NP families, and had shown sensitivity and specificity both > 94% using > 100 SFV+ and SFV− NP specimens [25]. Muniz et al. showed that SFV prevalence among captive specimens was 23% (61/267) versus 29% (19/65) in wild NPs [23]. The molecular prevalence found in this study is lower than that described for African OWP SFVs in wild monkeys (60–100%), including mandrills (*Mandrillus sphinx*), red colobus monkeys (*Piliocolobus badius badius*), baboons (*Papio cynocephalus*) and chimpanzees (*Pan troglodytes*) [35–38]. In comparison, the molecular prevalence of SFV in captive Asian macaques is 39% among rhesus macaque (*Macaca mulata*) [39], while a seroprevalence of 64–94% has been reported in captive cynomolgus macaque (*Macaca fascicularis*) [40]. The lower SFV prevalence in NPs may reflect a high number of specimens from juveniles, since SFV seroprevalence has been shown to be associated with age. For instance, in a study of a colony of tonkean macaques (*Macaca tonkeana*), SFV seroprevalence was shown to be lower in infants (5%), intermediate in sub-adults (44%) and high in adults (89%) [41]. The same age and seroprevalence relationship has been observed in baboons and cynomolgus macaques [1,40,42]. However, no age of specimens was available in Ref. [23], since that was a study conducted with retrospective samples.

In 2015, a new study estimated the SFV prevalence among Peruvian primates in zoos, rescue centers and the illegal trade market using both molecular and serological assays [25]. The seroprevalence of SFV in NPs from Peruvian zoos using both enzyme immunoassay (EIA) and Western blot (WB) was higher (47%) than those in rescue centers of free-living primates (19%; $p = 0.001$) and similar to those reported in NPs from U.S. zoos (45%). Noteworthy was the SFV prevalence of 43% in Peruvian zoos and 22% in rescue centers in *Lagothrix lagothicha* (wooly monkey), indicating an increased SFV infection in captivity. The lower prevalence in rescue centers could reflect testing of younger animals. Overall, the WB assay in that study showed a total prevalence of 78%, higher than those of the diagnostic PCR assay (19%) and for a PCR test that detected a 495-bp *pol* sequence (26%), indicating that WB more accurately detects previous or current SFV infection. The low efficiency of the diagnostic PCR method could be explained by the high genetic variability of NP SFVs. The *pol* genetic diversity between strains of SFV infecting genera within the same primate family is around 12% in the Cebidae and 31% in the Atelidae families. In contrast, a higher *pol* divergence (41%) occurs between SFV from the Atelidae and Cebidae [23]. The lower sensitivity of the PCR assay could also be explained by the low DNA proviral load (pVL) of NP SFVs in blood cells, with an average of 800 SFV copies/10^6 cells reported [43,44], very similar to that found in OWPs [45,46]. Furthermore, these findings suggest that SFV does not expand to significant levels in this compartment [46,47].

Another study in 2015 compared the serological and molecular prevalence of NP SFV at the Rio de Janeiro Zoo and the Center of Primatology of Rio de Janeiro state, confirming that WB is more sensitive for detecting SFV infection in NPs [24]. However, as some WB-seronegative animals in the study were PCR-positive, the use of both techniques for SFV detection is needed for epidemiologic studies. Monkeys testing positive with either or both tests would then be considered SFV-positive. In this study, the NP SFV prevalence was similar to that found in Peru, with a WB prevalence of 43% and a molecular prevalence of 29% in captive animals. Of the 140 specimens analyzed, 51% were positive in at least one test. Although serology in these recent studies was shown to be more sensitive for SFV detection, preparation of large amounts of antigens used in the serologic assays may be costly and is dependent on the laboratory having biosafety facilities and equipment for cultivating FV strains in cell culture [24,25]. Good alternatives to that limitation include cloning of SFV *gag* genes and expressing them in bacterial systems, or the use of synthesized peptides from *gag* gene sequences to detect antibodies, which have been used in feline foamy virus (FFV) and SFV research [48,49]. More recently, a new study developed a real-time PCR (qPCR) methodology to diagnose and measure SFV DNA pVL in NPs with a high sensitivity and specificity [43]. Of animals with detectable SFV DNA pVL, 90–96% were also WB-positive. NP SFV prevalence using the different methodologies is summarized in Table 2.

An important concern for detecting SFV in the blood of NPs is the small size of these animals, which limits the amount of blood collected. Consequently, there is typically only low amounts of genomic DNA available to be used for diagnostic PCR [23,24]. Considering this, qPCR can be used as a simpler alternative to SFV WB detection with the same sensitivity but using less DNA. Another alternative is the use of buccal swabs for PCR detection of NP SFVs. In addition to being a less invasive collection method, SFV replication is higher in the oral cavity of OWPs [45,50], which should increase the sensitivity of detecting SFV infection by using molecular methods [51,52]. For NPs, the SFV DNA pVL found in oral tissues ranges between 20–142 million copies/10^6 cells [43], which is higher than that reported for SFV-infected rhesus macaques (*Macaca mulatta*) using salivary gland, tonsil and tongue specimens (500–100,000 SFV copies/10^6 cells) [46]. A recent study showed that the DNA pVL found in oral tissues of NPs with matching PBMC samples was up to 8000 copies/10^6 cells higher than those observed in blood cells, showing that oral tissues are better specimens for SFV detection [43]. The authors of that NP study also showed that the DNA pVL in PBMC is a proxy for the detection of proviral DNA in PBMC by nested PCR with qPCR again being more sensitive. However, only 45% of NPs in that study had SFV detected in oral tissues, which could underestimate the true prevalence in NPs if only buccal swabs are used for diagnosis [43].

5. NP SFV Epidemiology and Transmission

In OWPs, SFV proviral DNA has been found in many tissues and cell types, including in oral-respiratory tissues and peripheral blood cells [47,53]. Nonetheless, viral expression and replication appear to be restricted to the oral mucosa, as studies have shown high levels of viral RNA only at this site [1,47]. It has also been reported that oral mucosa epithelial cells act as a virus reservoir [50]. Thus, scratches, bites and grooming constitute the main routes of horizontal OWP SFV transmission, mainly via parental care and aggressive behavior in territorial and sexual partner disputes [1].

For NPs, SFVs have been molecularly detected in liver specimens [23], oral tissues [43] and peripheral blood cells [23–25,43]. The SFV DNA proviral load (pVL) in oral mucosa is similar for NPs [43,44] and OWPs [45,46], indicating this compartment as a virus reservoir for FV infecting primates in general. The higher SFV DNA pVL found in oral tissues of SFV-infected NPs is compatible with horizontal transmission via contact with saliva in biting or grooming, as described for OWPs [1,50]. However, studies in NPs have not yet been conducted to determine SFV RNA levels in these compartments and their correlation with transmission. Since SFV isolates have been obtained from oral swabs of NPs, it would not be surprising that comparable SFV RNA levels are found in NPs as in OWPs [45].

Murray et al. proposed a model in which SFV primary infection occurs in blood and migratory cells, such as macrophages or leukocytes, which carry the virus to the basal epithelium of oropharyngeal tissues, with subsequent FV replication in differentiated epithelial cells [50]. A cynomolgus macaque (*Macaca fascicularis*) that was infected by SFV after a controlled blood transfusion from an SFV-infected donor macaque showed detectable DNA VLs in saliva 29 weeks after infection and detectable RNA VLs after 39 weeks [54]. In this scenario, it may take months for a newly infected animal to become capable of transmitting SFV. This model could explain why only 45% of SFV-infected NPs had DNA VL detectable in oral tissues [43]. Similar results were observed in free-ranging rhesus macaques (*Macaca mulatta*), of which about 30% of SFV-positive animals did not have detectable RNA VLs in saliva [45]. The RNA VLs in this study also correlated with the age of the macaques, with older monkeys having higher SFV RNA levels [45].

SFVs can also be transmitted vertically but studies have been limited to small numbers of species. Blasse et al. showed that mother-to-offspring transmission of SFV is frequent among Western chimpanzees (*Pan troglodytes verus*) [55]. However, vertical transmission was rare in a study of captive *Macaca tonkeana* [41]. Even less is known about vertical transmission in NPs. A five month-old *Chiropotes* infant in quarantine was SFV-positive by both WB and *pol*-integrase PCR testing, indicating a possible vertical transmission [24]. However, samples from the mother were not available for testing to confirm this hypothesis, as the infant was from a rescue center. Studies of specimens collected in utero, perinatally, and from breast milk are needed to better understand the risks of vertical transmission of SFV.

Sexual transmission occurs for animals infected with other retroviruses, like primate lentivirus (SIV), but is rare [56,57]. However, little is known about the potential for sexual transmission for SFV. Differences in the NP SFV prevalence in males and females have not been observed, suggesting that if sexual transmission occurs it is equally likely from male to female and vice versa [23–25]. Differences in the SFV prevalence among different age groups of NPs have been reported, suggesting that horizontal transmission is likely more common than vertical transmission. Ghersi et al. found that the SFV prevalence increased with age among captive NPs in Peru, with 0% in infants, 30–50% in juveniles, 50–58% in sub-adults and 55–64% in adults [25]. In NPs from Peruvian rescue centers in that study, the SFV seroprevalence was higher in adults (32%) than in juveniles (17%). These findings are congruent with the SFV prevalence found in different age groups of OWPs [1,40,41]. However, Muniz et al. did not find a significant difference in SFV prevalence between juveniles (73%) and adults (87%) in vivaria in Brazil [24]. This SFV prevalence disparity may reflect a more confined environment of the vivaria in Brazil, which can increase the stress of the animals and, consequently, viral transmission. Another explanation could be different transmission rates by primate species. For example, when SFV results of *Sapajus* were analyzed separately, as they represented one third of the samples in that study, infected NPs were on average 6.8 years older than the uninfected NPs [24]. Additional studies with NPs from other countries, environments, and with more species will help to better define NP SFV prevalence by age. Nonetheless, the finding of high VLs in the oral mucosa and in older animals, and the increased SFV prevalence in older monkeys, suggests that horizontal transmission likely occurs via aggressive behaviors, such as biting, as monkeys become adults [1].

Similar to SFV-infected OWPs, evidence of pathogenicity has not been reported in SFV-infected NPs, though systematic studies have not been conducted for both parvorders. In rhesus macaques, SIV and SFV co-infection was reported to accelerate immunodeficiency related death (75% of deaths in 39 weeks) in comparison to those infected with only SIV (37% of deaths in 39 weeks), suggesting SFV co-infection may affect pathogenicity [58]. Similar co-infection studies in SFV-infected NPs have not been done.

6. SFV Cross-Species Transmission

Episodes of SFV transmission between NP species seems rare with only a few reported cases. A captive yellow-breasted capuchin (*Sapajus xanthosternos*) of the Cebidae family was found to be infected with an SFV that was phylogenetically more similar with an SFV from a spider monkey (*Ateles* species) of the Atelidae family [23]. Most likely, this cross-species transmission occurred while these monkeys were in captivity, since both primate species are not sympatric in Brazil. *Sapajus xanthosternos* are naturally found in the Caatinga forest of northeastern Brazil, while all species of *Ateles* inhabit the Amazon forest in northern Brazil. Phylogenetic analysis has also shown divergent SFV in *Leontopithecus* (tamarins) that do not cluster together, as would be expected under the co-evolution of SFV and host hypothesis, indicating at least one cross-species transmission in captivity [24]. Studies with free-living *Leontopithecus* will have to elucidate this finding.

Ancient cross-species and cross-genus SFV transmission may also have occurred in NPs and could explain the extant phylogenetic relations observed for SFVs in squirrel monkeys (*Saimiri* sp.) in the Cebidae family [14,23,25]. Squirrel monkey SFVs are more similar to those from monkeys in the Atelidae family (Figure 3) instead of the Cebine family (capuchins) as expected with a stable co-speciation history. Phylogenetic dating suggests that this cross-species transmission may have occurred at least 17 MYA with one or more SFV lineages not yet characterized, or possibly from the *Aotus* genus [25]. SFV cross-species transmissions have also been described for OWPs and appear to be equally infrequent [36,59].

To date, all persistent SFV infections detected in humans with documented viral nucleic acids originated by zoonotic transmissions of SFV infecting OWPs [60–64]. Cases of zoonotic transmission have been reported among individuals with exposure to nonhuman primates (NHPs), including veterinarians, keepers, biologists, researchers, and pet owners. Butchers and hunters can also be infected with SFV as OWP hunting and meat consumption is common in African villages and indigenous communities [65]. These workers and hunters have been infected with many different divergent OWP SFVs, including macaques, African green monkeys, chimpanzees, gorillas, mandrills, colobus monkeys, and various *Cercopithecus* species [63,66–69]. Interestingly, studies have shown that between 18 and 36% of individuals who were severely bitten or injured from hunting wild chimpanzees and gorillas in Cameroon and Gabon were SFV-positive [60,70], further supporting bites as the major transmission route. Longitudinal studies of persons infected with OWP SFVs have yet to show strong evidence of diseases associated with their zoonotic infections [57–60]. One recent case-control study reported potential hematological abnormalities in apparently healthy SFV-infected persons from Cameroon [66]. More systematic longitudinal studies are required to investigate SFV disease associations, including in persons co-infected with other retroviruses such as human immunodeficiency and human T-cell leukemia viruses.

In contrast to OWPs, the potential for zoonotic transmission of NP SFVs to humans is less clear. A first study evaluated the presence of SFV among 116 primatologists, of which 69 were occupationally exposed to NPs [44]. While 12% (8/69) of the primatologists were positive for NP SFV by WB, no viral DNA was detected in the blood of these individuals, suggestive of exposure but not persistent infection or latent infection. Only four of the eight SFV-seropositive individuals reported accidents with NPs such as bites, scratches and injuries with contaminated sharp instruments. The other four workers reported contact with body fluids, but not parenterally, suggesting that contact with animal fluids without parenteral exposure may be sufficient for viral infection [44].

More recently, a study of persons occupationally exposed to SFV-infected NPs at a zoo and a primatology center in Brazil was reported. In this study, whole blood and oral swab samples were obtained from 56 individuals over three years (2011, 2012/2013 and 2014) [67]. A serological prevalence of 19% was found for NP anti-SFV antibodies, while—similar to the initial study described above—viral DNA was not detected in any of the sampled compartments. As issues related to the presence of PCR inhibitors in the DNA preparations were considered, the authors used different methods to clean the DNA from potential inhibitors, including the use of the OneStep PCR inhibitor removal kit (Zymo Research, Irvine, CA, USA) or of general column-based PCR purification kits after DNA extraction. However, even those measures failed to provide PCR-positive samples. Of the 12 SFV-seroreactive workers, 11 reported bites, scratches and/or direct contact with body fluids from NPs. Interestingly, for some of the workers more recently exposed to infected animals, a clearance of SFV antibodies was detected two years later compared to previous collection time points. WB-negative workers in this study reported contact with NPs for an average of 12 years, while the WB-positive workers reported NP contact for an average of only three years.

Combined, these findings in persons exposed to NPs suggest possible control of SFV infection and antibody clearance, in contrast to human infection with OWP SFV. In these NP exposure cases, it is not known whether the virus has been truly eliminated from the body or if it is still present in another body compartment or reservoir. Additional follow-up testing of these workers and additional studies of persons exposed to NPs will help to elucidate the potential for zoonotic transmission of NP SFVs to humans. Exposure to NPs in Brazil can be frequent in forest parks and in large urban centers where primates have been observed feeding on household waste [68]. Evidence for disease in these workers with SFV-reactive serology results was not reported and clear evidence of disease associations has not been found in persons infected with OWP SFVs [64,68].

Like OWP SFVs, studies have documented that different human cells can be infected with NP SFVs, including strains of SFVaxx and SFVssc, but the cell tropism was distinct between strains. SFVaxx infected HT1080 (fibrosarcoma), MDA (mammary adenocarcinoma) and C33A (cervical carcinoma), but not AGS (adenocarcinoma), LN (lymphoblastoid) and LoVo (adenocarcinoma), while SFVssc infected only HT1080 [44]. Another study showed that the human TRIM5α did not affect the replication of SFVcja and SFVaxx [69], but restricted the replication of SFVssc [20]. These latter findings may help to explain the seroreactive but PCR-negative results in humans exposed to NP SFVs.

7. Perspectives

While considerable progress has been made in recent years to better understand the epidemiology and evolutionary history of NP SFVs, more research is needed. Additional SFV genomes should be sequenced, with emphasis on those infecting species from the Pitheciidae family (titi, saki and uacari monkeys) and the *Aotus* genus (owl monkeys), in order to clarify the evolutionary relationships of SFV among NPs, especially the unusual relationships of SFV that infect squirrel monkeys (*Saimiri* sp). Studies published to date with NPs have used a large number of specimens of various captive genera and species, but few specimens of each species. Future work should focus on studies of the viral epidemiology of wild NPs, with a reasonable number of specimens per species. RNA VL in oral tissues needs to be determined, as well as which tissues are targeted by SFV infection in NPs. Follow-up studies of workers with direct or indirect contact with NPs should continue to clarify whether SFV infection is resolved or if the virus persists in certain cells or body compartments. Additional studies of persons naturally exposed to NPs and their SFV infections are needed to define zoonotic risks for these viruses.

Author Contributions: All authors contributed equally to this paper with the conception and design of the paper, literature review and analysis, drafting, critical revision and editing, and approval of the final version.

Funding: This research received no external funding.

Acknowledgments: Use of trade names is for identification only and does not imply endorsement by the U.S. Department of Health and Human Services, the Public Health Service, or the Centers for Disease Control and Prevention (CDC). The findings and conclusions in this report are those of the authors and do not necessarily represent the views of the CDC, or any of the authors' affiliated institutions.).

Conflicts of Interest: The authors declare no conflict of interest.

References

1. Murray, S.M.; Linial, M.L. Foamy virus infection in primates. *J. Med. Primatol.* **2006**, *35*, 225–235. [CrossRef] [PubMed]
2. Hooks, J.J.; Gibbs, C.J., Jr.; Chou, S.; Howk, R.; Lewis, M.; Gajdusek, D.C. Isolation of a new simian foamy virus from a spider monkey brain culture. *Infect. Immun.* **1973**, *8*, 804–813. [PubMed]
3. Estrada, A.; Garber, P.A.; Rylands, A.B.; Roos, C.; Fernandez-Duque, E.; Di Fiore, A.; Nekaris, K.A.; Nijman, V.; Heymann, E.W.; Lambert, J.E.; et al. Impending extinction crisis of the world's primates: Why primates matter. *Sci. Adv.* **2017**, *3*, e1600946. [CrossRef] [PubMed]
4. Perelman, P.; Johnson, W.E.; Roos, C.; Seuanez, H.N.; Horvath, J.E.; Moreira, M.A.; Kessing, B.; Pontius, J.; Roelke, M.; Rumpler, Y.; et al. A molecular phylogeny of living primates. *PLoS Genet.* **2011**, *7*, e1001342. [CrossRef] [PubMed]
5. Goodman, M.; Porter, C.A.; Czelusniak, J.; Page, S.L.; Schneider, H.; Shoshani, J.; Gunnell, G.; Groves, C.P. Toward a phylogenetic classification of Primates based on DNA evidence complemented by fossil evidence. *Mol. Phylogenet. Evol.* **1998**, *9*, 585–598. [CrossRef] [PubMed]
6. Brandon-Jones, D.; Eudey, A.A.; Geissmann, T.; Groves, C.P.; Melnick, D.J.; Morales, J.C.; Shekelle, M.; Stewart, C.-B. Asian Primate classification. *Int. J. Primatol.* **2004**, *25*, 67. [CrossRef]

7. Perez, S.I.; Tejedor, M.F.; Novo, N.M.; Aristide, L. Divergence times and the evolutionary radiation of new world monkeys (platyrrhini, primates): An analysis of fossil and molecular data. *PLoS ONE* **2013**, *8*, e68029. [CrossRef] [PubMed]
8. Rosenberger, A.L. Evolution of feeding niches in New World monkeys. *Am. J. Phys. Anthropol.* **1992**, *88*, 525–562. [CrossRef]
9. Carroll, S.B. *The Making of the Fittest: DNA and the Ultimate Forensic Record of Evolution*, 1st ed.; W.W. Norton & Co.: New York, NY, USA, 2006; p. 301.
10. Garber, P.A.; Leigh, S.R. Ontogenetic variation in small-bodied New World primates: Implications for patterns of reproduction and infant care. *Folia Primatol.* **1997**, *68*, 1–22. [CrossRef]
11. Amato, K.R.; Martinez-Mota, R.; Righini, N.; Raguet-Schofield, M.; Corcione, F.P.; Marini, E.; Humphrey, G.; Gogul, G.; Gaffney, J.; Lovelace, E.; et al. Phylogenetic and ecological factors impact the gut microbiota of two Neotropical primate species. *Oecologia* **2016**, *180*, 717–733. [CrossRef]
12. Boubli, J.P.; Byrne, H.; da Silva, M.N.F.; Silva-Junior, J.; Costa Araujo, R.; Bertuol, F.; Goncalves, J.; de Melo, F.R.; Rylands, A.B.; Mittermeier, R.A.; et al. On a new species of titi monkey (Primates: Plecturocebus Byrne et al., 2016), from Alta Floresta, southern Amazon, Brazil. *Mol. Phylogenet. Evol.* **2019**, *132*, 117–137. [CrossRef] [PubMed]
13. Peeters, M.; D'Arc, M.; Delaporte, E. Origin and diversity of human retroviruses. *AIDS Rev.* **2014**, *16*, 23–34. [PubMed]
14. Katzourakis, A.; Aiewsakun, P.; Jia, H.; Wolfe, N.D.; LeBreton, M.; Yoder, A.D.; Switzer, W.M. Discovery of prosimian and afrotherian foamy viruses and potential cross species transmissions amidst stable and ancient mammalian co-evolution. *Retrovirology* **2014**, *11*, 61. [CrossRef] [PubMed]
15. Khan, A.S.; Bodem, J.; Buseyne, F.; Gessain, A.; Johnson, W.; Kuhn, J.H.; Kuzmak, J.; Lindemann, D.; Linial, M.L.; Lochelt, M.; et al. Spumaretroviruses: Updated taxonomy and nomenclature. *Virology* **2018**, *516*, 158–164. [CrossRef]
16. Hooks, J.J.; Gibbs, C.J., Jr. The foamy viruses. *Bacteriol. Rev.* **1975**, *39*, 169–185.
17. Barahona, H.; Garcia, F.G.; Melendez, L.V.; King, N.W.; Ingalls, J.K. Isolation and characterization of lymphocyte associated foamy virus from a red uakari monkey (Cacajao rubicundus). *J. Med. Primatol.* **1976**, *5*, 253–265. [CrossRef]
18. Marczynska, B.; Jones, C.J.; Wolfe, L.G. Syncytium-forming virus of common marmosets (Callithrix jacchus jacchus). *Infect. Immun.* **1981**, *31*, 1261–1269.
19. Thumer, L.; Rethwilm, A.; Holmes, E.C.; Bodem, J. The complete nucleotide sequence of a New World simian foamy virus. *Virology* **2007**, *369*, 191–197. [CrossRef]
20. Pacheco, B.; Finzi, A.; McGee-Estrada, K.; Sodroski, J. Species-specific inhibition of foamy viruses from South American monkeys by New World Monkey TRIM5{alpha} proteins. *J. Virol.* **2010**, *84*, 4095–4099. [CrossRef]
21. Troncoso, L.L.; Muniz, C.P.; Siqueira, J.D.; Curty, G.; Schrago, C.G.; Augusto, A.; Fedullo, L.; Soares, M.A.; Santos, A.F. Characterization and comparative analysis of a simian foamy virus complete genome isolated from Brazilian capuchin monkeys. *Virus Res.* **2015**, *208*, 1–6. [CrossRef]
22. Muniz, C.P.; Cavalcante, L.T.F.; Dudley, D.M.; Pissinatti, A.; O'Connor, D.H.; Santos, A.F.; Soares, M.A. First complete genome sequence of a simian foamy virus infecting the neotropical primate brachyteles arachnoides. *Microbiol. Resour. Announc.* **2018**, *7*, 2. [CrossRef] [PubMed]
23. Muniz, C.P.; Troncoso, L.L.; Moreira, M.A.; Soares, E.A.; Pissinatti, A.; Bonvicino, C.R.; Seuanez, H.N.; Sharma, B.; Jia, H.; Shankar, A.; et al. Identification and characterization of highly divergent simian foamy viruses in a wide range of new world primates from Brazil. *PLoS ONE* **2013**, *8*, e67568. [CrossRef] [PubMed]
24. Muniz, C.P.; Jia, H.; Shankar, A.; Troncoso, L.L.; Augusto, A.M.; Farias, E.; Pissinatti, A.; Fedullo, L.P.; Santos, A.F.; Soares, M.A.; et al. An expanded search for simian foamy viruses (SFV) in Brazilian New World primates identifies novel SFV lineages and host age-related infections. *Retrovirology* **2015**, *12*, 94. [CrossRef] [PubMed]
25. Ghersi, B.M.; Jia, H.; Aiewsakun, P.; Katzourakis, A.; Mendoza, P.; Bausch, D.G.; Kasper, M.R.; Montgomery, J.M.; Switzer, W.M. Wide distribution and ancient evolutionary history of simian foamy viruses in New World primates. *Retrovirology* **2015**, *12*, 89. [CrossRef] [PubMed]
26. Han, G.Z.; Worobey, M. Endogenous viral sequences from the Cape golden mole (Chrysochloris asiatica) reveal the presence of foamy viruses in all major placental mammal clades. *PLoS ONE* **2014**, *9*, e97931. [CrossRef] [PubMed]

27. Aiewsakun, P.; Katzourakis, A. Marine origin of retroviruses in the early Palaeozoic Era. *Nat. Commun.* **2017**, *8*, 13954. [CrossRef]
28. Han, G.Z.; Worobey, M. An endogenous foamy-like viral element in the coelacanth genome. *PLoS Pathog.* **2012**, *8*, e1002790. [CrossRef]
29. Ruboyianes, R.; Worobey, M. Foamy-like endogenous retroviruses are extensive and abundant in teleosts. *Virus Evol.* **2016**, *2*, vew032. [CrossRef]
30. Han, G.Z. Extensive retroviral diversity in shark. *Retrovirology* **2015**, *12*, 34. [CrossRef]
31. Aiewsakun, P.; Simmonds, P.; Katzourakis, A. The first co-opted endogenous foamy viruses and the evolutionary history of reptilian foamy viruses. *Viruses* **2019**, *11*, 7. [CrossRef]
32. Switzer, W.M.; Salemi, M.; Shanmugam, V.; Gao, F.; Cong, M.E.; Kuiken, C.; Bhullar, V.; Beer, B.E.; Vallet, D.; Gautier-Hion, A.; et al. Ancient co-speciation of simian foamy viruses and primates. *Nature* **2005**, *434*, 376–380. [CrossRef] [PubMed]
33. Shankar, A.; Sibley, S.D.; Goldberg, T.L.; Switzer, W.M. Molecular analysis of the complete genome of a simian foamy virus infecting hylobates pileatus (pileated gibbon) reveals ancient co-evolution with lesser apes. *Viruses* **2019**, *11*, 605. [CrossRef] [PubMed]
34. Switzer, W.; Shanmugam, J.H.K.V.; Heneine, W. Seroprevalence of human infection with simian foamy virus from new world primates. In Proceedings of the 16th Conference on Retroviruses and Opportunistic Infection, Montreal, QC, Canada, 8–11 February 2009.
35. Mouinga-Ondeme, A.; Betsem, E.; Caron, M.; Makuwa, M.; Salle, B.; Renault, N.; Saib, A.; Telfer, P.; Marx, P.; Gessain, A.; et al. Two distinct variants of simian foamy virus in naturally infected mandrills (Mandrillus sphinx) and cross-species transmission to humans. *Retrovirology* **2010**, *7*, 105. [CrossRef] [PubMed]
36. Leendertz, S.A.; Junglen, S.; Hedemann, C.; Goffe, A.; Calvignac, S.; Boesch, C.; Leendertz, F.H. High prevalence, coinfection rate, and genetic diversity of retroviruses in wild red colobus monkeys (Piliocolobus badius badius) in Tai National Park, Cote d'Ivoire. *J. Virol.* **2010**, *84*, 7427–7436. [CrossRef] [PubMed]
37. Liu, W.; Worobey, M.; Li, Y.; Keele, B.F.; Bibollet-Ruche, F.; Guo, Y.; Goepfert, P.A.; Santiago, M.L.; Ndjango, J.B.; Neel, C.; et al. Molecular ecology and natural history of simian foamy virus infection in wild-living chimpanzees. *PLoS Pathog.* **2008**, *4*, e1000097. [CrossRef]
38. Broussard, S.R.; Comuzzie, A.G.; Leighton, K.L.; Leland, M.M.; Whitehead, E.M.; Allan, J.S. Characterization of new simian foamy viruses from African nonhuman primates. *Virology* **1997**, *237*, 349–359. [CrossRef]
39. Huang, F.; Wang, H.; Jing, S.; Zeng, W. Simian foamy virus prevalence in Macaca mulatta and zookeepers. *AIDS Res. Hum. Retroviruses* **2012**, *28*, 591–593. [CrossRef]
40. Hood, S.; Mitchell, J.L.; Sethi, M.; Almond, N.M.; Cutler, K.L.; Rose, N.J. Horizontal acquisition and a broad biodistribution typify simian foamy virus infection in a cohort of Macaca fascicularis. *Virol. J.* **2013**, *10*, 326. [CrossRef]
41. Calattini, S.; Wanert, F.; Thierry, B.; Schmitt, C.; Bassot, S.; Saib, A.; Herrenschmidt, N.; Gessain, A. Modes of transmission and genetic diversity of foamy viruses in a Macaca tonkeana colony. *Retrovirology* **2006**, *3*, 23. [CrossRef]
42. Blewett, E.L.; Black, D.H.; Lerche, N.W.; White, G.; Eberle, R. Simian foamy virus infections in a baboon breeding colony. *Virology* **2000**, *278*, 183–193. [CrossRef]
43. Muniz, C.P.; Zheng, H.; Jia, H.; Cavalcante, L.T.F.; Augusto, A.M.; Fedullo, L.P.; Pissinatti, A.; Soares, M.A.; Switzer, W.M.; Santos, A.F. A non-invasive specimen collection method and a novel simian foamy virus (SFV) DNA quantification assay in New World primates reveal aspects of tissue tropism and improved SFV detection. *PLoS ONE* **2017**, *12*, e0184251. [CrossRef] [PubMed]
44. Stenbak, C.R.; Craig, K.L.; Ivanov, S.B.; Wang, X.; Soliven, K.C.; Jackson, D.L.; Gutierrez, G.A.; Engel, G.; Jones-Engel, L.; Linial, M.L. New World simian foamy virus infections in vivo and in vitro. *J. Virol.* **2014**, *88*, 982–991. [CrossRef] [PubMed]
45. Soliven, K.; Wang, X.; Small, C.T.; Feeroz, M.M.; Lee, E.G.; Craig, K.L.; Hasan, K.; Engel, G.A.; Jones-Engel, L.; Matsen, F.A.; et al. Simian foamy virus infection of rhesus macaques in Bangladesh: Relationship of latent proviruses and transcriptionally active viruses. *J. Virol.* **2013**, *87*, 13628–13639. [CrossRef] [PubMed]
46. Murray, S.M.; Picker, L.J.; Axthelm, M.K.; Linial, M.L. Expanded tissue targets for foamy virus replication with simian immunodeficiency virus-induced immunosuppression. *J. Virol.* **2006**, *80*, 663–670. [CrossRef] [PubMed]

47. Falcone, V.; Leupold, J.; Clotten, J.; Urbanyi, E.; Herchenroder, O.; Spatz, W.; Volk, B.; Bohm, N.; Toniolo, A.; Neumann-Haefelin, D.; et al. Sites of simian foamy virus persistence in naturally infected African green monkeys: Latent provirus is ubiquitous, whereas viral replication is restricted to the oral mucosa. *Virology* **1999**, *257*, 7–14. [CrossRef]
48. Liu, Y.; Betts, M.J.; Lei, J.; Wei, G.; Bao, Q.; Kehl, T.; Russell, R.B.; Lochelt, M. Mutagenesis of N-terminal residues of feline foamy virus Gag reveals entirely distinct functions during capsid formation, particle assembly, Gag processing and budding. *Retrovirology* **2016**, *13*, 57. [CrossRef]
49. Lambert, C.; Couteaudier, M.; Gouzil, J.; Richard, L.; Montange, T.; Betsem, E.; Rua, R.; Tobaly-Tapiero, J.; Lindemann, D.; Njouom, R.; et al. Potent neutralizing antibodies in humans infected with zoonotic simian foamy viruses target conserved epitopes located in the dimorphic domain of the surface envelope protein. *PLoS Pathog.* **2018**, *14*, e1007293. [CrossRef]
50. Murray, S.M.; Picker, L.J.; Axthelm, M.K.; Hudkins, K.; Alpers, C.E.; Linial, M.L. Replication in a superficial epithelial cell niche explains the lack of pathogenicity of primate foamy virus infections. *J. Virol.* **2008**, *82*, 5981–5985. [CrossRef]
51. Smiley Evans, T.; Barry, P.A.; Gilardi, K.V.; Goldstein, T.; Deere, J.D.; Fike, J.; Yee, J.; Ssebide, B.J.; Karmacharya, D.; Cranfield, M.R.; et al. Optimization of a Novel Non-invasive Oral Sampling Technique for Zoonotic Pathogen Surveillance in Nonhuman Primates. *PLoS Negl. Trop. Dis.* **2015**, *9*, e0003813. [CrossRef]
52. Smiley Evans, T.; Gilardi, K.V.; Barry, P.A.; Ssebide, B.J.; Kinani, J.F.; Nizeyimana, F.; Noheri, J.B.; Byarugaba, D.K.; Mudakikwa, A.; Cranfield, M.R.; et al. Detection of viruses using discarded plants from wild mountain gorillas and golden monkeys. *Am. J. Primatol.* **2016**, *78*, 1222–1234. [CrossRef]
53. Schweizer, M.; Schleer, H.; Pietrek, M.; Liegibel, J.; Falcone, V.; Neumann-Haefelin, D. Genetic stability of foamy viruses: Long-term study in an African green monkey population. *J. Virol.* **1999**, *73*, 9256–9265. [PubMed]
54. Brooks, J.I.; Merks, H.W.; Fournier, J.; Boneva, R.S.; Sandstrom, P.A. Characterization of blood-borne transmission of simian foamy virus. *Transfusion* **2007**, *47*, 162–170. [CrossRef] [PubMed]
55. Blasse, A.; Calvignac-Spencer, S.; Merkel, K.; Goffe, A.S.; Boesch, C.; Mundry, R.; Leendertz, F.H. Mother-offspring transmission and age-dependent accumulation of simian foamy virus in wild chimpanzees. *J. Virol.* **2013**, *87*, 5193–5204. [CrossRef] [PubMed]
56. VandeWoude, S.; Apetrei, C. Going wild: Lessons from naturally occurring T-lymphotropic lentiviruses. *Clin. Microbiol. Rev.* **2006**, *19*, 728–762. [CrossRef]
57. Santiago, M.L.; Range, F.; Keele, B.F.; Li, Y.; Bailes, E.; Bibollet-Ruche, F.; Fruteau, C.; Noe, R.; Peeters, M.; Brookfield, J.F.; et al. Simian immunodeficiency virus infection in free-ranging sooty mangabeys (Cercocebus atys atys) from the Tai Forest, Cote d'Ivoire: Implications for the origin of epidemic human immunodeficiency virus type 2. *J. Virol.* **2005**, *79*, 12515–12527. [CrossRef]
58. Choudhary, A.; Galvin, T.A.; Williams, D.K.; Beren, J.; Bryant, M.A.; Khan, A.S. Influence of naturally occurring simian foamy viruses (SFVs) on SIV disease progression in the rhesus macaque (Macaca mulatta) model. *Viruses* **2013**, *5*, 1414–1430. [CrossRef]
59. Leendertz, F.H.; Zirkel, F.; Couacy-Hymann, E.; Ellerbrok, H.; Morozov, V.A.; Pauli, G.; Hedemann, C.; Formenty, P.; Jensen, S.A.; Boesch, C.; et al. Interspecies transmission of simian foamy virus in a natural predator-prey system. *J. Virol.* **2008**, *82*, 7741–7744. [CrossRef]
60. Betsem, E.; Rua, R.; Tortevoye, P.; Froment, A.; Gessain, A. Frequent and recent human acquisition of simian foamy viruses through apes' bites in central Africa. *PLoS Pathog.* **2011**, *7*, e1002306. [CrossRef]
61. Jones-Engel, L.; May, C.C.; Engel, G.A.; Steinkraus, K.A.; Schillaci, M.A.; Fuentes, A.; Rompis, A.; Chalise, M.K.; Aggimarangsee, N.; Feeroz, M.M.; et al. Diverse contexts of zoonotic transmission of simian foamy viruses in Asia. *Emerg. Infect. Dis.* **2008**, *14*, 1200–1208. [CrossRef]
62. Khan, A.S. Simian foamy virus infection in humans: Prevalence and management. *Exp. Rev. Anti Infect. Ther.* **2009**, *7*, 569–580. [CrossRef]
63. Switzer, W.M.; Bhullar, V.; Shanmugam, V.; Cong, M.E.; Parekh, B.; Lerche, N.W.; Yee, J.L.; Ely, J.J.; Boneva, R.; Chapman, L.E.; et al. Frequent simian foamy virus infection in persons occupationally exposed to nonhuman primates. *J. Virol.* **2004**, *78*, 2780–2789. [CrossRef] [PubMed]
64. Switzer, W.M.H. Foamy virus infection of humans. In *Molecular Detection of Human Viral Pathogens*; Liu, D., Ed.; CRC Press: Boca Raton, FL, USA, 2011.

65. Pinto-Santini, D.M.; Stenbak, C.R.; Linial, M.L. Foamy virus zoonotic infections. *Retrovirology* **2017**, *14*, 55. [CrossRef] [PubMed]
66. Brooks, J.I.; Rud, E.W.; Pilon, R.G.; Smith, J.M.; Switzer, W.M.; Sandstrom, P.A. Cross-species retroviral transmission from macaques to human beings. *Lancet* **2002**, *360*, 387–388. [CrossRef]
67. Wolfe, N.D.; Switzer, W.M.; Carr, J.K.; Bhullar, V.B.; Shanmugam, V.; Tamoufe, U.; Prosser, A.T.; Torimiro, J.N.; Wright, A.; Mpoudi-Ngole, E.; et al. Naturally acquired simian retrovirus infections in central African hunters. *Lancet* **2004**, *363*, 932–937. [CrossRef]
68. Calattini, S.; Betsem, E.B.; Froment, A.; Mauclere, P.; Tortevoye, P.; Schmitt, C.; Njouom, R.; Saib, A.; Gessain, A. Simian foamy virus transmission from apes to humans, rural Cameroon. *Emerg. Infect. Dis.* **2007**, *13*, 1314–1320. [CrossRef]
69. Switzer, W.M.; Tang, S.; Ahuka-Mundeke, S.; Shankar, A.; Hanson, D.L.; Zheng, H.; Ayouba, A.; Wolfe, N.D.; LeBreton, M.; Djoko, C.F.; et al. Novel simian foamy virus infections from multiple monkey species in women from the Democratic Republic of Congo. *Retrovirology* **2012**, *9*, 100. [CrossRef]
70. Mouinga-Ondeme, A.; Caron, M.; Nkoghe, D.; Telfer, P.; Marx, P.; Saib, A.; Leroy, E.; Gonzalez, J.P.; Gessain, A.; Kazanji, M. Cross-species transmission of simian foamy virus to humans in rural Gabon, Central Africa. *J. Virol.* **2012**, *86*, 1255–1260. [CrossRef]

viruses

MDPI

Article

Genome Analysis and Replication Studies of the African Green Monkey Simian Foamy Virus Serotype 3 Strain FV2014

Sandra M. Fuentes [1,†], Eunhae H. Bae [1,2,†], Subhiksha Nandakumar [1,3,†], Dhanya K. Williams [1,4] and Arifa S. Khan [1,*]

1 Laboratory of Retroviruses, Division of Viral Products, Office of Vaccines Research and Review, Center for Biologics Evaluation and Review, U.S. Food and Drug Administration, Silver Spring, MD 20993, USA; sandra.fuentes@fda.hhs.gov (S.M.F.); eunhaebae@gmail.com (E.H.B.); subhikshananda@gmail.com (S.N.); dhanya.williams@fda.hhs.gov (D.K.W.)

2 Current Address: Ross University School of Medicine, Miramar, FL 33027, USA

3 Current Address: Marie-Josée and Henry R. Kravis Center for Molecular Oncology, Memorial Sloan Kettering Cancer Center, New York, NY 10065, USA

4 Present Address: Office of Device Evaluation, Center for Devices and Radiological Health, U.S. Food and Drug Administration, Silver Spring, MD 20993, USA

* Correspondence: arifa.khan@fda.hhs.gov; Tel.: +1-240-402-9631

† These authors contributed equally to this work.

Received: 30 December 2019; Accepted: 1 April 2020; Published: 6 April 2020

Abstract: African green monkey (AGM) spumaretroviruses have been less well-studied than other simian foamy viruses (SFVs). We report the biological and genomic characterization of SFVcae_FV2014, which was the first foamy virus isolated from an African green monkey (AGM) and was found to be serotype 3. Infectivity studies in various cell lines from different species (mouse, dog, rhesus monkey, AGM, and human) indicated that like other SFVs, SFVcae_FV2014 had broad species and cell tropism, and in vitro cell culture infection resulted in cytopathic effect (CPE). In *Mus dunni* (a wild mouse fibroblast cell line), MDCK (Madin-Darby canine kidney cell line), FRhK-4 (a fetal rhesus kidney cell line), and MRC-5 (a human fetal lung cell line), SFVcae_FV2014 infection was productive resulting in CPE, and had delayed or similar replication kinetics compared with SFVmcy_FV21 and SFVmcy_FV34[RF], which are two Taiwanese macaque isolates, designated as serotypes 1 and 2, respectively. However, in Vero (AGM kidney cell line) and A549 (a human lung carcinoma cell line), the replication kinetics of SFVcae_FV2014 and the SFVmcy viruses were discordant: In Vero, SFVcae_FV2014 showed rapid replication kinetics and extensive CPE, and a persistent infection was seen in A549, with delayed, low CPE, which did not progress even upon extended culture (day 55). Nucleotide sequence analysis of the assembled SFVcae_FV2014 genome, obtained by high-throughput sequencing, indicated an overall 80–90% nucleotide sequence identity with SFVcae_LK3, the only available full-length genome sequence of an AGM SFV, and was distinct phylogenetically from other AGM spumaretroviruses, corroborating previous results based on analysis of partial *env* sequences. Our study confirmed that SFVcae_FV2014 and SFVcae_LK3 are genetically distinct AGM foamy virus (FV) isolates. Furthermore, comparative infectivity studies of SFVcae_FV2014 and SFVmcy isolates showed that although SFVs have a wide host range and cell tropism, regulation of virus replication is complex and depends on the virus strain and cell-specific factors.

Keywords: simian foamy virus; spumaretrovirus; serotype; high-throughput sequencing; replication kinetics; cytopathic effect; reverse transcriptase activity

1. Introduction

Early isolates of simian foamy viruses (SFVs), which belong to the recently described genus *Simiispumavirus* in the subfamily *Spumaretrovirinae* and family *Retroviridae* [1], were distinguished based on serotyping using neutralization assays. SFVcae_FV2014, previously known as SFV strain FV2014, isolated from the kidney tissue of an African green monkey (*Chlorocebus aethiops*), was designated as Type III [2] because it was serotypically distinct from other simian spumaretroviruses available at that time, which were SFV Type I and Type II, isolated from Taiwanese macaques (*Macaca cyclopis*) [3,4]. Subsequently, SFV strain LK3 was isolated from a lymphoblastoid cell line, established from a lymph node of a healthy *C. aethiops* [5] and designated as SFV serotype 3 based on sequence relatedness in hybridization experiments to the SFV Type III isolate FV2014 [6]. Unlike spumaretroviruses from macaque species, the number of reported foamy virus isolates from African green monkey (AGMs) are limited to FV2014 and LK3 [1]. The full-length sequence of SFV-3 strain LK-3 (referred to as SFV-3; [7]) was found to be more similar to SFV Type I than to the human foamy virus (subsequently found to be of chimpanzee origin [8]; current designation SFVpsc_huHSRV.13). Later, phylogenetic analysis based on short fragments in *env* obtained by DNA PCR amplification of 22 AGM spumaretrovirus sequences indicated diversity in AGM viruses and placed LK-3 and SFV-3/SFVcae_FV2014 on distinct branches of AGM spumaretroviruses [9]. It should be noted that in an earlier study [5], sera obtained from an SFVcae_LK3-infected AGM did not neutralize SFVcae_FV2014, and serum against the latter virus did not neutralize SFVcae_LK3. These results indicate that the serotype of SFVcae_LK3 needs to be further verified.

The high diversity of sequences in SFVs cocirculating with their host species is generally thought to be a result of intraspecies superinfection [10], and there is also evidence of interspecies virus infections and recombination. We have reported that the Taiwanese macaque isolate SFVmcy_2 (SFV serotype II, now referred to as SFVmcy_FV34[RF]), is a recombinant virus, which contains sequences in the *env*/SU region similar to SFVcae_LK3 (referred to as SFVagm-3; [11]). Additionally, Blochmann et al. reported isolation of SFVmac-R289hybAGM (currently designated as SFVmmu-R289hybAGM[RF]) from a rhesus macaque, which also had a similar recombination in *env* involving an AGM spumaretrovirus [12]. Since SFVs cocirculate and cospeciate with their hosts and are generally located in distinct geographical regions [8], foamy virus (FV) transmission and recombination may occur due to exposure of different NHP species in holding facilities during importation or handling in biomedical research facilitates and in zoos. Furthermore, human infections with FVs from various NHP species, including macaques and AGMs, have occurred due to occupational exposure in North America and in natural settings in Africa and Asia [8].

To study viral interactions of spumaretroviruses from different monkey species and potential for cross-species human infections, our laboratory previously developed well-characterized virus stocks of SFVs isolated from macaques [13,14]. In this study we describe the preparation and characterization of an SFVcae_FV2014 virus stock. Molecular and biological analysis showed that SFVcae_FV2014 is phylogenetically distinct from the AGM isolate SFVcae_LK3; furthermore, SFVcae_FV2014 had distinct replication kinetics from the macaque viruses, SFVmcy_FV21 and SFVmcy_FV34, based on infectivity studies using a variety of cell lines from different species.

2. Materials and Methods

2.1. Virus Preparation

SFV type 3 strain FV2014, an isolate from an African green monkey (grivet monkey kidney) [2], was obtained from American Type Culture Collection (ATCC, Manassas, VA, USA; catalogue number VR-218, lot 3W, titer $10^{4.25}$ per 0.2 mL in A-72 (canine tumor) cells; 8 days). The virus passage history provided by ATCC (host cells × number of passages) was: rabbit kidney (RabK) × 4, grivet monkey kidney (Grivet MkK) × 3, RabK × 10, primary rabbit kidney (PrRabK) × 1, and A-72 canine tumor cell line × 2 (ATCC CRL-1542).

A laboratory virus stock was prepared in *Mus dunni* cells, which were previously found to be highly susceptible to SFV replication [14]. Infected cells were grown until the cell culture was terminated due to extensive cytopathic effect (CPE) at passage 4 (day 11 after infection). Supernatant was collected and clarified by low speed centrifugation (1200 rpm for 10 min at 4 °C; GH-3.8 Swinging Bucket Rotor, Allegra 6KR Centrifuge, Beckman Coulter Life Sciences, Indianapolis, IN, USA) prior to filtration (0.45-µm-pore-size test tube top filter units; Corning, Cambridge, MA, USA). Aliquots were prepared for storage at −80 °C. The 50% tissue culture infective dose ($TCID_{50}$) of the SFVcae_FV2014 virus stock was determined in MRC-5 cells using ten-fold dilutions with read-out for CPE on day 14 [15].

SFVmcy_FV21 and SFVmcy_FV34[RF], which were originally isolated from *Macaca cyclopis* [3,4], were obtained from ATCC (catalogue number VR-276, FV21, lot 5 WE and catalogue number VR-277, FV-34, lot 5 WE, respectively). The passage history at ATCC (host cells × number of passages) for SFVmcy_FV21 was: PrRabK × 13, KB (subline of HeLa) × 1, LLC-MK2 (normal rhesus monkey kidney) × 7, KB × 1, normal rat kidney × 2, Hep2 × 3 and A-72 × 2; and for SFVmcy_FV34[RF] was: PrRabK × 13, KB × 2, normal rat kidney × 2, and A-72 × 2. Viruses were amplified with low passage (≤ 5 or about ≤ 15 days) in the *M. dunni* cell line [14]. Virus stocks were prepared when extensive CPE occurred, and reverse transcriptase (RT) activity was determined using a modified single-tube fluorescent product-enhanced RT assay (STF-PERT) [16], described in Section 2.3. The virus titer ($TCID_{50}$) was determined in MRC-5 cells at day 14: SFVmcy_FV21 virus stock was $10^{5.5}$ $TCID_{50}$ per mL and SFVmcy_FV34[RF] was $10^{5.03}$ $TCID_{50}$ per mL.

2.2. PCR Assays and Copy Number Standard

Detection of SFVmcy_FV21 and SFVmcy_FV34[RF] sequences was based on the previously described PCR assay using Set B outer and inner primer sets from the long terminal repeats (LTR) region [14]. The outer primer pair consisted of forward primer 5′-CAGTGAATTCCAGAATCTCTTC-3′ and reverse primer 5′-CACTTATCCCACTAGATGGTTC-3′, and the inner primer pair consisted of forward primer 5′-CCAGAATCTCTTCATACTAACTA-3′ and reverse primer 5′-GATGGTTCCCTAAGCAAGGC-3′. The PCR conditions were modified: 95 °C 3 min, 95 °C 3 min, 95 °C 1 min, 55 °C 1 min, and 72 °C 1 min, for 35 cycles with extension 72 °C 10 min and 4 °C hold.

For detection of SFVcae_FV2014 sequences, primers were selected from the LTR-gag region of the full-length genome (Genbank accession number MF582544) using Primer-Blast (NCBI, NLM, National Institutes of Health, Bethesda, MD, USA). The outer primers were designated as SFVcae-F3 (5′-TGTTTGAGTCTCTCCAGGCTT-3′ extending from nucleotide position 1365 to 1385) and SFVcae-R3 (5′-CCATCTGTCATGCGAAGTCC-3′; nucleotide position 1937 to 1918), which amplified a 573 bp fragment. The inner primers were designated as SFVcae-F2 (5′-TAATGGGCAATGGCAATGCTT-3′; nucleotide position 1452 to 1472) and SFVcae-R2 (5′-TCTCTGTGATTGGGTTGTCTAGC-3′; nucleotide position 1910 to 1888), which amplified a 459 bp fragment. The first amplification was performed in 100 µL volume using 3 U of the Taq DNA polymerase (Roche Applied Science, Mannheim, Germany, catalogue number 11647679001) with 0.5 µM final concentration of the outer primer set and 250 ng of total cell DNA (QIAamp DNA Blood Mini Kit, Qiagen, Germantown, MD, USA) or 2 ng cDNA, prepared using Superscript VILO cDNA synthesis kit (Life technologies, Cat no. 11754) and cleaned using Zymo Research's DNA clean and concentrator kit (catalogue number D4013). The second amplification was performed using the inner primer set and 10 µL PCR product from the first amplification in a total volume of 100 µL. For both amplifications, the conditions for the PCR were: 95 °C for 1 min, 55 °C for 1 min, and 72 °C for 1 min for 35 cycles. Initial denaturation was done at 95 °C for 3 min and the final extension at 72 °C for 10 min. Specificity of the LTR-gag PCR assays was determined by testing the three SFV isolates: The LTR PCR assay detected both SFVmcy_FV21 and SFVmcy_FV34[RF], whereas the LTR-gag PCR assay was specific for detection of SFVcae_FV2014.

The SFVcae_FV2014 LTR-*gag* fragment amplified using the outer primer pair was cloned and a copy number standard was made by spiking ten-fold dilutions of the DNA, ranging in the background of 0.25 µg cellular human genomic DNA (Roche, catalogue number 1169111200). Limit of detection for the second amplification was 10-100 copies.

Gag primers used for confirmation of sequence variants (described in Section 2.4.1) were SFV-3-F-1592 (5′-GTGAAAGGAATTGTGTA-3′) and SFV-3-R-2425 (5′-GAAGATGATGCAATAGG-3′) (covering the region extending from nucleotide positions 1592-2425). PCR amplification was performed in a total volume of 50 µL containing 2 ng cDNA, 0.5 µM of each oligo, 0.8mM dNTP mixture, 1× TaKaRa Ex Taq Buffer, and 5 U of TaKaRa Ex Taq (Clontech, catalogue number RR001A). PCR conditions were: 98 °C 3 min, 98 °C 10 s, 58 °C 1 min, and 72 °C 1 min, for 35 cycles with extension 72 °C 10 min and 4 °C hold.

2.3. Infectivity Analysis

Replication kinetics of SFVcae_FV2014, SFVmcy_FV21, and SFVmcy_FV34[RF] were compared using cell lines originating from different species and tissues shown in Table 1.

Table 1. Cell lines used in infectivity studies.

Cell Name	Source	Host Species	Tissue Origin	Cell Type
Mus dunni	[14]	wild mouse	tail	fibroblast
MDCK (NBL-2)	ATCC, CCL-34	dog	kidney	epithelial
FRhK-4	ATCC, CRL-1688	rhesus macaque	fetal, kidney	epithelial
Vero	ATCC, CCL-81	African green monkey	kidney	epithelial
MRC-5	ATCC, CCL-171	human	lung, fetal	fibroblast, diploid
A549	ATCC, CCL-185	human	lung, carcinoma	epithelial

Cells used in this study originated from cell banks used in our other SFV infectivity studies (unpublished; [14]). MDCK, MRC-5, and Vero were grown in Eagle's minimum essential medium (EMEM) and *M. dunni*, FhRK-4, and A549 were grown in Dulbecco's modified Eagle medium (DMEM). All media were supplemented with 10% fetal bovine serum (GE Healthcare Hyclone, Logan, Utah, catalogue number SH30071.03; heat inactivated 56 °C for 30 min), 100 U of penicillin per mL, 100 µg of streptomycin per mL (Quality Biological, Gaithersburg, MD, USA; catalogue number 120-095-721), and 2 mM L-glutamine (Quality Biological; catalogue number 118-084-721). In addition, EMEM was also supplemented with 1 mM sodium pyruvate (Quality Biological; catalogue number 116-079-721) and 0.1 mM minimum non-essential amino acids (MEM-NEAA, Quality Biologicals, catalogue number 116-078-721).

SFV infection was carried out according to our laboratory's standard protocol. Cells were planted in 25 cm^2 flasks 24 h prior to infection and virus (193 $TCID_{50}$) was added at 50–70% cell confluence. The number of cells planted were: *M. dunni*, 250,000; MDCK, 333,000; Vero, FRhK-4, A549; and MRC-5, 500,000. The cell passage at time of infection was: A549, p86; Vero, p129; MRC-5, p29; *M. dunni*, p45; FRhK-4, p45; and MDCK, p65). The optimum cell numbers were determined for each cell line and a low multiplicity of infection (approximate 0.0002–0.00045) was used. This was determined based on the most sensitive cell line in order to obtain differences in the replication kinetics for all of the viruses in the different cell lines. Cells were transferred to 75 cm^2 flasks upon reaching confluence and passaged every 3–4 days. Filtered supernatant (0.45-µm-pore-size test tube top filter units; Corning, Cambridge, MA, USA) was collected and stored at −80 °C at each passage. Cultures were terminated at 4+ CPE (>75% cell death) or at day 30 to day 55, in case of slow or no CPE. Virus replication was monitored by microscopic observation of CPE progression in the cell monolayer and by determining the RT activity in filtered supernatant using a modified STF-PERT assay [16], in which the RT and the PCR steps were done in two steps, instead of using the one-step published protocol due to the discontinuation of AmpliWax PCR Gem 50. The assay was performed as described previously except that the RT reaction was done in the first step and then the PCR reaction mix was added immediately for the second step in the assay. All the samples collected from infectivity studies in one cell line were tested in duplicate or triplicate in the modified STF-PERT assay to compare kinetics of virus replication. Uninfected cells were set-up in parallel as control.

2.4. *Preparation of Viral Nucleic Acid, Sequencing, and Bioinformatics Analysis*

2.4.1. High-Throughput Sequencing

Virus was concentrated by ultracentrifugation (45,000 rpm for 90 min at 4 °C; Rotor TLA-45, Beckman Coulter Optima MAX-XP Ultracentrifuge) or by using a Nanosep 30KD Omega Device (P/N OD030C33) with centrifugation at 5000× *g* for 20 min 4 °C. RNA was extracted using QIAamp Viral RNA Mini Kit (catalogue number 52904).

Viral nucleic acid prepared from SFVcae_FV2014 virus stock was sequenced using the MiSeq Illumina platform (CD Genomics, Shirley, NY, USA) as previously described [17], and a consensus virus sequence (SFVcae_FV2014 GenBank accession number MF582544) was generated by mapping the raw reads to the SFVcae_LK3 full-length genome as reference [7] (NCBI RefSeq accession number M74895). Default parameters were used for mapping: the length fraction (the minimum percentage of the total alignment length that must match the reference sequence at the selected similarity fraction) was set to be 0.5, and the similarity fraction (the minimum percentage identity between the aligned region of the read and the reference sequence) was set to be 0.8. The long terminal repeats (LTRs) were mapped separately using the same default mapping parameters to generate a complete and full-length consensus genome sequence of SFVcae_FV2014. Sequences in low-coverage regions were confirmed by virus-specific PCR assays. Open reading frames were identified using ORF Finder (https://www.ncbi.nlm.nih.gov/orffinder/).

Viral nucleic acid was prepared from filtered supernatant of SFVcae_FV2014-infected Vero cells at culture termination (day 15) for high-throughput sequencing using Illumina Hi-Seq (FDA/CBER Core Lab). The total numbers of quality, paired-end reads were 342,517,062 and the average read length was 99.2 bases. Sequence analysis was performed using CLC Genomics Workbench software, version 10.1.1 (CLC bio, Aarhus, Denmark). The sequence from SFVcae_FV2014 (accession number MF582544) was used as reference for the mapping. The default parameters were used, with the exception of length fraction and similarity fraction, which were set at 0.8 and 0.9, respectively.

To find virus variants, the reads were remapped using the SFVcae_FV2014 consensus sequence as the reference genome. Fixed ploidy variant detection analysis was done using the default setting with the noise threshold set at 10% and variant probability cutoff ≥35%, based on the known error rate of the Illumina sequencing platform [18]. Unaligned tail analysis helped to identify the previously reported splicing events in *tas, bet,* and *env* regions [19,20]. Ambiguous positions and splice sites were confirmed by PCR amplification and Sanger sequencing of gel-purified fragments (QIAquick gel extraction kit; Qiagen, catalogue number 28714).

2.4.2. Sanger Sequencing

Sanger sequencing was used to confirm virus infection and HTS sequence results. Viral nucleic acid was extracted from SFVcae_FV2014 virus stock and cDNA synthesis done as described in Section 2.4.1. Total DNA was extracted from virus supernatant to confirm virus infection by PCR amplifications as described in Section 2.2. PCR fragments were analyzed on a 0.6% agarose gel and the expected size fragment was extracted and purified using QIAquick gel extraction kit (Qiagen, catalogue number 28714) for Sanger sequencing (CBER Core Facility).

2.5. Sequence Comparison and Phylogenetic Analysis

Comparative nucleotide sequence analyses and amino acid analyses were done for full-length, individual viral genes, and LTR with MegAlign (DNASTAR Lasergene, Inc. Madison, WI, USA) using the ClustalW method. Accession numbers for SFV sequences used in the analysis are shown in Table 2.

Table 2. Simian foamy virus (SFV) isolates used for phylogenetic analysis and sequence alignments.

Virus	Previous Designation	Species of Virus Isolation	Accession Number [1]
SFVmcy_FV21	SFVmcy-1, (SFV serotype I)	Taiwanese macaque	NC_010819
SFVmcy_FV34[RF]	SFVmcy-2, (SFV serotype II)	Taiwanese macaque	KF026286
SFVmmu_K3T	SFVmmu-K3T	Rhesus macaque	KF026288
SFVmmu_R289HybAGM[RF]	SFV-R289HybAGM	Rhesus macaque	JN801175
SFVcae_FV2014	SFV 3 (SFV serotype III)	African green monkey	MF582544
SFVcae_LK3	SFVagm-3	African green monkey	NC_010820
SFVcae_agm4	agm4	African green monkey	AJ244075
SFVcae_agm5	agm5	African green monkey	AJ244067
SFVcae_agm20	agm20	African green monkey	AJ244091
SFVcae_agm24	agm24	African green monkey	AJ244090
SFVpve	SFVcpz	Chimpanzee	NC_001364
SFVpsc_huHRSV.13	HFV	Chimpanzee	KX08159
SFVggo	SFVgor	Gorilla	HM245790
BFVbta	BFV	Cow	NC_001831
EFVeca_1	EFVeca	Equine	AF201902
FFVfca_FUV7	FFVfca	Feline	Y08851

[1] GenBank or NCBI Reference Sequence.

To compare the amino acid sequence of the SFVcae_FV2014 Gag at nucleotide position 1857 with the Gag of other foamy viruses, the Gag amino acid sequences from SFVcae_LK3, SFVmmu_K3T, SFVmcy_FV21, SFVmcy_FV34[RF], SFVpsc_huHRSV.13, EFVeca_1, FFVfca_FUV7, and SFVcae_FV2014 (accession numbers in Table 2) were aligned using ClustalW (MegAlign Pro DNASTAR Lasergene v.15).

Phylogenetic trees were generated based upon the nucleotide sequences in the entire *env* gene and in the SU region of *env* using MEGA7.0.14 (Molecular Evolutionary Genetics Analysis; www.megasoftware.net) as previously described [11]. The list of viruses and accession numbers used in the analysis is shown in Table 2. Briefly, nucleotide sequences were aligned in MEGA using ClustalW. The maximum-likelihood method based on the general time reversible model was chosen because it had the lowest Bayesian information criteria score in a model test performed in MEGA. The bootstrap consensus tree inferred from 1000 replicates was taken to represent the evolutionary history of the taxa analyzed. Branches corresponding to partitions reproduced in less than 50% bootstrap replicates are collapsed. The initial tree for the heuristic search was obtained automatically by applying neighbor-joining and BioNJ algorithms to a matrix of pairwise distances estimated using the maximum-composite-likelihood (MCL) approach and then selecting the topology with the superior log likelihood value. A discrete gamma distribution was used to model evolutionary rate differences among sites. All positions containing gaps and missing data were eliminated.

3. Results

3.1. Characterization of SFVcae_FV2014 Virus Stock

A virus stock of SFVcae_FV2014 was prepared and characterized for molecular and biological studies. The original virus from ATCC was amplified, similar to our other laboratory stocks of SFVs, in *M. dunni* with low passage (<5) to avoid nucleotide sequence changes that could potentially occur due to extended virus passage. *M. dunni* cells were used for virus amplification since these were previously found to produce a large number of extracellular virus particles compared to other cell lines [14]. Virus titer was $10^{4.5}$ per mL in MRC-5 cells [21].

Illumina MiSeq was used to determine viral sequences in the SFVcae_FV2014 virus stock. The consensus sequence was published [17]. Further analysis indicated the presence of a variant in *gag* at nucleotide position 1857: the variant frequency of A was 52% (represented in the consensus sequence) and T was 48%. This result was confirmed by Sanger sequencing. Interestingly, further passage of virus by inoculating *M. dunni* cells with the SFVcae_FV2014 virus stock indicated increased frequency of the T variant (82%) at culture termination, which corresponded to extensive CPE and peak RT activity. The one nucleotide change resulted in a conservative amino acid mutation from isoleucine to leucine in the consensus sequence of SFVcae_FV2014 located in the coiled-coil CC1 domain of the Gag protein. It is noted that the leucine residue is highly conserved in spumaretroviruses (Figure 1).

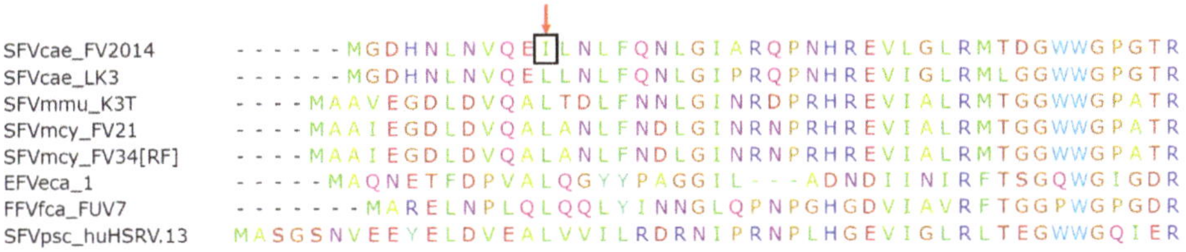

Figure 1. SFVcae_FV2014 variant. Amino acid sequence alignment for N-terminal Gag protein amino acids. The Gag sequences from different foamy viruses (FVs) were aligned using ClustalW. The first 50 amino acids of the alignment are shown. The red arrow points to the position of the conserved leucine in the CC1 domain of Gag; the change to isoleucine is indicated in the box.

The certificate of analysis for the original ATCC stock indicated that it was contaminated with *Mycoplasma hominis*. However, the bioinformatics analysis of the MiSeq data for our laboratory stock prepared in *M. dunni* did not show sequences mapping to *M. hominis* (NCBI accession number NC_013511; data not shown), thus indicating the absence of mycoplasma contamination in the SFVcae_FV2014 virus used in our infectivity studies.

3.2. Studies of SFVcae_FV2014 Replication

Infectivity studies were done to compare the biological properties of SFVcae_FV2014 and SFV macaque isolates, SFVmcy_FV21 and SFVmcy_FV34[RF]. To remove differences due to previous propagation of the viruses in different host species, all the virus stocks were generated by low-passage in *M. dunni* cells. The kinetics of virus replication were determined using a low virus amount (193 $TCID_{50}$), which was previously determined to allow virus propagation without early termination by extensive CPE. Cell lines from different host species and cell types were included to determine the influence of host on kinetics of SFV replication. Virus replication was evaluated based on development and progression of CPE in the cells and the increase in the RT activity produced in cell-free culture supernatant. The results from one of two studies are shown in Figure 2 (panels A–F): similar replication kinetics were seen in both.

In *M. dunni* (Figure 2A), SFVmcy_FV21 and SFVmcy_FV34[RF] showed similar and rapid replication: RT activity was initially seen in both SFVmcy isolates at day 4, which increased significantly (about 1000-fold) at day 8, resulting in culture termination due to extensive CPE. A delay in replication kinetics was seen with SFVcae_FV2014, where the initial RT activity and CPE was detected at day 8, which increased to a high level by day 15, and the culture was terminated due to extensive CPE. However, a similar level of RT activity was seen for the three viruses at culture termination (4–8 × 10^6 pU per µL). In MDCK cells, SFV viruses had similar kinetics as in *M. dunni* except virus production was about a log lower for SFVmcy viruses (Figure 2B).

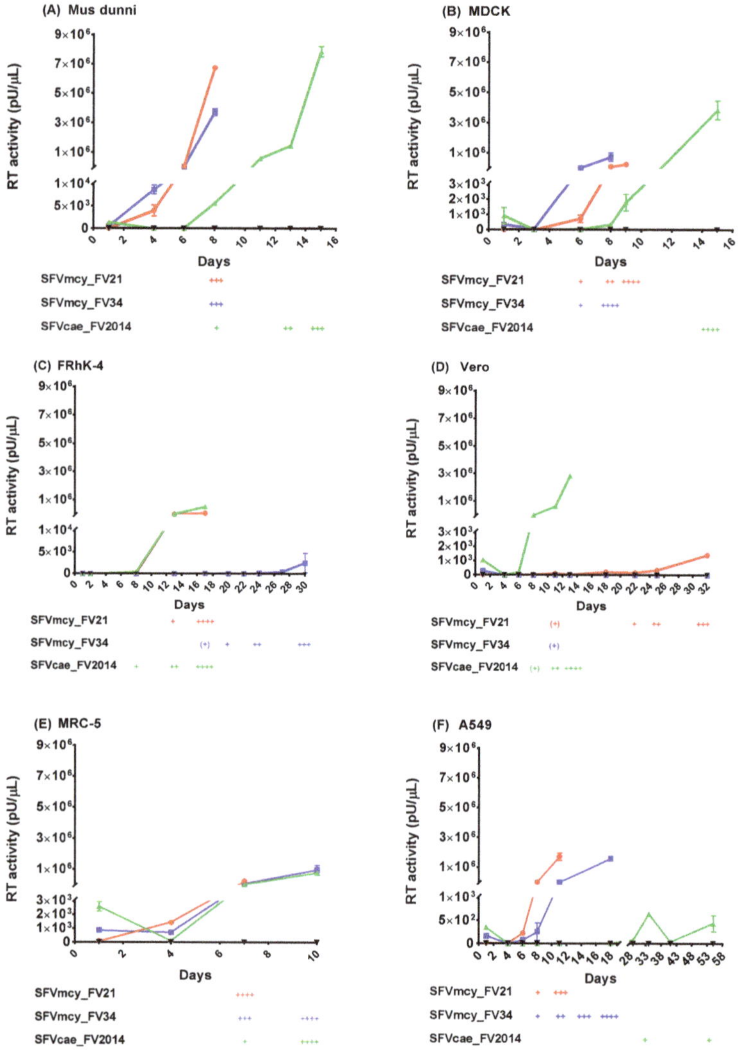

Figure 2. Kinetics of SFV replication. The kinetics of virus replication for SFVcae_FV2014 (▲) were compared with SFVmcy_FV21 (●) and SFVmcy_FV34 (■) in various cell lines from different species (**A**) *M. dunni*; (**B**) MDCK; (**C**) FRhK-4; (**D**) Vero; (**E**) MRC-5; and (**F**) A459 cells. Uninfected cells were the negative control (▼). Data from one of two independent studies are shown. Virus replication was determined based upon virus production in cell-free supernatant using the PERT assay (reported as pU/µL RT activity) and by visualization of cytopathic effect (CPE) development in the cells (reported as: + for up to 25% cell monolayer affected; ++, up to 50% monolayer affected; +++; up to 75% affected cells; and ++++, > 75% of cell monolayer affected). SFVmcy_FV21 infection in *M. dunni* was terminated at 3+ CPE due to insufficient cells for further passage. For comparison, the reverse transcriptase (RT) activity shown in the segmented Y-axis of the graph has the same Y-maximum value, although different cell lines had varied peak RT. The segmented, linear Y-axis shows the virus input and low-level RT activity on the bottom segment and the peak RT activity on the top segment. Error bars represent the SEM of virus supernatant samples tested in triplicate (*M. dunni*, MDCK, and MRC-5) or duplicate (Vero, FRhK-4, and A549) in the PERT assay. All samples from one cell line were tested in the same PERT assay.

Notable differences in replication of SFVmcy and SFVcae viruses were seen in the simian cell lines. In the FRhK-4 cells (Figure 2C), SFVmcy_FV21 and SFVcae_FV2014 had similar kinetics of replication with initial RT detection at day 8 and culture termination due to extensive CPE on day 17, with about similar levels of RT activity (1–5 × 10^5 pU per μL). Interestingly, SFVmcy_FV34[RF] had greatly delayed kinetics of replication: A very low level of RT activity was detected on day 8, which increased slowly but remained significantly low even at time of culture termination (about 75-fold lower); furthermore, there was also a delay in CPE progression, which was initially detected on day 17 but did not progress to extensive cell lysis even at day 30, when the experiment was terminated. In Vero cells (Figure 2D), the kinetics of replication for SFVcae_FV2014 were similar to *M. dunni cells*: with initial RT activity seen at day 6, with a fairly rapid and high increase in RT activity at time of culture termination on day 13 (about 3 × 10^6 pU per μL). Unexpectedly, the replication of the SFVmcy viruses was significantly delayed compared to SFVcae, with low RT and slow CPE progression: In the case of SFVmcy_FV21, RT activity could be initially detected on day 6 and progressed slowly, and was detected above input background on day 11, increasing at a low level until culture termination on day 32, with RT activity < 2 × 10^3 pU per μL. RT was not detected with infection of Vero using SFVmcy_FV34[RF]; although CPE was seen starting at day 11, no progression was seen during the culture period ending on day 32, at the time of experiment termination.

All three SFVs had rapid replication kinetics in MRC-5 cells (Figure 2E) although SFVmcy_FV21 had earlier culture termination at day 7 with 3- to 4-fold less RT activity compared with SFVmcy_FV34[RF] and SFVcae_FV2014, which had similar replication kinetics with culture termination on day 10 with high RT activity (about 10^6 pU per μL). SFV infection of A549 cells (Figure 2F) showed differences in replication kinetics between the different viruses: SFVmcy_FV21-induced CPE progressed more rapidly with culture termination on day 11, whereas CPE progressed slower with SFVmcy_FV34[RF] with culture termination on day 18, although for both viruses, CPE was seen at day 8 and the RT activity was initially detected on day 6. Very slow kinetics of replication were seen with SFVcae_FV2014: a low-level RT activity was seen at day 29 with a low peak on day 34, which decreased on day 41, the next time point tested, and again increased on day 55, at culture termination, and the RT activity above input was seen only at day 34 and also at day 55, when the experiment was terminated; low CPE was seen at day 39 and thereafter, but without progression.

Virus infection in Vero cells was confirmed for SFVmcy_FV21 and SFVmcy_FV34[RF] by PCR amplification of DNA prepared from cells collected on day 34 (Figure 3A, lane 1 and 2, respectively). Specific virus detection was verified by a second round of PCR amplification using internal primers, and virus identity was confirmed by nucleotide sequence analysis of the fragments from the first PCR amplification assays.

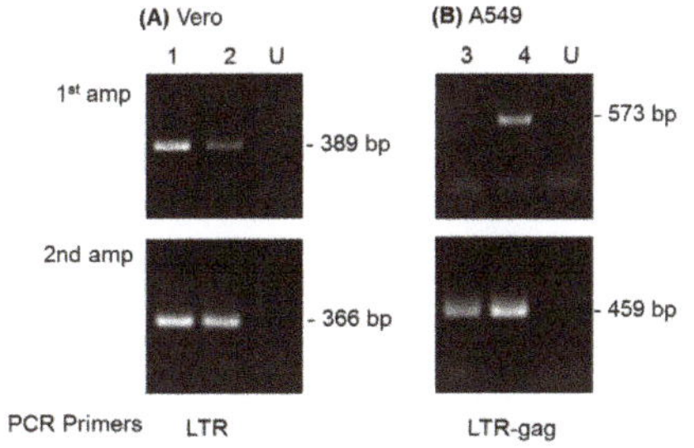

Figure 3. Detection of SFV sequences by DNA PCR analysis. DNA prepared at day 34 from SFVmcy_FV21- and SFVmcy_FV34[RF]-inoculated Vero cells (panel **A**, lanes 1 and 2, respectively) was analyzed using LTR primer sets (outer for 1st amplification and inner for second amplification). DNAs prepared from SFVcae-FV2014-inoculated A549 cells at day 34 and day 55 (panel **B**; lanes 3 and 4, respectively) were analyzed using LTR-gag outer and inner primer sets. DNA from uninoculated cells was obtained from each cell line (day 34) and included as negative control (lanes U).

Virus infection in A549 cells was investigated by DNA PCR analysis of cells collected at day 34 and day 55 (Figure 3B, lanes 3 and 4, respectively). The results indicated an increase in SFVcae_FV2014 sequences with passage due to detection in the first round of PCR at day 55 but only in the second amplification with the day 34 sample. Virus identity was confirmed by nucleotide sequence analysis of the fragment obtained in the first PCR amplification at day 55.

3.3. *SFVcae_FV2014 Genome Analysis*

3.3.1. Structure and Sequence Comparison

The genomic organization of the assembled SFVcae_FV2014 genome [17] was found to be similar to other SFVs: It had the expected structural genes (*gag*, *pol*, and *env*) and accessory (*tas* and *bet*) genes, an internal promoter, and long terminal repeats (LTRs) [8]. An 18-bp primer binding site (PBS) was identified at position 1713 to utilize the $tRNA^{Lys1,2}$ isoacceptor for initiation of minus-strand DNA synthesis of spumaviruses [22]. The complete genomic sequence of SFVcae_FV2014 with alignment to the SFVcae_LK3 sequence is shown in Figure S1 and summarized in Table 3. The size of the *gag* and *pol* regions in SFVcae_FV2014 were the same as those in SFVcae_LK3, encoding 643 amino acid Gag and 1143 amino acid Pol proteins, respectively. There was also a 52 bp overlap between *gag* and *pol* and between *pol* and *env* in both viruses. However, there were differences in the size of *env*, *tas*, and *bet*, which resulted in a difference in size of encoded proteins between SFVcae_FV2014 and SFVcae_LK3. The *env* encoded a protein containing four additional amino acids in SFVcae_FV2014, which did not affect the reading frame (986 aa). The *tas* region of SFVcae_FV2014 had an early stop codon resulting in a 296 aa protein as compared to 298 aa for the Tas in SFVcae_LK3. An insertion of nucleotide A in position 11703 resulted in SFVcae_FV2014 having a longer Bet (504 aa) compared to SFVcae_LK3 (469 aa) and to the SFVmcy_FV21 and SFVmcy_FV34[RF] (497 aa and 308 aa, respectively).

Table 3. Comparison of genomic structures of SFVcae isolates.

Viral Regions	Location [1]	SFVcae_FV2014 LTR/gene [2]	ORF [3]	Location [1]	SFVcae_LK3 LTR/gene [2]	ORF [3]
LTR	1–1710	1710		1–1708	1708	
gag	1827–3758	1932	643	1825–3756	1932	643
pol	3706–7137	3432	1143	3704–7135	3432	1143
env	7085–10045	2961	986	7083–10031	2949	982
tas	10,015–10,905	891	296	10,001–10,897	897	298
bet	10,015–10,285, 10,581–11,824	1515	504	10,001–10,271, 10,567–11,705	1410	469
LTR	11,418–13,127	1710		11,404–13,111	1708	

[1] nucleotide position; [2] number of nucleotides; [3] number of amino acids.

Comparative sequence analysis indicated that SFVcae_FV2014 and SFVcae_LK3 had an overall sequence identity of about 70% to 90%, with the highest identity in the LTR, *pol*, *tas*, and *bet* regions (Table 4). Interestingly, in *env* there was high nucleotide and amino acid sequence identity in LP and TM, but only about 71% nucleotide and 67% amino acid identity in the SU region. SFVcae_FV2014 sequences were also compared with SFVmcy_FV21 and recombinant viruses SFVmcy_FV34[RF] and SFVmmu_R289HybAGM, which were previously found to have 77% amino acid identity to SFVcae_LK3 in the SU region (designated as SFVagm-3 in previous study; [11]). An overall sequence identity of 50–85% was seen, with the lowest being in the LTR, *gag*, *tas*, and *bet* regions. In *env*, the lowest was observed in the SU region, however, interestingly, SFVmcy_FV21 had about 74% sequence identity with SFVcae_FV2014, which was slightly higher than that seen between the two SFVcae viruses. Similarity plot analysis (Simplot) and BootScan analysis in Simplot did not indicate recombination in sequences of SFVmcy_FV21 or SFVcae_FV2014 (data not shown).

Table 4. Sequence comparison of SFVcae_FV2014 and different SFV isolates.

SFV Isolates		% Sequence Identity								
		LTR	*gag*	*pol*	*env*	*env*-LP	*env*-SU	*env*-TM	*tas*	*bet*
SFVcae_LK3	nt	88.7[1]	81.5	86.3	79.1	79.6	71.1	86.6	90.2	88.8
	aa		85.4	91.6	81.5	86.5	67.3	93.9	91.3	88.5
SFVmcy_FV21	nt	66.9	68.1	81.7	75.0	71.4	73.8	77.0	66.1	61.8
	aa		65.8	86.1	78.2	73.0	73.5	84.8	52.2	51.4
SFVmcy_FV34(RF)	nt	65.8	68.8	81.9	75.0	72.2	69.1	76.6	65.4	64.4
	aa		66.7	86.3	78.2	73.8	63.2	83.9	52.5	50.9
SFVmmu_R289(RF)	nt	67.6	69.6	81.5	73.4	73.8	68.3	77.8	66.7	62.2
	aa		67.6	86.4	74.5	76.2	63.7	85.3	53.7	51.2

[1] Numbers are percent identity using the ClustalW alignment option in MegAlign (DNASTAR Lasergene).

To further analyze the relatedness of SFVcae_FV2014 in the SU region with other SFVs that are available only as a partial sequence, a BLASTN search of the GenBank nt/nr database was done. SFVcae_FV2014 had between 71–78% nucleotide sequence identity and between 68–81% amino acid similarity with the other SFV sequences from AGM (data not shown). Some of these (SFVcae_agm4, SFVcae_agm5, SFVcae_agm20, and SFVcae_agm24) were selected as representative sequences of clusters A–D [9] in the phylogenetic analysis discussed below.

3.3.2. Phylogenetic Analysis

Analysis of the evolutionary relatedness of the nucleotide sequences in LTR, *gag*, *pol*, *tas*, and *bet* showed that SFVcae_FV2014 and SFVcae_LK3 branched together and clustered with the macaque isolates, which included SFVmcy_FV21 and SFVmcy_FV34[RF] branched together, and the SFVmmu_R289HybAGM[RF] on a separate branch (data not shown). To evaluate the differences seen in SFV sequence identity in the LP, SU, and TM regions of *env* (Table 3), phylogenetic analyses were done in the full-length *env* and its subregions. This included SFVmmu_K3T, a naturally-occurring rhesus macaque virus isolated in our laboratory and in the SU region, also sequences from other AGM SFVs (SFVcae_agm4, SFVcae_agm5, SFVcae_agm20, and SFVcae_agm24). Constructed trees of the full-length *env*, SU, and TM regions are shown in Figure 4; results in the LP are not shown since they were similar to the TM. Analysis in *env* indicated the AGM viruses SFVcae_LK3 and SFVcae_FV2014 were branched together and clustered with the macaque isolates where SFVmcy_FV21 and SFVmmu_K3T branched together and SFVmcy_FV34[RF] and SFVmmu-R289HybAGM[RF] branched together. A difference in branch results was seen when analysis was done in the *env* subregions. In TM, SFVs branched with their monkey species: SFVmcy and SFVmmu were clustered on different branches and SFVcae isolates branched together. Similar results were seen in LP. However, in the SU region, although all of the SFVs from AGM were clustered together and the SFVs from macaques were clustered together, SFVcae-LK3 and SFVcae_FV2014 did not branch together and were grouped separately, along with different SFVcae_agm sequences: SFVcae_agm4 and SFVcae_agm6 with SFVcae_LK3 and SFVcae_agm20 and SFVcae_24 with SFVcae_FV2014 [9]. Interestingly, SFVmcy_FV34[RF] and SFVmmu-R289HybAGM[RF] branched together in a third group in the AGM cluster, further corroborating recombination in their SU region with SFV sequences from AGM [11,12].

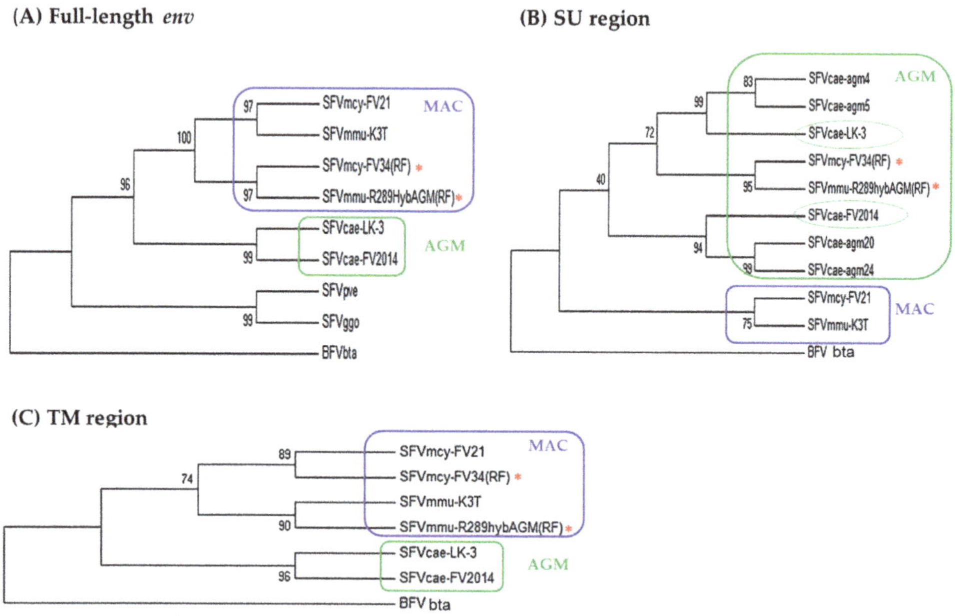

Figure 4. Phylogenetic analysis of SFV *env*. Results are shown for the nucleotide sequence in: (**A**) full-length *env*, using 2900 positions in the final dataset; (**B**) SU region using 1305 positions in the final dataset; and (**C**) TM region using 1242 positions in the final data set. The accession numbers of the virus sequences used for the analysis are shown in Table 2. BFVbta was used as the outgroup for all the trees. The percentage of replicate trees in which the associated taxa clustered together in the bootstrap test (1000 replicates) are shown next to the branches. Color indicates the clustering of AGM (green) and MAC (blue) isolates based on analysis of indicated regions in *env*. Recombinant virus is indicated with an asterisk.

4. Discussion

Previous analysis of spumaretroviruses in AGMs has focused on investigating intraspecies genetic diversity based on sequence analysis in the env/SU region [9]. The results showed prevalence of SFV strains that were divided into two phylogenetically diverged groups, each comprising distinct clusters (group 1 contained clusters A and B; group 2 contained clusters C and D). Furthermore, SFVcae_LK3 (designated as SFV-3/LK-3 in the reference paper) belonged to group 1 but was distinct from sequences in clusters A and B, whereas SFVcae_FV2014 (designated as SFV-3 in the reference paper) was an outlier and was divergent from both groups 1 and 2. In the present study we obtained the full-length genomic sequence of SFVcae_FV2014 and showed that it is a genetically distinct virus from SFVcae_LK3. The sequence differences between these SFV isolates might be due to distinct FV strains circulating in the AGMs in different geographical regions [23,24]. Although specific information about monkey origin is not available, it is reported that SFVcae_FV2014 was isolated from a grivet monkey kept in New York, USA [2], whereas other FV sequences in groups 1 and 2 were obtained from AGMs caught in the wild in Kenya and singly-housed in Freiburg, Germany [9]. Furthermore, SFVcae_LK3 was isolated from an AGM housed in Freiburg, Germany, but exposed to other AGMs and rhesus macaques during captivity [5]. Additionally, it is noted that SFVcae_LK3 was isolated from lymphoblastoid cells whereas the other sequences in groups 1 and 2 were PCR-amplified from kidney tissue. The phylogenetic differences in AGM SFV sequences from naturally-occurring viruses and the laboratory-isolates highlight the need for evaluating the biological properties of natural SFV isolates along with laboratory strains for developing relevant in vitro models to investigate SFV replication in NHPs and their potential for intra-, inter-, and cross-species virus transmission.

The large number of studies demonstrating broad distribution of SFVs in Old World and New World NHPs and species-specific prevalence of SFV strains have been based on sequence analysis of genomic regions [8,24–34]. Whole-genome analysis of some isolates has shown that genetically-diverse SFV strains circulating in different NHP species have contributed to the generation of recombinant viruses involving the SU region in *env* [11,12,35]. It is noted that sequence variation in SU was initially characterized in feline foamy viruses [36]. However, there is a lack of information regarding the biological properties of SFV strains that could be potential parent sequences involved in generation of recombinant viruses. We previously identified that SFVmcy_FV34[RF], isolated from *M. cyclopis*, was a recombinant virus with >90% overall nucleotide sequence identity to SFVmcy_FV21 (also isolated from the same monkey species), except in the SU region, which had about 76% nucleotide sequence identity to SFVcae_LK3, an AGM isolate [11]. Since recombination between viruses depends on the ability of two viruses to superinfect or coinfect the same species and replicate in the same cell type, we have investigated the biological properties of SFVmcy_FV34[RF] and its potential parent viruses SFVmcy_FV21 and SFVcae_FV2014, which had overall 80–90% nucleotide sequence identity to SFVcae_LK3. Cell lines from a range of different host species, tissues, and cell types were used to evaluate the host range and replication kinetics. To minimize variability in the virus preparations, the virus stocks were prepared in a similar manner and infectious titer obtained using the same assay. A low virus titer was used for infection to differentiate replication kinetics. As expected, there was productive infection with CPE in the fibroblastic cell lines [37,38], although higher virus production (RT activity) was seen in *M. dunni* [14] than in MRC-5. Furthermore, SFVcae_FV2014 had slightly slower replication kinetics in *M. dunni* compared with the SFVmcy viruses, whereas no difference was seen in MRC-5. Since all three viruses in the study were isolated from kidney tissue, kidney epithelial cell lines from rhesus monkey, AGM, and dog were included. Different kinetics of virus replication were seen: In MDCK cells, all three SFVs had rapid replication with CPE; in FRhK-4, SFVcae_FV2014 and SFVmcy_FV21 had similar rapid kinetics with CPE, whereas SFVmcy_FV34 had delayed kinetics ending in only 3+ CPE at day 30; in Vero only SFVcae_FV2014 showed rapid replication with CPE whereas SFVmcy_FV21 had delayed replication kinetics (3+ CPE at day 32) and SFVmcy_FV34 had a persistent infection without CPE progression (confirmed by PCR) until the culture was terminated on day 32. It should be noted that in our earlier study in Vero, SFVmcy_FV34 (then called SFV-2) showed low RT activity around day 30 but the lot of virus and infection titer used was different [14]. In the human lung carcinoma A549 epithelial cells, both SFVmcy viruses had productive infections with CPE, however, SFVcae_FV2014 had a persistent infection without CPE progression even on long-term culture (>50 days), although break-through low level RT activity was seen on day 33 and 55. It was noted that SFVcae_FV2014, SFVmcy_FV21, and SFVmcy_FV34[RF] had broad host ranges and infected all of the cell lines in the study, however, each had distinct replication kinetics except in MRC-5. This may be due to the MRC-5 cells being a diploid cell line whereas the others were continuous cell lines or because the viruses were titered in MRC-5. Further studies are needed to evaluate FV replication in primary tissues and cell cultures, diploid cells, and continuous cell lines to determine the relevant in vitro infectivity model that can accurately reflect in vivo infection.

The infectivity results in this study confirmed SFVs have a broad host range and further showed that regulation of virus replication post-entry is complex, depending on specific virus–host interactions. These results emphasize the need to study the biological properties of different SFV strains within a species to investigate their potential for replication and recombination as well as intra- and cross-species transmission. It is noted that a limitation of the current study is using SFVs that have an in vitro passage history in cell lines of different host species and cell types, however, FV genomes seem to be relatively stable and are therefore not expected to mutate in vitro or in vivo at a high rate like other retroviruses [9]. We are further investigating potential for SFV mutations in vitro by sequence analysis of viral genomes in productive and chronic infections.

Rapid replication of SFVcae_FV2014 was seen in Vero, however, a persistent infection was seen with SFVmcy_FV34[RF]. Since the SU region in the latter is related to the AGM viruses, the results suggest that sequences outside the SU may be involved in regulation of virus replication. We are currently investigating virus–host interactions to determine factors that could be important determinants of virus replication and virus latency. The overall results from the infectivity studies suggest a complex mechanism of regulation of SFV replication.

Transcription of SFVmcy_FV21 and SFVcae_LK3 (previously designated as SFV-1 and SFV-3) has been shown to be cell-line dependent [39] and productive, persistent infection of hematopoietic cells by SFV psc_huHRSV.13 (previously designated as HFV) has been reported [37]. Latently infected cultures with SFV have been established from epithelial cells [40–42] and lymphoblastoid cells [43]. Furthermore, in vivo SFV infection is widespread throughout the animal but remains generally latent except in the oral tissues [44]. Furthermore, recent in vivo studies have confirmed in vivo replication in oropharyngeal tissues [45] and further identified that it is limited to the short-lived differentiated epithelial cells [46]. Our infectivity studies analyzing the replication kinetics of three SFVs in different cell lines from various species indicates that virus replication is dependent on the virus strain and interaction of virus-specific sequences with host-specific factors is an important determinant of outcome of infection. Studies are underway with naturally-occurring SFV strains from rhesus macaques to identify the virus–host interactions involved in SFV replication.

Supplementary Materials: The following are available online at http://www.mdpi.com/1999-4915/12/4/403/s1, Figure S1. Nucleotide sequence alignment of SFVcae_FV2014 and SFVcae_LK3. Sequences were aligned using EMBOSS Stretcher version 6.6.0 using default parameters (http://www.ebi.ac.uk/Tools/psa/emboss_stretcher/help/index-nucleotide.html). Nucleotide positions are indicated. Vertical lines indicate identical bases and dots indicate different bases. The LTRs, *gag*, *pol*, *env*, *tas*, and *bet* regions are indicated. The TATA, poly A^+ signal, and poly A^+ sites are underlined in the LTRs. The 3 nucleotides for the start and termination codons of genes are shown in red. The TATA in tas is underlined and the start site of the internal promoter (IP) is indicated by an arrow. The regulatory signals are indicated based upon homology to the SFVcae_LK3 sequence [7].

Author Contributions: A.S.K. conceived and designed the experiments. E.H.B., S.N., S.M.F., and D.K.W. conducted the experiments. All authors contributed to writing and reviewing the manuscript. All authors have read and agreed to the published version of the manuscript.

Acknowledgments: All funding for the project was received by the U.S. Food and Drug Administration.

Conflicts of Interest: The authors declare no conflict of interest.

References

1. Khan, A.S.; Bodem, J.; Buseyne, F.; Gessain, A.; Johnson, W.; Kuhn, J.H.; Kuzmak, J.; Lindemann, D.; Linial, M.L.; Lochelt, M.; et al. Spumaretroviruses: Updated taxonomy and nomenclature. *Virology* **2018**, *516*, 158–164. [CrossRef] [PubMed]
2. Stiles, G.E.; Bittle, J.L.; Cabasso, V.J. Comparison of simian foamy virus strains including a new serological type. *Nature* **1964**, *201*, 1350–1351. [CrossRef] [PubMed]
3. Johnston, P.B. A second immunologic type of simian foamy virus: Monkey throat infections and unmasking by both types. *J. Infect. Dis.* **1961**, *109*, 1–9. [CrossRef] [PubMed]
4. Johnston, P.B. Strain fv-21 of simian foamy virus type 1 was cloned and sequenced after isolation from the taiwan monkey macaca cyclopsis. *J. Microbiol. Immunol. Infect.* **2000**, *33*, 60–61.
5. Neumann-Haefelin, D.; Rethwilm, A.; Bauer, G.; Gudat, F.; zur Hausen, H. Characterization of a foamy virus isolated from cercopithecus aethiops lymphoblastoid cells. *Med. Microbiol. Immunol.* **1983**, *172*, 75–86. [CrossRef]
6. Schweizer, M.; Corsten, B.; Neumann-Haefelin, D. Heterogeneity of primate foamy virus genomes. *Arch. Virol.* **1988**, *99*, 125–134. [CrossRef]
7. Renne, R.; Friedl, E.; Schweizer, M.; Fleps, U.; Turek, R.; Neumann-Haefelin, D. Genomic organization and expression of simian foamy virus type 3 (sfv-3). *Virology* **1992**, *186*, 597–608. [CrossRef]
8. Pinto-Santini, D.M.; Stenbak, C.R.; Linial, M.L. Foamy virus zoonotic infections. *Retrovirology* **2017**, *14*, 55. [CrossRef]

9. Schweizer, M.; Schleer, H.; Pietrek, M.; Liegibel, J.; Falcone, V.; Neumann-Haefelin, D. Genetic stability of foamy viruses: Long-term study in an african green monkey population. *J. Virol.* **1999**, *73*, 9256–9265. [CrossRef]
10. Liu, W.; Worobey, M.; Li, Y.; Keele, B.F.; Bibollet-Ruche, F.; Guo, Y.; Goepfert, P.A.; Santiago, M.L.; Ndjango, J.-B.; Neel, C.; et al. Molecular ecology and natural history of simian foamy virus infection in wild-living chimpanzees. *PLoS Pathog.* **2008**, *4*, e1000097. [CrossRef]
11. Galvin, T.A.; Ahmed, I.A.; Shahabuddin, M.; Bryan, T.; Khan, A.S. Identification of recombination in the envelope gene of simian foamy virus serotype 2 isolated from macaca cyclopis. *J. Virol.* **2013**, *87*, 8792–8797. [CrossRef] [PubMed]
12. Blochmann, R.; Curths, C.; Coulibaly, C.; Cichutek, K.; Kurth, R.; Norley, S.; Bannert, N.; Fiebig, U. A novel small animal model to study the replication of simian foamy virus In Vivo. *Virology* **2014**, *448*, 65–73. [CrossRef] [PubMed]
13. Nandakumar, S.; Bae, E.H.; Khan, A.S. Complete genome sequence of a naturally occurring simian foamy virus isolate from rhesus macaque (sfvmmu_k3t). *Genome Announc.* **2017**, *5*, e00827-17. [CrossRef] [PubMed]
14. Khan, A.S.; Sears, J.F.; Muller, J.; Galvin, T.A.; Shahabuddin, M. Sensitive assays for isolation and detection of simian foamy retroviruses. *J. Clin. Microbiol.* **1999**, *37*, 2678–2686. [CrossRef]
15. Karber, G. Beitrag zur kollektiven Behandlung pharmakologischer Reihenversuche. *Naunyn Schmiedebergs Arch. Exp. Pathol. Pharmakol.* **1931**, *162*, 480–483. [CrossRef]
16. Sears, J.F.; Khan, A.S. Single-tube fluorescent product-enhanced reverse transcriptase assay with ampliwax (stf-pert) for retrovirus quantitation. *J. Virol. Methods* **2003**, *108*, 139–142. [CrossRef]
17. Nandakumar, S.; Bae, E.H.; Khan, A.S. Complete genome sequence of the african green monkey simian foamy virus serotype 3 strain fv2014. *Genome Announc.* **2017**. [CrossRef]
18. Quail, M.A.; Smith, M.; Coupland, P.; Otto, T.D.; Harris, S.R.; Connor, T.R.; Bertoni, A.; Swerdlow, H.P.; Gu, Y. A tale of three next generation sequencing platforms: Comparison of ion torrent, pacific biosciences and illumina miseq sequencers. *BMC Genom.* **2012**, *13*, 341. [CrossRef]
19. Saib, A.; Koken, M.H.; van der Spek, P.; Peries, J.; de The, H. Involvement of a spliced and defective human foamy virus in the establishment of chronic infection. *J. Virol.* **1995**, *69*, 5261–5268. [CrossRef]
20. Giron, M.L.; de The, H.; Saib, A. An evolutionarily conserved splice generates a secreted env-bet fusion protein during human foamy virus infection. *J. Virol.* **1998**, *72*, 4906–4910. [CrossRef]
21. Khan, A.S.; Kumar, D. Simian foamy virus infection by whole-blood transfer in rhesus macaques: Potential for transfusion transmission in humans. *Transfusion* **2006**, *46*, 1352–1359. [CrossRef] [PubMed]
22. Maurer, B.; Bannert, H.; Darai, G.; Flugel, R.M. Analysis of the primary structure of the long terminal repeat and the gag and pol genes of the human spumaretrovirus. *J. Virol.* **1988**, *62*, 1590–1597. [CrossRef] [PubMed]
23. Aiewsakun, P.; Richard, L.; Gessain, A.; Mouinga-Ondeme, A.; Vicente Afonso, P.; Katzourakis, A. Modular nature of simian foamy virus genomes and their evolutionary history. *Virus Evol.* **2019**, *5*, vez032. [CrossRef] [PubMed]
24. Switzer, W.M.; Salemi, M.; Shanmugam, V.; Gao, F.; Cong, M.E.; Kuiken, C.; Bhullar, V.; Beer, B.E.; Vallet, D.; Gautier-Hion, A.; et al. Ancient co-speciation of simian foamy viruses and primates. *Nature* **2005**, *434*, 376–380. [CrossRef]
25. Feeroz, M.M.; Soliven, K.; Small, C.T.; Engel, G.A.; Andreina Pacheco, M.; Yee, J.L.; Wang, X.; Kamrul Hasan, M.; Oh, G.; Levine, K.L.; et al. Population dynamics of rhesus macaques and associated foamy virus in bangladesh. *Emerg. Microbes Infect.* **2013**, *2*, e29. [CrossRef]
26. Calattini, S.; Wanert, F.; Thierry, B.; Schmitt, C.; Bassot, S.; Saib, A.; Herrenschmidt, N.; Gessain, A. Modes of transmission and genetic diversity of foamy viruses in a macaca tonkeana colony. *Retrovirology* **2006**, *3*, 23. [CrossRef]
27. Ghersi, B.M.; Jia, H.; Aiewsakun, P.; Katzourakis, A.; Mendoza, P.; Bausch, D.G.; Kasper, M.R.; Montgomery, J.M.; Switzer, W.M. Wide distribution and ancient evolutionary history of simian foamy viruses in new world primates. *Retrovirology* **2015**, *12*, 89. [CrossRef]
28. Katzourakis, A.; Aiewsakun, P.; Jia, H.; Wolfe, N.D.; LeBreton, M.; Yoder, A.D.; Switzer, W.M. Discovery of prosimian and afrotherian foamy viruses and potential cross species transmissions amidst stable and ancient mammalian co-evolution. *Retrovirology* **2014**, *11*, 61. [CrossRef]
29. Betsem, E.; Rua, R.; Tortevoye, P.; Froment, A.; Gessain, A. Frequent and recent human acquisition of simian foamy viruses through apes' bites in central africa. *PLoS Pathog.* **2011**, *7*, e1002306. [CrossRef]

30. Calattini, S.; Nerrienet, E.; Mauclere, P.; Georges-Courbot, M.C.; Saib, A.; Gessain, A. Natural simian foamy virus infection in wild-caught gorillas, mandrills and drills from cameroon and gabon. *J. Gen. Virol.* **2004**, *85*, 3313–3317. [CrossRef]
31. Calattini, S.; Nerrienet, E.; Mauclere, P.; Georges-Courbot, M.C.; Saib, A.; Gessain, A. Detection and molecular characterization of foamy viruses in Central African chimpanzees of the *Pan troglodytes troglodytes* and *Pan troglodytes vellerosus* subspecies. *J. Med. Primatol.* **2006**, *35*, 59–66. [CrossRef] [PubMed]
32. Mouinga-Ondémé, A.; Betsem, E.; Caron, M.; Makuwa, M.; Sallé, B.; Renault, N.; Saïb, A.; Telfer, P.; Marx, P.; Gessain, A.; et al. Two distinct variants of simian foamy virus in naturally infected mandrills (*Mandrillus sphinx*) and cross-species transmission to humans. *Retrovirology* **2010**, *7*, 105. [CrossRef] [PubMed]
33. Rethwilm, A.; Bodem, J. Evolution of foamy viruses: The most ancient of all retroviruses. *Viruses* **2013**, *5*, 2349–2374. [CrossRef] [PubMed]
34. Leendertz, S.A.; Junglen, S.; Hedemann, C.; Goffe, A.; Calvignac, S.; Boesch, C.; Leendertz, F.H. High prevalence, coinfection rate, and genetic diversity of retroviruses in wild red colobus monkeys (*Piliocolobus badius badius*) in tai national park, cote d'ivoire. *J. Virol.* **2010**, *84*, 7427–7436. [CrossRef]
35. Richard, L.; Rua, R.; Betsem, E.; Mouinga-Ondémé, A.; Kazanji, M.; Leroy, E.; Njouom, R.; Buseyne, F.; Afonso, P.V.; Gessain, A. Cocirculation of two *env* molecular variants, of possible recombinant origin, in gorilla and chimpanzee simian foamy virus strains from central africa. *J. Virol.* **2015**, *89*, 12480–12491. [CrossRef]
36. Winkler, I.G.; Flugel, R.M.; Lochelt, M.; Flower, R.L. Detection and molecular characterisation of feline foamy virus serotypes in naturally infected cats. *Virology* **1998**, *247*, 144–151. [CrossRef]
37. Yu, S.F.; Stone, J.; Linial, M.L. Productive persistent infection of hematopoietic cells by human foamy virus. *J. Virol.* **1996**, *70*, 1250–1254. [CrossRef]
38. Mergia, A.; Leung, N.J.; Blackwell, J. Cell tropism of the simian foamy virus type 1 (sfv-1). *J. Med. Primatol.* **1996**, *25*, 2–7. [CrossRef]
39. Campbell, M.; Renshaw-Gegg, L.; Renne, R.; Luciw, P.A. Characterization of the internal promoter of simian foamy viruses. *J. Virol.* **1994**, *68*, 4811–4820. [CrossRef]
40. Schweizer, M.; Fleps, U.; Jackle, A.; Renne, R.; Turek, R.; Neumann-Haefelin, D. Simian foamy virus type 3 (sfv-3) in latently infected vero cells: Reactivation by demethylation of proviral DNA. *Virology* **1993**, *192*, 663–666. [CrossRef]
41. Clarke, J.K.; Samuels, J.; Dermott, E.; Gay, F.W. Carrier cultures of simian foamy virus. *J. Virol.* **1970**, *5*, 624–631. [CrossRef] [PubMed]
42. Hotta, J.; Loh, P.C. Enhanced production of a human spumavirus (retroviridae) in semi-permissive cell cultures after treatment with 5-azacytidine. *J. Gen. Virol.* **1987**, *Pt 4*, 1183–1186. [CrossRef]
43. Rhodes-Feuillette, A.; Mahouy, G.; Lasneret, J.; Flandrin, G.; Peries, J. Characterization of a human lymphoblastoid cell line permanently modified by simian foamy virus type 10. *J. Med. Primatol.* **1987**, *16*, 277–289. [PubMed]
44. Falcone, V.; Leupold, J.; Clotten, J.; Urbanyi, E.; Herchenroder, O.; Spatz, W.; Volk, B.; Bohm, N.; Toniolo, A.; Neumann-Haefelin, D.; et al. Sites of simian foamy virus persistence in naturally infected african green monkeys: Latent provirus is ubiquitous, whereas viral replication is restricted to the oral mucosa. *Virology* **1999**, *257*, 7–14. [CrossRef] [PubMed]
45. Murray, S.M.; Picker, L.J.; Axthelm, M.K.; Linial, M.L. Expanded tissue targets for foamy virus replication with simian immunodeficiency virus-induced immunosuppression. *J. Virol.* **2006**, *80*, 663–670. [CrossRef] [PubMed]
46. Murray, S.M.; Picker, L.J.; Axthelm, M.K.; Hudkins, K.; Alpers, C.E.; Linial, M.L. Replication in a superficial epithelial cell niche explains the lack of pathogenicity of primate foamy virus infections. *J. Virol.* **2008**, *82*, 5981–5985. [CrossRef] [PubMed]

viruses

MDPI

Article

Molecular Analysis of the Complete Genome of a Simian Foamy Virus Infecting *Hylobates pileatus* (pileated gibbon) Reveals Ancient Co-Evolution with Lesser Apes

Anupama Shankar [1], Samuel D. Sibley [2], Tony L. Goldberg [2] and William M. Switzer [1,*]

[1] Laboratory Branch, Division of HIV/AIDS Prevention, Center for Disease Control and Prevention, Atlanta, GA 30329, USA

[2] Department of Pathobiological Sciences, School of Veterinary Medicine, University of Wisconsin-Madison, Madison, WI 53706, USA

* Correspondence: bswitzer@cdc.gov; Tel.: +1-404-639-2019

Received: 1 April 2019; Accepted: 30 June 2019; Published: 3 July 2019

Abstract: Foamy viruses (FVs) are complex retroviruses present in many mammals, including nonhuman primates, where they are called simian foamy viruses (SFVs). SFVs can zoonotically infect humans, but very few complete SFV genomes are available, hampering the design of diagnostic assays. Gibbons are lesser apes widespread across Southeast Asia that can be infected with SFV, but only two partial SFV sequences are currently available. We used a metagenomics approach with next-generation sequencing of nucleic acid extracted from the cell culture of a blood specimen from a lesser ape, the pileated gibbon (*Hylobates pileatus*), to obtain the complete SFVhpi_SAM106 genome. We used Bayesian analysis to co-infer phylogenetic relationships and divergence dates. SFVhpi_SAM106 is ancestral to other ape SFVs with a divergence date of ~20.6 million years ago, reflecting ancient co-evolution of the host and SFVhpi_SAM106. Analysis of the complete SFVhpi_SAM106 genome shows that it has the same genetic architecture as other SFVs but has the longest recorded genome (13,885-nt) due to a longer long terminal repeat region (2,071 bp). The complete sequence of the SFVhpi_SAM106 genome fills an important knowledge gap in SFV genetics and will facilitate future studies of FV infection, transmission, and evolutionary history.

Keywords: simian foamy virus; gibbon; lesser apes; co-evolution; complete viral genome

1. Introduction

Foamy viruses (FVs) belong to the Retroviridae subfamily of Spumaretrovirinae, which have fundamentally different replication strategies compared to other complex retroviruses, such as human immunodeficiency virus (HIV). For example, FVs differ from other retroviruses in how they initiate infection. Like complex DNA viruses, FVs use two promoters for gene expression, one in the long terminal repeat (LTR) and one in the envelope (*env*) gene [1]. In addition, FVs complete reverse transcription within the virion before infection of a new host cell, such that the SFV genome can be double-stranded DNA or single-stranded RNA [2,3]. FVs infect a wide range of mammals, including cows, horses, cats, and nonhuman primates (NHPs) in which they are called simian foamy viruses (SFVs). SFVs have been identified in nearly every primate species examined across all continents where NHPs exist. Phylogenetic analyses show each of these NHPs to be infected with species-specific variants, reflecting a generally ancient co-evolution of SFVs and their hosts [3–15]. Like other simian retroviruses, SFVs can recombine and cross-species infections occur, both of which can complicate their evolutionary history [5,16–19]. Hence, analysis of complete genomes is necessary to fully understand the evolutionary trajectory of SFV.

SFVs received heightened public health attention following numerous reports of transmission of SFV from NHPs to humans across the globe via a variety of routes of exposure [3,12,20–22]. Many studies have documented SFV acquisition, both in persons working with NHPs in research facilities and zoos [20,21,23–28] and in humans exposed to NHPs in natural habitats, where hunting and butchering of primates and keeping NHPs as pets is common, especially in parts of Africa and Asia [24–27,29]. Although SFVs establish permanent infection of their primate hosts and in zoonotically infected humans, there has been no clear evidence of pathogenesis despite their ability to cause cytopathology in vitro [1,3,12,22,30–34]. Limited studies have also been unable to identify cases of person-to-person transmission [3,7,12,22,31]. As human populations expand and encroach upon NHP habitats, interaction among these species grows, increasing risks for SFV exposure and infection. Many areas of Asia, Africa, and South America have seen increases in deforestation with concomitant intensified incursions into NHP habitats [35,36]. The ensuing exposures to NHPs and their pathogens require continued monitoring, facilitated by the development and modification of new and existing assays for the detection of zoonotic viral agents, including SFV and other retroviruses.

The design of molecular methods for the accurate identification of SFV infection requires a database containing representative sequences from divergent SFV lineages. Although numerous partial nucleotide (nt) sequences (average length of about 500 nt, mostly in the polymerase (*pol*) gene), are available from a large number of SFVs from prosimians, Old World monkeys (OWMs), apes, and New World monkeys (NWMs), there remains a paucity of complete SFV genomes. Recently, the taxonomic classification of FVs has been standardized such that the SFV names include a lower case three-letter abbreviation, where the first letter is the first letter of the scientific name of the host genus and the next two letters are the first two letters of the species or subspecies they were isolated from [14]. Whole genome SFV sequences are currently available from one prosimian (SFVocr from a galago), four from NWMs (one each from a spider monkey (SFVaxx), marmoset (SFVcja), squirrel monkey (SFVssc), and capuchin (SFVsxa)), seven from OWMs (three from African green monkeys (SFVcae), four from macaques (SFVmcy, SFVmmu, SFVmfu, SFVmfa), one from a human infected with SFV from a spot-nosed guenon (SFVcni), and eight from great apes (four from chimpanzee (SFVpsc, SFVpve, SFVptr) species, including three from infected humans, three from gorilla (SFVggo), including two from infected humans, and one from an orangutan (SFVppy)) [14]. In contrast, there is a dearth of knowledge about SFV genomes of the smaller or "lesser" apes, family Hylobatidae (common name gibbons), despite their wide taxonomic diversity. Gibbons belong to the superfamily Hominoidea along with great apes and humans. Gibbons are found predominantly in tropical and sub-tropical forests of Southern and Southeast Asia from eastern Bangladesh and northeast India to southern China and Indonesia, including the islands of Sumatra, Borneo, and Java [37]. Unlike the great apes, which include about six species, gibbons are more diverse, with about 19 species identified depending on the classification source [38,39], most of which are endangered (www.iucnredlist.org) [40]. The Hylobatidae consists of five genera and 19 species (*Hoolock* species (n = 2), *Hylobates* sp. (n = 9), *Justitia* (n = 1), *Nomascus* sp. (n = 6), and *Symphalangus* sp. (n = 1).

A recent study reported a high seroprevalence of SFV in gibbons from Cambodia, although the seropositive samples were not SFV PCR-positive [41]. Like other NHPs, gibbons are frequently hunted or kept as pets, facilitating opportunities for human exposure to SFV; yet there is a lack of available sequences to optimize PCR assays for their detection. Considering these factors, elucidation of additional sequences from SFV-infected gibbons will provide the field with important molecular information for the development of diagnostic assays and will permit further examination of the biology and evolutionary history of SFV in apes, and in NHPs in general.

In a previous report [42], we described the isolation of a novel, highly divergent gibbon SFV strain (SFVhpi_SAM106) from a captive-born *Hylobates pileatus* (pileated gibbon) using blood cell co-culture, and the subsequent amplification of partial *pol* sequences. In this study, we used random hexamer-based deep-sequencing [43], a technique that uses random priming instead of relying on sequence-specific approaches, thus allowing molecular characterization of divergent viral sequences. In addition to *in silico* characterization of the full-length SFVhpi_SAM106 genome, we also analyzed evolutionary relationships to other complete monkey and ape SFVs by using non-simian FVs as outgroups.

2. Materials and Methods

2.1. Blood Sample Processing, Co-Culture, and PCR Identification of a Novel Divergent SFV in Gibbons

SFVhpi_SAM106 was previously isolated from peripheral blood mononuclear cells (PBMCs) prepared from whole blood from a *H. pileatus* (SAM106) co-cultured with canine thymocyte Cf2Th cells as described in detail elsewhere [42]. Briefly, frozen PBMCs were thawed, stimulated with interleukin-2 for three days at 37 °C, washed with media, and incubated with an equal number of Cf2Th cells. Cultures were monitored every 3 to 4 days for syncytial cytopathic effect (CPE) typical of FV. CPE was visible on day 38, whereupon infected Cf2Th cells and viral supernatants were collected and stored frozen in liquid nitrogen until use. This captive gibbon was wild-caught and was about 30 years old at the time of specimen collection. Previous PCR and sequence analysis of integrase sequences within the *pol* gene from this gibbon confirmed the presence of a highly divergent SFV distinct from other ape SFVs [42]. During that same study, we similarly isolated SFVhle from a *H. leucogenys* but were unable to recover virus from the stored tissue culture supernatants. As described in the initial publication, NHP blood specimens were obtained opportunistically in accordance with the animal care use committees at each participating institution [42].

2.2. Next Generation Sequencing and SFVhpi_SAM106 Genome Assembly

In total, 1 mL of tissue culture supernatant was centrifuged at 5000× *g* at 4 °C for 5 min with subsequent filtration through a 0.45 µm filter (Millipore, Billerica, MA, USA) to remove any residual host cells. Viral nucleic acids were then isolated using the Qiagen QIAamp MinElute virus spin kit (Qiagen, Hilden, Germany) according to the manufacturer's instructions, except that carrier RNA was omitted. The eluted nucleic acids were then treated with DNase I (DNA-free, Ambion, Austin, TX, USA) and cDNA was generated by priming with random hexamers using the Superscript double-stranded cDNA Synthesis kit (Invitrogen, Carlsbad, CA, USA). cDNA was purified using the Agencourt Ampure XP system (Beckman Coulter, Brea, CA, USA) and approximately 1 ng of cDNA was subjected to simultaneous fragmentation and adaptor ligation ("tagmentation") using the Nextera XT DNA Sample Prep Kit (Illumina Systems, San Diego, CA, USA). Briefly, fragmented DNA was PCR-amplified with Nextera index primers (15 cycles) and purified using the Agencourt Ampure XP system. The resulting DNA library was sequenced using an Illumina MiSeq (MiSeq Reagent Kit V3, 600 cycle, Illumina Systems, San Diego, CA, USA). To analyze sequence data, raw sequences were de-multiplexed and converted to FastQ format using the CASAVA v1.8.2 software (Illumina). The processed reads were then imported into the CLC Genomics Workbench v7 (CLC bio, Aarhus, Denmark), trimmed to remove Nextera-specific transposon sequences as well as short and low quality reads, and assembled using the CLC de novo assembler. Both singleton and assembled contiguous sequences (contigs) were queried against the GenBank database (http://www.ncbi.nlm.nih.gov/GenBank) using the basic local alignment search tools blastn and blastx [12], with a high e-value cut-off of 10 and word sizes of 11 and three for blastn and blastx queries, respectively. Contigs with significant homology to SFV were then mapped to SFVmcy (macaque SFV; GenBank accession number NC_010819) as the reference sequence to generate the consensus SFVhpi_SAM106 sequence.

2.3. Sanger Sequencing of LTR Region

We amplified the LTR region using primers specific to SFVhpi_SAM106 in order to confirm the LTR length. DNA was extracted from the tissue culture cells and 500 ng was used as template in two separate nested PCRs using SFVhpi_SAM106-specific primers. One assay spanned the 5′LTR and RU5 region while the second spanned the 3′end of *bet* and the 3′LTR. The primers for the

SFVhpi_SAM106_LTR-RU5 and SFVhpi_SAM106_*bet*-LTR fragments for the primary and secondary PCRs respectively are:

SFVhpi_SAM106_LTRF2 (5′ GCAGTAGGAGAACAACCTCCTT 3′) and FVRU5R1 (5′ CCCGACTT ATATTCGAGCCCCAC 3′) and

SFVhpi_SAM106_LTR_nestF2 (5′ GGAGGAATACTCCTCTCCCCCTCTC 3′); FVRU5R2 (5′ CACG TTGGGCGCCAAATTGTC 3′) and

SFVhpi_SAM106_*bet*_F1 (5′ GTGGGAGAAGGTAATATTAATCC 3′) and SFVhpi_SAM106_LTR_R1 (5′ GTGGAATATTCTGTGTTGATTATCC 3′) and

SFVhpi_SAM106_*bet*_nestF1 (5′ AGGCATATGGACCACCACAAG 3′) and SFVhpi_SAM 106_LTR_nestR1 (5′ CAACCTTGTTGATAAGGGCAAC 3′).

We performed an initial denaturation at 94 °C for 2 min. followed by 40 cycles of 94 °C for 1 min, 45 °C for 1 min; 72 °C for 2.5 min, with a final extension at 72 °C for 5 min. For both nested PCRs, we used 3 μL of the primary PCR product as template. Nested PCR products were electrophoresed in 1.0% agarose gels and visualized by ethidium bromide staining. For sequence analysis, the PCR products were purified using the Qiaquick gel extraction kit (Qiagen Inc., Valencia, CA) and then sequenced in both directions using a Big Dye terminator cycle kit (ThermoFisher Scientific, Waltham, MA) and additional internal SFVhpi_SAM106-specific sequencing primers to ensure sufficient coverage.

2.4. Complete SFVhpi_SAM106 Genome Sequence Analysis

Gene annotation tools in CLC Genomics Workbench were used to locate open reading frames (ORFs) within coding regions of the SFVhpi_SAM106 genome. Positions of the complete 5′ and 3′ long terminal repeats (LTRs) were determined manually using previously published ape SFV genomes as a reference. Potential splice donor and acceptor positions were inferred using neural network predictions implemented in NetGene2 (http://www.cbs.dtu.dk/services/NetGene2/). N-linked glycosylation sites were predicted using the N-GlycoSite tool at the HIV LANL website (https://www.hiv.lanl.gov/content/sequence/GLYCOSITE/glycosite.html) [44]. Potential nuclear localization signals in the Tas protein were predicted using NucPred (https://nucpred.bioinfo.se/cgi-bin/single.cgi) and PSORTII (https://psort.hgc.jp/form2.html). Coiled-coil motifs were inferred using the website https://embnet.vital-it.ch/software/COILS_form.html. Nuclear export signals (NESs) were inferred using neural networks and hidden Markov models at http://www.cbs.dtu.dk/services/NetNES/.

Using Geneious v7.0.6, we extracted the five coding regions, *gag*, *pol*, *env*, *tas*, and *bet*, and aligned them with representative SFVs with complete genomes from four other apes, two OWMs, four NWMs, one prosimian, and one FV each from equine, bovine, and feline hosts (Table 1). We also created a concatamer of the major FV coding regions (group-specific antigen (*gag*), polymerase (*pol*), and envelope (*env*)) to enable maximally robust phylogenetic analysis. Concatamers of major coding regions of other slowly evolving cell-associated retroviruses are commonly used for evolutionary analyses [45–47]. Finally, since recombination was reported recently in the surface protein (SU) region of *env*, we also prepared an alignment of the complete SFV *env* sequences of species in Table 1 and those from chimpanzee, gorilla, humans, and macaques used in the analyses by Galvin et al. and Richard et al. consisting of 48 taxa [19,48] All alignments were checked for evidence of potential recombination events using first a 400-nt window and a 40-nt step, and then a 200-nt window and 20-nt step, using the Kimura-2 parameter nucleotide substitution model with gap stripping in Simplot v 3.5.1 [49]. We also checked for recombination by using the Recombination Detection Program (RDP) v4 with the default parameters [50].

Table 1. Foamy virus complete genomes analyzed.

Foamy Virus	Mammalian Host	Host Scientific Name	Family	GenBank Accession Number
SFVhpi_SAM106	Pileated gibbon	*Hylobates pileatus*	*Hylobatidae*	M621235
SFVpve	Western chimpanzee	*Pan troglodytes verus*	*Hominidae*	U04327
SFVpsc	Eastern chimpanzee	*Pan troglodytes schweinfurthii*	*Hominidae*	Y07725
SFVppy	Bornean orangutan	*Pongo pygmaeus*	*Hominidae*	AJ544579
SFVggo	Lowland gorilla	*Gorilla gorilla gorilla*	*Hominidae*	NC_039029
SFVcae	African green monkey	*Cercopithecus aethiops*	*Cercopithecidae*	M74895
SFVmcy	Formosan rock macaque	*Macaca cyclopsis*	*Cercopithecidae*	X54482
SFVcja	Common marmoset	*Callithrix jacchus*	*Callitrichinae*	GU356395
SFVsxa	Yellow-breasted capuchin	*Sapajus xanthosternos*	*Cebinae*	KP143760
SFVaxx	Spider monkey	*Ateles* species	*Atelinae*	EU010385
SFVssc	Common squirrel monkey	*Saimiri sciureus*	*Saimirinae*	GU356394
SFVocr	Brown greater galago	*Otolemur crassicaudatus*	*Galagidae*	KM233624
EFVeca	Horse	*Equus caballus*	*Equidae*	AF201902
BFVbta	Cow	*Bos taurus*	*Bovidae*	U94514
FFVfca	Cat	*Felis catus*	*Felidae*	Y08851

We performed codon-based nucleotide alignments using MAFFT v 7.017 [51], followed by manual adjustments and gap stripping. We used the model selection algorithm in MEGA v6 [52] to determine the best fitting nucleotide substitution model, which was inferred to be the general time reversible (GTR) model with gamma (Γ) distribution and invariable sites (GTR+Γ+I). Likelihood mapping of quartet topologies implemented in IQ-TREE v1.6.8 was used to check for evidence of good phylogenetic signal in the alignment [53]. We also checked the phylogenetic signal and evidence of nucleotide substitution saturation in the alignments with the program DAMBE v7.0.35 (http://dambe.bio.uottawa.ca/DAMBE/dambe.aspx).

Phylogenies and divergence dating were simultaneously inferred using Bayesian inference with the program BEAST v.1.8.4 [54]. For BEAST analysis, we created six taxon groups, including Hominoidae (great apes), *Pan/Gorilla*, NWMs, OWMs, OWM/Hominoidae, and all simians. We used the MAFFT alignments and enforced monophyly for both simian and non-simian taxon groups in the analyses. To evaluate the potential effect of nucleotide heterogeneity sometimes observed at third codon positions of RNA viruses on the phylogeny, we also conducted phylogenetic analysis after stripping the third codon positions (cdp) from the alignment. We used an uncorrelated lognormal relaxed molecular clock, a birth-death speciation tree prior, and 100 million Markov Chain Monte Carlo (MCMC) iterations with a 10% burn-in. To more accurately estimate divergence dates, we set priors for the time to the most recent ancestor (TMRCA) dates across the FV phylogeny using normal distribution priors and nuclear DNA split estimates for NHPs and other matching non-simian placental mammals from www.timetree.org [55,56] as follows: 18.6–20.2 million years ago (mya), standard deviation (SD) 0.82 for Hominoidae; 8.44–9.06 mya, SD 0.33 for the *Pan troglodytes/Gorilla* split; 27.61–29.44 mya, SD 0.94 for the OWM/Hominoidae split; 74–78 mya, SD 2.0 for the *Equs caballus/Bos taurus* split; and 91–96 mya, SD 3.1 for *Boreoutheria* (placental mammals).

We used Tracer v1.6 to ensure all parameters converged with effective sampling size (ESS) values >250. Trees were logged every 10,000 generations. Two independent BEAST runs were performed to ensure convergence and reliability of the results. We used TreeAnnotator v1.8.3 to choose the maximum clade credibility tree from the posterior distribution of 10,001 sampled trees with a burn-in value of 1000 trees. The inferred trees were visualized using FigTree v1.4.2 http://tree.bio.ed.ac.uk/software/figtree/).

2.5. Comparison of FV tRNA Binding Motifs

tRNA primer binding site sequences for SFVhpi_SAM106 were identified using tRNAdb (http://trnadb.bioinf.uni-leipzig.de), a database that can be queried for tRNA binding motifs and outputs consensus and features of conservation for any selected set of tRNAs. FV tRNA motifs were compared to investigate potentially divergent primer binding sites.

2.6. Nucleotide Sequence Accession Number

The complete genome of SFVhpi_SAM106 has been deposited in GenBank with the accession number M621235.

3. Results

3.1. SFVhpi_SAM106 Genome Assembly

Assembly of 38,000 paired-end reads yielded the complete SFVhpi_SAM106 coding genome with 380× coverage. The longest contig obtained by *de novo* assembly was 11,815 nt. The read lengths ranged from 175 to 250 bp. The average read length was 203.59 bp. The sequence of the complete genome was determined by manual alignment of overlapping 5′ and 3′ LTR regions to give a final length of 13,885 nt.

3.2. Organization of the SFVhpi_SAM106 Genome and Comparison with Other Ape SFVs

The SFVhpi_SAM106 genome consists of all expected structural, enzymatic and auxillary gene coding regions, including *gag*, *pol*, *env*, *tas*, and *bet*, together flanked by two LTRs (Figure 1).

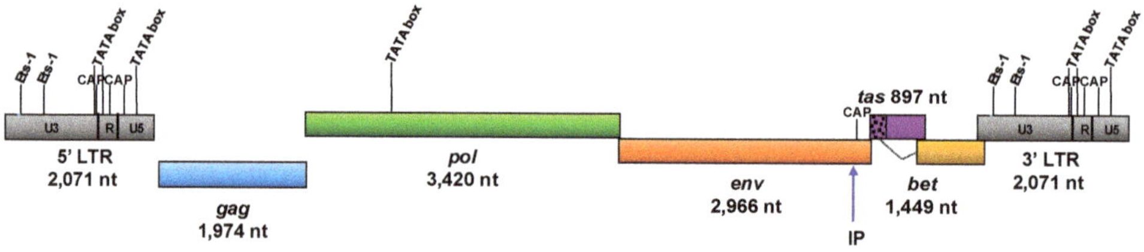

Figure 1. Genomic structure of SFVhpi_SAM106. Ets-1, ETS proto-oncogene 1 transcription factor motif; CAP, catabolite activator protein transcription motif; TATA box, promoter region motif; LTR, long terminal repeat; IP, internal promoter; *gag*, group-specific antigen; *pol*, polymerase; *env*, envelope; *tas*, transactivator gene; *bet*, between *env* and *tas* genes; U3, unique 3′ region of the LTR; R, repeat region of the LTR; U5, unique 5′ region of the LTR. The Bet protein is translated from a spliced RNA and residues from the 5′ part of *tas* indicated by the speckled region and dotted line.

Gene and genome length comparisons with other ape SFVs are provided in Table 2. SFVhpi_SAM106 has the longest recorded genome among ape SFVs owing to its longer LTRs, whereas the lengths of the five coding regions are comparable in size to those from other ape SFVs.

Table 2. Ape simian foamy virus (SFV) gene and genome nucleotide length comparison.

Virus [1]	LTR	*gag*	*pol*	*env*	*tas*	*bet*	Genome
SFVhpi_SAM106	2071	1974	3420	2966	897	1449	13,885
SFVpve	1760	1959	3438	2964	900	1470	13,246
SFVpsc	1767	1944	3431	2964	900	1446	13,242
SFVggo	1283	1964	3154	2963	897	1443	12,258
SFVppy	1621	1987	3236	2965	834	1392	12,823

[1]. SFVhpi_SAM106, pileated gibbon (M621235); SFVpve, chimpanzee (U04327); SFVpsc, chimpanzee (Y07725); SFVppy, orangutan (AJ544579); SFVggo, gorilla (JQ867465); LTR, long terminal repeat; *gag*, group-specific antigen; *pol*, polymerase; *env*, envelope; *tas*, transactivator gene; *bet*, between *env* and *tas* genes.

Nucleotide and amino acid identity comparisons of the major genes and proteins, respectively, of SFVhpi_SAM106 to those of other ape FVs are provided in Table 3. Sequence analysis showed the SFVhpi_SAM106 genome was nearly equidistant from other ape SFVs, sharing approximately 65% nucleotide identity across the *gag–pol–env* region of the coding genome. The highest gene and protein identities were seen with *pol*/Pol followed by *env*/Env, *gag*/Gag, *tas*/Tas, and *bet*/Bet.

Table 3. Percent nucleotide and amino acid identity comparisons of SFVhpi_SAM106 compared to SFVs of other ape hosts.

Virus [1]	*gag*/Gag	*pol*/Pol	*env*/Env	*tas*/Tas	*bet*/Bet	Concatamer [2]
SFVpve	49.2/38.9	74.3/75.9	67.0/66.2	49.2/31.3	49.2/27.9	65.6/63.4
SFVpsc	49.6/38.3	73.4/75.2	67.3/67.1	49.7/38.5	50.3/29.6	65.7/63.5
SFVggo	48.0/40.2	74.1/76.6	67.8/67.5	48.3/29.7	48.0/30.7	65.7/64.7
SFVppy	48.7/40.6	73.2/76.1	65.8/63.8	48.0/32.7	41.3/22.2	64.7/63.3

[1]. SFVhpi_SAM106, pileated gibbon; SFVpve, chimpanzee (U04327); SFVpsc, chimpanzee, (Y07725); SFVppy, orangutan (AJ544579); SFVggo, gorilla (JQ867465). *gag*, group-specific antigen; *pol*, polymerase; *env*, envelope; *tas*, transactivator protein; Bet, between *env* and *tas* protein. [2]. Concatenation of *gag*/Gag, *pol*/Pol, and *env*/Env nucleotide/proteins.

The LTR, at 2071 nt (positions 1–2071), was found to be the longest among the ape SFVs by about 300 to 800 nucleotides. We confirmed the LTR length by PCR using SFVhpi_SAM106 PCR primers and Sanger sequencing. Both the SFVhpi_SAM106_LTR-RU5 and *bet*-LTR fragments were 100% identical to the LTR obtained by NGS and were 1968 bp and 2029 bp in length after removing the primer sequences. The U3 region extends from positions 1 to 1704, which is about 300 nt longer than that of other ape SFVs; followed by the R region (positions 1705 to 1911), which is about 20 nt longer than that of other ape SFVs; and the U5 region (positions 1912 to 2071), which is about the same length as that in other ape SFVs. Three TATA box motifs were found at nucleotide positions 76, 239, and 396 upstream of the primer binding site (PBS), which is in turn 104 nt upstream of the start codon for *gag*. The poly A motif (AATAAA) is located at position 1889, the conserved 3′ and central polypurine tracts (AGGAGAGGG) are located at positions 7973 and 11,813, respectively. The first two dimerization signals (DS) were highly conserved and are located at positions 2081 and 2140, but a potential third DS was not strictly conserved and consisted of AAAAGTC instead of AAAATGG found in other SFVs [57]. There are two Ets-1 transcription factor binding domains in the 5′ LTR at positions 402 and 766. There are also three CAP (catabolite activator protein transcription motif) sites at positions 1647, 1692, and 1808. We also identified a polypurine tract (PPT) at positions 11,795, just upstream of the start of the 3′ LTR. The conserved tRNAlys PBS motif 5′-TGG CGC CCA ACG TGG GGC-3′ at positions 2074 to 2091 in SFVhpi_SAM106 is present in all available complete ape SFV genomes. The relatively conserved SFV Env/Orf-2 splice donor (AG**TTG^GTAA**TTT) and acceptor (TTTTA**AG^A**TAAT) sites are located at positions 10,292 and 10,411, respectively, and were predicted by NetGene2. The nucleotide identity of the SFVhpi_SAM106 LTR to other ape SFV LTRs ranged from 30% to 45%, with the closest identity to LTRs from chimpanzee SFVs.

The internal promoter (IP) was identified by comparison with other FVs and is located at *env* nucleotide positions 10,142 to 10,198 (5′-CAA GAG AA **CATAAA** AGA TCA AAT CGA GAG AGC AAC CGC AGA GC-3′) (Figure 1). However, unlike the TATAAA box consensus motif of exogenous FV IPs, the SFVhpi_SAM106 TATA promoter box is more similar to that of two endogenous FVs (sloth and coelacanth) in that it starts with a cytosine (highlighted in the IP sequence in bold and italics) instead of a thymine [58]. A potential CAP site was identified 48 nucleotides downstream of the IP. Fifteen N-linked glycosylation sites were identified, of which one is in the LP region, 11 are in SU, and three are in TM. Ten of these are NXT variants and five are NXS. In comparison, SFVppy has 13 N-linked glycosylation sites of which one is in LP, nine are in SU, and three are in TM. Nine of these are NXT variants and four are NXS.

The number, position, and composition of potential *tas*-response elements (TREs) varies among SFVs and requires in vivo experiments for confirmation [58]. By comparison with other SFVs, we identified a potential TRE upstream of the IP at position 10,021 (CTTAAAGGCAGAAGAGAAA). TREs in the LTR region could not be readily identified.

We observed that *gag* (1974 nt; positions 2178–4151), *pol* (3420 nt; positions 4102–7521), *env* (2966 nt; positions 7481–10,446), and *tas* (897 nt; positions 10,420–11,316) ORF lengths are similar to other ape SFVs (Tables 2 and 3). To identify the potential splice/acceptor sites for the *bet* gene, we used an online neural network prediction tool. Although we found evidence of a splice donor site in SFVhpi_SAM106 at positions 10,693 to 10,702 (5′-GAGGAATGA^TAAGTTAAT-3′) and a splice acceptor site at positions 10,991 to 11,010 (5′-CTCCTATTAG^GTACACTGGG-3′) indicating possible bet splicing, support was not strong (0.54 and 0.30, respectively). We also found a splice acceptor site within the bet ORF (positions 11,375–11,395, 5′-AATTCTCAG^ATGATGAGGAT-3′) with strong support (0.96), which could potentially give rise to an alternate *tas-bet* fusion transcript 1065 nucleotides and 355 amino acids in length.

Notable motifs identified *in silico* in Gag include the cytoplasmic retention and targeting signal (CTRS) (GEWGFGD**R**YNVVQIVLQD) located at aa positions 39 to 56 with the highly conserved arginine (R) at position 46 essential for intracytoplasmic particle formation. The YXXL motif involved in particle assembly was highly conserved at positions 77 to 80. The P3-cleavage site (RSFN/TVSQ) is located at aa positions 624 to 631 in the carboxyl terminus. Analysis of the Gag sequence did not identify conserved P(T/S)AP late domain motifs in the center of the protein, but we did find two PPAP motifs at aa positions 269 to 272 and 296 to 299. These motifs are similar in number and location to those in SFVpve and SFVggo, but not SFVppy, in which the single PSAP motif is located near the end of Gag. We also identified an assembly domain (YEMLGL) at aa positions 462 to 467. Examination of Gag for glycine-arginine (GR) rich boxes involved in viral replication identified four potential GR-boxes at aa positions 485 to 509 (GGRGRGRNNRNAASGNTQGGNQRQSR), 515 to 534 (GRQSQGGRGRGSNNNTNSRQ), 538 to 562 (QNSSGYNLRPRTYNQRYGGGQGRR), and 595 to 612 (RGDQPRRSGAGRGQGGNR) compared to the three such motifs found in other SFVs. The highly conserved chromatin binding motif was located in the third GR at AA positions 542 to 548 (underlined above), which for other FVs is in GRII [59]. However, a nuclear localization signal (NLS) present in GRII of SFVpsc was not identified in the SFVhpi_SAM106 GRIII by using PSORTII and NucPred [59]. An NES at the N-terminus of Gag has been shown to be critical for the late stages of virus replication of SFVpsc (formerly HFV) and is partially conserved in SFVmcy and SFVcae [60]. Comparison with other SFVs identified a potential NES at aa positions 91 to 108 (LAFNGIGPAEGALRFGPL); however, NetNES predicted in the SFVhpi_SAM106 Gag a leucine-rich NES around aa positions 8 to 20 (LDVQELVLLMQDL), which is relatively conserved in other ape SFV Gag proteins. NetNes correctly predicted the reported NES in SFVpsc, SFVpve, and SFVggo, but not in SFVppy, SFVmcy, SFVcae, SFVocr, SFVcja, SFVaxx, SFVssc, SFVsxa, BFVbta, and EFVeca. An NES similar to that in SFVhpi_SAM106 was predicted for FFVfca.

Within the Pro-Pol polypeptide, the highly conserved protease catalytic center (DTGA) and reverse transcriptase (RT) catalytic site (YVDD) were located at aa positions 24 to 26 and 312 to 315, respectively. The DSF motif required for RNAse H activity located at positions 670 to 672 was also conserved. The viral protease cleavage site for the integrase (IN) protein (YTVN/NIQN) was partially conserved (YVNN/XNXX) and located at aa positions 749 to 756, potentially coding for a 388 aa IN peptide. The IN catalytic center (DD35E) was found at $D^{898}D^{936}E^{972}$ and the zinc-finger motif at $H^{813}H^{817}C^{847}C^{850}$. Interestingly, we also identified a highly conserved TATA box motif at positions 4840 to 4846 in *pol* present in the RT region of all FVs with the consensus sequence (T(A/T)(T/C)AA(A/G) (Figure 2). In SFVhpi_SAM106, this TATAAA motif is 80 nucleotides upstream of the RT active site.

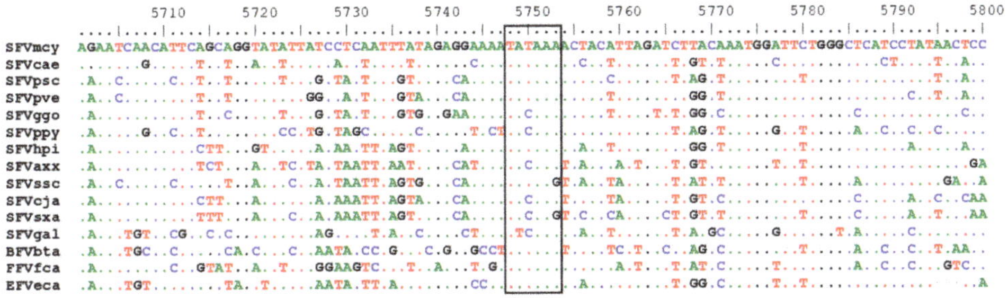

Figure 2. Conserved TATA box in alignment of foamy virus polymerase sequences. Dots represent conserved nucleotides relative to the first sequence. Nucleotide positions are after alignment using MAFFT. Old World apes (OWA): SFVpve, *Pan troglodytes verus* (chimpanzee), GenBank accession number U04327; SFVpsc, *Pan troglodytes schweinfurthii* (chimpanzee), Y07725; SFVppy, *Pongo pygmaeus* (orangutan), AJ544579; SFVggo, *Gorilla gorilla* (gorilla), NC_039029; SFVhpi_SAM106, *Hylobates pileatus*, (pileated gibbon) M621235. Old World monkeys (OWMs): SFVcae, *Cercopithecus aethiops* (African green monkey), M74895; SFVmcy, *Macaca cyclopsis* (macaque), X54482. New World monkeys (NWM): SFVcja, *Callithrix jacchus* (common marmoset), GU356395; SFVsxa, *Sapajus xanthosternos* (capuchin), KP143760; SFVaxx, *Ateles* species (spider monkey), EU010385; SFVssc, *Saimiri sciureus* (squirrel monkey), GU356394. Prosimian (Pro): SFVocr, *Otolemur crassicaudatus* (brown greater galago), KM233624. Non-simian mammals (NSM): EFVeca, *Equus caballus* (equine), AF201902; BFVbta, *Bos taurus* (bovine), U94514; and FFVfca, *Felis catus* (feline), Y08851.

For the 989-aa Env protein, the highly conserved WXXW motif required for Gag interaction and budding is located at aa positions 10 to 13 (WLIW). The cellular furin protease cleavage sites, which cleave the N-terminal leader peptide (LP) from the SU and the SU from the transmembrane (TM) protein, are located at aa positions 125 to 131 (RLAR/RSLR) and 570 to 577 (RKRA/TSSN) to generate three potential Env proteins of lengths 127 (LP), 446 (SU), and 416 (TM), respectively. The highly conserved hydrophobic WXXW motif in the LP required for Env incorporation and particle release is located at aa positions 10 to 13. The membrane-spanning domain located at aa positions 945 to 980 (AKGIFGTAFSLVAYVKPILIGIGVIILLVVIFKIIS) is partially conserved. The consensus KKK endoplasmic reticulum retrieval signal located at aa positions 694 to 696 of the TM (or positions 985 to 987 of Env) is partially conserved and has the sequence KAK, whereas SFVppy, SFVaxx, SFVggo_BAK74, and SFVssc motifs have the sequence KRK. A putative receptor-binding domain (RBD) is located in SU at aa positions 227 to 552 and the relatively conserved fusion peptide (LRSMGYALTGGIQTVSQI) is located in the TM at aa positions 581 to 598 of Env [61].

The ape SFV Tas proteins are highly divergent (Table 3) and hence identification of the poorly defined acidic activation and DNA binding domains was not possible. Tas is a nuclear protein involved in transcriptional transactivation with a partially conserved NLS at the 3′ end of the protein. In SFVhpi_SAM106, the NLS GTGRKRRTN is located at aa positions 216 to 224 with a strong NucPred score of 0.87, whereas PSORT II identified RKRR in this motif as an NLS, but with a low score (−0.16). Neither prediction program found a bipartite NLS in SFVhpi_SAM106 or other ape SFV Tas proteins. PSORT II predicted with high reliability (94.1) that the SFVhpi_SAM106 Tas was a nuclear protein, similar to the Tas protein of SFVppy (reliability score = 94.1), but more likely than those from SFVggo and SFVpve/psc (reliability score = 89). The PSORT II predictor uses a heuristic algorithm, including neural networks, to identify nuclear proteins are rich in basic residues. The SFVhpi_SAM106 Tas includes 41 basic amino acids (R = 25, K = 12, H = 4), or about 13.7% of the protein, compared to 12.2% (34; R = 15, K = 15, H = 4) for SFVppy, 14.1% (42; R = 14, K = 20, H = 8) for SFVggo, 16.6% (50; R = 16, K = 22, H = 12) for SFVpve, and 15.3% (46; R = 18, K = 17, H = 11) for SFVpsc. A leucine-rich NES was predicted to be at aa positions 97 to 107 (LICERLILLAL).

Although the *bet* splice acceptor site described above was not strong, the SFVhpi_SAM106 Bet protein length of 483 aa was similar to that of other ape SFVs (SFVpve = 490 aa, SFVpsc = 482 aa, SFVggo = 481 aa, SFVppy = 464). Comparison with these other ape SFV Bet proteins identified a potential integrin-binding motif (K/RGD) at aa positions 306 to 308 that was partially conserved (KGT), with SFVpve, SFVggo, and SFVppy having a KGD motif and SFVpsc having an RGD motif. The tripeptide RGD domain has been shown to be required for cell membrane binding, so it will be important to examine the functionality of the D > T mutation at the third aa position in the SFVhpi_SAM106 Bet. One study has proposed the SFVpve Bet is secreted in both the cytoplasm and nucleus of infected cells and contains a bipartite NLS in the C-terminus [62]. PSORT II does detect the bipartite NLS RKIRTLTEMTQDEIRKR at aa positions 463 to 479 of SFVpsc Bet, but with a cytoplasmic protein reliability prediction of 70.6% rather than a nuclear one. NucPred did not predict a NLS in the SFVpsc Bet. Neither NucPred nor PSORT II identified any putative NLS in the SFVhpi_SAM106, SFVpve, SFVggo, and SFVppy Bet proteins.

3.3. *Absence of Evidence of Genetic Recombination in the SFVhpi_SAM106 Genome*

Simplot analyses on the *gag-pol-env* concatamer alignment did not show any evidence of genetic recombination at a threshold of 70% of permuted trees, a cutoff commonly used for the analysis of other retroviruses (data not shown). These results were consistent across two window and step sizes in the analysis. We also found no significant evidence of recombination using the recombination detection program RDP4 using eight methods (RDP, GENCONV, Chimaera, MaxChi, BootScan, SiScan, 3Seq, and LARD). We did not find any evidence of recombination of the SFVhpi_SAM106 env using the 48 taxa dataset by phylogenetic and RDP analysis, but we did confirm the two different SU RBD SFV clades as previously reported (Supplementary Figure S1) [19,48]. Phylogenetic analysis of the two alignments encompassing the complete *env* and the region without the RBD in SU showed the typical co-evolutionary history of FV with SFVhpi_SAM106 ancestral to SFVppy, SFV OWMs, and then chimpanzees and gorillas with strong support. In the analysis of only the BD region of SU, SFVhpi_SAM106 was ancestral to the chimpanzee and gorilla SFVs, but with no support. In addition, SFVppy clustered FFVfca with good support between the NWM SFV and the other OWMA SFVs. Combined, these results suggest an absence of recombination in SFVhpi_SAM106 and that genetic recombination did not affect our phylogenetic results when using the *gag-pol-env* concatamer.

3.4. *Evolutionary Relationships and Divergence Dating of SFVhpi_SAM106 and Other FVs*

Likelihood mapping of the 15 taxa 7,412 position *gag-pol-env* concatamer alignment showed an equal distribution of the majority of possible quartets across the tree of which 98.4% were fully resolved, i.e., tree-like, with only 1.68% of unresolved quartets. These results suggest an overall dataset with very good phylogenetic signal and very little "noise" and hence suitable for phylogenetic reconstruction. Excellent phylogenetic signal was also found in both *gag-pol-env* alignments with scores >99.3 using DAMBE. Little nucleotide substitution saturation was found in the alignments using the method of Xia in DAMBE [63]. Together, our results indicate the alignments were satisfactory for phylogenetic analysis.

Phylogenetic trees generated using Bayesian inference of the *gag-pol-env* concatamer showed that FV sequences from a broad range of genetically diverse NHPs and non-simians formed monophyletic lineages and distinct clusters that mirrored host taxonomic relationships (Figure 3). SFVhpi_SAM106 clustered with other ape SFVs with strong posterior probability (PP > 1) support (Figure 3). The FV phylogeny was similar to that seen in our previous study, where SFVhpi_SAM106 is a sister taxa of but ancestral to the great ape SFVs, mirroring the phylogeny of the host mitochondrial and nuclear sequences in which the lesser apes are an outgroup to the great apes [6,42]. An identical phylogeny was obtained with the *gag-pol-env* first and second cdp alignment, indicating the absence of substitution saturation at the third cdp in the analysis of the unstripped alignment (Figure 3). As expected, the representative prosimian FV sequence from a galago (SFVocr) was ancestral to all other SFVs.

The three non-simian FVs from equine, feline, and bovine formed a clade separate from the SFVs, with BFV and EFV clustering together with strong support (PP = 1). All BEAST analyses had standard deviation values of the uncorrelated lognormal relaxed clock (ucld.stdev) greater than zero but less than one, indicating that variation in substitution rates across branches was not consistent with a strict molecular clock but also was not so great as to bias the analyses (Table 4). The absence of site-to-site variation was also supported by alpha parameters of the gamma distribution above 1.0 (Table 4).

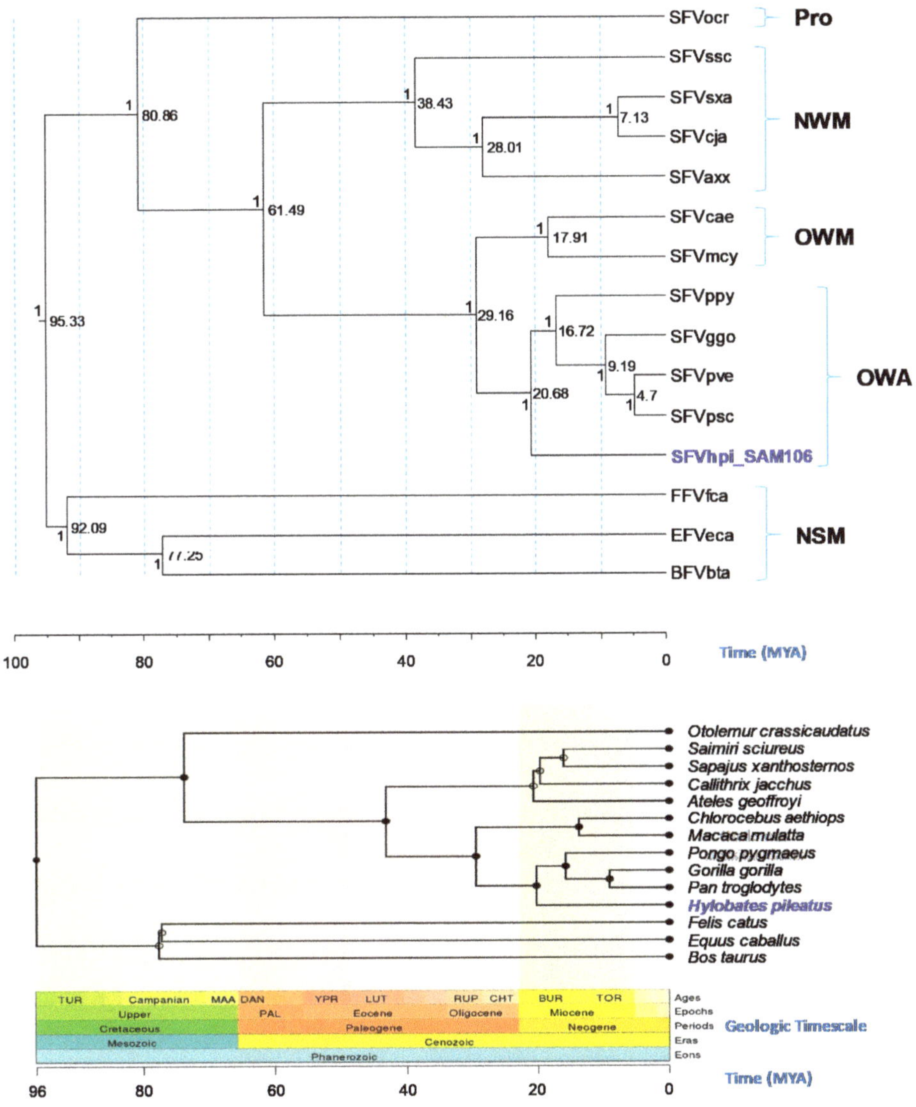

(A)

Figure 3. *Cont.*

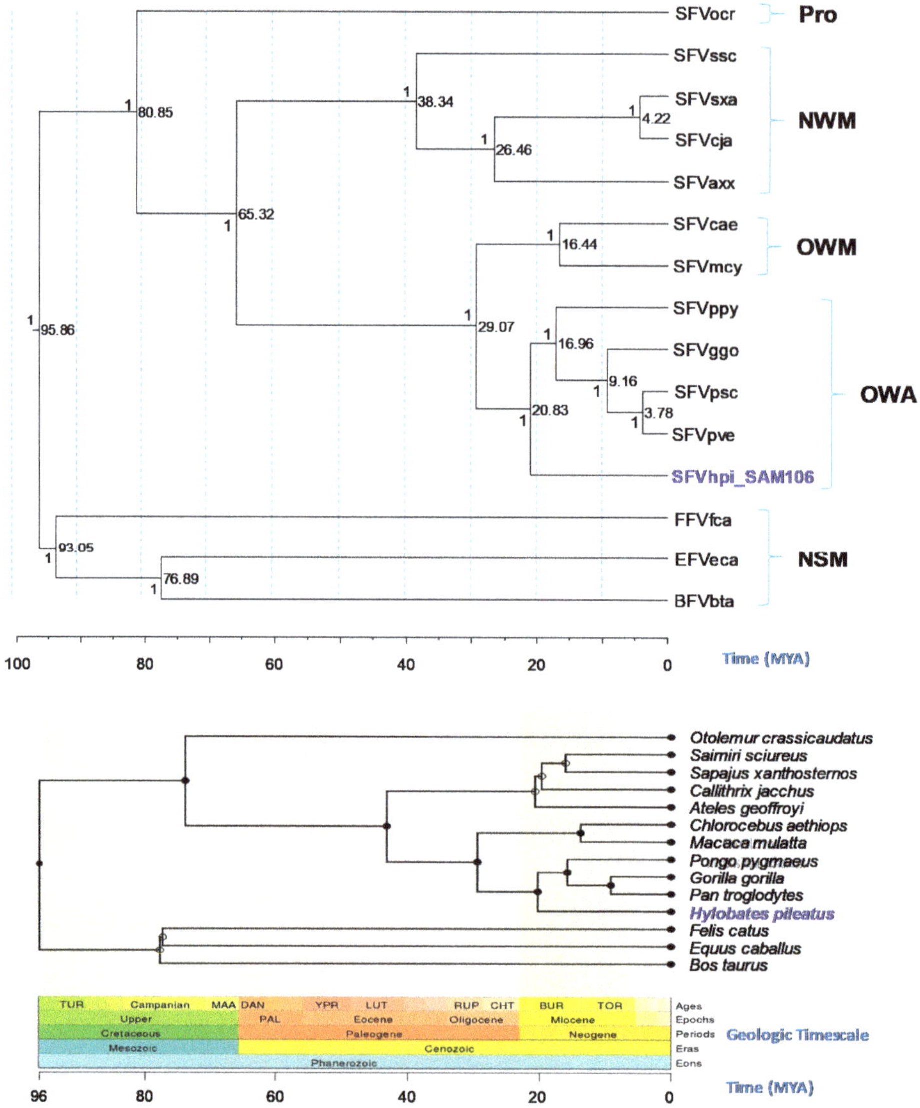

(B)

Figure 3. Evolutionary relationships and divergence dates of foamy viruses (FVs) and their mammalian hosts. (**A**) FV phylogeny inferred using *gag-pol-env* concatamer (~7.4 kb). (**B**) FV phylogeny inferred using the first and second coding positions of the *gag-pol-env* concatamer (~4.9-kb). Phylogeny inferred using BEAST and mammalian host phylogeny inferred at Timetree.org as well as the corresponding geologic timescale. Old World apes (OWAs): SFVpve, *Pan troglodytes verus* (chimpanzee), GenBank accession number U04327; SFVpsc, *Pan troglodytes schweinfurthii* (chimpanzee), Y07725; SFVppy, *Pongo pygmaeus* (orangutan), AJ544579; SFVggo, *Gorilla gorilla* (gorilla), NC_039029; SFVhpi_SAM106, *Hylobates pileatus*, (pileated gibbon) M621235. Old World monkeys (OWMs): SFVcae, *Cercopithecus aethiops* (African green monkey), M74895; SFVmcy, *Macaca cyclopsis* (macaque), X54482. New World monkeys (NWM): SFVcja, *Callithrix jacchus* (common marmoset), GU356395; SFVsxa, *Sapajus xanthosternos* (capuchin), KP143760; SFVaxx, *Ateles* species (spider monkey), EU010385; SFVssc, *Saimiri sciureus* (squirrel monkey), GU356394. Prosimian (Pro): SFVocr, *Otolemur crassicaudatus* (brown greater galago), KM233624. Non-simian mammals (NSMs): EFVeca, *Equus caballus* (equine), AF201902; BFVbta, *Bos taurus* (bovine), U94514; and FFVfca, *Felis catus* (feline), Y08851). Posterior probabilities (on the branch left of the node) and time to most recent ancestors in millions of years (right of node) are provided at each node of the FV phylogeny. Solid circles in the Timetree.org mammalian phylogeny indicate nodes that map directly to the NCBI taxonomy and open circles indicate nodes that were created during the polytomy resolution process. TOR, Tortonian; BUR, Burdigalian; CHT, Chattian; RUP, Rupelian; LUT, Lutetian; YPR, Ypresian; DAN, Danian; MAA, Maastrichtian; TUR, Turonian ages. PAL, Paleogene epoch.

Bayesian dating analyses showed that for the *gag-pol-env* concatamer alignment, the TMRCA for SFVhpi_SAM106 and the Hominoidea was 20.69 mya with a 95% highest posterior density (HPD) interval of 19.13 to 22.19 mya (Table 4). This divergence date occurs during the Miocene epoch (Figure 3). The TMRCA for the SFV OWM/ape split (Crown Catarrhini) was 27.28 mya with a 95% HPD interval of 27.28 to 30.09 mya. The SFVpsc, SFVpve/SFVggo split (Crown Homininae) had a TMRCA of 9.18 mya with a 95% HPD interval of 8.54 to 9.8 mya. For the OWM SFV (Crown Cercopithecinae), a TMRCA of 18.05 mya was inferred with a 95% HPD interval of 11.29 to 24.7 mya. In contrast, TRMCAs for the non-simian FVs were much older, estimated to be 92.4 mya (95% HPD interval of 85.03–98.69 mya). The TMRCA for the Boreoutherian (placental mammals) at the root of the FV phylogeny was estimated to be 95.46 mya (95%HPD interval of 90.08 to 101.19 mya) during the Upper epoch and Mesozoic era. Similar TMRCAs were inferred for the 12 cdp alignment (Table 4). Our inferred FV and host divergence dates were similar to those inferred by others using different methods, supporting the robustness of our dating methods (Table 4). The inferred mean substitution rates ranged from 5.05×10^{-9} to 9.82×10^{-9} nucleotides/site/year across the *gag-pol-env* coding region (Table 4).

Table 4. Time to most recent common ancestor (TMRCA) estimates in millions of years ago and nucleotide substitution rates for foamy viruses (FVs) [1].

FV [2], Host or Analysis Parameter	FV *gag-pol-env*	FV *gag-pol-env (12cdp)* [3]	FV Pol [4]	Host [5]
SFVhpi_SAM106/SFVgreat ape split (Crown Hominoidea)	20.69 (19.13–22.19)	20.83 (19.32–22.45)	N/A [6]	22.32 (20.54–23.85
SFV OWM/ape split (Crown Catarrhini)	29.13 (27.28–30.09)	29.07 (27.37–30.96)	31.60 (25.36–37.85)	32.12 (29.44–33.82)
SFVpve, SFVpsc/SFVggo split (Crown Homininae)	9.18 (8.54–9.8)	9.16 (8.53–9.8)	8.29 (6.52–10.05)	10.63 (10.02–11.68)
SFV OWM (Crown Cercopithecinae)	18.05 (11.29–24.77)	16.44 (10.18–22.81)	N/A	14.09 (12.24–15.82)
Prosimian SFV (Crown Primates)	82.53 (64.77–96.82)	80.85 (65.25–95.16)	86.92 (76.34–97.22)	74.11 (68.17–81.20)
Non-simian FV (horse/cat split)	92.4 (85.03–98.69)	93.05 (86.2–99.12)	N/A	80.6 (63.0–115.4)
BFV/EFV split (cow/horse split)	77.2 (73.26–80.85)	76.89 (73.11–80.61)	N/A	105.7 (74.1–130.8)
Root FV placental mammals (Crown Boreotheria)	95.46 (90.08–101.19)	95.86 (90.47–101.36)	98.59 (95.94–100.78)	120.5 (97.8–136.6)
Mean rate [7]	8.68×10^{-9} (7.88×10^{-9}–9.48×10^{-9})	5.05×10^{-9} (4.62×10^{-9}–5.51×10^{-9})	N/A	N/A[9]
ucld.stdev [8]	0.5524 (0.4084, 0.7252)	0.435 (0.2931–0.5911)	N/A	N/A
α-parameter (Γ-distribution) [9]	1.079 (0.9704, 1.1858)	1.064 (0.8954, 1.2586)	N/A	N/A
ESS [10]	>258	>1063	N/A	N/A

[1]. Median TMRCAs; 95% high posterior density values are shown in parentheses. [2]. SFVhpi_SAM106, SFV from *Hylobates pileatus;* OWM, old world monkeys; SFVpve, SFV from *Pan troglodytes verus;* SFVpsc, SFV from *Pan troglodytes schweinfurthii;* SFVggo, SFV from *Gorilla gorilla*, non-simian foamy viruses include bovine foamy virus (BFV), equine foamy virus (EFV), and feline foamy virus (FFV). [3]. 12 cdp, first and second codon positions. Length is 4.942 kb versus 7.412 kb for the complete coding concatamer. [4]. FV Pol amino acid divergence dates were inferred with Bayesian phylogenetic inference and a time-dependent rate phenomenon, which is a power-law decay function [64]. [5]. Primate and non-primate divergence dates from Pozzi et al. (complete mitochondrial genomes) and dos Reis et al. (nuclear genomes and mitochondrial genomes) [65,66]. [6]. N/A, not available. [7]. Mean evolutionary rate in nucleotide substitutions/site/year. [8]. Standard deviation (stdev) of the uncorrelated lognormal (ucld) relaxed clock, BEAST analysis parameter indicating the amount of variation in the substitution rate across branches. Values close to zero indicate little substitution rate variation and the presence of a molecular clock, whereas values >1 indicate substantial rate heterogeneity amongst lineages. [9]. Shape parameter of the gamma (Γ) distribution of rate heterogeneity among sites. [10]. ESS, effective sampling size values for all BEAST parameters.

4. Discussion

Using a metagenomics approach, we obtained the first complete genome of an SFV from a lesser ape, the pileated gibbon (*Hylobates pileatus*). Next generation sequencing is a powerful molecular method and has been used to obtain complete genomes of other SFV isolates recently [13,67,68]. We characterized the SFVhpi_SAM106 genome by detailed sequence analysis and provided a deeper understanding of the evolutionary history of FVs, especially within the Hominoidea. Most of the important genomic structures and functional domains were conserved in SFVhpi_SAM106 with some exceptions. While the organization of the SFVhpi_SAM106 genome is similar to that of other FVs, it has several unique features, including an LTR at ~2 kb that is 1.2 to 1.6 times longer than that in other FVs, attributable mostly to longer U3 and R regions. Given that the 5′ LTR U3 and R regions of FVs contain transcriptional start control elements, including the *tas* response elements (TREs) and cellular transcription factors, it will be important to conduct transcription-mapping experiments to determine the functional significance of the longer LTRs of SFVhpi_SAM106 for replication and regulation. Since the number and location of FV TREs are not conserved, we were unable to locate the SFVhpi_SAM106 TREs within the LTRs or *env* sequences *in silico*. Others have shown that tissue culture of chimpanzee SFV in diploid human fibroblasts isolated from an infected human selects for isolates with substantial nonrandom nucleotide deletions in the U3 region can increase viral replication [69]. The U3 deletion variant was also present as the majority variant in the infected human but was absent from naturally-infected chimpanzees [69]. However, SFVhpi_SAM106 was isolated from infected PBMCs using canine thymocyte cells [42], which have not been shown to impact SFV LTR length or functionality in this dog cell line or in other non-human cells, including SFVggo and SFVcpz isolates from zoonotically-infected humans grown in baby hamster kidney cells (BHK-21) [57]. Comparisons of SFVhpi_SAM106 LTRs directly from PBMCs from the pileated gibbon and those obtained by culture may be needed to further evaluate this unusually long LTR.

Additional differences from other FV prototypes included four instead of three potential GR boxes in Gag and a TATA box promoter motif in the IP in *env*, which is more similar to those of two endogenous FVs from the sloth and coelacanth by starting with a cytosine instead of a thymine present in other FVs [58]. Since the GR and TATA box motifs are important for viral replication, studies are needed to determine the effect of these genetic differences on SFVhpi_SAM106 replication and growth. Some subtypes of human and simian immunodeficiency viruses (HIVs and SIVs) have the CATAAA TATA box sequence in their LTRs, which have not been shown to decrease LTR promoter activity by the HIV-1 transcription activator (Tat) protein in vitro [70]. Examination of the SFVhpi_SAM106 genome for additional TATA promoters identified a highly conserved TATA box upstream of the RT active site promoter in the FV genome and its possible effect on viral replication is needed.

FVs have been shown to have co-evolved with their hosts for millions of years as vertebrates diversified in the Paleozoic Era [5,6,64]. Our results expand knowledge of the evolutionary history of FVs and show for the first time that SFVhpi_SAM106 from the lesser ape, *Hylobates pileatus*, follows this same ancient co-speciation trajectory. The phylogenetic position of SFVhpi_SAM106 mirrors that of the gibbon host, with a divergence date of about 21 mya (95% HPD 19.13–22.19 mya) during the Miocene Epoch of the Cenozoic Era. The FV divergence dates inferred with our methods are strongly congruent with those of Aiewsakun and Katzourakis, who used Bayesian phylogeny and a time-dependent rate power-law decay function that is independent of archaeological calibrators [64]. Our Hylobatidae/Hominidae divergence dates are also consistent with those of Matsudaira et al. (20.3 mya, 95% CI 17.5–23.6 mya) and Chan et al. (19.25 mya, 95% HPD 15.54–22.99), who examined ape complete mitochondrial sequences [71,72]. The Hylobatidae/Hominidae divergence dates are slightly older than those of reported by Thinh et al. (16.26, 95% HPD 14.69–18.16 mya), who used only complete cytochrome B mitochondrial sequences [38]. In addition, our inferred SFV divergence dates are also highly consistent with those reported for the evolutionary histories of NHPs and other placental mammals examined in our study and had very close divergence dates with overlapping confidence intervals (Table 4). Together, these results show that our use of multiple host divergence calibration points provided a robust inference of FV evolutionary histories. As with all evolutionary studies, the inferred divergence dates represent minimum ages that are younger than true ages, because the fossil record is incomplete.

Given the strong evidence of FVs co-diverging with their hosts, both FVs and their mammalian hosts [73] should have very similar evolutionary rates. Indeed, FVs have extremely low rates of evolution, similar to rates observed for mitochondrial protein-coding genomes of about 1×10^{-8} substitutions/site/year [4,6,11]. However, our estimates were a log lower and are more similar to those of the mammalian neutral substitution rate for nuclear genes and for endogenous retroviruses of 1×10^{-9} substitutions/site/year [74,75]. Our lower inferred FV nucleotide substitution rates may reflect the use of older calibration dates for the *Equs caballus/Bos Taurus* split and for Boreoutheria in the phylogenetic analyses.

Genetic recombination did not appear to affect our phylogenetic results. Phylogenetic analysis of only the FV *env* region with additional SFV taxa from the gorilla, chimpanzee, and macaque with evidence of a variant RBD from a potential recombination event showed that SFVhpi_SAM106 was ancestral to SFVppy and then all other OWMA SFVs instead of ancestral to only the apes as we found for the *gag-pol-env* concatamer alignments. Similar results were inferred even after removal of the putative recombination region in the RBD of SU, whereas in the RBD-only alignment, placement of the SFVhpi_SAM106 and SFVppy taxa were not resolved. Similar genetic relationships were observed by Richard et al. in SFVppy when examining complete gorilla and chimpanzee *env* sequences [19]. One exception in their analysis of the variant RBD region is that SFVppy clustered ancestral to chimpanzee and gorilla clade 1 instead of with FFVfca as in our analysis since non-simian FVs were not included in their analysis [19,48]. Such nonconforming FV co-evolutionary phylogenetic relationships may reflect the phenomenon called long branch attraction (LBA), which can occur when highly divergent lineages are included in the phylogenetic analysis [73]. LBA can potentially be resolved by the addition of additional sequence information [73], which we have done by using the *gag-pol-env* concatamer, or by inclusion of more SFV sequences from gibbons and orangutans when they become available.

As with other NHPs, gibbons are threatened by habitat encroachment for forest clearance, road construction, and changes in agriculture resources. Gibbons are also hunted for food, medicine, or for exportation for the pet trade (see also the International Union for Conservation of Nature's Red List at www.iucnredlist.org) [40,76]. Gibbons are also common members of zoological exhibits. All of these activities can lead to human exposures to gibbons and their microbial communities, including SFVs, which have crossed into humans from many NHP species [12]. Until now, only two short SFV integrase sequences were available to inform the design of sensitive PCR assays for the detection of human infection [42]. More sensitive molecular assays are needed to detect the low copies of integrated genomes typically found in SFV infection. The small number of complete SFV genomes from all available NHPs has also limited the design of generic SFV PCR primers. These limitations may help explain the inability to detect SFV sequences in seropositive pileated gibbons from Cambodia using generic PCR assays [28]. The availability of the complete SFVhpi_SAM106 genome from our study will facilitate the design of more sensitive and specific PCR assays for the detection of gibbon SFVs and fills an important knowledge gap in the SFV database, facilitating future studies of FV infection, transmission, and the evolutionary history of FVs.

5. Conclusions

By using a metagenomics approach, we obtained the complete SFVhpi_SAM106 genome from a pileated gibbon (*Hylobates pileatus*). Bayesian analysis showed that SFVhpi_SAM106 is ancestral to other ape SFVs with a divergence date of ~20.6 million years ago, reflecting ancient co-evolution of the host and virus. Our molecular analysis also showed that the SFVhpi_SAM106 genome has the longest genome (13,885 nt) of all SFVs with complete genomes available, due to a much longer LTR

(2071 bp). The complete sequence of the SFVhpi_SAM106 genome will provide invaluable information for further understanding the epidemiology and evolutionary history of SFVs.

Supplementary Materials: The following are available online at http://www.mdpi.com/1999-4915/11/7/605/s1. Supplementary Figure S1.

Author Contributions: W.M.S. and T.L.G. conceived and designed the study; A.S., W.M.S., and S.D.S. performed the experiments; A.S., S.D.S., T.L.G., and W.M.S. analyzed the data; A.S. prepared the draft manuscript and all authors contributed to the final version, which was approved by all authors for submission.

Funding: This work was supported by intramural CDC funding and by NIH grant TW009237 as part of the joint NIH-NSF Ecology of Infectious Disease program and the UK Economic and Social Research Council (grant ES/J011266/1).

Acknowledgments: Use of trade names is for identification only and does not imply endorsement by the U.S. Centers for Disease Control and Prevention (CDC). The findings and conclusions in this report are those of the authors and do not necessarily represent the views of the CDC.

Conflicts of Interest: The authors declare no conflict of interest. The funding sponsors had no role in the design of the study; in the collection, analyses, or interpretation of data; in the writing of the manuscript, and in the decision to publish the results.

References

1. Linial, M.L. Foamy viruses are unconventional retroviruses. *J. Virol.* **1999**, *73*, 1747–1755. [PubMed]
2. Rethwilm, A. Molecular biology of foamy viruses. *Med. Microbiol. Immunol.* **2010**, *199*, 197–207. [CrossRef] [PubMed]
3. Pinto-Santini, D.M.; Stenbak, C.R.; Linial, M.L. Foamy virus zoonotic infections. *Retrovirology* **2017**, *14*, 55. [CrossRef] [PubMed]
4. Ghersi, B.M.; Jia, H.; Aiewsakun, P.; Katzourakis, A.; Mendoza, P.; Bausch, D.G.; Kasper, M.R.; Montgomery, J.M.; Switzer, W.M. Wide distribution and ancient evolutionary history of simian foamy viruses in new world primates. *Retrovirology* **2015**, *12*, 89. [CrossRef] [PubMed]
5. Katzourakis, A.; Aiewsakun, P.; Jia, H.; Wolfe, N.D.; LeBreton, M.; Yoder, A.D.; Switzer, W.M. Discovery of prosimian and afrotherian foamy viruses and potential cross species transmissions amidst stable and ancient mammalian co-evolution. *Retrovirology* **2014**, *11*, 61. [CrossRef] [PubMed]
6. Switzer, W.M.; Salemi, M.; Shanmugam, V.; Gao, F.; Cong, M.E.; Kuiken, C.; Bhullar, V.; Beer, B.E.; Vallet, D.; Gautier-Hion, A.; et al. Ancient co-speciation of simian foamy viruses and primates. *Nature* **2005**, *434*, 376–380. [CrossRef] [PubMed]
7. Betsem, E.; Rua, R.; Tortevoye, P.; Froment, A.; Gessain, A. Frequent and recent human acquisition of simian foamy viruses through apes' bites in central africa. *PLoS Pathog.* **2011**, *7*, e1002306. [CrossRef] [PubMed]
8. Calattini, S.; Nerrienet, E.; Mauclere, P.; Georges-Courbot, M.C.; Saib, A.; Gessain, A. Natural simian foamy virus infection in wild-caught gorillas, mandrills and drills from cameroon and gabon. *J. Gen. Virol.* **2004**, *85*, 3313–3317. [CrossRef]
9. Calattini, S.; Nerrienet, E.; Mauclere, P.; Georges-Courbot, M.C.; Saib, A.; Gessain, A. Detection and molecular characterization of foamy viruses in central african chimpanzees of the pan troglodytes troglodytes and pan troglodytes vellerosus subspecies. *J. Med. Primatol.* **2006**, *35*, 59–66. [CrossRef]
10. Mouinga-Ondeme, A.; Betsem, E.; Caron, M.; Makuwa, M.; Salle, B.; Renault, N.; Saib, A.; Telfer, P.; Marx, P.; Gessain, A.; et al. Two distinct variants of simian foamy virus in naturally infected mandrills (*Mandrillus sphinx*) and cross-species transmission to humans. *Retrovirology* **2010**, *7*, 105. [CrossRef]
11. Schulze, A.; Lemey, P.; Schubert, J.; McClure, M.O.; Rethwilm, A.; Bodem, J. Complete nucleotide sequence and evolutionary analysis of a gorilla foamy virus. *J. Gen. Virol.* **2011**, *92*, 582–586. [CrossRef] [PubMed]
12. Switzer, W.M.; Heneine, W. Foamy virus infection of humans. In *Molecular Detection of Human Viral Pathogens*; Liu, D., Ed.; CRC Press, Taylor & Francis Group: Boca Raton, FL, USA, 2011; Volume 1, pp. 131–146.
13. Troncoso, L.L.; Muniz, C.P.; Siqueira, J.D.; Curty, G.; Schrago, C.G.; Augusto, A.; Fedullo, L.; Soares, M.A.; Santos, A.F. Characterization and comparative analysis of a simian foamy virus complete genome isolated from brazilian capuchin monkeys. *Virus Res.* **2015**, *208*, 1–6. [CrossRef] [PubMed]

14. Khan, A.S.; Bodem, J.; Buseyne, F.; Gessain, A.; Johnson, W.; Kuhn, J.H.; Kuzmak, J.; Lindemann, D.; Linial, M.L.; Lochelt, M.; et al. Spumaretroviruses: Updated taxonomy and nomenclature. *Virology* **2018**, *516*, 158–164. [CrossRef] [PubMed]
15. Rethwilm, A.; Bodem, J. Evolution of foamy viruses: The most ancient of all retroviruses. *Viruses* **2013**, *5*, 2349–2374. [CrossRef] [PubMed]
16. Leendertz, F.H.; Zirkel, F.; Couacy-Hymann, E.; Ellerbrok, H.; Morozov, V.A.; Pauli, G.; Hedemann, C.; Formenty, P.; Jensen, S.A.; Boesch, C.; et al. Interspecies transmission of simian foamy virus in a natural predator-prey system. *J. Virol.* **2008**, *82*, 7741–7744. [CrossRef]
17. Leendertz, S.A.; Junglen, S.; Hedemann, C.; Goffe, A.; Calvignac, S.; Boesch, C.; Leendertz, F.H. High prevalence, coinfection rate, and genetic diversity of retroviruses in wild red colobus monkeys (*Piliocolobus badius badius*) in Tai National Park, Cote D'ivoire. *J. Virol.* **2010**, *84*, 7427–7436. [CrossRef] [PubMed]
18. Liu, W.; Worobey, M.; Li, Y.; Keele, B.F.; Bibollet-Ruche, F.; Guo, Y.; Goepfert, P.A.; Santiago, M.L.; Ndjango, J.B.; Neel, C.; et al. Molecular ecology and natural history of simian foamy virus infection in wild-living chimpanzees. *PLoS Pathog.* **2008**, *4*, e1000097. [CrossRef]
19. Richard, L.; Rua, R.; Betsem, E.; Mouinga-Ondeme, A.; Kazanji, M.; Leroy, E.; Njouom, R.; Buseyne, F.; Afonso, P.V.; Gessain, A. Cocirculation of two env molecular variants, of possible recombinant origin, in gorilla and chimpanzee simian foamy virus strains from central Africa. *J. Virol.* **2015**, *89*, 12480–12491. [CrossRef]
20. Heneine, W.; Switzer, W.M.; Sandstrom, P.; Brown, J.; Vedapuri, S.; Schable, C.A.; Khan, A.S.; Lerche, N.W.; Schweizer, M.; Neumann-Haefelin, D.; et al. Identification of a human population infected with simian foamy viruses. *Nat. Med.* **1998**, *4*, 403–407. [CrossRef]
21. Switzer, W.M.; Bhullar, V.; Shanmugam, V.; Cong, M.E.; Parekh, B.; Lerche, N.W.; Yee, J.L.; Ely, J.J.; Boneva, R.; Chapman, L.E.; et al. Frequent simian foamy virus infection in persons occupationally exposed to nonhuman primates. *J. Virol.* **2004**, *78*, 2780–2789. [CrossRef]
22. Khan, A.S. Simian foamy virus infection in humans: Prevalence and management. *Expert Rev. Anti-Infect. Ther.* **2009**, *7*, 569–580. [CrossRef] [PubMed]
23. Murphy, H.W.; Miller, M.; Ramer, J.; Travis, D.; Barbiers, R.; Wolfe, N.D.; Switzer, W.M. Implications of simian retroviruses for captive primate population management and the occupational safety of primate handlers. *J. Zoo Wildl. Med.* **2006**, *37*, 219–233. [CrossRef] [PubMed]
24. Gessain, A.; Rua, R.; Betsem, E.; Turpin, J.; Mahieux, R. Htlv-3/4 and simian foamy retroviruses in humans: Discovery, epidemiology, cross-species transmission and molecular virology. *Virology* **2013**, *435*, 187–199. [CrossRef] [PubMed]
25. Smith, K.M.; Anthony, S.J.; Switzer, W.M.; Epstein, J.H.; Seimon, T.; Jia, H.; Sanchez, M.D.; Huynh, T.T.; Galland, G.G.; Shapiro, S.E.; et al. Zoonotic viruses associated with illegally imported wildlife products. *PLoS ONE* **2012**, *7*, e29505. [CrossRef] [PubMed]
26. Switzer, W.M.; Tang, S.; Ahuka-Mundeke, S.; Shankar, A.; Hanson, D.L.; Zheng, H.; Ayouba, A.; Wolfe, N.D.; LeBreton, M.; Djoko, C.F.; et al. Novel simian foamy virus infections from multiple monkey species in women from the Democratic Republic of Congo. *Retrovirology* **2012**, *9*, 100. [CrossRef] [PubMed]
27. Wolfe, N.D.; Switzer, W.M.; Carr, J.K.; Bhullar, V.B.; Shanmugam, V.; Tamoufe, U.; Prosser, A.T.; Torimiro, J.N.; Wright, A.; Mpoudi-Ngole, E.; et al. Naturally acquired simian retrovirus infections in central African hunters. *Lancet* **2004**, *363*, 932–937. [CrossRef]
28. Muniz, C.P.; Cavalcante, L.T.F.; Jia, H.; Zheng, H.; Tang, S.; Augusto, A.M.; Pissinatti, A.; Fedullo, L.P.; Santos, A.F.; Soares, M.A.; et al. Zoonotic infection of Brazilian primate workers with new world simian foamy virus. *PLoS ONE* **2017**, *12*, e0184502. [CrossRef]
29. Feeroz, M.M.; Soliven, K.; Small, C.T.; Engel, G.A.; Andreina Pacheco, M.; Yee, J.L.; Wang, X.; Kamrul Hasan, M.; Oh, G.; Levine, K.L.; et al. Population dynamics of rhesus macaques and associated foamy virus in Bangladesh. *Emerg. Microbes Infect.* **2013**, *2*, 1–14. [CrossRef]
30. Mergia, A.; Blackwell, J.; Papadi, G.; Johnson, C. Simian foamy virus type 1 (sfv-1) induces apoptosis. *Virus Res.* **1997**, *50*, 129–137. [CrossRef]
31. Boneva, R.S.; Switzer, W.M.; Spira, T.J.; Bhullar, V.B.; Shanmugam, V.; Cong, M.E.; Lam, L.; Heneine, W.; Folks, T.M.; Chapman, L.E. Clinical and virological characterization of persistent human infection with simian foamy viruses. *AIDS Res. Hum. Retroviruses* **2007**, *23*, 1330–1337. [CrossRef]

32. Buseyne, F.; Betsem, E.; Montange, T.; Njouom, R.; Bilounga Ndongo, C.; Hermine, O.; Gessain, A. Clinical signs and blood test results among humans infected with zoonotic simian foamy virus: A case-control study. *J. Infect. Dis.* **2018**, *218*, 144–151. [CrossRef] [PubMed]
33. Linial, M. Why aren't foamy viruses pathogenic? *Trends Microbiol.* **2000**, *8*, 284–289. [CrossRef]
34. Murray, S.M.; Linial, M.L. Foamy virus infection in primates. *J. Med. Primatol.* **2006**, *35*, 225–235. [CrossRef] [PubMed]
35. Vieira, I.C.; Toledo, P.M.; Silva, J.M.; Higuchi, H. Deforestation and threats to the biodiversity of Amazonia. *Braz. J. Biol.* **2008**, *68*, 949–956. [CrossRef] [PubMed]
36. Wolfe, N.D.; Eitel, M.N.; Gockowski, J.; Muchaal, P.K.; Nolte, C.; Prosser, A.T.; Torimiro, J.N.; Weise, S.; Burke, D.S. Deforestation, hunting and the ecology of microbial emergence. *Glob. Chang. Hum. Health* **2000**, *1*, 10–25. [CrossRef]
37. Cunningham, C.; Mootnick, A. Gibbons. *Curr. Biol.* **2009**, *19*, R543–R544. [CrossRef]
38. Thinh, V.N.; Rawson, B.; Hallam, C.; Kenyon, M.; Nadler, T.; Walter, L.; Roos, C. Phylogeny and distribution of crested gibbons (genus *Nomascus*) based on mitochondrial cytochrome b gene sequence data. *Am. J. Primatol.* **2010**, *72*, 1047–1054. [CrossRef] [PubMed]
39. Kim, S.K.; Carbone, L.; Becquet, C.; Mootnick, A.R.; Li, D.J.; de Jong, P.J.; Wall, J.D. Patterns of genetic variation within and between gibbon species. *Mol. Biol. Evol.* **2011**, *28*, 2211–2218. [CrossRef] [PubMed]
40. Fan, P.; Bartlett, T.Q. Overlooked small apes need more attention! *Am. J. Primatol.* **2017**, *79*, e22658. [CrossRef]
41. Ayouba, A.; Duval, L.; Liegeois, F.; Ngin, S.; Ahuka-Mundeke, S.; Switzer, W.M.; Delaporte, E.; Ariey, F.; Peeters, M.; Nerrienet, E. Nonhuman primate retroviruses from cambodia: High simian foamy virus prevalence, identification of divergent stlv-1 strains and no evidence of siv infection. *Infect. Genet. Evol.* **2013**, *18*, 325–334. [CrossRef]
42. Hussain, A.I.; Shanmugam, V.; Bhullar, V.B.; Beer, B.E.; Vallet, D.; Gautier-Hion, A.; Wolfe, N.D.; Karesh, W.B.; Kilbourn, A.M.; Tooze, Z.; et al. Screening for simian foamy virus infection by using a combined antigen western blot assay: Evidence for a wide distribution among old world primates and identification of four new divergent viruses. *Virology* **2003**, *309*, 248–257. [CrossRef]
43. Lauck, M.; Hyeroba, D.; Tumukunde, A.; Weny, G.; Lank, S.M.; Chapman, C.A.; O'Connor, D.H.; Friedrich, T.C.; Goldberg, T.L. Novel, divergent simian hemorrhagic fever viruses in a wild ugandan red colobus monkey discovered using direct pyrosequencing. *PLoS ONE* **2011**, *6*, e19056. [CrossRef] [PubMed]
44. Zhang, M.; Gaschen, B.; Blay, W.; Foley, B.; Haigwood, N.; Kuiken, C.; Korber, B. Tracking global patterns of n-linked glycosylation site variation in highly variable viral glycoproteins: Hiv, siv, and hcv envelopes and influenza hemagglutinin. *Glycobiology* **2004**, *14*, 1229–1246. [CrossRef] [PubMed]
45. Calattini, S.; Betsem, E.; Froment, A.; Bassot, S.; Chevalier, S.A.; Mahieux, R.; Gessain, A. Identification and complete sequence analysis of a new htlv-3 strain from South Cameroon. In Proceedings of the 13th International Conference on Human Retrovirology: HTLV and Related Viruses, Hakone, Japan, 21–25 May 2007.
46. Switzer, W.M.; Qari, S.H.; Wolfe, N.D.; Burke, D.S.; Folks, T.M.; Heneine, W. Ancient origin and molecular features of the novel human t-lymphotropic virus type 3 revealed by complete genome analysis. *J. Virol.* **2006**, *80*, 7427–7438. [CrossRef] [PubMed]
47. Switzer, W.M.; Salemi, M.; Qari, S.H.; Jia, H.; Gray, R.R.; Katzourakis, A.; Marriott, S.J.; Pryor, K.N.; Wolfe, N.D.; Burke, D.S.; et al. Ancient, independent evolution and distinct molecular features of the novel human T-lymphotropic virus type 4. *Retrovirology* **2009**, *6*, 9. [CrossRef] [PubMed]
48. Galvin, T.A.; Ahmed, I.A.; Shahabuddin, M.; Bryan, T.; Khan, A.S. Identification of recombination in the envelope gene of simian foamy virus serotype 2 isolated from *Macaca cyclopis*. *J. Virol.* **2013**, *87*, 8792–8797. [CrossRef] [PubMed]
49. Lole, K.S.; Bollinger, R.C.; Paranjape, R.S.; Gadkari, D.; Kulkarni, S.S.; Novak, N.G.; Ingersoll, R.; Sheppard, H.W.; Ray, S.C. Full-length human immunodeficiency virus type 1 genomes from subtype c-infected seroconverters in india, with evidence of intersubtype recombination. *J. Virol.* **1999**, *73*, 152–160.
50. Martin, D.P.; Murrell, B.; Golden, M.; Khoosal, A.; Muhire, B. Rdp4: Detection and analysis of recombination patterns in virus genomes. *Virus Evol.* **2015**, *1*, vev003. [CrossRef]
51. Katoh, K.; Toh, H. Recent developments in the MAFFT multiple sequence alignment program. *Brief. Bioinform.* **2008**, *9*, 286–298. [CrossRef]

52. Tamura, K.; Stecher, G.; Peterson, D.; Filipski, A.; Kumar, S. Mega6: Molecular evolutionary genetics analysis version 6.0. *Mol. Biol. Evol.* **2013**, *30*, 2725–2729. [CrossRef]
53. Nguyen, L.T.; Schmidt, H.A.; von Haeseler, A.; Minh, B.Q. Iq-tree: A fast and effective stochastic algorithm for estimating maximum-likelihood phylogenies. *Mol. Biol. Evol.* **2015**, *32*, 268–274. [CrossRef] [PubMed]
54. Drummond, A.J.; Rambaut, A. Beast: Bayesian evolutionary analysis by sampling trees. *BMC Evol. Biol.* **2007**, *7*, 214. [CrossRef] [PubMed]
55. Perelman, P.; Johnson, W.E.; Roos, C.; Seuanez, H.N.; Horvath, J.E.; Moreira, M.A.; Kessing, B.; Pontius, J.; Roelke, M.; Rumpler, Y.; et al. A molecular phylogeny of living primates. *PLoS Genet.* **2011**, *7*, e1001342. [CrossRef] [PubMed]
56. Hedges, S.B.; Marin, J.; Suleski, M.; Paymer, M.; Kumar, S. Tree of life reveals clock-like speciation and diversification. *Mol. Biol. Evol.* **2015**, *32*, 835–845. [CrossRef] [PubMed]
57. Rua, R.; Betsem, E.; Calattini, S.; Saib, A.; Gessain, A. Genetic characterization of simian foamy viruses infecting humans. *J. Virol.* **2012**, *86*, 13350–13359. [CrossRef] [PubMed]
58. Kehl, T.; Tan, J.; Materniak, M. Non-simian foamy viruses: Molecular virology, tropism and prevalence and zoonotic/interspecies transmission. *Viruses* **2013**, *5*, 2169–2209. [CrossRef] [PubMed]
59. Yu, S.F.; Edelmann, K.; Strong, R.K.; Moebes, A.; Rethwilm, A.; Linial, M.L. The carboxyl terminus of the human foamy virus gag protein contains separable nucleic acid binding and nuclear transport domains. *J. Virol.* **1996**, *70*, 8255–8262.
60. Renault, N.; Tobaly-Tapiero, J.; Paris, J.; Giron, M.L.; Coiffic, A.; Roingeard, P.; Saib, A. A nuclear export signal within the structural gag protein is required for prototype foamy virus replication. *Retrovirology* **2011**, *8*, 6. [CrossRef]
61. Wang, G.; Mulligan, M.J. Comparative sequence analysis and predictions for the envelope glycoproteins of foamy viruses. *J. Gen. Virol.* **1999**, *80*, 245–254. [CrossRef]
62. Lecellier, C.H.; Vermeulen, W.; Bachelerie, F.; Giron, M.L.; Saib, A. Intra- and intercellular trafficking of the foamy virus auxiliary bet protein. *J. Virol.* **2002**, *76*, 3388–3394. [CrossRef]
63. Xia, X.; Xie, Z.; Salemi, M.; Chen, L.; Wang, Y. An index of substitution saturation and its application. *Mol. Phylogenet. Evol.* **2003**, *26*, 1–7. [CrossRef]
64. Aiewsakun, P.; Katzourakis, A. Marine origin of retroviruses in the early Palaeozoic Era. *Nat. Commun.* **2017**, *8*, 13954. [CrossRef] [PubMed]
65. Pozzi, L.; Hodgson, J.A.; Burrell, A.S.; Sterner, K.N.; Raaum, R.L.; Disotell, T.R. Primate phylogenetic relationships and divergence dates inferred from complete mitochondrial genomes. *Mol. Phylogenet. Evol.* **2014**, *75*, 165–183. [CrossRef]
66. dos Reis, M.; Inoue, J.; Hasegawa, M.; Asher, R.J.; Donoghue, P.C.; Yang, Z. Phylogenomic datasets provide both precision and accuracy in estimating the timescale of placental mammal phylogeny. *Proc. Biol. Sci.* **2012**, *279*, 3491–3500. [CrossRef]
67. Nandakumar, S.; Bae, E.H.; Khan, A.S. Complete genome sequence of a naturally occurring simian foamy virus isolate from rhesus macaque (sfvmmu_k3t). *Genome Announc.* **2017**, *5*. [CrossRef]
68. Nandakumar, S.; Bae, E.H.; Khan, A.S. Complete genome sequence of the African green monkey simian foamy virus serotype 3 strain fv2014 (sfvcae_fv2014). *Genome Announc.* **2018**, *6*. [CrossRef]
69. Schmidt, M.; Herchenroder, O.; Heeney, J.; Rethwilm, A. Long terminal repeat u3 length polymorphism of human foamy virus. *Virology* **1997**, *230*, 167–178. [CrossRef] [PubMed]
70. van Opijnen, T.; Kamoschinski, J.; Jeeninga, R.E.; Berkhout, B. The human immunodeficiency virus type 1 promoter contains a cata box instead of a tata box for optimal transcription and replication. *J. Virol.* **2004**, *78*, 6883–6890. [CrossRef]
71. Matsudaira, K.; Ishida, T. Phylogenetic relationships and divergence dates of the whole mitochondrial genome sequences among three gibbon genera. *Mol. Phylogenet. Evol.* **2010**, *55*, 454–459. [CrossRef]
72. Chan, Y.C.; Roos, C.; Inoue-Murayama, M.; Inoue, E.; Shih, C.C.; Pei, K.J.; Vigilant, L. Mitochondrial genome sequences effectively reveal the phylogeny of Hylobates gibbons. *PLoS ONE* **2010**, *5*, e14419. [CrossRef]
73. Bergsten, J. A review of long-branch attraction. *Cladistics* **2005**, *21*, 163–193. [CrossRef]
74. Kumar, S.; Subramanian, S. Mutation rates in mammalian genomes. *Proc. Natl. Acad. Sci. USA* **2002**, *99*, 803–808. [CrossRef] [PubMed]

75. Johnson, W.E.; Coffin, J.M. Constructing primate phylogenies from ancient retrovirus sequences. *Proc. Natl. Acad. Sci. USA* **1999**, *96*, 10254–10260. [CrossRef] [PubMed]
76. Rawson, B.M.; Insua-Cao, P.; Ha, N.M.; Thinh, V.N.; Duc, H.M.; Mahood, S.; Geissmann, T.; Roos, C. *The Conservation Status of Gibbons in Vietnam*; Fauna & Flora International Vietnam Programme: Hanoi, Vietnam, 2011; p. 155.

viruses

MDPI

Article

The First Co-Opted Endogenous Foamy Viruses and the Evolutionary History of Reptilian Foamy Viruses

Pakorn Aiewsakun [1,*], Peter Simmonds [2] and Aris Katzourakis [3,*]

[1] Department of Microbiology, Faculty of Science, Mahidol University, Bangkok 10400, Thailand
[2] Nuffield Department of Medicine, University of Oxford, South Parks Road, Oxford OX1 3SY, UK
[3] Department of Zoology, University of Oxford, South Parks Road, Oxford OX1 3SY, UK
* Correspondence: Pakorn.Aiewsakun@gmail.com (P.A.); Aris.Katzourakis@zoo.ox.ac.uk (A.K.)

Received: 9 May 2019; Accepted: 4 July 2019; Published: 12 July 2019

Abstract: A recent study reported the discovery of an endogenous reptilian foamy virus (FV), termed ERV-Spuma-Spu, found in the genome of tuatara. Here, we report two novel reptilian foamy viruses also identified as endogenous FVs (EFVs) in the genomes of panther gecko (ERV-Spuma-Ppi) and Schlegel's Japanese gecko (ERV-Spuma-Gja). Their presence indicates that FVs are capable of infecting reptiles in addition to mammals, amphibians, and fish. Numerous copies of full length ERV-Spuma-Spu elements were found in the tuatara genome littered with in-frame stop codons and transposable elements, suggesting that they are indeed endogenous and are not functional. ERV-Spuma-Ppi and ERV-Spuma-Gja, on the other hand, consist solely of a foamy virus-like *env* gene. Examination of host flanking sequences revealed that they are orthologous, and despite being more than 96 million years old, their *env* reading frames are fully coding competent with evidence for strong purifying selection to maintain expression and for them likely being transcriptionally active. These make them the oldest EFVs discovered thus far and the first documented EFVs that may have been co-opted for potential cellular functions. Phylogenetic analyses revealed a complex virus–host co-evolutionary history and cross-species transmission routes of ancient FVs.

Keywords: foamy virus; spumavirus; reptile foamy virus; endogenous foamy virus; endogenous retrovirus; ancient retroviruses; co-evolution; co-speciation; foamy virus-host interactions

1. Introduction

Foamy viruses (FV; the *Spumaretrovirinae* subfamily) are a unique subgroup of retroviruses (family *Retroviridae*) comprising an independent lineage basal to all other exogenous retroviruses [1]. FV surveillance and the discovery of their endogenous retrovirus (ERV) counterparts revealed that the host range of FVs covers a wide range of vertebrates, including mammals [2,3], amphibians [4], lobe-finned fish [5], bony fish [4,6], and cartilaginous fish [4,7], considerably wider than those of other retrovirus groups. Owing to the wealth of sequence data and the identification of multiple instances of endogenization for FVs, the longer-term evolutionary history of FVs can be investigated in great detail. For example, analysis of endogenous and modern-day viral sequences revealed that FVs have been broadly co-diversifying with their hosts since the origin of vertebrates, dating back almost half a billion years ago to the early Palaeozoic Era [4].

A recent study reported the discovery of the first reptilian endogenous FV (EFV) in the tuatara genome, namely ERV-Spuma-Spu [8]. Phylogenetic analysis showed that ERV-Spuma-Spu is basal to the clade of mammalian FVs. Based on this finding, the authors speculated that the reptilian FV lineage may have diverged from the mammalian FV linage more than 320 million years ago under the virus–host co-speciation assumption. Nevertheless, since there was effectively only one reptilian FV linage in the study, the inferred co-speciation could not be verified, and a history of viral cross-species transmissions might have been overlooked. Indeed, this was shown to be the case before for the lobe-finned fish EFV, CoeEFV [4].

Here, we further characterize ERV-Spuma-Spu and report two additional reptilian EFVs found in the genomes of panther gecko (*Paroedura picta*) and Schlegel's Japanese gecko (*Gekko japonicus*), designated ERV-Spuma-Ppi and ERV-Spuma-Gja, respectively. Evolutionary analyses together with other currently available FV and EFV sequences suggest that these reptile EFVs do not form a monophyletic clade and that they are significantly younger than their hosts. This in turn suggests that, in contrast to what was previously suggested, their ancestors likely originated from cross-species transmissions, where one gave rise to ERV-Spuma-Spu and the other gave rise to the two gecko EFVs. Our results improve our understanding of how FVs evolved and interacted with their hosts in the distant past.

2. Materials and Methods

2.1. ERV-Spuma-Spu Mining

The tuatara genome (*Sphenodon punctatus*; accession number: QEPC01000000) was searched using tBLASTn and a CoeEFV Pol protein query with an E-value cut off of 1×10^{-6}. This returned 20,581 hits from 2370 contigs (Table S1). These hits were then combined together (including the sequence between the two hits) if they were ≤ 5000 base pairs apart or overlapping and were in the same orientation. This resulted in 12,520 merged Pol hits (Table S2).

These hits were subsequently subjected to reciprocal BLASTx against a database of retrovirus proteins one by one with an E-value cut off of 1×10^{-6} (Table S2). If the best match protein did not belong to a member of the *Spumaretrovirinae* subfamily or the *Spumavirus* genus, the hit was then excluded from the downstream analyses. Ultimately, 87,387 retrovirus proteins were retrieved from the National Center for Biotechnology Information (NCBI) protein database on the 7th of June 2018 using 3 search queries. The first query was 'txid11632[Organism:exp] NOT "partial" AND 500:100000[SLEN]', which retrieved proteins that belong to the members of the *Retroviridae* family [NCBI: txid11632] with a length between 500 and 100,000 amino acids and were not annotated as partial (86,662 sequences). The second query was 'txid186534[Organism:exp] NOT "partial" AND 500:100000[SLEN]', which retrieved proteins that belong to the members of the *Caulimoviridae* family [NCBI: txid186534] with a length between 500 and 100,000 amino acids and were not annotated as partial (720 sequences). The last query was 'txid186665[Organism:exp]', which retrieved proteins that belong to the members of the *Metaviridae* family [NCBI: txid186665] (5 sequences). Out of 12,520 Pol hits, only 2757 exhibited the greatest similarity to FV proteins (Table S2). The rest were removed from the subsequent dataset.

We noted that some of these 2757 Pol sequence candidates, nevertheless, may actually have been those of Class III ERVs and not actually of EFVs. To further exclude false positive hits, we used them as queries in a BLASTx search against 194 retrovirus and ERV Pol protein sequences, publicly available from the database held at http://bioinformatics.cvr.ac.uk/paleovirology/site/html/retroviruses.html. Those with the best hit protein that did not belong to the *Spumavirus* genus at an E-value cut off of 1×10^{-6} were further excluded from the dataset. Only 1959 sequence candidates remained after this procedure (Table S2).

To recover potentially full elements, we extracted these 1959 Pol hits from the tuatara genome with 10,000 base pairs extended on both ends. They were then searched against the CoeEFV Env protein query using tBLASTn. The analysis showed that only 165 out of 1959 sequences exhibited similarity to CoeEFV Env protein at the 1×10^{-6} E-value cut off (Table S3). These 165 endogenous viral elements were designated ERV-Spuma-Spu elements.

2.2. Consensus Sequence Reconstruction

The top 20 elements of the 165 ERV-Spuma-Spu elements that exhibited the greatest similarity to the concatenated CoeEFV Pol-Env protein sequence were aligned and used to reconstruct a consensus sequence. At the time of analysis, the quality of the tuatara genome was low, however, containing many large strings of undetermined nucleotides ('N's). Furthermore, the majority of the identified ERV-Spuma-Spu elements were also interrupted by transposable elements. Because of this, the standard protocol of consensus sequence reconstruction (or ancestral sequence reconstruction) inferred false gaps where they should not have been. To overcome this problem, we only allowed gaps in the consensus sequence if there were more than 15 sequences containing gaps in that particular position; otherwise, a consensus base pair from non-gap sequences would be inferred. Standard ambiguous bases were used in the case of base count ties. The consensus sequence of the virus internal region was inferred separately from the LTR portion (Data S1), and the consensus LTR sequence was inferred from both 5′ and 3′ LTRs (Data S2). Only 16 LTR sequences from 11 elements could be aligned with confidence. ORFfinder (https://www.ncbi.nlm.nih.gov/orffinder/) was used to identify open reading frames, and tRNAScan (http://lowelab.ucsc.edu/tRNAscan-SE/) was used to identify the primer binding site. We also attempted to identify the internal promoter in ERV-Spuma-Spu by comparing its sequence to those of mammalian FVs. The consensus sequence is in Figure 1, Figure S1, and Data S3. As previously reported [8], reciprocal BLASTp searches showed that the proteins identified from the consensus sequence were most similar to those of modern-day FVs, supporting that these ERV-Spuma-Spu elements are indeed FVs.

2.3. EFVs in Other Reptiles

Pol and Env protein sequences of the consensus ERV-Spuma-Spu and CoeEFV were used in a tBLASTn search against the NCBI Whole Genome Shotgun database restricted to reptiles and excluding the tuatara genome to examine if other reptile genomes had any EFVs.

Numerous tBLASTn hits were returned from six reptile genomes showing similarity to the Pol protein sequences. From each genome, we selected one to five top hits (19 hits in total) and examined if they were most similar to modern-day FVs. Reciprocal BLASTx analysis suggested that none of them were FV-like, however (Table S4). We thus did not analyze these sequences any further.

In contrast, only two FV-like *env* elements were found. One was found in the genome of the panther gecko (*Paroedura picta*; BDOT01000314.1:c548029-545198), and the other was found in the genome of Schlegel's Japanese gecko (*Gekko japonicus*; LNDG01066615.1:c46188-43360). Neither elements contained in-frame stop codons or transposable elements. Results from reciprocal BLASTx searchers (Table S4) suggested that they were indeed EFVs, showing the greatest similarity to modern-day FVs. They were designated ERV-Spuma-Ppi and ERV-Spuma-Gja, respectively.

The contigs containing ERV-Spuma-Ppi and ERV-Spuma-Gja were co-linear, suggesting that they may be orthologs. Genes surrounding the EFVs were determined and compared to confirm orthology. While LNDG01066615.1 was annotated with genes, BDOT01000314.1 was not. We thus used the gene prediction program AUGUSTUS [9] to annotate the contig. Homologous regions in other reptiles, including the European green lizard (*Lacerta viridis*, OFHU01003482.1), the brown spotted pitviper (*Protobothrops mucrosquamatus*, BCNE02010247.1), and the green anole (*Anolis carolinensis*, NW_003339653.1), were identified based on the genes found on LNDG01066615.1 and BDOT01000314.1 by using tBLASTn. AUGUSTUS [9] was used to annotate the genes on these contigs when gene annotations were not available. The results are shown in Figure 2.

To determine the type of selection that ERV-Spuma-Ppi and ERV-Spuma-Gja were under, their nucleotide sequences were aligned, and a dN/dS ratio was computed by using CodeML implemented in PAML 4.9e [10]. The run mode was set to the "pairwise" mode (runmode = −2). No clock was assumed (clock = 0: no clock) with all sites assumed to have evolved under the same rate (fixed α = 1 and α = 0), and the equilibrium codon frequencies were assumed to be equal to those that were observed (CodonFreq = 3: code table; estFreq = 0: use observed freqs). The universal genetic code (icode = 0: universal) was used to determine the number of synonymous and non-synonymous sites and changes. The basic model of selection (model = 0: one dN/dS ratio; NSsites = 0: one ω) was used to compute an overall dN/dS ratio for the entire *env* like gene.

To investigate the possibility that ERV-Spuma-Ppi and ERV-Spuma-Gja might be transcriptionally active, we used them to query the Reptilian Transcriptomes v2.0 Database [11], using both BLASTn and tBLASTn searches. One very significant hit was returned from the transcriptomic sequence database of common leopard Gecko (*Eublepharis macularius*), named "EMA_Contig_Illumina_8645". It was a consensus contig that was estimated from 499 raw transcript reads.

2.4. Recombination Analyses

A concatenated alignment of *pol-env* nucleotide sequences of mammalian, tuatara, amphibian, and lobe-finned fish FVs/EFVs was prepared for recombination analyses. Their *gag* sequences were not included, as they could not be aligned among these viruses. To obtain ERV-Spuma-Spu's *pol* and *env* sequences, we used BLASTn to query the 165 ERV-Spuma-Spu elements with the consensus ERV-Spuma-Spu's *pol* and *env* sequences with an E-value cut off of 1×10^{-6}. Hits that were found in the same ERV-Spuma-Spu element and that were in the same orientation were concatenated according to their hit locations to obtain contiguous viral sequences without transposable elements. We only included those with both *pol* and *env* gene coverage of ≥ 80% in the alignment. The final alignment contained 45 sequences, 27 of which were ERV-Spuma-Spu elements and were 4695 nucleotides (nt) long (*pol*: 2685 nt; *env*: 2010 nt) (Data S4).

Potential recombination events were detected using 7 programs: RDP, GENECONV, Chimaera, MaxChi, BootScan, SiScan, and 3Seq, implemented in Recombination Detection Program 4 [12] with their default settings. Only those detected with >4 programs were considered significant.

2.5. Phylogenetic Analyses

Recombination analyses suggested that FVs' *pol* and *env* genes might have different evolutionary histories (see Results). We thus estimated Pol and Env protein phylogenies separately under the Bayesian phylogenetic framework by using MrBayes 3.2.6 [13] to better understand how they evolved (Figure 3). The Env protein alignment was derived from the *env* nucleotide alignment used in the recombination analyses with the addition of sequences from the two gecko EFVs (Data S5). For the Pol protein alignment, sequences from fish EFVs and non-FV class III ERVs were included as an outgroup (Data S6). This alignment (containing only the reverse transcriptase and integrase coding domain portions) was based on the one we used in our previous study, allowing the results to be compared. The best-fit amino acid substitution models were determined to be JTT+I+Γ(4)+F for the Env alignment and JTT+Γ(4)+F for the Pol alignment by ProtTest 3.4.2 [14] under the sample size corrected Akaike information criterion. Two Markov chain Monte Carlo chains were run for 10,000,000 steps with a sampling frequency of 1 per 1000 steps. The metropolis coupling algorithm (3 hot chains and 1 cold chain) was used to improve the sampling. The first 25% of sampled parameter values were discarded as burn-in. Potential scale reduction factors of all parameters were ~1.000 in both analyses, indicating that they were all well sampled from their posterior distributions and had converged.

2.6. Evolutionary Timescale Inference

Many studies have shown that mammalian FVs have a long-term co-speciation history with their hosts throughout the entire evolution of the eutheria [2,15–17]. This extraordinarily evolutionary feature has led to the observation that the relationship between the virus total per-lineage substitution numbers (s) and the evolutionary timescales (t) can be approximated very well by a power-law function: $log(t) = \alpha log(s) + \beta$ [18]. We used this relationship, the so-called time-dependent rate phenomenon (TDRP) model, to estimate evolutionary timescales of reptile EFVs.

For each of the trees in the posterior distribution obtained from the Bayesian phylogenetic analyses, we traced the simian foamy virus Pan troglodytes verus (SFVpve) backwards in time to various virus–host co-speciation nodes to obtain various s estimates, of which the corresponding t estimates could be inferred directly under the co-speciation assumption (Table S5). Based on virus–host tree topology comparison, seven co-speciation nodes could be inferred in the Pol phylogeny (Figure 3A, labeled with black Roman numerals), and five were inferred in the Env tree (Figure 3B, labeled with black Roman numerals) down the SFVpve lineage. These corresponding s and t estimates were used to calibrate the TDRP model. The model fitting was performed by using the *lm* function implemented in R 3.1.2 [19], and the *t* and the *s* estimates were log-transformed (base 10) prior to the linear model fitting. The model was then extrapolated to estimate the timescales of other nodes from their *s* estimates.

3. Results

3.1. Characterisation of ERV-Spuma-Spu

By using a series of BLAST searches (see Materials and Methods for details), we identified 165 FV-like endogenous viral elements (EVEs) in the genome of tuatara (*Sphenodon punctatus*; accession number: QEPC01000000). All of these EVEs showed the greatest similarity to modern FV Pol protein sequences (and not to those of other retroviruses) and harbored FV-like *env* sequences (Tables S1–S3). We observed that most of these EVEs contained transposable elements, interrupting their protein coding regions, indicating that they are genuine non-functional and old endogenous viruses and not contamination of extant virus sequences in the sequence of the tuatara genome. Due to the poor quality of the tuatara genome at the time of analysis, many EVE sequences contained large strings of "N", representing undetermined nucleotide sequences. We treated them as gaps in the downstream analyses in this study.

A consensus sequence of these FV-like EVEs (Figure 1A) was reconstructed for genome annotation (see Materials and Methods for details). Twenty out of the 165 elements that showed the greatest similarity to the concatenated CoeEFV's Pol and Env protein sequence were aligned and curated and subsequently used to reconstruct a consensus sequence. The consensus sequence of the virus body was inferred separately from the long terminal repeat (LTR) portion (Data S1), and the consensus LTR sequence was inferred from both 5′- and 3′-LTR sequences (Data S2). An average pairwise distance between these 20 elements was estimated to be only 0.118 substitutions per site (body portion), and they could be aligned with high confidence, indicating that they are of the same virus lineage. See Figure S1 and Data S3 for the full consensus sequence. Sequence comparison revealed that this virus is highly similar to the ERV-Spuma-Spu previously reported in [8]. They exhibit 97.17% nucleotide percentage identity and 97% coverage (with the one in [8] being 3% shorter), suggesting they are the same virus. The slight differences are likely due to the different methods we used to reconstruct the sequences.

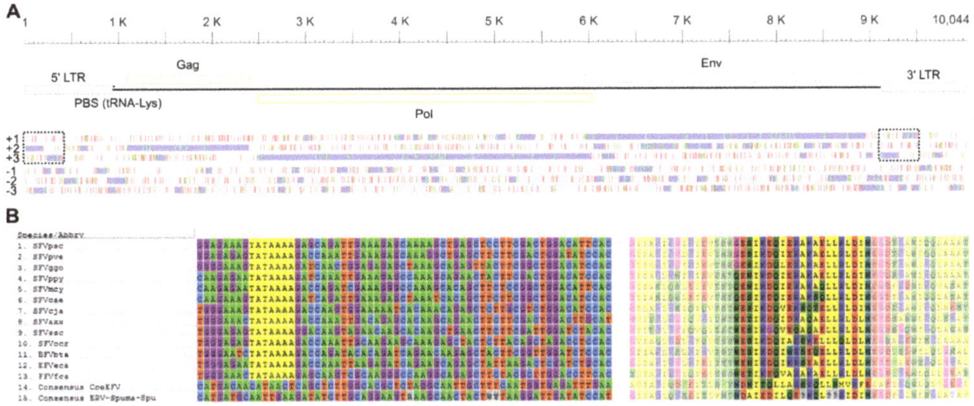

Figure 1. Reconstructed, putative, ERV-Spuma-Spu genome (**A**) and foamy virus (FV) internal promoters (**B**). Top-A, scale bar indicates nucleotide position. Middle-A, schematic diagram representing the genomic organisation of ERV-Spuma-Spu. LTR: long terminal repeat (grey); PBS: primer binging site; Gag: *group antigen* gene (green); Pol: *polymerase* gene (yellow); Env: *envelope* gene (blue). Bottom-A, start (green) and stop (red) codon positions in the six translation frames (+1, +2, +3, −1, −2, and −3). Potential open reading frames are shown in purple. The dotted boxes indicate the two open reading

frames identified as a single accessory gene in [8]. The nucleotide sequences of consensus ERV-Spuma-Spu can be found in Figure S1 and Data S3. Left-B, internal promoters (TATAAAA) towards the 3′ end of the *env* gene could be identified in all mammalian FVs (highlighted in yellow) but were absent from CoeEFV (endogenous FVs) and ERV-Spuma-Spu. Right-B, protein sequences used to guide the nucleotide alignment. Those corresponding to the sequences on the left are shown in brighter colors.

In summary, the consensus sequence was 10,044 nucleotides (nt) long. The LTRs were 935 nt in length (5′-LTR: nt 1–935, 3′-LTR: nt 9110–10,044), which were longer than those of other retroviruses such as alpharetroviruses (~350 nt), gammaretroviruses (~600 nt), deltaretroviruses (~550–750 nt), and lentiviruses (~600 nt), but were typical for FVs (~950–1700 nt) [20]. We noted that our LTRs were longer than those reported in [8] (694 nt); a sequence comparison showed that the consensus sequence reported in [8] was missing ~240 nt corresponding to the beginning (i.e., the 5′ end) of the LTRs (Data S2). A lysine tRNA utilizing primer binding site (PBS) was identified downstream of the 5′-LTR (TGGCGCCCAAYGTGGGGCTCGA, nt 938–959), which is typical of mammalian FVs [21,22]. The *gag* gene was predicted to be 1308 nt long (nt 1085–2392) to generate a 435 amino acid (aa) protein. This was markedly shorter than those of mammalian FVs (~550–650 aa). The *pol* and *env* genes were determined to be 3540 nt (nt: 2487–6026; 1179 aa) and 3003 nt (nt: 5956–8958; 1000 aa) long, respectively, which are typical lengths of mammalian FV *pol* and *env* genes. Results from reciprocal BLAST analyses revealed that all three protein products were most similar to those of mammalian FVs (Table 1), consistent with previously reported results [8]. Phylogenetic analysis also showed that these EVEs clustered with other FVs and EFVs (see below), supporting that this consensus sequence is indeed derived from EFV elements.

Table 1. Reciprocal BLASTp analyses of ERV-Spuma-Spu against the National Center for Biotechnology Information (NCBI) non-redundant retroviral protein database.

Protein	Best reciprocal BLASTp Hit	Accession Number	Query Coverage	E-Value	% Identity
Gag	Gag polyprotein [Feline foamy virus]	AAC58530.1	95%	5×10^{-33}	27%
Pol	Pol [Rhesus macaque simian foamy virus]	YP_009513242.1	96%	0.0 *	44%
Env	Env protein [Japanese macaque simian foamy virus]	YP_009508557.1	91%	1×10^{-101}	28%

* as explicitly reported by the program.

One hypothetical open reading frame (ORF) was identified as an accessory gene in the previous study [8]. This ORF could be mapped to nt 9114–9498 in our consensus sequence, corresponding to the LTR portion (Data S2). In our consensus sequence, the identified ORF appeared to be broken into two separate ORFs of different frames (nt 9114–9305, frame +3 and nt 9343–9498, frame +1; Figure 1A). The crucial difference was that the Wei et al. sequence missed a nucleotide, causing the two ORFs to merge as one (Data S2; 10049th column in the alignment; 196th nt in our consensus LTR sequence). Indeed, we failed to locate any accessory genes between the *env* gene and the 3′-LTR, typical of a mammalian FV (Figure 1A). In addition, as previously noted, the hypothetical accessory protein did not exhibit significant similarity to any known FV proteins [8] or indeed any molecular sequences in the National Center for Biotechnology Information (NCBI) non-redundant (nr) nucleotide collection database. Furthermore, we could not identify an internal promoter towards the 3′ end of the *env* gene (Figure 1B) required for efficient accessory gene expression [23,24]. All these results suggest that ERV-Spuma-Spu may actually lack accessory genes and that the previously identified accessory gene was an artifact.

3.2. The Discovery and Characterisation of Gecko EFVs

In addition to ERV-Spuma-Spu elements, we were able to recover two FV-like elements from two gecko genomes, namely panther gecko (*Paroedura picta*; accession number: BDOT01000000) and Schlegel's Japanese gecko (*Gekko japonicus*; accession number: LNDG01000000). They were found on contig BDOT01000314.1 (nt: c548,029–545,198; 943 aa) and contig LNDG01066615.1 (nt: c46,188–43,360; 942 aa), respectively. Both elements consisted solely of a full-length FV-like *env* gene, and no other FV-like elements could be identified. Interestingly, neither of them contained any in-frame stop codons or transposable elements. Reciprocal BLAST analyses showed that both elements were most similar to modern mammalian FVs (Table S4). Consistent with this finding, phylogenetic analysis revealed that they clustered with other FVs and EFVs (see below). Combined, these results strongly suggest that they are EFVs. We designated the two elements ERV-Spuma-Ppi and ERV-Spuma-Gja, respectively.

We determined that BDOT01000314.1 and LNDG01066615.1 were co-linear, suggesting that ERV-Spuma-Ppi and ERV-Spuma-Gja might be orthologous. ERV-Spuma-Gja was found in the intronic region of the predicted endoplasmic reticulum membrane protein complex subunit 1 gene (EMC1: XM_015412627.1) between exon 21 and 22 in the antisense orientation. Further examination revealed three other genes in the same vicinity of ERV-Spuma-Gja, namely ubiquitin protein ligase E3 component n-recognin 4 gene (UBR4: XM_015412557.1), MRT4 homolog, ribosome maturation factor gene (MRTO4: XM_015412607.1), and aldo-keto reductase family 7 member A2 gene (AKR7A2: XM_015412595-6.1). At the time of analysis, the contig BDOT01000314.1 (of the panther gecko genome) was not annotated with genes; nevertheless, we were able to confirm that ERV-Spuma-Ppi had the same genomic location as ERV-Spuma-Gja and was surrounded by the same set of genes in the same order, confirming that they are orthologs. Moreover, we were able to identify corresponding homologous genomic regions in the genomes of European green lizard (*Lacerta viridis*, OFHU01003482.1), brown spotted pitviper (*Protobothrops mucrosquamatus*, BCNE02010247.1), and green anole (*Anolis carolinensis*, NW_003339653.1) based on the presence of these genes. However, none of these reptile genomes had homologs of ERV-Spuma-Ppi and ERV-Spuma-Gja. The results are shown in Figure 2. We thus could infer that ERV-Spuma-Ppi and ERV-Spuma-Gja are at least 96 (83–98) million years (myr) old based on the speciation date of panther gecko and Schlegel's Japanese gecko [25]. Furthermore, a pairwise nucleotide sequence comparison of ERV-Spuma-Ppi and ERV-Spuma-Gja estimated its dN/dS ratio to be 0.14 (0.08–0.54), strongly suggesting that they were under strong purifying selection pressure.

Remarkably, when we queried the Reptilian Transcriptomes V2.0 Database [11] with ERV-Spuma-Ppi and ERV-Spuma-Gja, we recovered a transcript consensus contig from the transcriptome of common leopard gecko (*Eublepharis macularius*), which is closely related to panther gecko and Schlegel's Japanese gecko. The sequence exhibited 82.2 and 93.0 aa percentage identity (E-value = 4×10^{-66} and 2×10^{-74}) and 81.6 and 86.94 nt percentage identity (E-value = 1×10^{-93} and 4×10^{-118}) to ERV-Spuma-Ppi and ERV-Spuma-Gja, respectively. The contig was 626 bases long and constructed from 499 raw reads. We could not check for the homolog of ERV-Spuma-Ppi and ERV-Spuma-Gja in the leopard gecko genome, as it is currently not available. However, this finding suggests that ERV-Spuma-Ppi and ERV-Spuma-Gja might be transcriptionally active.

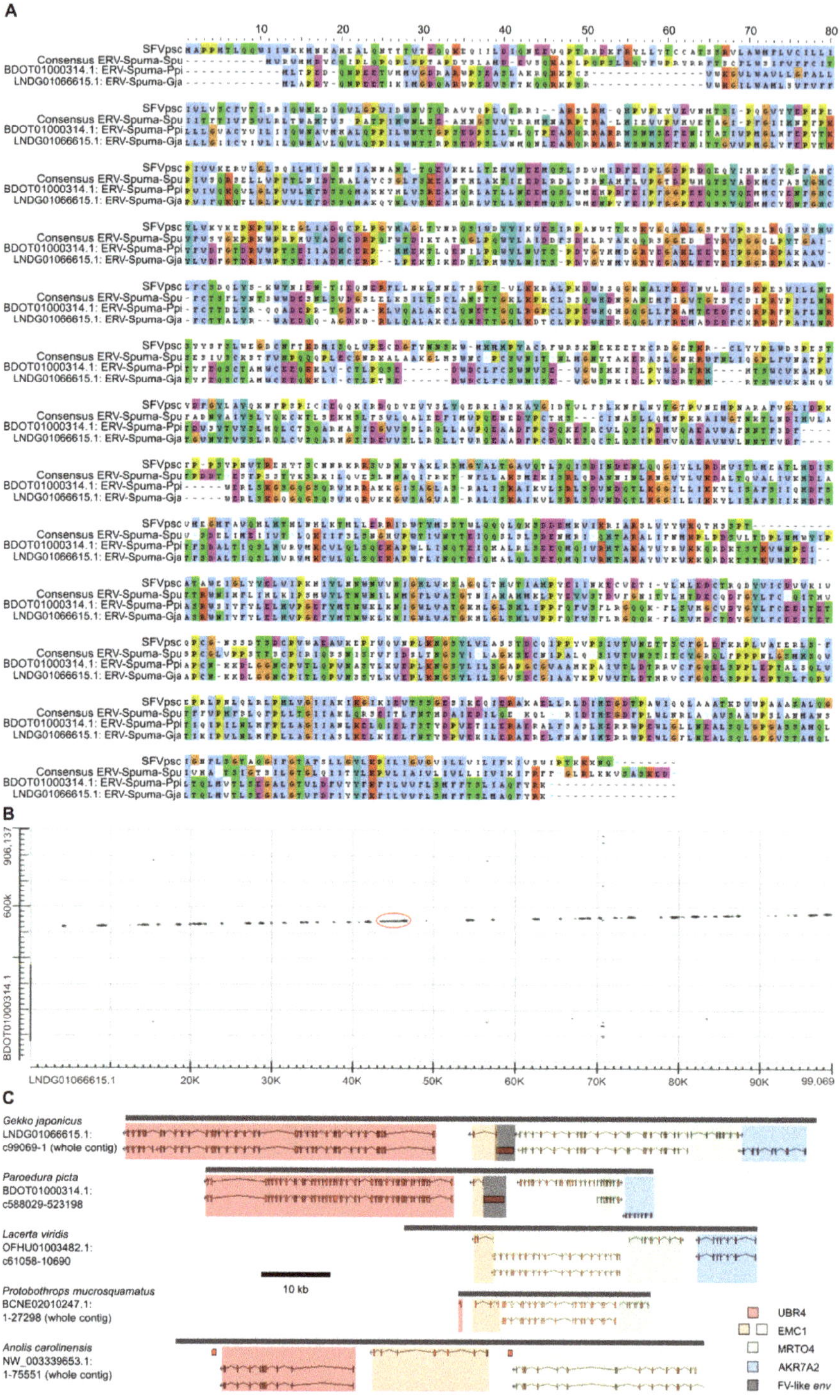

Figure 2. FV-like *env* sequences in panther gecko (*Paroedura picta*, BDOT01000314.1) and Schlegel's Japanese gecko (*Gekko japonicus*, LNDG01066615.1). (**A**) Alignment of Env protein sequences of prototype

FV (SFVpsc), consensus ERV-Spuma-Spu, and the two gecko FV-like endogenous viral elements, BDOT01000314.1: ERV-Spuma-Ppi, and LNDG01066615.1: ERV-Spuma-Gja. (**B**) BLASTn dot matrix between LNDG01066615.1 and BDOT01000314.1. The red circle indicates the location of the FV-like *env* sequences. (**C**) Homologous regions in three other reptiles, namely European green lizard (*Lacerta viridis*, OFHU01003482.1), brown spotted pitviper (*Protobothrops mucrosquamatus*, BCNE02010247.1), and green anole (*Anolis carolinensis*, NW_003339653.1). Genes were predicted by AUGUSTUS [9]. Four eukaryotic genes are shown on the diagram from left to right: ubiquitin protein ligase E3 component n-recognin 4 (UBR4, red), ER membrane protein complex subunit 1 (EMC1, orange and yellow), MRT4 homolog, ribosome maturation factor (MRTO4, green), and aldo-keto reductase family 7 member A2 (AKR7A2, blue). Gene homology at the protein level was examined by using BLASTp. FV-like env genes are highlighted in grey. Grey bars represent the contigs, and the scale bar (black) represents a length of 10 kb.

3.3. Recombination Analyses

A concatenated nucleotide alignment of *pol* and *env* sequences of ERV-Spuma-Spu elements together with those of mammalian, amphibian, and lobe-finned fish FVs and EFVs was checked for potential recombination events by Recombination Detection Program 4 (RDP4) [12]; *gag* sequences were not included, as they could not be aligned among these viruses. We found that, out of 165 ERV-Spuma-Spu elements, 138 of them (83.6%) had coverage of either *pol* or *env* genes of < 80% (see Methods and Materials for details), likely due to the poor genome quality at the time of analysis. We thus decided to exclude them from any further downstream analyses. The alignment contained 45 sequences, 27 of which were those of ERV-Spuma-Spu elements, and was 4695 nt (*pol*: 2685 nt; *env*: 2010 nt) long after curation (Data S4).

The analysis first identified two ERV-Spuma-Spu elements as recombinants (QEPC01002018.1: 1489335–1511987, and QEPC01002018.1: 1489335–1511987), harboring an integrase coding domain of unknown origin at the same genomic locations (position in the alignment: nt 2038–2596; Figure S2). We removed the recombinant regions (nt 2152–2432 after manual inspection) and performed the analysis again to further examine for other potential recombination events.

The results from the second round of analysis suggested that the *pol* and the *env* genes have different evolutionary histories. Based on the default dendrogram outputs from RDP4 [12] estimated using the unweighted pair group method with arithmetic mean, we found that, while ERV-Spuma-Spus' *pol* genes are more closely related to those of CoeEFV, their *env* genes are more similar to those of mammalian FVs (Figure S3). No recombination could be detected in either of the individual *pol* and *env* nucleotide alignments after that.

3.4. Phylogenetic Analyses and Evolutionary Timescale Estimation

To better understand how the *pol* and *env* genes evolved, their evolutionary histories were estimated from their corresponding protein alignments by using a Bayesian phylogenetic method (Figure 3). The Env protein alignment was derived from the *env* nucleotide alignment used in the recombination analyses with the addition of the two gecko EFVs to investigate how they relate to other FVs (Data S5). For the Pol protein alignment, we included sequences from fish EFVs and non-FV class III ERVs as an outgroup. This Pol alignment (Data S6) was based on the one we used previously in the study reporting the discovery of amphibian and fish EFVs [4], allowing the results to be compared.

Overall, the well-established broad co-speciation pattern between mammalian FVs and their hosts could be recovered from both the Pol and the Env phylogenies (Figure 3), and the topology of the Pol tree was comparable to that previously published in [4]. Our analyses suggested that ERV-Spuma-Spus' Pol is sister to that of CoeEFV (Bayesian posterior probability clade support = 0.99), while their Env is more closely related to those of mammalian FVs (Bayesian posterior probability clade support = 0.97). These results were consistent with those obtained from the recombination analysis (Figure S3). In addition, we found that the Env proteins of ERV-Spuma-Spu elements did not cluster with gecko EFVs; they instead formed two separate lineages, with gecko EFVs being closer to mammalian FVs (Bayesian posterior probability clade support = 1.00). In addition, we noted that, while our Pol protein analysis strongly supports the sister taxon relationship between ERV-Spuma-Spu and CoeEFV, the previous Pol protein analysis showed that ERV-Spuma-Spu is a sister taxon of mammalian FVs, inferred under the maximum likelihood framework with 89% bootstrap support [8]. This could be due to the differences in the methods (Bayesian vs. maximum likelihood) and/or the alignments used (reversed transcriptase + RNase-H + integrase domain vs. reversed transcriptase + RNase-H).

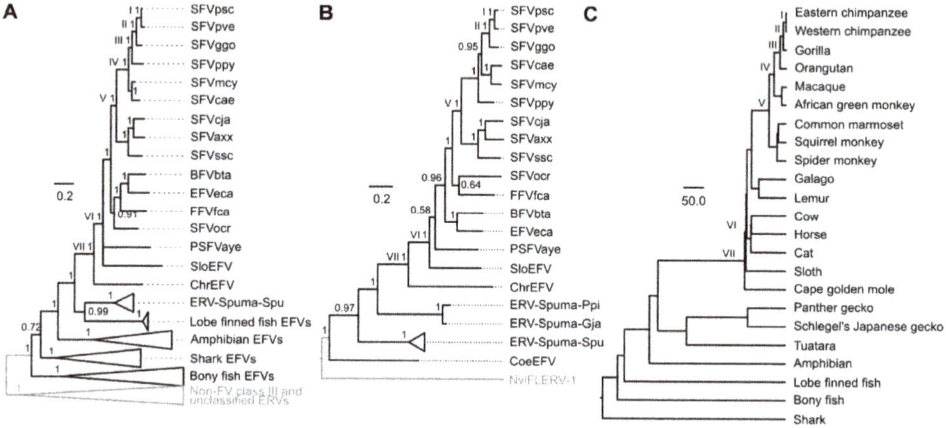

Figure 3. Foamy virus Pol, Env, and host phylogenies. Bayesian Pol (**A**) and Env (**B**) phylogenies were estimated by using MrBayes 3.2.6 [13], and their scale bars are in the units of amino acid substitutions per site. Both Pol and Env trees were rooted by the mid-point rooting method, and the determined outgroups are shown in grey. Arabic numerals on nodes are Bayesian posterior probability clade support values. The topologies of the Pol and the Env trees were compared to that of the host phylogeny (**C**) to identify virus–host co-speciation events labeled with Roman numerals. Nodes on different phylogenies that are labeled with the same Roman numeral are those corresponding to the same co-speciation event. The timescale of the identified co-speciation nodes, directly inferred from their hosts (Table S5), was used to calibrate the timescales of other nodes. The host tree topology was estimated elsewhere [26], and its scale bar is in units of millions of years. The virus–host association can be found in Table S6. SFV: simian foamy virus; psc, *Pan troglodytes schweinfurthii* chimpanzee; pve, *Pan troglodytes verus* chimpanzee; ggo, *Gorilla gorilla* gorilla; *ppy*, *Pongo pygmaeus* orangutan; mcy, *Macaca cyclopis* macaque; cae, *Chlorocebus aethiops* Grivet; cja, *Callithrix jacchus* marmoset; axx, Ateles spider monkey; scc, *Saimiri sciureus* squirrel monkey; ocr, *Otolemur crassicaudatus* brown greater galago; BFVbta, bovine foamy virus Bos taurus; EFVeca, equine foamy virus Equus caballus; FFVfca, feline foamy virus Felis catus; PSFVaye, prosimian foamy virus aye-aye; EFV, endogenous foamy virus; SloEFV, sloth EFV; ChrEFV, Cape golden mole EFV; CoeEFV, Coelacanth EFV; NviFLERV-1, Notophthalmus viridescens foamy virus-like endogenous retrovirus - 1.

Evolutionary timescales of reptile EFVs were estimated using the time dependent rate phenomenon (TDRP) model [18,27]. The TDRP model is a model that describes the relationship between total per lineage substitutions (*s* estimates) and their associated evolutionary timescales (*t* estimates) using a power law function ($t = \alpha s^{\beta}$), and this relationship can be used to estimate a *t* value for an arbitrary node given its *s* (node height in the units of substitutions per site) [18,27]. We traced simian foamy virus Pan troglodytes verus (SFVpve) down the trees to obtain total per lineage substitutions across various timescales for the TDRP model estimation. Based on virus–host tree topology comparison, we inferred seven virus–host co-speciation events in the Pol phylogeny (Figure 3A, labeled with Roman numerals) and five in the Env tree (Figure 3B, labeled with Roman numerals) that lie along the SFVpve lineage, and the timescales of these nodes were inferred directly from those of their hosts (Table S5). Two TDRP models were estimated based on the *t* and the *s* estimates of these identified co-speciation nodes, one for the Pol protein [α = 364.08 (242.33–533.43), β = 1.59 (1.34–1.86), Adjusted R^2 = 0.95 (0.90–0.99)], which was comparable to the one previously reported {α = 407.89 (264.32–583.97), β = 1.63 (1.38–1.90), Adjusted R^2 = 0.95 (0.91–0.99) [4]}, and the other for the Env protein [α = 124.18 (100.42–152.36), β = 1.41 (1.21–1.60), Adjusted R^2 = 0.96 (0.91–0.99)]. They were then used to extrapolate in order to calculate the timescales of other nodes based on their *s* estimates.

Analyses of the Pol protein sequences suggested that the ERV-Spuma-Spu lineage diverged 232.50 (173.70–303.33) myr ago (mya), which was comparable to that estimated based on the Env protein sequences, which was 257.15 (202.49–324.05) mya. These age estimates were, however, significantly lower than those of their hosts, which were estimated to be 324.7 (318–331.4) mya [28]. The age of the gecko EFV lineage was estimated to be 208.54 (171.59–250.91) myr old based on phylogenetic analysis of the Env protein sequences. This was consistent with their minimum age estimate of ~96 myr old. In addition, based on the Pol phylogeny, we also estimated the age of the amphibian EFV lineage and the entire clade of vertebrate FVs/EFVs to be 326.40 (229.14–448.65) myr old and 479.08 (298.31–718.86) myr old, respectively. These estimates were comparable to those previously reported {amphibian FVs: 348 (251–478) myr old and vertebrate FVs: 455 (304–684) myr old [4]} and those of their hosts (amphibians: ~335 myr old [29], and vertebrates: ~465 myr old [29]). Our results are thus consistent with those previously reported and support the long-term co-evolution between FVs and their hosts since the origin of vertebrates.

4. Discussion

This study reports two novel reptile EFVs that reside in the genomes of panther gecko (ERV-Spuma-Ppi) and Schlegel's Japanese gecko (ERV-Spuma-Gja) and further characterizes ERV-Spuma-Spu [8]. Together with ERV-Spuma-Spu [8], we analyzed the evolutionary history of reptilian FVs in detail, filling in the gap in our knowledge of the deep history of FV-host co-evolution.

ERV-Spuma-Ppi and ERV-Spuma-Gja are not full length ERVs, comprising only a full-length FV-like *env* gene, and are present in only a single copy in each genome. We showed that they are orthologous, being present in the same host genomic location in both species. Based on the speciation date of their gecko hosts, we inferred that these EFVs are at least 96 (83–98) myr old [25], making them the oldest EFVs ever discovered to date. The two gecko EFVs are located in the intronic region of the EMC1 gene in an antisense orientation typical of an old fixed intronic ERV; antisense integrations are favored because they are likely minimally disruptive to the host's gene transcription processes [30]. Remarkably, they do not contain any in-frame stop codons or transposable elements despite being almost 100 myr old and have been under strong purifying selection with a dN/dS estimate of 0.14 (0.08–0.54). Furthermore, by searching the transcriptomic sequence database of the common leopard gecko in the Reptilian Transcriptomes v2.0 Database [11], we discovered a transcript consensus sequence constructed from 499 reads that is highly similar to ERV-Spuma-Ppi and ERV-Spuma-Gja, exhibiting more than 80 percent identity both at the protein and the nucleotide levels. Combined, these findings suggest that they might be transcriptionally active and have been maintained for potential cellular functions, making them the first ever known co-opted EFVs. We, however, noted that the transcript we retrieved was distinct from the two gecko EFVs obtained from a different host species and mapped to only a small portion of the 3′ end of the *env* genes. Additional analyses of transcriptomic data obtained directly from *Gekko japonicas* and *Paroedura picta* are thus required to confirm that the two gecko EFVs are transcriptionally active.

Retroviral *env* genes are known to have been co-opted many times by various vertebrate hosts for a wide range of functions. The most well-known one is perhaps the *syncytin* genes, which was captured for a function in placental formation numerous times by various mammals (see [31,32] for reviews). A recent study identified (for the first time) a functionally active *syncytin* gene outside mammals, namely *syncytin-Mab1*, in a lizard *Mabuya* [33,34]. The reptilian *syncytin* gene was identified as a gammaretrovirus *env* gene, however, which belongs to a different group to our two gecko EFVs. Furthermore, *Mabuya* is a viviparous placental lizard, while geckos are not. Thus, the functions of ERV-Spuma-Ppi and ERV-Spuma-Gja might differ from that of *syncytin-Mab1*.

The fact that the *env* reading frames are still intact and under purifying selection despite their old age suggests that ERV-Spuma-Ppi and ERV-Spuma-Gja are functional at the protein level. BLASTp analyses against the NCBI nr protein database failed to identify cellular proteins that are related to ERV-Spuma-Ppi and ERV-Spuma-Gja. Therefore, their functions still remain elusive. Nonetheless, the two gecko EFVs are inserted in the EMC1 gene, which intriguingly shows greatest expression level in placenta tissues in human [35]. One could thus imagine that the two genetic elements might be co-expressed and are in turn functionally associated, as has been repeatedly shown in several organisms [36–38]. Although geckos lay eggs and do not possess true placenta tissues such as *Mabuya* lizards, the physical association of EMC1 with co-opted retroviral *env* sequences suggests their possible involvement in the reproductive system of geckos, analogous to the *syncytin* gene in mammals [31,32] and viviparous placental lizards [33,34]. Furthermore, the EMC1 protein influences virus cross-membrane transportation and infectivity via direct physical contact with viral particles [39]. The two gecko EFVs might thus play an active role in the host immune systems as well, if their functions are indeed associated with those of EMC1. Indeed, studies have shown that retroviral *env* genes can be co-opted and exapted for host anti-viral defense, acting as restriction factors against related retroviruses [40,41]. Our finding warrants further functional investigation to confirm the potential involvement of ERV-Spuma-Ppi and ERV-Spuma-Gja in gecko reproductive and/or immune systems.

We were able to identify 165 ERV-Spuma-Spu elements in the tuatara genome. Examination of their consensus sequence revealed that ERV-Spuma-Spu only possessed the three main retroviral core genes, namely *gag*, *pol*, and *env*, flanked by two LTRs. A previous study identified one short hypothetical open reading frame (192 nt) as an accessory gene [8]; however, we found that the sequence was actually part of the 3'-LTR. On the other hand, we could not identify any accessory genes located between the *env* gene and the 3' LTR, which is typical for a mammalian FV [4,6,42]. The authors of the previous study also noted that the identified accessory gene did not exhibit similarity to any known foamy accessory genes. Further examination revealed that the hypothetical protein was not intact and did not exhibit significant similarity to any known molecular sequences in the NCBI nr database. In addition, we could not identify a potential internal promoter towards the 3' end of the *env* gene. It is thus possible that the previously identified accessory gene in ERV-Spuma-Spu might have been an artifact. At face value, the observed lack of accessory genes is suggestive of ancient gene losses in ancestral exogenous reptile FVs. Alternatively, it could be that the ancestral exogenous tuatara FVs did possess accessory genes but lost them after becoming endogenous. This observation is also consistent with multiple acquisitions of accessory genes in other FVs at the same genomic location, which is perhaps less parsimonious but nevertheless possible. Discovery of other reptilian FVs or EFVs will help elucidate this issue.

Furthermore, we found that the ERV-Spuma-Spu *gag* gene was markedly shorter than those of typical simian FVs. Protein sequence comparison showed that the putative ERV-Spuma-Spu Gag protein had a full matrix domain essential for Gag–Gag interaction [43,44], Gag–Env interaction [44], and Gag–microtubular network interaction [45]. The conserved central region, which is evolutionarily related to orthoretroviral capsid proteins [46], could also be found. The regions between the matrix and the capsid domain (aa ~180–~300 of the SFVpsc Gag protein) were missing, however, containing the late domain (P_{284}SAP domain), which mediates viral particle release [47]. Nevertheless, this region was not highly conserved; indeed, non-primate FVs including bovine, equine, and feline FVs also lack this region and the late domain [48].

Moreover, a region homologous to the C-terminus of the nucleocapsid domain (corresponding to aa 549–648 in the SFVpsc Gag protein) containing part of the glycine/arginine rich box (GR) II and the entire GR-III was also missing from the putative ERV-Spuma-Spu Gag protein. GR-I, a nucleolar localization signal [49] that mediates nucleic acid binding [50] and is important for Pol packaging [51] and particle formation [52], could still be found. Sequence examination revealed that the chromatin-binding sequence (CBS) in GR-II (aa 534–546 in the SFVpsc Gag protein [53]) required for a direct physical contact between FV Gag protein and host nucleosomes [54] was still intact (Figure 4). The conserved tyrosine and arginine residues in the CBS (Y405 and R408) could also be found (Figure 4), and are essential for Gag chromosome binding and nuclear accumulation of Gag and genomic DNA [49,54,55]. The arginine-tyrosine-glycine (RYG) residues following the CBS (Figure 4) are crucial for nuclear accumulation of FV Gag and DNA, and, perhaps most importantly, DNA integration [55]. Mutagenesis of these residues causes significant reduction in all three activities, even if the CBS is complete [55]. Intriguingly, the RYG domain is absent from both ERV-Spuma-Spu and CoeEFV (Figure 4), which are incidentally the only two EFVs known to be present in high copy numbers in the host genomes [5,8]. In addition, the missing GR-III box was shown to be a nucleolar localization signal similar to GR-I [49]. Studies have shown that the deletion of GR-III only marginally affects viral budding [52,56], intracellular localization [52,57], reverse transcription [52], RNA packaging/binding [50,52,56,58], and particle morphology [52] but significantly reduces DNA packaging [52] and thus infectivity [52,56]. The lack of GR-III box and the RYG residues might help with the virus retrotransposition process by allowing their DNA to accumulate in the host cell and subsequently re-integrate into the host chromosomes in a steady and non-aggressive manner. As previously reported [8], a number of ERV-Spuma-Spu elements of different ages with paired-LTRs could be recovered. This means that at least some of the ERV-Spuma-Spu elements originated from the re-integration process and not via host genomic copying or LINE-mediated retrotransposition of viral mRNA, supporting our hypothesis. These observations might underlie the high copy number of ERV-Spuma-Spu and CoeEFV elements found in the tuatara [8] and the coelacanth genomes [5], respectively.

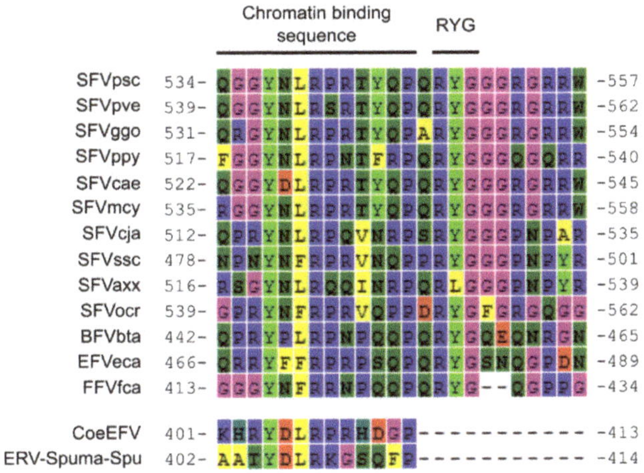

Figure 4. An alignment of chromatin-binding sequences (CBS) and surrounding regions. CBSs of CoeEFV and ERV-Spuma-Spu are intact. The conserved tyrosine (Y; 4th column) and arginine (R; 7th column) residues in the CBS, which are essential for Gag mitotic chromosome binding and nuclear accumulation of Gag and genomic DNA [49,54,55], could be found in all viruses. The arginine-tyrosine-glycine (RYG) residues, which are also important for nuclear accumulation of FV Gag and DNA [55], were absent from CoeEFV and ERV-Spuma-Spu but could be found in all mammalian FVs.

Based on their observation that ERV-Spuma-Spu is more closely related to mammalian FVs than CoeEFV, Wei et al. proposed an ancient co-speciation of ERV-Spuma-Spu and mammalian FVs dating back more than 320 million years ago [8]. This study, on the other hand, estimated the dates directly based on molecular analyses of Pol and Env protein sequences and the more well-established history of mammalian FV-host co-speciation. Our evolutionary analyses of Pol and Env proteins showed that the

ERV-Spuma-Spu lineage is only 232.50 (173.70–303.33) and 257.15 (202.49–324.05) myr old, respectively, comparable to one another in age. These estimates are much lower than those of their hosts, ~324.7 myr old [28]. This finding rejects the ancient co-speciation hypothesis previously proposed and instead suggests that the ancestral virus that gave rise to ERV-Spuma-Spu elements arose from (potentially a series of) cross species transmission(s) from an unknown, non-reptilian host. This result also highlights the pitfall of using tree topologies alone to infer a virus–host co-speciation history, especially when there are only a few lineages in the investigation.

Our phylogenetic analyses of Env proteins revealed that, while ERV-Spuma-Ppi and ERV-Spuma-Gja form a clade, they do not form a monophyletic clade with ERV-Spuma-Spu elements, with the two gecko EFVs being closer to mammalian FVs than ERV-Spuma-Spu (Bayesian posterior probability clade support = 1.00). We estimated the age of the gecko EFV lineage to be 208.54 (171.59–250.91) myr old. Again, this low age estimate is suggestive of a cross-species transmission origin for the gecko EFVs' ancestor, one that is broadly contemporary but independent from the transmission that gave rise to the ancestor of ERV-Spuma-Spu elements.

The phylogenetic placement of CoeEFV with respect to that of the ERV-Spuma-Spu lineage also suggests an evolutionary history of cross-species transmission. While the Pol protein of CoeEFV exhibits a sister relationship with that of ERV-Spuma-Spu viruses (Figure 3A), its Env protein does not, instead being basal to the clade of mammalian and reptile FVs (Figure 3B). Since CoeEFV forms a clade with ERV-Spuma-Spu viruses in the Pol phylogeny, their branching dates from mammalian FVs are hence the same, estimated to be 232.50 (173.70–303.33) mya. This is indeed comparable to the previously reported estimate of 262.76 (195.00–342.08) mya [4] and further supports the complex evolutionary history of FVs that might have transmitted several times between terrestrial and aquatic animals in the distant past [4].

On the other hand, we estimated CoeEFV's Env protein (and thus its *env* gene) to share a most recent common ancestor with that of mammalian FVs 332.68 (236.13–451.42) mya. This age estimate is drastically older than that of the *pol* gene, suggesting that CoeEFV's *pol* and *env* genes might have different evolutionary histories. We note however that this age estimate is conditioned on how the Env tree is rooted. In this study, we chose the mid-point rooting method, which placed NviFLERV-1 (the amphibian EFV) as the most basal lineage in the Env tree (Figure 3B), consistent with the topology of the Pol tree (Figure 3A). However, if the *pol* and the *env* genes can have different evolutionary histories, then there would be no intrinsic reasons for the Pol and the Env tree topologies to closely resemble each other. Another possibility is to subjectively place CoeEFV as the most basal linage in the Env tree, in which case the estimated date would be the divergence date of NviFLERV-1 instead, which in turn would make it a lower bound estimate for the branching date of CoeEFV's *env* gene. This nonetheless still supports the hypothesis that CoeEFV's *pol* and *env* genes have different evolutionary histories.

This finding mirrors observations from primate [59] and feline FVs [60,61]. Studies at the population level identified the surface domain of their *env* genes to have evolutionary histories that are strikingly different from the rest of the *env* gene and the *pol* gene [59–62], segregating into two variants that co-circulate in the same host populations while other genomic regions are not phylogenetically distinguishable. This domain carries the receptor binding domain and is targeted by neutralizing antibodies [60,63], which may help explain its greater diversity. Our analyses could not detect this evolutionary feature, since our dataset comprises only one sequence from each FV species. Nonetheless, it is remarkable that a similar evolutionary pattern could still be observed at the species level focusing on different timescales. Our results thus further support the modular nature of FV genomes and that this might be a widespread evolutionary feature of FVs.

Our analyses reveal a complex evolutionary history and ancient transmission routes of ancient FVs, likely involving host switches across the boundary between water and land, as well as the modular nature of their genomes. Our work also highlights the importance and the value of recombination analysis and temporal information in evolutionary inference as well as the pitfalls of tree-topology based virus–host co-speciation analysis. Discovery of additional EFVs will undoubtedly further our understanding and improve our knowledge of the complex and rich natural history of FVs.

Supplementary Materials: The following are available online at http://www.mdpi.com/1999-4915/11/7/641/s1, Figure S1: ERV-Spuma-Spu consensus sequence, Figure S2: Recombination detection in *pol-env* alignment, first round, Figure S3: Recombination detection in *pol-env* alignment, second round, Table S1: tBLASTn using CoeEFV Pol as probe against the tuatara genome, Table S2: Merged Pol hits and reciprocal BLASTx results, Table S3: tBLASTn using CoeEFV Env as probe against the extended Pol hits, Table S4: foamy virus-like endogenous viral elements in other reptiles, Table S5: host evolutionary timescales, Table S6: foamy virus-host association, Data S1: alignment of ERV-Spuma-Spu sequences – virus body portion, Data S2: alignment of ERV-Spuma-Spu sequences – long terminal repeat portion, Data S3: ERV-Spuma-Spu consensus sequence, Data S4: *pol-env* alignment, Data S5: Env alignment, Data S6 Pol alignment.

Author Contributions: P.A. and A.K. conceived the project. P.A. and A.K. researched the data for the article. P.A., P.S., and A.K. substantially contributed to discussion of content. P.A. performed analyses and wrote the article. P.A., P.S., and A.K. reviewed and edited the manuscript before submission.

Acknowledgments: This work is funded by Wellcome Trust.

Conflicts of Interest: The authors declare no conflict of interest.

References

1. Hayward, A.; Cornwallis, C.K.; Jern, P. Pan-vertebrate comparative genomics unmasks retrovirus macroevolution. *Proc. Natl. Acad. Sci. USA* **2015**, *112*, 464–469. [CrossRef]
2. Katzourakis, A.; Aiewsakun, P.; Jia, H.; Wolfe, N.D.; LeBreton, M.; Yoder, A.D.; Switzer, W.M. Discovery of prosimian and afrotherian foamy viruses and potential cross species transmissions amidst stable and ancient mammalian co-evolution. *Retrovirology* **2014**, *11*, 61. [CrossRef] [PubMed]
3. Han, G.-Z.; Worobey, M. Endogenous viral sequences from the Cape golden mole (Chrysochloris asiatica) reveal the presence of foamy viruses in all major placental mammal clades. *PLoS ONE* **2014**, *9*, e97931. [CrossRef] [PubMed]
4. Aiewsakun, P.; Katzourakis, A. Marine origin of retroviruses in the early Palaeozoic Era. *Nat. Commun.* **2017**, *8*, 13954. [CrossRef]
5. Han, G.-Z.; Worobey, M. An endogenous foamy-like viral element in the coelacanth genome. *PLoS Pathog.* **2012**, *8*, e1002790. [CrossRef]
6. Ruboyianes, R.; Worobey, M. Foamy-like endogenous retroviruses are extensive and abundant in teleosts. *Virus Evol.* **2016**, *2*, vew032. [CrossRef]
7. Han, G.Z. Extensive retroviral diversity in shark. *Retrovirology* **2015**, *12*, 34. [CrossRef] [PubMed]
8. Wei, X.; Chen, Y.; Duan, G.; Holmes, E.C.; Cui, J. A reptilian endogenous foamy virus sheds light on the early evolution of retroviruses. *Virus Evol.* **2019**, *5*, vez001. [CrossRef]
9. Stanke, M.; Morgenstern, B. AUGUSTUS: A web server for gene prediction in eukaryotes that allows user-defined constraints. *Nucleic Acids Res.* **2005**, *33*, W465–W467. [CrossRef]
10. Yang, Z. PAML 4: Phylogenetic analysis by maximum likelihood. *Mol. Biol. Evol.* **2007**, *24*, 1586–1591. [CrossRef]
11. Tzika, A.C.; Ullate-Agote, A.; Grbic, D.; Milinkovitch, M.C. Reptilian transcriptomes v2.0: An extensive resource for sauropsida genomics and transcriptomics. *Genome Biol. Evol.* **2015**, *7*, 1827–1841. [CrossRef] [PubMed]
12. Martin, D.P.; Murrell, B.; Golden, M.; Khoosal, A.; Muhire, B. RDP4: Detection and analysis of recombination patterns in virus genomes. *Virus Evol.* **2015**, *1*, vev003. [CrossRef] [PubMed]
13. Ronquist, F.; Teslenko, M.; Mark, P.; Ayres, D.L.; Darling, A.; Hohna, S.; Larget, B.; Liu, L.; Suchard, M.A.; Huelsenbeck, J.P. MrBayes 3.2: Efficient Bayesian phylogenetic inference and model choice across a large model space. *Syst. Biol.* **2012**, *61*, 539–542. [CrossRef] [PubMed]
14. Abascal, F.; Zardoya, R.; Posada, D. ProtTest: Selection of best-fit models of protein evolution. *Bioinformatics* **2005**, *21*, 2104–2105. [CrossRef] [PubMed]
15. Katzourakis, A.; Gifford, R.J.; Tristem, M.; Gilbert, M.T.P.; Pybus, O.G. Macroevolution of complex retroviruses. *Science* **2009**, *325*, 1512. [CrossRef] [PubMed]

16. Switzer, W.M.; Salemi, M.; Shanmugam, V.; Gao, F.; Cong, M.-E.; Kuiken, C.; Bhullar, V.; Beer, B.E.; Vallet, D.; Gautier-Hion, A.; et al. Ancient co-speciation of simian foamy viruses and primates. *Nature* **2005**, *434*, 376–380. [CrossRef] [PubMed]
17. Ghersi, B.M.; Jia, H.; Aiewsakun, P.; Katzourakis, A.; Mendoza, P.; Bausch, D.G.; Kasper, M.R.; Montgomery, J.M.; Switzer, W.M. Wide distribution and ancient evolutionary history of simian foamy viruses in New World primates. *Retrovirology* **2015**, *12*, 89. [CrossRef] [PubMed]
18. Aiewsakun, P.; Katzourakis, A. Time dependency of foamy virus evolutionary rate estimates. *BMC Evol. Biol.* **2015**, *15*, 119. [CrossRef] [PubMed]
19. R Core Team. R: A Language and environment for statistical computing. *R Found. Stat. Comput.* **2014**, *1*, 409.
20. Stoye, J.P.; Blomberg, J.; Coffin, J.M.; Fan, H.; Hahn, B.; Neil, J.; Quackenbush, S.; Rethwilm, A.; Tristem, M. Family-Retroviridae. In *Virus Taxonomy: Ninth Report of the International Committee on Taxonomy of Viruses;* King, A.M.Q., Lefkowitz, E.J., Adams, M.J., Carstens, E.B., Eds.; Elsevier Academic Press: San Diego, CA, USA, 2011; pp. 477–495. ISBN 978-0-12-384684-6.
21. Linial, M.L. Foamy viruses are unconventional retroviruses. *J. Virol.* **1999**, *73*, 1747–1755. [PubMed]
22. Lee, E.G.; Stenbak, C.R.; Linial, M.L. Foamy virus assembly with emphasis on pol encapsidation. *Viruses* **2013**, *5*, 886–900. [CrossRef] [PubMed]
23. Löchelt, M.; Yu, S.F.; Linial, M.L.; Flügel, R.M. The human foamy virus internal promoter is required for efficientgene expression and infectivity. *Virology* **1995**, *206*, 601–610. [CrossRef]
24. Campbell, M.; Renshaw-Gegg, L.; Renne, R.; Luciw, P.A. Characterization of the internal promoter of simian foamy viruses. *J. Virol.* **1994**, *68*, 4811–4820. [PubMed]
25. Kumar, S.; Stecher, G.; Suleski, M.; Hedges, S.B. TimeTree: A resource for timelines, timetrees, and divergence times. *Mol. Biol. Evol.* **2017**, *34*, 1812–1819. [CrossRef] [PubMed]
26. Bininda-Emonds, O.R.P.; Cardillo, M.; Jones, K.E.; MacPhee, R.D.E.; Beck, R.M.D.; Grenyer, R.; Price, S.A.; Vos, R.A.; Gittleman, J.L.; Purvis, A. The delayed rise of present-day mammals. *Nature* **2007**, *446*, 507–512. [CrossRef] [PubMed]
27. Aiewsakun, P.; Katzourakis, A. Time-dependent rate phenomenon in viruses. *J. Virol.* **2016**, *90*, 7184–7195. [CrossRef] [PubMed]
28. Dos Reis, M.; Thawornwattana, Y.; Angelis, K.; Telford, M.J.; Donoghue, P.C.J.; Yang, Z. Uncertainty in the timing of origin of animals and the limits of precision in molecular timescales. *Curr. Biol.* **2015**, *25*, 2939–2950. [CrossRef] [PubMed]
29. Broughton, R.E.; Betancur-R, R.; Li, C.; Arratia, G.; Ortí, G. Multi-locus phylogenetic analysis reveals the pattern and tempo of bony fish evolution. *PLoS Curr.* **2013**, *5*. [CrossRef]
30. Brady, T.; Lee, Y.N.; Ronen, K.; Malani, N.; Berry, C.C.; Bieniasz, P.D.; Bushman, F.D. Integration target site selection by a resurrected human endogenous retrovirus. *Genes Dev.* **2009**, *23*, 633–642. [CrossRef]
31. Lavialle, C.; Cornelis, G.; Dupressoir, A.; Esnault, C.; Heidmann, O.; Vernochet, C.; Heidmann, T. Paleovirology of "syncytins", retroviral env genes exapted for a role in placentation. *Philos. Trans. R. Soc. B Biol. Sci.* **2013**, *368*, 20120507. [CrossRef]
32. Denner, J. Expression and function of endogenous retroviruses in the placenta. *APMIS* **2016**, *124*, 31–43. [CrossRef] [PubMed]
33. Cornelis, G.; Funk, M.; Vernochet, C.; Leal, F.; Tarazona, O.A.; Meurice, G.; Heidmann, O.; Dupressoir, A.; Miralles, A.; Ramirez-Pinilla, M.P.; et al. An endogenous retroviral envelope syncytin and its cognate receptor identified in the viviparous placental Mabuya lizard. *Proc. Natl. Acad. Sci. USA* **2017**, *114*, E10991–E11000. [CrossRef] [PubMed]
34. Denner, J. Function of a retroviral envelope protein in the placenta of a viviparous lizard. *Proc. Natl. Acad. Sci. USA* **2017**, *114*, 13315–13317. [CrossRef] [PubMed]
35. Fagerberg, L.; Hallström, B.M.; Oksvold, P.; Kampf, C.; Djureinovic, D.; Odeberg, J.; Habuka, M.; Tahmasebpoor, S.; Danielsson, A.; Edlund, K.; et al. Analysis of the human tissue-specific expression by genome-wide integration of transcriptomics and antibody-based proteomics. *Mol. Cell. Proteom.* **2014**, *13*, 397–406. [CrossRef] [PubMed]
36. Szczepińska, T.; Pawłowski, K. Genomic positions of co-expressed genes: Echoes of chromosome organisation in gene expression data. *BMC Res. Notes* **2013**, *6*, 229. [CrossRef] [PubMed]
37. Williams, E.J.B.; Bowles, D.J. Coexpression of neighboring genes in the genome of Arabidopsis thaliana. *Genome Res.* **2004**, *14*, 1060–1067. [CrossRef] [PubMed]

38. Lee, J.M.; Sonnhammer, E.L.L. Genomic gene clustering analysis of pathways in eukaryotes. *Genome Res.* **2003**, *13*, 875–882. [CrossRef] [PubMed]
39. Bagchi, P.; Inoue, T.; Tsai, B. EMC1-dependent stabilization drives membrane penetration of a partially destabilized non-enveloped virus. *Elife* **2016**, *5*, e21470. [CrossRef] [PubMed]
40. Malfavon-Borja, R.; Feschotte, C. Fighting fire with fire: Endogenous retrovirus envelopes as restriction factors. *J. Virol.* **2015**, *89*, 4047–4050. [CrossRef] [PubMed]
41. Blanco-Melo, D.; Gifford, R.J.; Bieniasz, P.D. Co-option of an endogenous retrovirus envelope for host defense in hominid ancestors. *Elife* **2017**, *6*, e22519. [CrossRef] [PubMed]
42. Lindemann, D.; Rethwilm, A. Foamy virus biology and its application for vector development. *Viruses* **2011**, *3*, 561–585. [CrossRef] [PubMed]
43. Tobaly-Tapiero, J.; Bittoun, P.; Giron, M.L.; Neves, M.; Koken, M.; Saib, A.; De, T.H. Human foamy virus capsid formation requires an interaction domain in the N terminus of Gag. *J. Virol* **2001**, *75*, 4367–4375. [CrossRef] [PubMed]
44. Goldstone, D.C.; Flower, T.G.; Ball, N.J.; Sanz-Ramos, M.; Yap, M.W.; Ogrodowicz, R.W.; Stanke, N.; Reh, J.; Lindemann, D.; Stoye, J.P.; et al. A unique spumavirus Gag N-terminal domain with functional properties of orthoretroviral matrix and capsid. *PLoS Pathog.* **2013**, *9*, e1003376. [CrossRef] [PubMed]
45. Matthes, D.; Wiktorowicz, T.; Zahn, J.; Bodem, J.; Stanke, N.; Lindemann, D.; Rethwilm, A. Basic residues in the foamy virus Gag protein. *J. Virol.* **2011**, *85*, 3986–3995. [CrossRef] [PubMed]
46. Ball, N.J.; Nicastro, G.; Dutta, M.; Pollard, D.J.; Goldstone, D.C.; Sanz-Ramos, M.; Ramos, A.; Müllers, E.; Stirnnagel, K.; Stanke, N.; et al. Structure of a spumaretrovirus Gag central domain reveals an ancient retroviral capsid. *PLoS Pathog.* **2016**, *12*, e1005981. [CrossRef] [PubMed]
47. Pincetic, A.; Leis, J. The mechanism of budding of retroviruses from cell membranes. *Adv. Virol.* **2009**, *2009*, 623969. [CrossRef]
48. Stange, A.; Mannigel, I.; Peters, K.; Heinkelein, M.; Stanke, N.; Cartellieri, M.; Göttlinger, H.; Rethwilm, A.; Zentgraf, H.; Lindemann, D. Characterization of prototype foamy virus gag late assembly domain motifs and their role in particle egress and infectivity. *J. Virol.* **2005**, *79*, 5466–5476. [CrossRef]
49. Paris, J.; Tobaly-Tapiero, J.; Giron, M.L.; Burlaud-Gaillard, J.; Buseyne, F.; Roingeard, P.; Lesage, P.; Zamborlini, A.; Saïb, A. The invariant arginine within the chromatin-binding motif regulates both nucleolar localization and chromatin binding of Foamy virus Gag. *Retrovirology* **2018**, *15*, 48. [CrossRef]
50. Yu, S.F.; Edelmann, K.; Strong, R.K.; Moebes, A.; Rethwilm, A.; Linial, M.L. The carboxyl terminus of the human foamy virus Gag protein contains separable nucleic acid binding and nuclear transport domains. *J. Virol* **1996**, *70*, 8255–8262.
51. Lee, E.-G.; Linial, M.L. The C Terminus of Foamy Retrovirus Gag Contains Determinants for Encapsidation of Pol Protein into Virions. *J. Virol.* **2008**, *82*, 10803–10810. [CrossRef]
52. Mullers, E.; Uhlig, T.; Stirnnagel, K.; Fiebig, U.; Zentgraf, H.; Lindemann, D. Novel Functions of Prototype Foamy Virus Gag Glycine- Arginine-Rich Boxes in Reverse Transcription and Particle Morphogenesis. *J. Virol.* **2011**, *85*, 1452–1463. [CrossRef] [PubMed]
53. Tobaly-Tapiero, J.; Bittoun, P.; Lehmann-Che, J.; Delelis, O.; Giron, M.L.; de Thé, H.; Saïb, A. Chromatin tethering of incoming foamy virus by the structural Gag protein. *Traffic* **2008**, *9*, 1717–1727. [CrossRef] [PubMed]
54. Lesbats, P.; Serrao, E.; Maskell, D.P.; Pye, V.E.; O'Reilly, N.; Lindemann, D.; Engelman, A.N.; Cherepanov, P. Structural basis for spumavirus GAG tethering to chromatin. *Proc. Natl. Acad. Sci. USA* **2017**, *114*, 5509–5514. [CrossRef] [PubMed]
55. Wei, G.; Kehl, T.; Bao, Q.; Benner, A.; Lei, J.; Löchelt, M. The chromatin binding domain, including the QPQRYG motif, of feline foamy virus Gag is required for viral DNA integration and nuclear accumulation of Gag and the viral genome. *Virology* **2018**, *524*, 56–68. [CrossRef] [PubMed]
56. Stenbak, C.R.; Linial, M.L. Role of the C terminus of foamy virus Gag in RNA packaging and Pol expression. *J. Virol.* **2004**, *78*, 9423–9430. [CrossRef] [PubMed]
57. Schliephake, A.W.; Rethwilm, A. Nuclear localization of foamy virus Gag precursor protein. *J. Virol.* **1994**, *68*, 4946–4954.
58. Hamann, M.V.; Müllers, E.; Reh, J.; Stanke, N.; Effantin, G.; Weissenhorn, W.; Lindemann, D. The cooperative function of arginine residues in the Prototype Foamy Virus Gag C-terminus mediates viral and cellular RNA encapsidation. *Retrovirology* **2014**, *11*, 87. [CrossRef]

59. Richard, L.; Rua, R.; Betsem, E.; Mouinga-Ondémé, A.; Kazanji, M.; Leroy, E.; Njouom, R.; Buseyne, F.; Afonso, P.V.; Gessain, A. Cocirculation of two env molecular variants, of possible recombinant origin, in gorilla and chimpanzee simian foamy virus strains from Central Africa. *J. Virol.* **2015**, *89*, 12480–12491. [CrossRef]
60. Winkler, I.G.; Flügel, R.M.; Löchelt, M.; Flower, R.L.P. Detection and molecular characterisation of feline foamy virus serotypes in naturally infected cats. *Virology* **1998**, *247*, 144–151. [CrossRef]
61. Phung, H.T.T.; Ikeda, Y.; Miyazawa, T.; Nakamura, K.; Mochizuki, M.; Izumiya, Y.; Sato, E.; Nishimura, Y.; Tohya, Y.; Takahashi, E.; et al. Genetic analyses of feline foamy virus isolates from domestic and wild feline species in geographically distinct areas. *Virus Res.* **2001**, *76*, 171–181. [CrossRef]
62. Galvin, T.A.; Ahmed, I.A.; Shahabuddin, M.; Bryan, T.; Khan, A.S. Identification of recombination in the envelope gene of simian foamy virus serotype 2 isolated from Macaca cyclopis. *J. Virol.* **2013**, *87*, 8792–8797. [CrossRef]
63. Lambert, C.; Couteaudier, M.; Gouzil, J.; Richard, L.; Montange, T.; Betsem, E.; Rua, R.; Tobaly-Tapiero, J.; Lindemann, D.; Njouom, R.; et al. Potent neutralizing antibodies in humans infected with zoonotic simian foamy viruses target conserved epitopes located in the dimorphic domain of the surface envelope protein. *PLoS Pathog.* **2018**, *14*, e1007293. [CrossRef]

viruses

MDPI

Review

Simian Foamy Virus Co-Infections

Shannon M. Murray * and Maxine L. Linial

Division of Basic Sciences, Fred Hutchinson Cancer Research Center, 1100 Fairview Ave N, Seattle, WA 98109, USA; mlinial@fredhutch.org

* Correspondence: smurray@fredhutch.org

Received: 8 July 2019; Accepted: 21 September 2019; Published: 27 September 2019

Abstract: Foamy viruses (FVs), also known as spumaretroviruses, are complex retroviruses that are seemingly nonpathogenic in natural hosts. In natural hosts, which include felines, bovines, and nonhuman primates (NHPs), a large percentage of adults are infected with FVs. For this reason, the effect of FVs on infections with other viruses (co-infections) cannot be easily studied in natural populations. Most of what is known about interactions between FVs and other viruses is based on studies of NHPs in artificial settings such as research facilities. In these settings, there is some indication that FVs can exacerbate infections with lentiviruses such as simian immunodeficiency virus (SIV). Nonhuman primate (NHP) simian FVs (SFVs) have been shown to infect people without any apparent pathogenicity. Humans zoonotically infected with simian foamy virus (SFV) are often co-infected with other viruses. Thus, it is important to know whether SFV co-infections affect human disease.

Keywords: foamy virus; spumaretrovirus; co-infections; NHP; pathogenesis; zoonoses

1. Introduction

Foamy viruses (FVs) comprise the *Spumaretrovirinae* subfamily of the family *Retroviridae* and are also designated spumaretroviruses [1]. FVs are ancient complex retroviruses that have co-evolved with their nonhuman primate (NHP) hosts for at least 60 million years [2]. Interestingly, recent sequencing of an ancient marine fish, the coelacanth, revealed an endogenous foamy virus (FV) [3]. The coelacanth is an ancient marine four-lobed fish believed to be the organism that first became terrestrial and is the ancestor of all terrestrial organisms. This indicates that FVs have existed for an estimated 400 million years [3], making *Spumaretrovirinae* the oldest known extant vertebrate virus subfamily.

FVs are apparently nonpathogenic in their natural hosts, which include NHPs (reviewed in [4]), felines [5], bovines [6], and equines [7]. FVs have also been found in bats, although the physiological consequences were not stated [8]. In non-primate hosts, FV prevalence is reported to be between ca. 30–70% in adults, depending on age, host, and location (reviewed in [9]). FVs were first identified by their cytopathicity in tissue culture cells ([10–12], reviewed in [13]). Thus, there have been many efforts to determine whether these viruses are pathogenic in vivo. To date, there have been no reports demonstrating clear-cut pathogenicity in natural or accidental hosts (reviewed in [14]). However, in research settings, there is some evidence that FVs can exacerbate the pathogenesis of other viruses. This phenomenon cannot be well studied in natural infections, as finding FV uninfected adult animals is difficult.

Simian FVs (SFVs) replicate primarily in tissues of the oral mucosa [15,16], and transmission most likely occurs through transfer of saliva from one individual to the next. Often, infected saliva transfer occurs through grooming, biting, or sharing food (reviewed in [4]). It is also thought that SFVs from saliva enters the blood or oral cavity of the recipient [17]. In NHP blood transfusion studies, SFV can be transmitted through blood [17,18]. However, it is not known whether this occurs in natural settings. In natural FV-infected felines, FV DNA has been detected in buccal swabs and in the blood [19].

While humans have contacts with felines and bovines, there is no evidence for actual infection of humans with FVs from these species (reviewed in [14]). Zoonotic infections with SFVs are frequent among animal caretakers, zoo keepers, bushmeat hunters, and others in direct contact with NHPs [20–23]. For example, ca. 2–5% of individuals in North America who report contact with NHPs are FV-infected, as determined by SFV polymerase chain reaction (PCR) (reviewed in [14]). There is no evidence for human-to-human transmission. The underlying reason(s) as to why the virus has not adapted to humans, but to all other primate species, is unknown.

Interestingly, SFV replication takes place in the most terminally differentiated superficial epithelial cells of the oral mucosa—those about to slough off into saliva [15]. The lack of pathogenicity of FV infections may be a result of this replicative niche in a cell type that turns over rapidly and is relatively dispensable to the host [15]. If this cellular niche for SFV replication is altered as described below for experimental simian immunodeficiency virus (SIV) infections, there may be potential for pathogenic effects.

2. FVs and the Virome

Each organism is host to a multitude of microbes, known as the microbiome. Organisms are also host to a collection of viruses, known as the virome (reviewed in [24]). Since, in natural species, FVs infect the majority of adults, FVs are considered part of the virome. It is well established that the virome plays a role in health and disease and that co-infecting viruses can affect each other and the microbiome [24]. In this review, we will consider the effect of FVs on infections by other viruses, in some cases, pathogens, and we will also consider the effects of other viruses upon FV infections, summarized in Table 1.

Table 1. Foamy virus (FV) and retrovirus co-infections: their effects on the host.

Co-Infecting Retrovirus	Genus	Host Species	Effects on FV	Effects of FV	References
Simian Immunodeficiency Virus (SIV)	*Lentivirus*	*Macaca mulatta* (rhesus macaque)	FV replication expanded to the jejunum	Increased SIV RNA loads in the blood Decreased survival and greater CD4+ T cell loss	[25] [26]
Simian T cell-Lymphotropic Virus (STLV-1)	*Deltaretrovirus*	*Papio anubis* (baboon)	FV proviral load increased in the peripheral blood, but not in saliva	Not determined	[27]
Feline Leukemia Virus (FeLV)	*Gammaretrovirus*	*Felis catus* (domestic cat)	Higher FFV DNA loads in PBMC correlated with increased FeLV viremia and disease progression FFV DNA in the oral cavity was detected in more cats with progressive FeLV disease compared to regressive FeLV disease	Not determined	[28] [19]

3. SFV Zoonotic Infections

There is evidence for zoonotic transmission of SFVs to humans (reviewed in [14]). Many of the zoonotically infected people are those with direct contact with NHPs, including bushmeat hunters in Africa as well as zoo and laboratory workers [20–23,29]. People whose interactions with NHPs are less direct but who are SFV-infected have been found in Asia [30]. There are small numbers of individuals identified who are infected with both SFV and human immunodeficiency virus (HIV) [31,32]. Moreover, as there is interest in using FV as a vector for gene therapy [33,34], the questions surrounding FV co-infections are becoming more relevant.

4. SFV and Other Retrovirus Co-Infections

SFVs are endemic in all NHP species examined to date in Africa, Asia, and the Americas [13,35]. In Africa, there are at least three other endemic complex retroviruses that infect NHPs. These are SIV, simian T-cell lymphotropic virus-1 (STLV-1), and simian retrovirus type D (SRV D). SIV had been thought to be nonpathogenic in its natural African monkey hosts [36], but there are reports of an acquired immunodeficiency syndrome (AIDS)-like illness in some SIV-infected natural hosts [37,38]. Additionally, when SIV infects other NHP species, such as chimpanzees and gorillas, it can be pathogenic in some cases [39–41].

STLV-1 has not been as extensively studied in its natural NHP hosts as human T-cell lymphotropic virus-1 (HTLV-1) has been in humans. HTLV-1 is pathogenic in only a small fraction of infected humans (reviewed in [42]), and STLV-1 infection in NHPs has been associated with a number of T cell abnormalities, including lymphomas and leukemias (reviewed in [43]). Many Asian NHPs are infected with another retrovirus, SRV D [44,45]. Thus, it is likely that many macaques are co-infected with SRV D and SFV. In NHPs, SFV as well as cytomegalovirus (CMV), a herpesvirus, are endemic and therefore many adult animals are co-infected with both viruses [46]. However, whether these CMV or SRV D co-infections alter animal health has not been reported.

4.1. SFV and SIV Co-Infections

Researchers have used the rhesus macaque (RM), also known as *Macaca mulatta*, as a model for HIV infections. In the wild, SIV is not known to exist in Asia [47,48], the natural habitat of RM. SIV sooty mangabey (SIVsm) has been found to be pathogenic in RM [49] and has become the virus used to infect RM to recapitulate HIV infections. SFV infection is latent in most tissues, including the blood. SFV replication is only detected in oropharyngeal tissues [16,25]. A key question concerning FV–host interactions is whether FV replication is controlled by the host immune system. To address this question, RM infected with pathogenic SIV strains (SIVmac239 and SIVmac155T3) that lead to CD4+ T cell depletion were studied, and SFV replication was assessed in the blood and other tissues [25]. In SIV/SFV co-infected RM, SFV replication was expanded to include the small intestine, the jejunum [25], which is a site of SIV-induced CD4+ T cell depletion [50]. However, other tissues that were CD4+ T cell depleted were not permissive for SFV replication [25]. Thus, it is not only CD4+ T cell depletion per se that is responsible for the expansion of SFV replication to the jejunum. Overall, this indicates that the host immune system is not limiting systemic SFV replication. It is important to note that the strains of SIV used in this study were lab-adapted, highly pathogenic strains that are HIV infection models in NHPs and are unlike SIV strains in natural hosts, which are usually poorly pathogenic.

It is also possible that SFV can affect the pathogenicity of other viruses, such as SIV. In natural settings, most adult NHPs are naturally infected with SFV. Therefore, this issue was addressed using RM individually housed in primate center facilities. The researchers examined SFV− and SFV+ RM infected with a pathogenic SIV strain (SIVmac239) [26]. The SFV+ animals had increased SIV viral loads in the blood and died more rapidly than SFV− RM. Thus, SFV infection does exacerbate SIV pathogenesis in experimentally SIV-infected RM.

The mechanism by which SFV increases SIV pathogenesis is unknown. One tissue target of SIV pathogenesis in RM is the jejunum [50]. Whether SFV replication in the jejunum contributes to this pathogenicity is an outstanding question. Because the SIV RM model commonly uses SFV+ animals, the RM model might not totally recapitulate HIV pathogenesis in people who are SFV−. There is evidence of HIV/SFV co-infections in humans [29,32]. Bushmeat hunters often get bitten by NHPs and become SFV-infected [29]. The number of bushmeat hunters co-infected with SFV and HIV is small. It would be of interest to compare HIV infections of bushmeat hunters who are SFV-infected or uninfected.

Free-living chimpanzees (cpz) in multiple countries of Africa, such as Cameroon and Gabon, have been analyzed for infection with SFVcpz and SIVcpz [51]. The researchers found that 15/70 (~21%) of SFV-infected animals were co-infected with SIV. This indicates that co-infection of these two viruses is common in chimpanzees. In another study, in the monkey the Ugandan red colobus [52], SFV/SIV co-infections were also common, with 23% of individuals co-infected. The routes of transmission of these two viruses are apparently different, with SFV transmission primarily through saliva. In the case of SIV, both sexual transmission and aggressive behavior have been implicated (reviewed in [53]). The effects of these two viruses on the health of free-living NHPs was not noted in either study, but this would be of great interest because these are clear examples of natural co-infections.

4.2. SFV and STLV-1 Co-Infections

A cohort of naturally SFV-infected baboons were studied. Some of the baboons were also naturally infected with STLV-1, while others were not, with 18 baboons studied per group. It was found that SFV DNA levels in the blood, but not in the saliva, were increased in the STLV-1-infected baboons [27]. It is not known why there is increased SFV DNA in the blood after STLV-1 infection. Two possibilities are (1) increased integrated SFV proviruses, or (2) increased numbers of SFV viral particles in the blood. The authors show that, in tissue culture cells, the related HTLV-1 transcriptional activator protein (Tax) can stimulate the FV long terminal repeat (LTR). They suggest that this could be a mechanism that explains the in vivo results [27]. However, it is also possible that since STLV-1 increases the number of lymphoid cells in the blood, this could result in more SFV in the blood as well. Overall, STLV-1 infection is unlikely to alter SFV transmission, since SFV transmission is mostly through saliva rather than blood. It is not known whether SFV infection alters the pathogenicity of STLV-1, since all of the STLV-1-infected animals were also SFV-infected. There is also concern about SFV/HTLV-1 co-infection in humans [54], as discussed further below.

4.3. SFV and SRV D Co-Infections

SRV D infections in Asian primates such as macaques sometimes causes an immunodeficiency-like syndrome [44,45]. SRV D appears to be transmitted through saliva as well as urine and feces [55]. There is a report of one worker who is seropositive for both SFV and SRV D [56]. It should be noted that this individual was both seropositive and PCR positive for SFV, but could not be shown to be PCR positive for SRV D. Thus, this person may have been exposed to both viruses, producing antibodies, but may not be actively SRV D infected. There is no evidence that this SRV D/SFV seropositive human has any retroviral-related pathogenesis.

5. SFV Zoonotic Co-Infections and Hematological Changes

One study identified HTLV-1 and SFV co-infected hunters in Central Africa [54]. Fifty-six percent of the hunters bitten by NHPs and infected with HTLV-1 were also infected with SFV, suggesting that these two viruses may have been co-transmitted via the bites [54]. However, the pathogenic effects of the co-infection were not evaluated.

There is a publication presenting evidence that SFV-infected bushmeat hunters from Cameron seem to have different levels of hematological markers, including hemoglobin, creatine phosphokinase, and bilirubin, than SFV-uninfected bushmeat hunters [57]. The SFV-infected group had a higher incidence of HTLV-1 infections, and all participants except for one were infected with hepatitis B virus (HBV). Thus, it is hard to ascribe the differences in hematological markers to SFV infection alone. These differences could result from SFV co-infection with either HTLV-1 or HBV. In fact, as described in baboons infected with STLV-1 [27], FV DNA levels were increased in the blood of co-infected animals. Another publication reports no hematological differences in SFV-infected North American research and zoo workers occupationally exposed to NHPs [58]. Since these individuals were unlikely to be infected with HTLV-1 and/or HBV, this supports the notion that hematological changes from SFV infection are a result of co-infections. In natural hosts, there is no evidence that SFV alone leads to any hematological changes. However, hematological changes in natural hosts infected with FV have not been thoroughly investigated.

6. Non-Primate FV Co-Infections

Most work on FV transmission has been done in NHPs. This has served as the general model for FV transmission in other natural species. While the transmission route for non-primate FVs has been speculated to include saliva, other transmission modes seem to occur. For example, bovine foamy virus (BFV) has been detected in bovine breast milk [59]. In fact, BFV has been shown to be transmitted from mothers' milk to calves [60].

6.1. BFV and Herpesvirus Co-Infections

A serious illness of unknown origin in dairy cows is non-responsive post-partum metritis (NPPM). It is thought to be caused by a virus, as it is unresponsive to antibiotics. There is some evidence that bovine gammaherpesviruses (BoHVs) are associated with this disease (M. Materniak-Kornas, personal communication, 2019). Since many cows are infected by BFV [60], it is possible that co-infection of BFV and BoHV-4 or BoHV-6 is a factor in the disease. However, the researchers found that is not the case, since as many healthy cows as sick cows were infected with BFV (M. Materniak-Kornas, personal communication, 2019).

6.2. FFV and Other Retrovirus Co-Infections in Cats

Feline leukemia virus (FeLV), a retrovirus of cats, often leads to fatal diseases, including lymphomas [61]. One study examined FeLV and FFV co-infections in domestic cats [28]. Natural FeLV infections can have two outcomes; these are progressive infections leading to disease, or regressive infections. Regressive infections are characterized by a transient production of viral structural proteins and a persistence of low levels of integrated viral DNA. Cats that are progressively infected have detectable FeLV RNA and infectious virions. It was found that higher levels of FFV DNA in the blood correlated with increased FeLV viremia and disease progression [28]. In another feline study, the researchers examined FeLV regressive versus progressive infections [19]. In cats with regressive infections, there were lower levels of FFV DNA in the oral cavity. This suggests the possibility that innate or adaptive immunity to FeLV in the regressors could affect FFV as well.

There are cats co-infected with FFV and feline immunodeficiency virus (FIV), a lentivirus causing decreases in CD4+ T cells and feline acquired immune deficiency syndrome (FAIDS) [62]. In one study, a small number of cats were experimentally infected with FIV alone or with FIV and FFV. In this study, FFV co-infection did not enhance the pathogenesis of FIV [63]. This is in contrast with what was seen in RM infected with SFV and SIV, as described above [26]. However, in a study of FFV experimental infection, FFV RNA was rarely seen in saliva samples (in only 1 of 80 samples) [64]. Thus, the FIV/FFV co-infection study might be flawed, since it is possible that FFV experimental infection does not mirror natural FFV infections. More studies are needed to assay viral RNA in tissues of naturally FV-infected non-primates, including cats.

7. Conclusions

In natural hosts, FVs are highly prevalent and therefore finding uninfected adult animals is difficult. Thus, all information about the effect of FVs on other viral infections in these species involves artificial situations in which some animals are kept FV-free. Most of the studies on FV effects on other viral infections use lab-adapted pathogenic viruses. In research laboratory settings, there is clear indication that FV infections exacerbate lentiviral outcomes. There is also evidence that SFV has an expanded tissue tropism in lentiviral co-infected NHPs. The prevalence of FV co-infected individuals has been described in natural hosts. However, these studies did not report whether FV co-infection affects pathogenesis induced by other viruses. Therefore, it is not known whether the results from lab settings are relevant to what occurs in natural settings. The mechanism of how FV infections may affect other viral infections is not clear.

Humans can be zoonotically infected with SFVs from NHPs. While it has been reported that there are people co-infected with SFV and HIV or HTLV-1, there are almost no data about whether SFV infection of humans can exacerbate other viral infections. Overall, more studies in natural settings and of human zoonotic FV co-infections would be important to understand whether FVs contribute to the pathogenicity of other microorganisms. One example of a FV pathogenic effect on hosts is in RM, using lab-adapted strains of a lentivirus, SIV. In the future, it will be important to see whether HIV pathogenesis is worse in humans co-infected with SFV. It is also possible that in humans, FV infections could exacerbate other viral infections such as HTLV-1, HBV, or even CMV or other herpesviruses. The understanding of how SFVs affect other human viruses is important, given the potential use of FV vectors for gene therapy to treat human diseases.

Author Contributions: S.M.M. and M.L.L. both contributed to the writing of this review article.

Acknowledgments: We would like to acknowledge Delia Pinto-Santini for helpful comments on the manuscript and Magdalena Materniak-Kornas for sharing unpublished data. We also would like to thank the Fred Hutchinson Cancer Research C for financial support.

Conflicts of Interest: The authors declare no conflict of interest. The funders had no role in the writing of the manuscript, or in the decision to publish the article.

References

1. Khan, A.S.; Bodem, J.; Buseyne, F.; Gessain, A.; Johnson, W.; Kuhn, J.H.; Kuzmak, J.; Lindemann, D.; Linial, M.L.; Lochelt, M.; et al. Spumaretroviruses: Updated taxonomy and nomenclature. *Virology* **2018**, *516*, 158–164. [CrossRef] [PubMed]
2. Switzer, W.M.; Salemi, M.; Shanmugam, V.; Gao, F.; Cong, M.E.; Kuiken, C.; Bhullar, V.; Beer, B.E.; Vallet, D.; Gautier-Hion, A. Ancient co-speciation of simian foamy viruses and primates. *Nature* **2005**, *434*, 376–380. [CrossRef] [PubMed]
3. Han, G.Z.; Worobey, M. An Endogenous Foamy-like Viral Element in the Coelacanth Genome. *PLoS Pathog.* **2012**, *8*, e1002790. [CrossRef] [PubMed]
4. Linial, M.L. Foamy viruses. In *Fields Virology*, 5th ed.; Knipe, D.M., Howley, P.M., Eds.; Wolters Kluwer/Lippincott Williams & Wilkins: Philadelphia, PA, USA, 2007; pp. 2245–2263.
5. Riggs, J.L.; Oshirls, L.S.; Taylor, D.O.; Lennette, E.H. Syncytium-forming agent isolated from domestic cats. *Nature* **1969**, *222*, 1190–1191. [CrossRef] [PubMed]
6. Malmquist, W.A.; Van der Maaten, M.J.; Boothe, A.D. Isolation, immunodiffusion, immunofluorescence, and electron microscopy of a syncytial virus of lymphosarcomatous and apparently normal cattle. *Cancer Res.* **1969**, *29*, 188–200. [PubMed]
7. Tobaly-Tapiero, J.; Bittoun, P.; Neves, M.; Guillemin, M.C.; Lecellier, C.H.; Puvion-Dutilleul, F.; Gicquel, B.; Zientara, S.; Giron, M.L.; de The, H.; et al. Isolation and characterization of an equine foamy virus. *J. Virol.* **2000**, *74*, 4064–4073. [CrossRef] [PubMed]
8. Wu, Z.; Ren, X.; Yang, L.; Hu, Y.; Yang, J.; He, G.; Zhang, J.; Dong, J.; Sun, L.; Du, J.; et al. Virome Analysis for Identification of Novel Mammalian Viruses in Bat Species from Chinese Provinces. *J. Virol.* **2012**, *86*, 10999–11012. [CrossRef]
9. Saib, A. Non-primate foamy viruses. In *Current Topics in Microbiology and Immunology*; Rethwilm, A., Ed.; Springer: Berlin, Germany, 2003; Volume 277, pp. 197–212.
10. Enders, J.; Peebles, T. Propagation in tissue culture of cytopathogenic agents from patients with measles. *Proc. Soc. Exp. Biol. Med.* **1954**, *86*, 277–287. [CrossRef]
11. Achong, B.G.; Mansell, W.A.; Epstein, M.A.; Clifford, P. An unusual virus in cultures from a human nasopharyngeal carcinoma. *J. Natl. Cancer Inst.* **1971**, *46*, 299–307.
12. Rustigian, R.; Johnston, P.; Reihart, H. Infection of monkey kidney tissue cultures with virus-like agents. *Proc. Soc. Exp. Med.* **1955**, *88*, 8–16. [CrossRef]
13. Meiering, C.D.; Linial, M.L. Historical perspective of foamy virus epidemiology and infection. *Clin. Microbiol. Rev.* **2001**, *14*, 165–176. [CrossRef] [PubMed]
14. Pinto-Santini, D.M.; Stenbak, C.R.; Linial, M.L. Foamy virus zoonotic infections. *Retrovirology* **2017**, *14*, 55. [CrossRef] [PubMed]

15. Murray, S.M.; Picker, L.J.; Axthelm, M.K.; Hudkins, K.; Alpers, C.E.; Linial, M.L. Replication in a superficial epithelial cell niche explains the lack of pathogenicity of primate foamy virus infections. *J. Virol.* **2008**, *82*, 5981–5985. [CrossRef] [PubMed]
16. Falcone, V.; Leupold, J.; Clotten, J.; Urbanyi, E.; Herchenröder, O.; Spatz, W.; Volk, B.; Bölm, N.; Toniolo, A.; Neumann-Haefelin, D.; et al. Sites of simian foamy virus persistence in naturally infected African green monkeys: Latent provirus is ubiquitous, whereas viral replication is restricted to the oral mucosa. *Virology* **1999**, *257*, 7–14. [CrossRef] [PubMed]
17. Khan, A.S.; Kumar, D. Simian foamy virus infection by whole-blood transfer in rhesus macaques: Potential for transfusion transmission in humans. *Transfusion* **2006**, *46*, 1352–1359. [CrossRef] [PubMed]
18. Brooks, J.I.; Merks, H.W.; Fournier, J.; Boneva, R.S.; Sandstrom, P.A. Characterization of blood-borne transmission of simian foamy virus. *Transfusion* **2007**, *47*, 162–170. [CrossRef] [PubMed]
19. Cavalcante, L.T.F.; Muniz, C.P.; Jia, H.; Augusto, A.M.; Troccoli, F.; Medeiros, S.O.; Dias, C.G.A.; Switzer, W.M.; Soares, M.A.; Santos, A.F. Clinical and Molecular Features of Feline Foamy Virus and Feline Leukemia Virus Co-Infection in Naturally-Infected Cats. *Viruses.* **2018**, *10*, 702. [CrossRef]
20. Engel, G.A.; Small, C.T.; Soliven, K.; Feeroz, M.M.; Wang, X.; Hasan, K.; Gunwha, O.; Alam, S.; Craig, K.; Jackson, D.; et al. Zoonotic simian foamy virus in Bangladesh reflects diverse patterns of transmission and co-infections among humans. *Emerg. Microbes Infect.* **2013**, *2*, e58. [CrossRef]
21. Betsem, E.; Rua, R.; Tortevoye, P.; Froment, A.; Gessain, A. Frequent and recent human acquisition of simian foamy viruses through apes' bites in central Africa. *PLoS Pathog.* **2011**, *7*, e1002306. [CrossRef]
22. Heneine, W.; Switzer, W.M.; Sandstrom, P.; Brown, J.; Vedapuri, S.; Schable, C.A.; Khan, A.S.; Lerche, N.W.; Schweizer, M.; Neumann-Haefelin, D.; et al. Identification of a human population infected with simian foamy viruses. *Nat. Med.* **1998**, *4*, 403–407. [CrossRef]
23. Brooks, J.I.; Rud, E.W.; Pilon, R.G.; Smith, J.M.; Switzer, W.M.; Sandstrom, P.A. Cross-species retroviral transmission from macaques to human beings. *Lancet* **2002**, *360*, 387–388. [CrossRef]
24. Cadwell, K. The virome in host health and disease. *Immunity* **2015**, *42*, 805–813. [CrossRef]
25. Murray, S.M.; Picker, L.J.; Axthelm, M.K.; Linial, M.L. Expanded tissue targets for foamy virus replication with simian immunodeficiency virus-induced immunosuppression. *J. Virol.* **2006**, *80*, 663–670. [CrossRef] [PubMed]
26. Choudhary, A.; Galvin, T.A.; Williams, D.K.; Beren, J.; Bryant, M.A.; Khan, A.S. Influence of naturally occurring simian foamy viruses (SFVs) on SIV disease progression in the Rhesus macaque (*Macaca mulatta*) model. *Viruses* **2013**, *5*, 1414–1430. [CrossRef] [PubMed]
27. Alais, S.; Pasquier, A.; Jegado, B.; Journo, C.; Rua, R.; Gessain, A.; Tobaly-Tapiero, J.; Lacoste, R.; Turpin, J.; Mahieux, R. STLV-1 co-infection is correlated with an increased SFV proviral load in the peripheral blood of SFV/STLV-1 naturally infected non-human primates. *PLoS Negl. Trop. Dis.* **2018**, *12*, e0006812. [CrossRef] [PubMed]
28. Powers, J.; Chiu, E.; Kraberger, S.; Roelke-Parker, M.; Lowery, I.; Erbeck, K.; Troyer, R.; Carver, S.; VandeWoude, S. Feline leukemia virus disease outcomes in a domestic cat breeding colony: Relationship to endogenous FeLV and other chronic viral infections. *J. Virol.* **2018**. [CrossRef] [PubMed]
29. Wolfe, N.D.; Switzer, W.M.; Carr, J.K.; Bhullar, V.B.; Shanmugam, V.; Tamoufe, U.; Prosser, A.T.; Torimiro, J.N.; Wright, A.; Mpoudi-Ngole, E.; et al. Naturally acquired simian retrovirus infections in central African hunters. *Lancet* **2004**, *363*, 932–937. [CrossRef]
30. Jones-Engel, L.; Steinkraus, K.A.; Murray, S.M.; Engel, G.A.; Grant, R.; Aggimarangsee, N.; Lee, B.P.Y.-H.; May, C.; Schillaci, M.A.; Somgird, C.; et al. Sensitive assays for simian foamy viruses reveal a high prevalence of infection in commensal, free-ranging, Asian monkeys. *J. Virol.* **2007**, *81*, 7330–7337. [CrossRef]
31. Switzer, W.M.; Tang, S.; Zheng, H.; Shankar, A.; Sprinkle, P.S.; Sullivan, V.; Granade, T.C.; Heneine, W. Dual Simian Foamy Virus/Human Immunodeficiency Virus Type 1 Infections in Persons from Cote d'Ivoire. *PLoS ONE* **2016**, *11*, e0157709. [CrossRef]
32. Switzer, W.M.; Garcia, A.D.; Yang, C.; Wright, A.; Kalish, M.L.; Folks, T.M.; Heneine, W. Coinfection with HIV-1 and simian foamy virus in West Central Africans. *J. Infect. Dis.* **2008**, *197*, 1389–1393. [CrossRef]
33. Trobridge, G.D.; Horn, P.A.; Beard, B.C.; Kiem, H.-P. Large Animal Models for Foamy Virus Vector Gene Therapy. *Viruses* **2012**, *4*, 3572–3588. [CrossRef]

34. Kiem, H.P.; Wu, R.A.; Sun, G.; von, L.D.; Rossi, J.J.; Trobridge, G.D. Foamy combinatorial anti-HIV vectors with MGMTP140K potently inhibit HIV-1 and SHIV replication and mediate selection in vivo. *Gene* **2010**, *17*, 37–49. [CrossRef]
35. Stenbak, C.R.; Craig, K.L.; Ivanov, S.B.; Wang, X.; Soliven, K.C.; Jackson, D.L.; Gutierrez, G.A.; Engel, G.; Jones-Engel, L.; Linial, M.L. New World simian foamy virus infections in vivo and in vitro. *J. Virol.* **2014**, *88*, 982–991. [CrossRef]
36. Sharp, P.M.; Shaw, G.M.; Hahn, B.H. Simian immunodeficiency virus infection of chimpanzees. *J. Virol.* **2005**, *79*, 3891–3902. [CrossRef]
37. Ling, B.; Apetrei, C.; Pandrea, I.; Veazey, R.S.; Lackner, A.A.; Gormus, B.; Marx, P.A. Classic AIDS in a sooty mangabey after an 18-year natural infection. *J. Virol.* **2004**, *78*, 8902–8908. [CrossRef]
38. Pandrea, I.; Silvestri, G.; Apetrei, C. AIDS in african nonhuman primate hosts of SIVs: A new paradigm of SIV infection. *Curr. Hiv. Res.* **2009**, *7*, 57–72. [CrossRef]
39. Keele, B.F.; Jones, J.H.; Terio, K.A.; Estes, J.D.; Rudicell, R.S.; Wilson, M.L.; Li, Y.; Learn, G.H.; Beasley, T.M.; Schumacher-Stankey, J.; et al. Increased mortality and AIDS-like immunopathology in wild chimpanzees infected with SIVcpz. *Nature* **2009**, *460*, 515–519. [CrossRef]
40. Etienne, L.; Nerrienet, E.; LeBreton, M.; Bibila, G.T.; Foupouapouognigni, Y.; Rousset, D.; Nana, A.; Djoko, C.F.; Tamoufe, U.; Aghokeng, A.F.; et al. Characterization of a new simian immunodeficiency virus strain in a naturally infected Pan troglodytes troglodytes chimpanzee with AIDS related symptoms. *Retrovirology* **2011**, *8*, 4.
41. D'arc, M.; Furtado, C.; Siqueira, J.D.; Seuanez, H.N.; Ayouba, A.; Peeters, M.; Soares, M.A. Assessment of the gorilla gut virome in association with natural simian immunodeficiency virus infection. *Retrovirology* **2018**, *15*, 19. [CrossRef]
42. Peeters, M.; Delaporte, E. Simian retroviruses in African apes. *Clin. Microbiol. Infect.* **2012**, *18*, 514–520. [CrossRef]
43. Murphy, H.W.; Miller, M.; Ramer, J.; Travis, D.; Barbiers, R.; Wolfe, N.D.; Switzer, W.M. Implications of simian retroviruses for captive primate population management and the occupational safety of primate handlers. *J. Zoo Wildl. Med.* **2006**, *37*, 219–233. [CrossRef]
44. Lerche, N.W.; Osborn, K.G. Simian retrovirus infections: Potential confounding variables in primate toxicology studies. *Toxicol. Pathol.* **2003**, *31* (Suppl. 1), 103–110. [CrossRef]
45. Brody, B.A.; Hunter, E.; Kluge, J.D.; Lasarow, R.; Gardner, M.; Marx, P.A. Protection of macaques against infection with simian type D retrovirus (SRV-1) by immunization with recombinant vaccinia virus expressing the envelope glycoproteins of either SRV-1 or Mason-Pfizer monkey virus (SRV-3). *J. Virol.* **1992**, *66*, 3950–3954.
46. Blewett, E.L.; Lewis, J.; Gadsby, E.L.; Neubauer, S.R.; Eberle, R. Isolation of cytomegalovirus and foamy virus from the drill monkey (*Mandrillus leucophaeus*) and prevalence of antibodies to these viruses amongst wild-born and captive-bred individuals. *Arch. Virol.* **2003**, *148*, 423–433. [CrossRef]
47. Klatt, N.R.; Silvestri, G.; Hirsch, V. Nonpathogenic simian immunodeficiency virus infections. *Cold Spring Harb. Perspect. Med.* **2012**, *2*, a007153. [CrossRef]
48. Ayouba, A.; Duval, L.; Liegeois, F.; Ngin, S.; Ahuka-Mundeke, S.; Switzer, W.M.; Delaporte, E.; Ariey, F.; Peeters, M.; Nerrienet, E. Nonhuman primate retroviruses from Cambodia: High simian foamy virus prevalence, identification of divergent STLV-1 strains and no evidence of SIV infection. *Infect. Genet. Evol.* **2013**, *18*, 325–334. [CrossRef]
49. Apetrei, C.; Kaur, A.; Lerche, N.W.; Metzger, M.; Pandrea, I.; Hardcastle, J.; Falkenstein, S.; Bohm, R.; Koehler, J.; Traina-Dorge, V.; et al. Molecular epidemiology of simian immunodeficiency virus SIVsm in U.S. primate centers unravels the origin of SIVmac and SIVstm. *J. Virol.* **2005**, *79*, 8991–9005. [CrossRef]
50. Veazey, R.S.; DeMaria, M.; Chalifoux, L.V.; Shvetz, D.E.; Pauley, D.R.; Knight, H.L.; Rosenzweig, M.; Johnson, R.P.; Desrosiers, R.C.; Lackner, A.A. Gastrointestinal tract as a major site of CD4+ T cell depletion and viral replication in SIV infection. *Science* **1998**, *280*, 427–431. [CrossRef]
51. Liu, W.; Worobey, M.; Li, Y.; Keele, B.F.; Bibollet-Ruche, F.; Guo, Y.; Goepfert, P.A.; Santiago, M.L.; Ndjango, J.B.; Neel, C.; et al. Molecular ecology and natural history of simian foamy virus infection in wild-living chimpanzees. *PLoS Pathog.* **2008**, *4*, e1000097. [CrossRef]

52. Goldberg, T.L.; Sintasath, D.M.; Chapman, C.A.; Cameron, K.M.; Karesh, W.B.; Tang, S.; Wolfe, N.D.; Rwego, I.B.; Ting, N.; Switzer, W.M. Coinfection of Ugandan red colobus (Procolobus [Piliocolobus] rufomitratus tephrosceles) with novel, divergent delta-, lenti-, and spumaretroviruses. *J. Virol.* **2009**, *83*, 11318–11329. [CrossRef]
53. VandeWoude, S.; Apetrei, C. Going Wild: Lessons from Naturally Occurring T-Lymphotropic Lentiviruses. *Clin. Microbiol. Rev.* **2016**, *19*, 728–762. [CrossRef] [PubMed]
54. Filippone, C.; Betsem, E.; Tortevoye, P.; Cassar, O.; Bassot, S.; Froment, A.; Fontanet, A.; Gessain, A. A Severe Bite From a Nonhuman Primate Is a Major Risk Factor for HTLV-1 Infection in Hunters From Central Africa. *Clin. Infect. Dis.* **2015**, *60*, 1667–1676. [CrossRef] [PubMed]
55. Hara, M.; Sata, T.; Kikuchi, T.; Nakajima, N.; Uda, A.; Fujimoto, K.; Baba, T.; Mukai, R. Isolation and characterization of a new simian retrovirus type D subtype from monkeys at the Tsukuba Primate Center, Japan. *Microbes Infect.* **2005**, *7*, 126–131. [CrossRef] [PubMed]
56. Lerche, N.W.; Switzer, W.M.; Yee, J.L.; Shanmugam, V.; Rosenthal, A.N.; Chapman, L.E.; Folks, T.M.; Heneine, W. Evidence of infection with simian type D retrovirus in persons occupationally exposed to nonhuman primates. *J. Virol.* **2001**, *75*, 1783–1789. [CrossRef] [PubMed]
57. Buseyne, F.; Betsem, E.; Montange, T.; Njouom, R.; Bilounga, N.C.; Hermine, O.; Gessain, A. Clinical Signs and Blood Test Results Among Humans Infected With Zoonotic Simian Foamy Virus: A Case-Control Study. *J. Infect. Dis.* **2018**, *218*, 144–151. [CrossRef]
58. Boneva, R.S.; Switzer, W.M.; Spira, T.J.; Bhullar, V.B.; Shanmugam, V.; Cong, M.E.; Lam, L.; Heneine, W.; Folks, T.M.; Chapman, L.E. Clinical and virological characterization of persistent human infection with simian foamy viruses. *Aids Res. Hum. Retrovir.* **2007**, *23*, 1330–1337. [CrossRef]
59. Romen, F.; Backes, P.; Materniak, M.; Sting, R.; Vahlenkamp, T.W.; Riebe, R.; Pawlita, M.; Kuzmak, J.; Lochelt, M. Serological detection systems for identification of cows shedding bovine foamy virus via milk. *Virology* **2007**, *364*, 123–131. [CrossRef]
60. Johnson, R.H.; de la Rosa, J.; Abher, I.; Kertayadnya, I.G.; Entwistle, K.W.; Fordyce, G.; Holroyd, R.G. Epidemiological studies of bovine spumavirus. *Vet. Microbiol.* **1988**, *16*, 25–33. [CrossRef]
61. Hartmann, K. Clinical aspects of feline retroviruses: A review. *Viruses* **2012**, *4*, 2684–2710. [CrossRef]
62. Winkler, I.G.; Löchelt, M.; Flower, R.L. Epidemiology of feline foamy virus and feline immunodeficiency virus infections in domestic and feral cats: A seroepidemiological study. *J. Clin. Microbiol.* **1999**, *37*, 2848–2851.
63. Zenger, E.; Brown, W.C.; Song, W.; Wolf, A.M.; Pedersen, N.C.; Longnecker, M.; Li, J.; Collisson, E.W. Evaluation of cofactor effect of feline syncytium-forming virus on feline immunodeficiency virus infection. *Am. J. Vet. Res.* **1993**, *54*, 713–718. [PubMed]
64. Ledesma-Feliciano, C.; Troyer, R.M.; Zheng, X.; Miller, C.; Cianciolo, R.; Bordicchia, M.; Dannemiller, N.; Gagne, R.; Beatty, J.; Quimby, J.; et al. Feline Foamy Virus Infection: Characterization of Experimental Infection and Prevalence of Natural Infection in Domestic Cats with and without Chronic Kidney Disease. *Viruses* **2019**, *11*, 662. [CrossRef] [PubMed]

viruses

MDPI

Article

Eco-Epidemiological Profile and Molecular Characterization of Simian Foamy Virus in a Recently-Captured Invasive Population of *Leontopithecus chrysomelas* (Golden-Headed Lion Tamarin) in Rio de Janeiro, Brazil

Thamiris S. Miranda [1], Cláudia P. Muniz [1,2], Silvia B. Moreira [3], Marina G. Bueno [4,5], Maria Cecília M. Kierulff [4,6], Camila V. Molina [4], José L. Catão-Dias [7], Alcides Pissinatti [3], Marcelo A. Soares [1,2] and André F. Santos [1,*]

1 Departamento de Genética, Universidade Federal do Rio de Janeiro, Rio de Janeiro 21941-617, Brazil; thamirismiranda02@gmail.com (T.S.M.); claudia.muniz16@gmail.com (C.P.M.); masoares@biologia.ufrj.br (M.A.S.)

2 Programa de Oncovirologia, Instituto Nacional de Câncer, Rio de Janeiro 20231-050, Brazil

3 Centro de Primatologia do Rio de Janeiro, Instituto Estadual do Ambiente, Guapimirim 25948-395, Brazil; silviabm.inea@gmail.com (S.B.M.); alcidespissinatti@gmail.com (A.P.)

4 Instituto Pri-Matas para a Conservação da Biodiversidade, Belo Horizonte 31160-250, Brazil; buenomg@gmail.com (M.G.B.); ceciliakierulff@gmail.com (M.C.M.K.); camolina.vet@gmail.com (C.V.M.)

5 Laboratório de Virologia Comparada e Ambiental—LVCA, Instituto Oswaldo Cruz—IOC, Fundação Oswaldo Cruz-Fiocruz, Rio de Janeiro 21040-360, Brazil

6 Instituto Nacional da Mata Atlântica—INMA, 29650,000, Santa Teresa, Espírito Santo 29932-540, Brazil

7 Laboratório de Patologia Comparada de Animais Selvagens—LAPCOM, Departamento de Patologia, Faculdade de Medicina Veterinária e Zootecnia, Universidade de São Paulo, São Paulo 05508-270, Brazil; jlcataodias@gmail.com

* Correspondence: andre.santos@ufrj.br; Tel.: 55-21-3839-6383

Received: 6 August 2019; Accepted: 29 September 2019; Published: 10 October 2019

Abstract: Simian foamy viruses (SFV) infect a wide range of Old World and Neotropical primates (NP). Unlike Old World primates, little is known about the diversity and prevalence of SFV in NP, mainly from a free-living population. Phylogenetic analyses have shown that SFV coevolved with their hosts. However, viral strains infecting *Leontopithecus chrysomelas* did not behave as expected for this hypothesis. The purpose of this study was to determine the eco-epidemiological profile and molecular characterization of SFV in a recently captured invasive population of *L. chrysomelas* located in Niteroi/RJ using buccal swab as an alternative collection method. A prevalence of 34.8% (32/92) and a mean viral load of 4.7 log copies of SFV/10^6 cells were observed. With respect to time since capture, SFV prevalence was significantly higher in the group of animals sampled over 6 months after capture (55.2%) than in those more recently captured (25.4%) ($p = 0.005$). Infected solitary animals can contribute to SFV transmission between different groups in the population. SFV strains formed two distinct clades within the SFV infecting the Cebidae family. This is the first study to use buccal swabs as a tool to study SFV diversity and prevalence in a recently free-living NP population upon recent capture.

Keywords: spumavirus; viral prevalence; epidemiology; Neotropical primates; free-living primates; Brazil

---

1. Introduction

Simian foamy viruses (SFV) are complex retroviruses that naturally infect a wide range of non-human primates, including Neotropical primates (NP) [1–3]. Phylogenetic analyses have indicated that SFV coevolved with nonhuman primates for at least 60 million years [4], contributing to the lack of pathogenicity observed in these animals [5]. In NP, the prevalence is generally higher in animals in captivity (45–51%) compared to animals in the wild (14–30%) [2,3]. Although SFV has been described in at least 23 species of NP [3], there are only five complete genomes sequenced [6–9], a small number considering the high diversity of NP, distributed in at least 176 species, 17–21 genera and three to five families according to distinct classification systems [10,11]. Although the first NP SFV has been identified over four decades ago in cell cultures of spider monkey (*Ateles sp.*) saliva [12], very little is known about the distribution, prevalence, and genetic variability of SFVs that infect this group, and most studies have been conducted with captive animals. Although there are two studies reporting SFV prevalence in free-ranging NP, they are restricted to a limited number of available specimens and species [2,3]. Therefore, the epidemiological profile of SFV for a given NP species and/or genera in the wild is at least an inaccurate estimate since it has never been evaluated at the population level.

Leontopithecus chrysomelas (golden-headed lion tamarin) is a small size NP belonging to the Cebidae family [13] categorized as *EN-Endangered* by The International Union for Conservation of Nature (IUCN) [14] and it is endemic in the south of Bahia state, Brazil [15]. However, a few *L. chrysomelas* individuals have been introduced into an urban Atlantic Forest fragment in Niterói city (Rio de Janeiro state, Brazil) by a private collector in the mid-90s, being considered as an exotic invasive species in this region [16]. This invasive population have had close contact with humans and domestic animals, entering at human houses and being fed by them, increasing the risk of virus transmission in both directions [17–20]. Moreover, the few introduced animals reproduced, becoming hundreds of animals, estimated in excess of 700 in late 2015 [21], and could be a threat to the local golden lion tamarin (*Leontopithecus rosalia*), an endangered species endemic to Rio de Janeiro state, with risks of disease transmission [14–16], competition by habitat and hybridization [16]. For those reasons, many *L. chrysomelas* family groups were captured as part of a conservation project to remove this introduced species, administered and conducted by the non-governmental organization Pri-Matas Institute since 2012. The captured animals were kept in quarantine at *Centro de Primatologia do Rio de Janeiro* (CPRJ; Guapimirim, RJ, Brazil) and between 2012 and 2013 some were translocated to an area in southern Bahia without *L. chrysomelas* and others groups were maintained in captivity [16].

Yet retroviruses have a close phylogenetic relationship with their hosts [22], the dynamics of infection can be influenced by ecological and behavioral factors, impacting their prevalence, virus–host interactions, within- and between-species transmission [23,24], and also transmission to the surrounding human population [25–27]. SFV transmission occurs mainly through bites and grooming [28]. Therefore, social behaviors that increase contact between individuals may potentiate the likelihood of SFV transmission, impacting SFV prevalence rates. In NP, there are different complex social and behavioral structures [29,30]; however, little is known about how these structures and anthropogenic actions impact the viral ecology of SFV in free-living animals. In a phylogenetic analysis early study by our group, the only SFV sequences obtained from a *L. chrysomelas* and a *L. rosalia* did not cluster to form a single clade for *Leontopithecus* [3]. Here, for the first time in NP, a large number of recently-captured *L. chrysomelas* specimens were analyzed, allowing us to deepen our knowledge on SFV prevalence, circulating viral genetic diversity, and how social behaviors and the environment may influence SFV transmission in this population.

2. Materials and Methods

2.1. Study Population and Ethics Statement

Buccal swab samples were collected from of 92 *L. chrysomelas* captured in Niterói city (Rio de Janeiro state, Brazil) in the period from December 2014 to September 2017. The captured specimens were distributed in 29 family groups and 4 were found to be solitary (captured alone). Each *L. chrysomelas* family group and solitary specimen was kept separated after their capture and have their material collected from two to fourteen months. Specimens were classified as two groups, those collected from two to six months after their capture and those collected from seven to fourteen months after their capture. The sexual maturity was classified according to size, dentition and weight of the specimens and these data, as well as gender, geographic location of capture and family groups were made available. The material and information were collected by the CPRJ and Pri-Matas veterinarians.

All procedures were conducted in full compliance with Federal permits issued by the Brazilian Ministry of the Environment (SISBIO 30939-12) and samples were collected following the national guidelines and provisions of IBAMA (Instituto Brasileiro do Meio Ambiente e dos Recursos Naturais Renováveis, Brazil; permanent license number 11375–1). The project was approved by the Ethics Committee on the Use of Animals (CEUA/CCS) of Universidade Federal do Rio de Janeiro, under the reference number 037-14.

2.2. Sample Collection, Processing and Confirmation of Genomic DNA Integrity

Buccal swabs were collected using sterile cotton swabs with a plastic shaft that was then placed into a sterile tube containing 500 μL of saline solution (0.9% NaCl), transported to the Genetics Department of Universidade Federal do Rio de Janeiro on ice and were stored at −80 °C until processing. Genomic DNA (gDNA) was extracted from buccal swab samples using the PureLink®Genomic DNA kit (ThermoFisher Scientific, Grand Island, NY, USA) according to the manufacturer's specifications. After extraction, samples had their contaminants (PCR inhibitors) removed using the OneStep™ PCR Inhibitor Removal Kit (Zymo Research, Irvine, CA, USA). Shortly thereafter, samples were quantified using Nanodrop and stored at −20 °C. The integrity of the gDNA for PCR analysis was checked by PCR amplification of a mitochondrial constitutive gene (*cytB*) as previously described [1]. All DNA samples testing positive for *cytB* sequences were further considered suitable for SFV PCR detection.

2.3. Detection and Quantification of SFV

To detect NP SFV proviral DNA, we first performed a screening semi-nested PCR for short integrase sequences of 192 bp using generic primers and standard PCR conditions as previously described [1] as a diagnostic PCR test for NP SFV using 12 ng of buccal gDNA. In addition to the conventional diagnostic PCR for SFV detection, a real-time PCR assay was also performed to detect and quantify SFV viral copies in buccal swab samples, targeting a 124 bp region of the *pol* gene as previously described [31]. Primers and probes were designed using an alignment of available *pol* sequences from NP SFV, including representatives from all three NP families [1]. Briefly, one forward and one reverse primer were used (QSIP4Nmod (for) 5′-TGC ATT CCG ATC AAG GAT CAG C-3′ and QSIR1Nmod2 (rev) 5′- TTC CTT TCC ACY WTY CCA CTA CT-3′), with the probe DIAPR2 5′-FAM-TGG GGI TGG TAA GGA GTA CTG WAT TCC A-SpC6-3′. Following a 10 min incubation at 95 °C to activate Taq polymerase, a three-step PCR was performed at 95 °C for 15 sec, 50 °C for 15 sec, and 62 °C for 15 sec for 55 cycles using the 7500 Real-Time PCR platform (Applied Biosystems, Foster City, CA, USA). The sensitivity of the assay was 100 copies of SFV/reaction, as determined in [31].

To normalize the amount of diploid cells per reaction, the mean number of housekeeping gene ribonuclease P/MRP 30 kDa subunit (*RPP30*) copies of five *L. chrysomelas* swab samples (284 copies/ng) was used, as described previously [31]. Thus, since each cell has two copies of the RPP30 gene, the mean used was 142 cells/ng of DNA in buccal swab samples of *L. chrysomelas*.

2.4. Amplification of a Larger SFV Fragment from the Cebidae Family

For the positive samples in at least one of the SFV detection tests (diagnostic PCR or real-time PCR), one additional PCR was carried out to amplify a larger SFV subgenomic region for phylogenetic analysis. Despite the controversy about the number of NP families, the *Leontopithecus* genera was classified as part of the Cebidae family in the present report [11]. Primers were then designed using a conserved region of *pol* in an alignment of two SFV complete genomes representing the Cebidae family available at GenBank from marmoset and yellow-breasted capuchin (accession numbers GU356395 and KP143760, respectively) [7,9] and *pol* sequences generated by the diagnostic PCR test in this study as describe above. Briefly, the new nested PCR was performed using primers: (1° Round: *pol*5474 5′ GCCAAACATGAGAAAGGATG 3′ and *pol*5960 5′ TACCACTTTGTAGGTCTTCC 3′ with annealing temperature of 53.4 °C) and (2° Round: *pol*5500 5′ GTCATATCCGTAYGTGCAAAC 3′ and *pol*5878 5′CTTTGGGGGTGGTAAGG 3′ with annealing temperature of 56 °C), amplifying a 378 bp fragment.

In addition, primer combinations were tested in the 2° round above to analyze the amplification efficiency of the viral fragments. The *pol*5474 *and pol*5878 primers (annealing temperature of 54 °C), and *pol*5500 with *pol*5960 (annealing temperature of 56 °C) were combined, amplifying fragments of 404 bp and 460 bp, respectively. PCR were performed with an initial temperature of 94 °C, followed by 35 cycles of 94 °C for 30 seconds, primer annealing at temperatures varying according to the combination of primers for 30 sec and 72 °C for 90 sec. Products were sequenced by the Sanger method using and ABI 3130 XL automatic sequencer (Applied Biosystems) and primers of the second round.

2.5. Sequence Analysis

Generated sequences were submitted to the BLASTn tool (http://blast.ncbi.nlm.nih.gov) for similarity analysis with SFV sequences deposited at Genbank. SFV sequences were edited using the SeqMan program v.7.0 (DNASTAR, Madison, WI, USA) and aligned with NP SFV reference sequences deposited in GenBank using the BioEdit Sequence Alignment Editor v.7.0.4 [32]. From the alignment, a phylogenetic tree was generated with Mega7 [33], using the maximum likelihood method and the Tamura 3-parameter correction model with discrete gamma rate variation. The bootstrap method was used with 1000 replicates to estimate the reliability of the phylogenetic clusters. Values above 70% were considered significant [3]. A similarity analysis between SFVlcm strains in the *pol* sequence was conducted using the Maximum Composite Likelihood model. The analysis involved 13 nucleotide sequences. All positions containing gaps and missing data were stripped. There was a total of 263 nucleotide positions in the final dataset. Evolutionary analyses were conducted in MEGA7. The geographical distribution of the *L. chrysomelas* family groups was plotted using the coordinates of family groups using program RStudio [34] using package Leaflet OpenStreetMap® contributors under license Open Data Commons Open Database License (ODbL).

2.6. Statistical Analyses

To understand better the epidemiology of SFV in *L. chrysomelas*, differences in SFV prevalence were evaluated with Chi Square trend analysis for the following categories: males and females; and infants, juveniles and adults. We also divided the familiar groups according to the time elapsed between capture and collection: one group between 1 and 6 months of captivity time ($n = 63$) and another group between 7 and 14 months in captivity ($n = 29$). After logarithmic transformation of SFV viral load data, T-tests were performed to test for associations between viral loads and all the characteristics mentioned above. For low sample numbers ($n < 20$), the Fisher Exact Test was used to evaluate epidemiological prevalence between groups with different captivity times and the efficiency of amplification by the diagnostic PCR between the two strains of SFVlcm described in this study. For all these tests, p-values ≤ 0.05 were considered significant.

2.7. Data Availability

All SFV sequences generated herein have been deposited at GenBank with the accession numbers MN178627 to MN178637.

3. Results

3.1. Population Profile

Samples of 29 golden-headed lion tamarin family groups were collected in this study. The mean number of specimens captured was eight per group, ranging from three to 12, while the mean number of specimens collected was three by group, ranging from one to seven animals. Of the 92 animals collected at CPRJ, we found a higher proportion of males (56.5%) than females (43.5%) (Table 1). With respect to sexual maturity, the specimens analyzed were constituted largely by adults ($n = 45$; 49%), followed by juveniles ($n = 32$; 35%) and infants ($n = 15$; 16%). All gDNA samples extracted from buccal swabs were positive for the constitutive mitochondrial *cytB* gene, and therefore were considered suitable to the molecular tests for SFV detection and quantification.

Table 1. Comparison of simian foamy virus (SFV) prevalence estimates by quantitative PCR (qPCR) and conventional PCR (cPCR) in relation to sex and the sexual maturity of *L. chrysomelas*.

Characteristic	N (%)	qPCR+/cPCR+	qPCR+/cPCR-	qPCR-/cPCR+	qPCR-/cPCR-	SFV Prevalence (%)
Total	92	11 (12%)	17 (18.5%)	4 (4,3%)	73 (58%)	32/92 (34.8%)
Sex						
Male	52 (56.5%)	6 (11.5%)	8 (15.3%)	2 (4%)	36 (66.2%)	16/61 (30.7%)
Female	40 (43.5%)	5 (12.5%)	9 (22.5%)	2 (5%)	24 (60%)	16/40 (40%)
Sexual maturation						
Infants	15 (16%)	1 (6.7%)	3 (20%)	2 (13.3%)	9 (60%)	6/15 (40%)
Juveniles	32 (35%)	3 (9.4%)	7 (22%)	1 (3%)	21 (65.6%)	11/32 (34.4%)
Adults	45 (49%)	7 (15.5%)	7 (15.5%)	1 (2.2%)	30 (66.7%)	15/45 (33.3%)

3.2. SFV Molecular Detection and Quantification

A sample was considered positive for SFV infection when it tested positive in either one of the two molecular tests used (conventional diagnostic PCR and/or qPCR). Using this criterion, 15 samples (16.3%) were positive by diagnostic PCR and 28 (30.4%) were positive by qPCR (Table 1). When comparing the two assays, the results were 70% concordant. Of the discordant results, qPCR was more sensitive (17%) than the conventional diagnostic PCR (4%) ($p = 0.006$). Thus, 32/92 (34.8%) of the animals were considered infected with SFV (Table 1). Females and males presented similar SFV prevalence (40%) and (30.7%), respectively ($p = 0.483$). Regarding sexual maturity, no statistical difference was observed in the prevalence of SFV infection between different groups ($p = 0.502$) (Table 1). By grouping infants with juvenile specimens and comparing with adults, the SFV prevalence between immature and mature animals was very similar, 17/47 (36.2%) and 15/45 (33.3%), respectively ($p = 0.946$).

We sought to address whether the low sensitivity of the conventional diagnostic PCR was related to the lower number of SFV DNA copies of the negative samples for diagnostic PCR, but positive for qPCR, but there was no correlation between those conditions ($p = 0.175$). Among the 28 samples that had detectable SFV DNA VL, after normalization with the mean RPP30 copies in buccal swab cells, the mean VL was 4.7 log copies of SFV/10^6 cells, ranging from 3.47 to 5.98 log copies/10^6 cells. No differences were found between oral SFV DNA VL of males ($n = 14$) and females ($n = 14$) (mean of 4.7 log and 4.8 log copies/10^6 cells, respectively; $p = 0.735$). Regarding sexual maturity, the mean DNA VL were also similar between the different groups: infants ($n = 4$), juveniles ($n = 10$) and adults ($n = 14$) with means of 4.7, 4.6 and 4.7 log copies/10^6 cells, respectively ($p = 0.254$).

With respect to time in captivity, SFV prevalence was lower in animals kept in captivity within 1–6 months (25.4%; 16/63) than in animals that stay in captivity more than seven months (55.2%; 16/29) ($p = 0.005$) (Table 2). The SFV prevalence among females also differed in the two groups with 32% (9/28) in the former group and 66.6% (8/12) in the latter ($p = 0.042$). The same was observed to male infections, with 20% (7/35) in the shorter captivity group and 47.1% (8/17) in the longer captivity group ($p = 0.043$). The SFV prevalence was also higher in the longer captivity group among all different age groups. However, only in juveniles had SFV prevalence reached a borderline statistical significance ($p = 0.055$; Table 2).

Table 2. Comparison of SFV prevalence in relation to sex and sexual maturity of groups classified according to captivity time at Centro de Primatologia do Rio de Janeiro (CPRJ).

	1–6 Months	7–14 Months	p-Value
Gender			
Male	7/35 (20%)	8/17 (47%)	0.043
Female	9/28 (32%)	8/12 (67%)	0.042
Sexual Maturity			
Infants	4/12 (33%)	2/3 (67%)	0.525
Juveniles	4/19 (21%)	7/13 (54%)	0.055
Adults	8/32 (25%)	7/13 (54%)	0.062
Total	16/63(25%)	16/29 (55%)	0.005

3.3. Phylogenetic Analysis and Similarity of SFV from L. Chrysomelas

To perform a phylogenetic analysis and to infer the evolutionary history of the SFV that infect this population of *L. chrysomelas*, it was necessary to amplify larger PCR fragments. Of the 32 SFV previously positive samples, three samples amplified a 378 bp fragment with the 5500 and 5878 primer combination (see Methods); another six samples amplified a 404 bp fragment with the 5474 and 5878 primer combination and two additional samples amplified a 460 bp fragment with the 5500 and 5960 combination of primers tested in the second round PCR. Only two samples amplified for two different primer combinations (5500 and 5878; 5474 and 5878). However, for one of the samples (specimen 780), the two primer combinations amplified two distinct variants (Figure 1). In total, 10 animals amplified for larger region of *pol*. Due to a short sequence overlap of our generated sequences with the SFV *pol* sequences available from Genbank, the phylogenetic analysis was limited only to the five complete NP SFV genomes available in the literature. The analysis suggests there are two distinct lineages of SFV co-circulating in the population of *L. chrysomelas* analyzed; a major lineage, herein named SFVlcm-1 (described in red; Figure 1), formed a single clade that branches out of the other SFVs infecting the Cebidae family, and another lineage (SFVlcm-2; described in blue), formed a clade with SFV infecting *Sapajus xanthosternos* and *Callithrix jacchus* (Figure 1). As expected, both strains clustered within the viruses infecting the Cebidae family. When analyzing the PCR amplification efficiency of NP SFV between the two strains found, we observe that among SFVlcm-1 strain only 25% (2/8) amplified by the conventional diagnostic PCR, whereas SFVlcm-2 strain had 100% (2/2) of the strain PCR-amplified ($p = 0.520$).

The pairwise distance analysis showed that the sequences within each strain are similar to each other, with an average divergence of 1% within strain 1 and of 2.6% within strain 2. When comparing SFVlcm-1 to -2, the mean divergence between them was 11%, higher than when compared strain 1 to sequences of other representatives of the Cebidae family, 8.5% and 8.8% for *Sapajus* and *Callithrix*, respectively (Table 3).

3.4. Evaluation of SFV Transmission among Groups of L. chrysomelas

To investigate the eco-epidemiological profile of the SFV infection among the *L. chrysomelas* groups, a map was plotted using the GPS coordinates obtained during specimens' captures in the forest area of Niteroi city to analyze SFV distribution (Figure 2). The viral distribution among the family groups was widely disseminated in the population. The SFVlcm-1 strain was present in three spatially separated groups and the SFVlcm-2 strain was limited to a single group. All groups belonged to the central forest area (Figure 2).

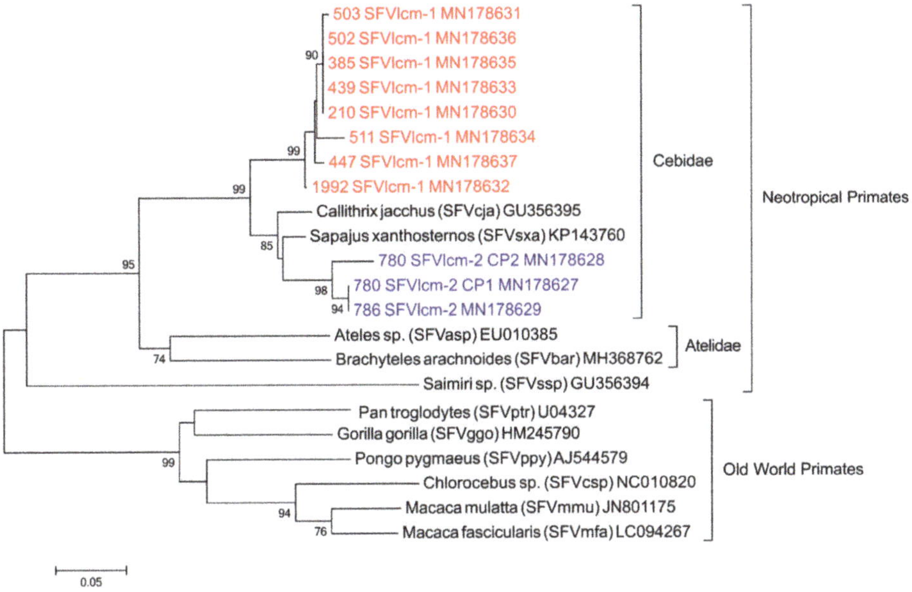

Figure 1. Platyrrhini SFV: phylogeny tree inferred using maximum likelihood analysis with a fragment of viral polymerase (360 bp). New sequences generated in the current study are marked in red (cluster SFVlcm-1) and in blue (cluster SFVlcm-2), all deposited at GenBank under the accession numbers MN178627 to MN178637. Bootstrap support was determined using 1000 nonparametric resampling replicates and values ≥ 70% are provided at nodes.

Table 3. Evolutionary divergence estimates between SFV sequences from Cebidae.

	1	2	3	4	5	6	7	8	9	10	11	12
1.210 SFVlcm-1												
2.385 SFVlcm-1	0.000											
3.439 SFVlcm-1	0.000	0.000										
4.447 SFVlcm-1	0.012	0.012	0.012									
5.502 SFVlcm-1	0.000	0.000	0.000	0.012								
6.503 SFVlcm-1	0.004	0.004	0.004	0.015	0.004							
7.511 SFVlcm-1	0.023	0.023	0.023	0.027	0.023	0.027						
8.1992 SFVlcm-1	0.011	0.011	0.011	0.015	0.011	0.015	0.035					
9.780 SFVlcm-2_CP1	0.116	0.116	0.116	0.107	0.116	0.121	0.106	0.103				
10.780 SFVlcm-2_CP2	0.125	0.125	0.125	0.116	0.125	0.130	0.120	0.121	0.039			
11.786 SFVlcm-2	0.116	0.116	0.116	0.107	0.116	0.121	0.106	0.103	0.000	0.039		
12.SFVsxa	0.090	0.090	0.090	0.077	0.090	0.094	0.076	0.077	0.051	0.081	0.051	
13.SFVcja	0.090	0.090	0.090	0.090	0.090	0.094	0.085	0.081	0.064	0.094	0.064	0.039

The number of nucleotide substitutions per site between sequences is shown. Standard error estimates are shown above the diagonal. Analyses were conducted using the Maximum Composite Likelihood model. The analysis involved 13 nucleotide sequences. Codon positions included were 1st + 2nd + 3rd. All positions containing gaps and missing data were stripped. There were a total of 263 nucleotide positions in the final dataset. Evolutionary analyses were conducted in MEGA7. The colors represent the viral strains: in red SFVlcm -1; blue SFVlcm-2 and gray the complete genomes of SFVsxa and SFVcja.

Interestingly, we observed that of the four solitary animals, three were infected by SFV (Figure 2). Three were males and one was female, with an SFV prevalence of SFV of 67% (2/3) and 100% (1/1), respectively. All the solitary animals were adults. These data suggest that errant males and females can contribute to the spread of SFV infection within this free-ranging primate population.

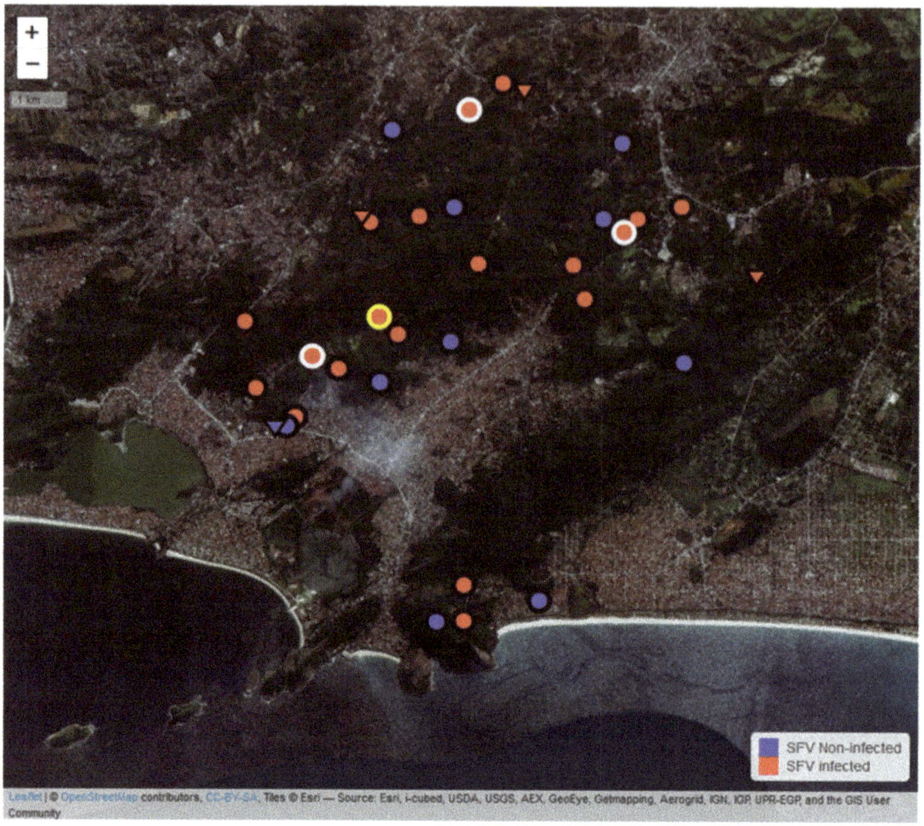

Figure 2. Eco-epidemiology of SFV in the *L. chrysomelas* family groups in the city of Niteroi/RJ. The location of each *L. chrysomelas* family group is represented by circles and of solitary animals by triangle. The red color represents infected animals or groups (when at least one animal is infected in the group), while the blue color represents the uninfected animals measured by conventional diagnostic PCR and/or quantitative PCR. Gray halos around the circles depict the presence of the SFVlcm-1 strain, while the yellow halo represents the SFVlcm-2 strain. The absence of halos indicates lack of amplification of the larger pol fragment, not allowing the classification in SFVlcm-1 or 2.

4. Discussion

The study of SFV in NP can be specially challenging due to the difficult access to free-living primates and limited volumes of blood that can be collected, since many specimens have a small size [29]. Moreover, of the 176 species of NP that circulate in Brazil, many are threatened to extinction [35]. To detect the SFV provirus, a high mass of genomic DNA (250–500 ng) is necessary from peripheral blood mononuclear cells [1], since blood cells are a recognized site of foamy virus latency [36]. Therefore, the use of buccal swabs is an important tool for SFV detection, since it preserves the animal's health and provides a higher viral load since the oral mucosa is a major SFV replication site [28,31]. Thus, alternative stress-relieving methods, such as buccal swab, are attractive sample sources for the study of SFV, mainly in small primates threatened to extinction.

In the more recently-captured subgroup studied here, an SFV prevalence of 25.4% was observed, similar to the one found in previous studies with free-living primates (14–30%) [2]. However, the SFV prevalence of the subgroup with longer time in captivity was much higher (55.2%), in agreement to the observed in captive Peruvian and Brazilian primates (45–51%) [2,3]. This increase in SFV prevalence among animals kept in captivity for longer occurred for both sexes and mainly among juveniles. Although this population of *L. chrysomelas* lived in a restricted fragment of Atlantic forest, favoring the contact between groups, the captivity environment clearly contributed to increased transmission of SFV. It is known that an environment that does not promote the welfare and interest of the animal can generate stress, which can be reflected in behavioral changes such as increased aggressiveness [37], but likely also in the susceptibility to infectious agents. Transmission of SFV can happen through blood transfusion [38], maternal milk [39] and mainly by biting and grooming [5]. Thus, stressful environments can collaborate for a higher dissemination of SFV between captive animals.

The area where these animals have occupied is very fragmented (Figure 2), and some areas are very close to urban areas, where many of these animals were seen close to household waste to feed [18]. The proximity between non-human primates and humans can contribute to a risk of SFV zoonotic transmission to the latter [25–27]. Although until now SFV is not known to cause disease in its natural hosts [5], the association of SFV infection with mild anemia was observed in humans [40]. Little yet is known about the transmissibility of SFV from NP to humans and their consequences, but, previous work by our group has shown prevalence rates of SFV zoonotic transmission to primate handlers using serological assays [25]. We are currently working with primate handler samples to deepen our knowledge of NP SFV zoonotic transmission.

When conventional diagnostic PCR was standardized, there were only three complete NP SFV genomes available at Genbank, and the sensitivity of the assay was measured at 100% in seven NP genera studied (*Cebus, Alouatta, Callithrix, Aotus, Ateles, Saimiri, Cacajao* and *Pithecia*) [1]. However, sensitivity drops too much for detecting SFV from other genera such as *Leontopithecus*. Therefore, a quantitative PCR was developed using all available NP SFV *pol* sequences as references for degenerate primer design that amplifies a smaller and more conserved *pol* gene region. This assay was able to detect SFV in two additional species of *Leontopithecus*, and in one species each of *Callimico* and *Saguinus* previously found to be SFV-negative using the conventional diagnostic PCR assay [31]. As demonstrated previously [31], the qPCR was shown to be more sensitive than the conventional diagnostic PCR for detection of NP SFV, When correlating the number of SFV copies with the sensitivity of conventional diagnostic PCR, similar to what has been observed for feline FV [41], no association was found. These results suggest that the false negatives in the conventional PCR may be due to a high genetic heterogeneity of NP SFV sequences at primer locations determined previously to be 41% in the virus *pol* region [1].

SFV DNA VL comprises both the integrated virus (provirus) and the genomic DNA of the virus particle, since SFV can produce both DNA and RNA particles [5]. Little is known about the standards of the DNA VL in the oral mucosa of NP. A recent study [31] found a mean viral load of 4.7 log SFV copies/10^6 cells among 23 NP specimens of 12 different species in captivity, including four *L. chrysomelas* specimens [31], similar to that has been found in this study. However, when comparing the VL of only four *L. chrysomelas* and one *L. rosalia* quantifiable for SFV of the previous study (range 2.9–7.3 log SFV copies/10^6 cells), the variation was much higher than the one observed in this study (standard deviation 0.62), which can be explained by differences in sample size. In addition, no association was found regarding the viral load and the sex of the animal, also as observed in the previous study. Finally, also as in the previous study [31], we could not observe any age-related viral load trends in buccal swab samples. These results differ from those reported for rhesus macaques, in which viral load increases with age in the oral cavity of the animals [36]. However, it should be noted that we quantified VL DNA instead of VL RNA, as reported in the rhesus study, and that may explain such lack of correlation observed here. Another important issue is that Liu et al. [24] tested 173 fecal samples from wild chimpanzees (including 87 SFVcpz RNA-positive samples), and none of them detected viral DNA. DNA genome particle production may not reflect replication *in vivo*, and may represent an *in vitro* artifact when using tumor cells with high dNTP levels. Thus, it is unclear whether the viral detection tests (conventional diagnostic PCR and quantitative PCR) in this study are also detecting viral DNA but only proviral DNA.

When comparing the impact of different demographic factors on SFV prevalence, either in the population or in subgroups according to the captivity time, we observed that, as described by others [1–3], the animal sex does not seem to influence SFV acquisition. Yet it has been reported that SFV prevalence increases with age [3,39], no such correlation was observed here. This homogenization in the prevalence between the age groups can be explained, at least in part, by the social behavior of *Leontopithecus*. Group members do social grooming, all members of the family groups help to carry the offspring of the alpha couple and in nature (or captivity), all individuals sleep together, often in the hollows of trees [42], intensifying the contact between them and consequently the chance of SFV transmission. Another interesting ecological characteristic of many NP like *L. chrysomelas*, upon reaching maturity and especially males, is to leave their groups to form a new family group to avoid consanguinity [42]. Interestingly, of the four solitary animals, three were infected, even though they were kept isolated after months at CPRJ since their capture in the wild, showing that these animals may contribute to the dissemination of SFV in the population by entering into existing groups or forming new groups. Our results demonstrate for the first time a new SFV transmission dynamics in primates, on an ecological scale, highlighting the importance of molecular and ecological virology studies in free-living primates.

The use of primers for PCR amplification of larger fragments of the SFV LTR-*gag* region and the *pol* region from previous studies showed a low efficiency to amplify SFV from *L. chrysomelas* [1,3], indicating that SFVlcm can harbor a high nucleotide heterogeneity, at least in the region of primer annealing. To amplify larger DNA fragments, we developed new PCR primers only using sequences of representative SFV genomes infecting primates of Cebidae family to increase specificity. However, the new PCR amplified only 24% of samples diagnosed as SFV-positive, suggesting that there may be more variants circulating in the population, requiring more sensitive techniques, such as shotgun next-generation sequencing, to amplify the complete genomes of these viruses [6].

Phylogenetic analysis showed that, unlike a previous study [3] where a SFV sequence of *L. chrysomelas* clustered with SFV infecting Pitheciidae family members, all SFV sequences from *L. chrysomelas* here in generated grouped into the Cebidae family, which is expected according to the co-speciation hypothesis [4]. However, two distinct lineages of SFVlcm were observed. The most frequent, which formed a separate clade, was named SFVlcm-1, while the other, SFVlcm-2, formed a clade with SFVsxa and SFVcja, infecting *Sapajus xanthosternos* and *Callithrix jacchus*, respectively (Figure 1). The nucleotide divergence between the two strains was 11%, although this refers to a small fragment of the viral *pol* gene, which is conserved among SFVs. Since an earlier study has reported the occurrence of cross-species transmission between *L. chrysomelas*, *Sapajus xanthosthernos* and Pitheciidae species [3], cross-species transmission between species may have occurred in the Atlantic forest fragment where *L. chrysomelas* lives, where there are reports of other PN species, such as *Callithrix jacchus*. Another possibility could indicate that these variants came from cross-species transmission events prior to the arrival of the specimens in Niteroi/RJ, since in the endemic area of Bahia there are also other species of primates, as black-tufted marmoset (*Callithrix penicillata*) and yellow-breasted capuchin monkey (*Sapajus xanthosthernos*). However, as the phylogenetic inference of the two lineages was limited to only five complete NP SFV genomes available in the literature, of only two NP families, and was based on short *pol* sequences, we cannot assess whether the SFVlcm-2 clade was derived from a recombination event between SFVlcm-1 and an SFV from another species, as it has been already described in SFV-Infected Old World monkeys [43]. These alternative scenarios turn the understanding of the complete evolutionary history of the SFV infecting *L. chrysomelas* a difficult task at the moment. This issue will only be clarified with the amplification of larger SFV sequences or complete genomes from *L. chrysomelas* derived from the native population of Bahia and other NP SFV representatives.

In conclusion, we have demonstrated here for the first time an increase in the SFV prevalence of recently-captive *L. chrysomelas*, including the characterization of two novel SFV strains, SFVlcm-1 and -2, by using oral swab as an efficient alternative non-invasive method. We also present new ecological dynamics of SFV transmission from infected solitary animals that dispersed to form new groups or joined existing groups. Further studies are needed to fully characterize the SFV variants in this species, only preliminarily described here, which will improve our understanding of retroviral infections in the Platyrrhini parvorder, covering all primates of the Americas.

Author Contributions: Conceptualization, A.F.S., M.A.S., A.P.; methodology, T.S.M., C.P.M., S.B.M., M.G.B.; validation, S.B.M., M.G.B., M.C.K.; formal analysis, T.S.M., C.V.M., M.A.S., A.F.S.; investigation, T.S.M., C.V.M., M.S., A.F.S.; resources, J.L.C.-D., M.A.S., A.F.S.; data curation, T.S.M., C.V.M., S.B.M., M.G.B., M.C.M.K.; writing—original draft preparation, T.S.M., M.A.S., A.F.S.; writing—review and editing, T.S.M., S.B.M., M.G.B., M.C.M.K., A.P., M.A.S., A.F.S.; supervision, M.A.S., A.F.S.; project administration, M.A.S., A.F.S.; funding acquisition, M.C.M.K., J.L.C.-D., A.P., M.A.S., A.F.S.

Funding: This study was supported by the Brazilian Research Council (CNPq; grant 312903/2017-0 to A.F.S.) and by the Rio de Janeiro State Science Foundation (FAPERJ; grant E-26/112.647/2012 to MAS and grant E-26/202.738/2018 to A.F.S.).

Acknowledgments: We are grateful to Pri-Matas team and CPRJ/INEA collaborators who assisted in providing samples and biogeographical data. We would also like to thank all the institutions and organizations which provided financial support for the Tamarins Translocation Project including the Fundação Grupo O Boticario, the Lion Tamarin of Brazil Fund, the Primate Action Fund, the Margot Marsh Foundation, The Mohamed bin Zayed Species Conservation Fund, Câmara de Compensação Ambiental/ Secretaria de Estado do Ambiente e Sustentabilidade - SEAS (RBO Energia e Porto Sudeste, the Tropical Forest Conservation Act/ Fundo Brasileiro para Biodiversidade (TFCA/FUNBIO)—Rio de Janeiro.

Conflicts of Interest: We declare no conflicts of financial or personal interests.

References

1. Muniz, C.P.; Troncoso, L.L.; Moreira, M.A.; Soares, E.A.; Pissinatti, A.; Bonvicino, C.R.; Seuánez, H.N.; Sharma, B.; Jia, H.; Shankar, A.; et al. Identification and Characterization of Highly Divergent Simian Foamy Viruses in a Wide Range of New World Primates from Brazil. *PLoS ONE* **2013**, *8*, e67568. [CrossRef] [PubMed]
2. Ghersi, B.M.; Jia, H.; Aiewsakun, P.; Katzourakis, A.; Mendoza, P.; Bausch, D.G.; Kasper, M.R.; Montgomery, J.M.; Switzer, W.M. Wide distribution and ancient evolutionary history of simian foamy viruses in New World primates. *Retrovirology* **2015**, *12*, 89. [CrossRef] [PubMed]
3. Muniz, C.P.; Jia, H.; Shankar, A.; Troncoso, L.L.; Augusto, A.M.; Farias, E.; Pissinatti, A.; Fedullo, L.P.; Santos, A.F.; Soares, M.A.; et al. An expanded search for simian foamy viruses (SFV) in Brazilian New World primates identifies novel SFV lineages and host age-related infections. *Retrovirology* **2015**, *12*, 94. [CrossRef] [PubMed]
4. Switzer, W.M.; Salemi, M.; Shanmugam, V.; Gao, F.; Cong, M.E.; Kuiken, C.; Bhullar, V.; Beer, B.E.; Vallet, D.; Gautier-Hion, A.; et al. Ancient co-speciation of simian foamy viruses and primates. *Nature* **2005**, *434*, 376. [CrossRef] [PubMed]
5. Pinto-Santini, D.M.; Stenbak, C.R.; Linial, M.L. Foamy virus zoonotic infections. *Retrovirology* **2017**, *14*, 55. [CrossRef] [PubMed]
6. Muniz, C.P.; Cavalcante, L.T.F.; Dudley, D.M.; Pissinatti, A.; O'Connor, D.H.; Santos, A.F.; Soares, M.A. First Complete Genome Sequence of a Simian Foamy Virus Infecting the Neotropical Primate Brachyteles arachnoides. *Microbiol. Resour. Announc.* **2018**, *7*, e00839-18. [CrossRef] [PubMed]
7. Troncoso, L.L.; Muniz, C.P.; Siqueira, J.D.; Curty, G.; Schrago, C.G.; Augusto, A.; Fedullo, L.; Soares, M.A.; Santos, A.F. Characterization and comparative analysis of a simian foamy virus complete genome isolated from Brazilian capuchin monkeys. *Virus Res.* **2015**, *208*, 1–6. [CrossRef]
8. Thümer, L.; Rethwilm, A.; Holmes, E.C.; Bodem, J. The complete nucleotide sequence of a New World simian foamy virus. *Virology* **2007**, *369*, 191–197. [CrossRef]
9. Pacheco, B.; Finzi, A.; McGee-Estrada, K.; Sodroski, J. Species-Specific Inhibition of Foamy Viruses from South American Monkeys by New World Monkey TRIM5 Proteins. *J. Virol.* **2010**, *84*, 4095–4099. [CrossRef] [PubMed]
10. Rylands, A.B.; Mittermeier, R.A. *Taxonomic Listing of the New World Primates*; IUCN Species Survival Commission (SSC) Primate Specialist Group (PSG): Austin, TX, USA, 2019.
11. Perelman, P.; Johnson, W.E.; Roos, C.; Seuánez, H.N.; Horvath, J.E.; Moreira, M.A.M.; Kessing, B.; Pontius, J.; Roelke, M.; Rumpler, Y.; et al. A molecular phylogeny of living primates. *PLoS Genet.* **2011**, *7*, e1001342. [CrossRef]

12. Hooks, J.J.; Gibbs, C.J.; Chou, S.; Howk, R.; Lewis, M.; Gajdusek, D.C. Isolation of a new simian foamy virus from a spider monkey brain culture. *Infect. Immun.* **1973**, *8*, 804–813. [PubMed]
13. Moreira, M.A.M.; Bonvicino, C.R.; Soares, M.A.; Seuánez, H.N. Genetic diversity of neotropical primates: Phylogeny, population genetics, and animal models for infectious diseases. *Cytogenet. Genome Res.* **2010**, *128*, 88–98. [CrossRef] [PubMed]
14. IUCN. *IUCN Red List of Threatened Species. Version 2016-2. Fourth Quart*; IUCN: Gland, Switzerland, 2016.
15. Moraes, A.M.; Grativol, A.D.; De Vleeschouwer, K.M.; Ruiz-Miranda, C.R.; Raboy, B.E.; Oliveira, L.C.; Dietz, J.M.; Galbusera, P.H.A. Population Genetic Structure of an Endangered Endemic Primate (Leontopithecus chrysomelas) in a Highly Fragmented Atlantic Coastal Rain Forest. *Folia Primatol.* **2018**, *89*, 365–381. [CrossRef] [PubMed]
16. Kierulf, C. Golden-headed lion tamarins invaders in Niteroi – when an endangered species became a threat. *Tamarin Tales* **2015**, *13*, 1–3.
17. Dos Santos, A.V.P.; de Souza, A.M.; de Machado, C.S.C.; Bueno, M.G.; Catao-Dias, J.L.; Campos, S.D.E.; Knackfuss, F.B.; Pissinatti, A.; Kierulff, M.C.M.; Silva DG de, F.; et al. Hematological evaluation of free-living golden-headed lion tamarins (Leontopithecus chrysomelas) from an Urban Atlantic Forest. *J. Med. Primatol.* **2019**, *48*, 106–113. [CrossRef] [PubMed]
18. Molina, C.V.; Heinemann, M.B.; Kierulff, C.; Pissinatti, A.; da Silva, T.F.; de Freitas, D.G.; de Souza, G.O.; Miotto, B.A.; Cortez, A.; de Semensato, B.P.; et al. Leptospira spp., rotavirus, norovirus, and hepatitis E virus surveillance in a wild invasive golden-headed lion tamarin (Leontopithecus chrysomelas; Kuhl, 1820) population from an urban park in Niterói, Rio de Janeiro, Brazil. *Am. J. Primatol.* **2019**, *81*, e22961. [CrossRef] [PubMed]
19. Dos Santos, A.V.P.; de Souza, A.M.; Bueno, M.G.; Catao-Dias, J.L.; Toma, H.K.; Pissinati, A.; Molina, C.V.; Kierulff, M.C.M.; Silva, D.G.F.; Almosny, N.R.P. Molecular detection of Borrelia burgdorferi in free-living golden headed lion tamarins (Leontopithecus chrysomelas) in Rio de Janeiro, Brazil. *Rev. Inst. Med. Trop. Sao Paulo* **2018**, *60*. [CrossRef]
20. Aitken, E.H.; Bueno, M.G.; Dos Santos Ortolan, L.; Alvaréz, J.M.; Pissinatti, A.; Kierulff, M.C.M.; Catão-Dias, J.L.; Epiphanio, S. Survey of Plasmodium in the golden-headed lion tamarin (Leontopithecus chrysomelas) living in urban Atlantic forest in Rio de Janeiro, Brazil. *Malar J.* **2016**, *15*, 93. [CrossRef]
21. Feistner, A.T.C.; Askew, J.A.; Hyde Roberts, S.; Radford, L.; Williamson, E. Book Review: The International Encyclopedia of Primatology. *Folia Primatol.* **2018**. [CrossRef]
22. Gogarten, J.F.; Akoua-Koffi, C.; Calvignac-Spencer, S.; Leendertz, S.A.J.; Weiss, S.; Couacy-Hymann, E.; Koné, I.; Peeters, M.; Wittig, R.M.; Boesch, C.; et al. The ecology of primate retroviruses—An assessment of 12 years of retroviral studies in the Taï national park area, Côte d'Ivoire. *Virology* **2014**, *460*, 147–153. [CrossRef]
23. Leendertz, F.H.; Zirkel, F.; Couacy-Hymann, E.; Ellerbrok, H.; Morozov, V.A.; Pauli, G.; Hedemann, C.; Formenty, P.; Jensen, S.A.; Boesch, C.; et al. Interspecies Transmission of Simian Foamy Virus in a Natural Predator-Prey System. *J. Virol.* **2018**, *82*, 7741–7744. [CrossRef] [PubMed]
24. Liu, W.; Worobey, M.; Li, Y.; Keele, B.F.; Bibollet-Ruche, F.; Guo, Y.; Goepfert, P.A.; Santiago, M.L.; Ndjango, J.B.N.; Neel, C.; et al. Molecular ecology and natural history of Simian foamy virus infection in wild-living chimpanzees. *PLoS Pathog.* **2008**, *4*, e1000097. [CrossRef] [PubMed]
25. Muniz, C.P.; Cavalcante, L.T.F.; Jia, H.; Zheng, H.Q.; Tang, S.; Augusto, A.M.; Pissinatti, A.; Fedullo, L.P.; Santos, A.F.; Soares, M.A.; et al. Zoonotic infection of Brazilian primate workers with New World simian foamy virus. *PLoS ONE* **2017**, *12*, e0184502. [CrossRef] [PubMed]
26. Mouinga-Ondeme, A.; Caron, M.; Nkoghe, D.; Telfer, P.; Marx, P.; Saib, A.; Leroy, E.; Gonzalez, J.-P.; Gessain, A.; Kazanji, M. Cross-Species Transmission of Simian Foamy Virus to Humans in Rural Gabon, Central Africa. *J. Virol.* **2012**, *86*, 1255–1260. [CrossRef] [PubMed]
27. Khan, A.S. Simian foamy virus infection in humans: Prevalence and management. *Expert Rev. Anti Infect. Ther.* **2009**, *7*, 569–580. [CrossRef] [PubMed]
28. Murray, S.M.; Picker, L.J.; Axthelm, M.K.; Hudkins, K.; Alpers, C.E.; Linial, M.L. Replication in a Superficial Epithelial Cell Niche Explains the Lack of Pathogenicity of Primate Foamy Virus Infections. *J. Virol.* **2008**, *82*, 5981–5985. [CrossRef]
29. Rylands, A.B.; Anzenberger, G. Introduction: New World Primates. *Int. Zoo Yearb.* **2012**, *46*. [CrossRef]
30. Pinto, L.P.S.; Rylands, A.B. Geographic distribution of the golden-headed lion tamarin, leontopithecus chrysomelas: Implications for its management and conservation. *Folia Primatol.* **1997**, *68*, 161–180. [CrossRef]

31. Muniz, C.P.; Zheng, H.Q.; Jia, H.; Cavalcante, L.T.F.; Augusto, A.M.; Fedullo, L.P.; Pissinatti, A.; Soares, M.A.; Switzer, W.M.; Santos, A.F. A non-invasive specimen collection method and a novel simian foamy virus (SFV) DNA quantification assay in New World primates reveal aspects of tissue tropism and improved SFV detection. *PLoS ONE* **2017**, *12*, e0184251. [CrossRef]
32. Phillips, J.L.; Gnanakaran, S. BioEdit: An important software for molecular biology. *Proteins Struct Funct Bioinforma.* **2015**, *2*, 60–61.
33. Kumar, S.; Stecher, G.; Tamura, K. MEGA7: Molecular Evolutionary Genetics Analysis Version 7.0 for Bigger Datasets Brief communication. *Mol. Biol. Evol.* **2016**, *33*, 1870–1874. [CrossRef] [PubMed]
34. RStudio Team. *RStudio: Integrated Development for R [Computer Software]*; RStudio, Inc.: Boston, MA, USA, 2015.
35. Estrada, A.; Garber, P.A.; Mittermeier, R.A.; Wich, S.; Gouveia, S.; Dobrovolski, R.; Nekaris, K.A.I.; Nijman, V.; Rylands, A.B.; Maisels, F.; et al. Primates in peril: The significance of Brazil, Madagascar, Indonesia and the Democratic Republic of the Congo for global primate conservation. *PeerJ* **2018**, *6*, e4869. [CrossRef] [PubMed]
36. Soliven, K.; Wang, X.; Small, C.T.; Feeroz, M.M.; Lee, E.-G.; Craig, K.L.; Hasan, K.; Engel, G.A.; Jones-Engel, L.; Matsen, F.A.; et al. Simian Foamy Virus Infection of Rhesus Macaques in Bangladesh: Relationship of Latent Proviruses and Transcriptionally Active Viruses. *J. Virol.* **2013**, *87*, 13628–13639. [CrossRef]
37. Ceballos, M.C.; Sant'Anna, A.C. Evolução da ciência do bem-estar animal: Uma breve revisão sobre aspectos conceituais e metodológicos. *Rev. Acad. Ciênc. Anim.* **2018**, *16*, 1–24. [CrossRef]
38. Brooks, J.I.; Merks, H.W.; Fournier, J.; Boneva, R.S.; Sandstrom, P.A. Characterization of blood-borne transmission of simian foamy virus. *Transfusion* **2007**, *47*, 162–170. [CrossRef]
39. Blasse, A.; Calvignac-Spencer, S.; Merkel, K.; Goffe, A.S.; Boesch, C.; Mundry, R.; Leendertz, F.H. Mother-Offspring Transmission and Age-Dependent Accumulation of Simian Foamy Virus in Wild Chimpanzees. *J. Virol.* **2013**, *87*, 5193–5204. [CrossRef]
40. Buseyne, F.; Betsem, E.; Montange, T.; Njouom, R.; Bilounga Ndongo, C.; Hermine, O.; Gessain, A. Clinical Signs and Blood Test Results among Humans Infected with Zoonotic Simian Foamy Virus: A Case-Control Study. *J. Infect. Dis.* **2018**, *218*, 144–151. [CrossRef]
41. Cavalcante, L.T.F.; Muniz, C.P.; Jia, H.; Augusto, A.M.; Troccoli, F.; de Medeiros, S.O.; Dias, C.G.A.; Switzer, W.M.; Soares, M.A.; Santos, A.F. Clinical and molecular features of feline foamy virus and feline leukemia virus co-infection in naturally-infected cats. *Viruses* **2018**, *10*, 702. [CrossRef]
42. Review, B. Lion Tamarins-Biology and Conservation. *Folia Primatol.* **2004**, *75*, 383–384.
43. Richard, L.; Rua, R.; Betsem, E.; Mouinga-Ondémé, A.; Kazanji, M.; Leroy, E.; Njouom, R.; Buseyne, F.; Afonso, P.V.; Gessain, A. Cocirculation of Two env Molecular Variants, of Possible Recombinant Origin, in Gorilla and Chimpanzee Simian Foamy Virus Strains from Central Africa. *J. Virol.* **2015**, *89*, 12480–12491. [CrossRef]

viruses

MDPI

Article

Infection with Foamy Virus in Wild Ruminants—Evidence for a New Virus Reservoir?

Magdalena Materniak-Kornas [1,*], Martin Löchelt [2], Jerzy Rola [3] and Jacek Kuźmak [1]

1. Department of Biochemistry, National Veterinary Research Institute, 24-100 Pulawy, Poland; jkuzmak@piwet.pulawy.pl
2. German Cancer Research Center DKFZ, Program Infection, Inflammation and Cancer, Division of Viral Transformation Mechanisms, 69120 Heidelberg, Germany; m.loechelt@dkfz.de
3. Department of Virology, National Veterinary Research Institute, 24-100 Pulawy, Poland; jrola@piwet.pulawy.pl

* Correspondence: magdalena.materniak@piwet.pulawy.pl; Tel.: +48-81-889-3116

Received: 18 October 2019; Accepted: 31 December 2019; Published: 3 January 2020

Abstract: Foamy viruses (FVs) are widely distributed and infect many animal species including non-human primates, horses, cattle, and cats. Several reports also suggest that other species can be FV hosts. Since most of such studies involved livestock or companion animals, we aimed to test blood samples from wild ruminants for the presence of FV-specific antibodies and, subsequently, genetic material. Out of 269 serum samples tested by ELISA with the bovine foamy virus (BFV) Gag and Bet antigens, 23 sera showed increased reactivity to at least one of them. High reactive sera represented 30% of bison samples and 7.5% of deer specimens. Eleven of the ELISA-positives were also strongly positive in immunoblot analyses. The peripheral blood DNA of seroreactive animals was tested by semi-nested PCR. The specific 275 bp fragment of the *pol* gene was amplified only in one sample collected from a red deer and the analysis of its sequence showed the highest homology for European BFV isolates. Such results may suggest the existence of a new FV reservoir in bison as well as in deer populations. Whether the origin of such infections stems from a new FV or is the result of BFV inter-species transmission remains to be clarified.

Keywords: foamy viruses; BFV; wild ruminants; European bison; red deer; roe deer; fallow deer; seroreactivity; inter-species transmission

---

1. Introduction

Foamy viruses (FVs), also known as spumaviruses, are the least known subfamily of *Retroviridae* [1]. Some features of their replication pathway and complex genomic organization distinguish them from other retroviruses [2,3]. Infections with FVs are persistent with sustained antibody response against viral antigens and the presence of viral DNA in leukocytes [4]. The most likely routes of FV transmission are via the transfer of blood and saliva and social interactions [3,5–7]. Over the last 60 years, FVs have been isolated and described in different species of non-human primates (Simian FVs (SFVs)) [8], as well as in cattle (Bovine FV (BFV), in the past also called bovine syncytial virus (BSV)) [9,10], cats (Feline FV (FFV)) and horses (Equine FV (EFV)) [3,11]. Several other non-primate FVs have been reported as having been isolated or simply described in sea lions, leopards, sheep, goats, hamsters, and American bison on the basis of cross-antigenicity with known FV, specific cytopathic effects or electron microscopy analyses [10,12–16]. Although FVs can be commonly isolated from infected animals, no disease has been associated with infections and, therefore, FVs are recognized as apathogenic on their own [17,18]. This lack of pathogenicity contrasts strongly with the cytopathic effects seen in vitro in infected cell cultures, with the appearance of "foamy-like" syncytia [17,19]. Based on the detection of diverse SFVs in simian-exposed humans, many studies have been focused on the inter-species transmission of FVs from simian and non-simian FVs [18,19]. While infections of humans by FVs from different simians and non-human primates are well evidenced, little is presently known about the possibility of such inter-species transmission caused by FVs of live-stock animals. Since BFV is highly prevalent within cattle populations [3,7,20], special attention should be paid to the possible involvement of BFV in inter-species transmission, especially regarding free-ranging wild ruminants. This is a very important and pertinent issue, owing to increasing human impact on the environment, globalization, and the establishment of breeding of some wild ruminants posing new threats including the uncontrolled transmission of infectious agents into wildlife [21,22]. There are many examples of highly prevalent life-stock viral pathogens crossing species barriers into wild ruminants, including bovine respiratory viruses like parainfluenza virus (BPIV-3), bovine adenovirus (BAdV), or bovine respiratory syncytial virus (BRSV) infecting European bison (*Bison bonasus*) in Poland [23]. The most important alphaherpesvirus, bovine herpesvirus 1 (BoHV) have also been reported to infect almost 40% of cervids in Poland [24], and a low percentage of the bison population [25]. Inter-species infections with ruminant retroviruses have been also reported previously: Bovine leukemia virus (BLV) infections have occasionally been described in European bison [25] or alpaca (*Vicugna pacos*) [26], while small ruminant lentiviruses (SRLV) infections have been found in Rocky Mountain goats (*Oreamnos americanus*) [27], Passirian goat in northen Italy [28] and recently in red deer (*Cervus elaphus*) and muflon (*Ovis aries musimon*) in Spain [29]. All reported cases are most likely due to the spill-over from domestic animals, acquired similarly to the well documented case of SRLV infection of endangered wild ibex (*Capra ibex*) in the French Alps, which was probably a result of sharing grazing grounds with a small herd of heavily infected goats [30].

The goal of the current study was the detection of antibodies and genetic material of BFV or a related FV in blood samples collected from free-ranging wild ruminants in Poland in order to address questions related to inter-species transmissions and altered pathogenicity in the new host or as part of a changed virome/microbiome.

2. Materials and Methods

2.1. Animal Samples

The samples used in this study came from 269 wild ruminants (suborder: *Ruminantia*, within the order of even-toed ungulates, *Artiodactyla*). Out of those, 256 samples were collected from cervids (family of *Cervidae*) including red deer (*Cervus elaphus*, n = 134), roe deer (*Capreolus capreolus*, n = 103), or fallow deer (*Dama dama*, n = 19), and 13 from free-ranging bovides (family of *Bovidae*), the highly endangered European bison (*Bison bonasus*). The serum samples of European bison and 18 fallow deer had been deposited as archival samples in the Departments of Biochemistry and Virology, NVRI, respectively. Whole blood samples were collected from the main vein or aorta of red deer and roe deer mainly as blood clots during seasonal hunting. All specimens were collected during the 2009/2010 hunting season. Blood clots were squeezed through sterile gauze and centrifuged for 15 min. at 3000 rpm. Obtained supernatants were collected for serological testing and pellets containing blood cells were washed twice with PBS and frozen at −70 °C until DNA preparation.

2.2. DNA Preparation

Total DNA was extracted from pelleted blood cells using the DNeasy Blood & Tissue Kit (Qiagen, Hilden, Germany) following the manufacturer's instructions. DNA concentrations and the 260 nm/280 nm ratio were measured spectrophotometrically using GeneQuant (GE Healthcare, Warsaw, Poland) and stored at −20 °C until use. The DNA quality of selected samples was tested using capillary electrophoresis with highly sensitive gel (Fragment Analyser, Agilent).

2.3. Antibody Detection

GST (glutathione S-transferase) capture ELISAs were performed to examine the antibody response to BFV proteins in sera of wild ruminants using a well-established and validated generic GST-ELISA for domestic cattle as described by Romen and co-workers [7]. In short, 96-well microtiter plates (Thermo Labsystems, Dreieich, Germany) were coated with glutathione casein, blocked with 0.2% (*w/v*) casein and 0.05% (*v/v*) Tween 20 in PBS (blocking buffer), and then incubated with cleared *E. coli* lysates at a concentration of 0.25 µg/µL (total lysate in blocking buffer) containing the GST-tag or GST-X-tag fusion proteins (X = BFV-Gag, BFV-Bet, or BFV-Env). For pre-absorption of GST-binding antibodies, all sera were incubated at a dilution of 1:100 in a blocking buffer containing 2 µg/µL total lysate of a GST-tag expressing *E. coli* culture prior to application on the coated plates. After pre-absorption serum samples were incubated for 1 h at RT in the coated ELISA plate wells, washed, and incubated for 1 h at RT with Protein G—peroxidase conjugate (Sigma, 1:10,000 dilution). Protein G has a broad binding capacity for ruminant IgG [31]. TMB (Tetramethylbenzidine, Sigma, Poznan, Poland) was added as a substrate. For each serum, the absorbance of the GST-tag was determined and subtracted from the absorbance with the GST-X-tag protein to calculate the specific reactivity against the BFV antigens. Optical density (OD) measurements were done in duplicates and antibody levels were expressed as average net OD. As positive and negative internal controls, the pool of serum samples from five BFV naturally infected cows and five uninfected animals, diagnosed by GST-ELISA and PCR tests [32], were used at 1:100 dilutions.

Due to the lack of positive and negative controls from wild ruminants, cut-off values were calculated from the ELISA results for BFV Gag and Bet antigens obtained for cervids and European bison, excluding 3 outliers of bison origin and 9 outliers of cervid origin. These criteria resulted in 10 samples from European bison and 247 from cervids. The calculation was done in two ways: a less stringent cut-off was calculated as 1 × (mean + 3SD) and a highly stringent one as 2 × (mean + 3SD), which provided two cut-off values for each antigen, both methods are commonly used for diagnostic ELISA tests where defined negative and positive controls from the species tested are not available [33].

2.4. Western Blotting Analysis

Cf2Th cells (canine fetal thymus cells, Cat. No. 90110521, European Collection of Authenticated Cell Cultures (ECACC), UK) were co-cultured with BFV100-infected Cf2Th cells in a proportion of 10 to 1 and grown in DMEM, supplemented with 10% fetal bovine serum in the 5% CO_2 atmosphere. Three days after infection, when the cytopathic effect appeared, cells were lysed using a CHAPS buffer (0.5 M EDTA, 1 M Tris HCL pH 8.8, 100 mM NaCl, 0.5 M CHAPS, 0.5 M sodium deoxycholate; Sigma, Poznan, Poland). Uninfected Cf2Th cells were grown under the same condition. Of the total cell lysates, 10 µg of infected and uninfected control cells were separated by SDS-PAGE and served as the antigen for western blotting analyses (WB) [4]. Wild ruminant sera were used at 1:100 dilutions (*v/v* in 3% bovine albumin, 0.01% Tween 20, PBS) and Protein G–peroxidase conjugate (Sigma, Poznan, Poland) at 1:10,000 dilution. As positive and negative controls, the pools of serum samples from five BFV naturally infected cows and five uninfected animals, diagnosed by GST-ELISA and PCR tests [32], were used at 1:100 dilutions. ECL Plus reagents (GE Healthcare, Warsaw, Poland) were used for the detection of specifically bound antibodies.

2.5. FVs DNA Detection, Cloning, and Sequencing

Semi-nested polymerase chain reaction (PCR) was performed using genomic DNA from blood cells of 16 red and roe deer selected based on high reactivity in ELISA and the availability of high DNA quality, which was confirmed using a capillary system with highly sensitive gel (Fragment Analyser, Agilent). A set of external primers: BFVpolF1: TGGGAAAACCAGGTCGGACATC, BFVpolR: TACGACATCTGCTGTAAACAATGC, FFVpolF1: TGGGGAGAATCAGGTGGGTCATA and FFVpolR: TACAACATCTCCAGTAAACAACCC,

EFVpolF1: TGGGAAAATCAAGTGGGACATA, EFVpolR: TACAACATCTGCAGTAAATAAGGC and internal primers: BFVpolF2: ATGGACGCTGGAGGATGGTGTTAGAC, FFVpolF2: ATGGTCGCTGGAGAATGGTACTGGAC and EFVpolF2: ATGGACGATGGAGAATGGTACTGGAT (Genomed, Warsaw, Poland) were designed to 100% match the corresponding part of the *pol* gene encoding for reverse transcriptase of all known non-primates FVs, i.e., BFV (GenBank accession no.: NC_001831.1), FFV (GenBank accession no.: NC_039242.1), and EFV (GenBank accession no.: AF201902.1). The first amplification included 2 U of DyNazyme DNA polymerase (Thermo Fisher Scientific), 1× PCR buffer with 1.5 mM MgCl2, 0.2 µM of each primer, 0.4 mM of dNTP-mix (Thermo Fisher Scientific) and 1 µg of genomic DNA. The temperature profile was as follows: initial denaturation at 94 °C for 3 min, denaturation at 94 °C for 45 s, annealing at 54 °C for 45 s, elongation at 72 °C for 1 min, and final elongation at 72 °C for 5 min. Semi-nested amplification was completed in similar conditions using 1/10 volume of the first PCR as a template. The expected size of the amplicon was 275 bp.

Another semi-nested PCR was performed using DNA from the blood of one selected red deer. The following primers (Genomed, Warsaw, Poland) were used to amplify the sequence located in the BFV *gag* gene (1139-1381 nt): Gag-1: GACGCAACAAACCAACCAC; Gag-2: GTTCTTGTCCGTATCGTTGTG [34] and BFVpolR: TACGACATCTGCTGTAAACAATGC. The first amplification was performed in the same conditions as described for the BFV *pol* reaction, but included Gag-1 and BFVpolR primers, while the semi-nested PCR was performed as described previously with Gag-1 and Gag-2 primers [4], but using 1/10 volume of first PCR as a template. The expected size of the semi-nested PCR product was 243 bp.

Nested PCR for BFV LTR-derived sequences was performed using genomic DNA from blood cells of selected deer (see earlier in this section). The following primers (MWG Biotech) within the BFV LTR region, mostly covering the U3 region and the beginning of the R region, were used in this study: BFV-LTR-1_S: TTACTTGCCCGGAGGATTGG, BFV-LTR-1_AS: TAGTGATCTGGAAGGTAAGC, BFV-LTR-2_S: CTTATGGATGGAGCCTTATGG, BFV-LTR-2_AS: CTTACCACAGCCTGGAAGTC. All primers were designed to 100% match all known BFV sequences (GenBank accession no.: U94514, GI 9629644, GI 22947830). The first reaction of the amplification included 2.5 U of *Taq* DNA polymerase (ThermoFisher Scientific), 1× PCR buffer with 1.5 mM MgCl2, 0.2 µM of each primer, 0.1 mM of dNTP-mix (ThermoFisher Scientific), and 1 µg of genomic DNA. The first PCRs were performed with the following temperature profile: initial denaturation at 94 °C for 3 min, denaturation at 94 °C for 45 s, annealing at 52 °C for 45 s, elongation at 72 °C for 2 min, and final elongation at 72 °C for 10 min. Nested amplification was done at similar conditions, with the exception of the annealing step where the temperature was 54 °C for 45 s and using 1/10 volume of the first PCR as a template. The expected size of the amplicon was 874 bp.

The resulting amplicons were analyzed on 1% agarose gels, cloned into the pCR2.1-TOPO vector (Invitrogen), and sequenced from both sides according to the method of Sanger [35] by Genomed, Warsaw, Poland for the *pol* sequence and GATC (Konstanz, Germany) for the LTR sequences.

For bioinformatics analyses, primer sequences were removed from the cloned amplicons, which were aligned to the reference sequences of non-primate FVs available in GenBank (EFV—LC_381046.1, AF201902.1, NC_002201.1, BFV-US—NC_001831.1, BFV-3026—AY134750.1, BFV-100—JX307861.1, and BFV Riems—JX307862.1, as well as all available isolates of FFV—accession numbers are listed on the phylogenetic tree in Figure 5) using the Geneious alignment module within the Geneious Pro 5.3 software (Biomatters Ltd., Auckland, New Zealand). The alignment was submitted to the MEGA 6.0 version for the best model selection measured by the the Bayesian information criterion (BIC) and the corrected Akaike information criterion (AICc). According to the results Tamura 3-parameter with Gamma distribution [36] substitution model was applied in MEGA 6.0 to infer a phylogenetic tree using maximun likelihood method. The statistical confidence limits of the phylogram topologies were assessed with 1000 bootstrap replicates. The sequences obtained in this study were deposited in the GenBank database with the following accession numbers: MN630606-MN630611 for *pol* and MN630602–MN630605 for LTR sequences.

2.6. Statistical Analysis

Scatter plot analyses were performed to calculate the linear correlations of the net OD values obtained for Gag and Bet antigens in ELISA tests. Calculations and the generation of graphs were done using STATISTICA ver. 10 (StatSoft, part of Dell Software, USA).

3. Results

3.1. Serological Screening of Wild Ruminants Samples

The study included 269 serum samples from wild ruminants collected in different parts of Poland (Figure 1). The samples originated from cervids such as red deer (*Cervus elaphus*, n = 134), roe deer (*Capreolus capreolus*, n = 103), and fallow deer (*Dama dama*, n = 19), as well as free-ranging bovides, the highly endangered European bison (*Bison bonasus*, n = 13). Serum samples were assayed for the reactivity toward BFV Gag, Bet, and Env-SU antigens using GST-capture ELISA as previously described [7]. The observed net OD values for the Gag antigen ranged between 0.001–1.246 and between 0.001–1.339 for Bet in cervid samples. The overall reactivity of bison samples was lower and ranged between 0.056–0.660 for Gag and 0.087–0.590 for Bet. The reactivity to the Env-SU antigen was very low, comparable with the background, and was therefore not further considered as the GST-tagged Env has also been shown in previous studies to be of low diagnostic value [7].

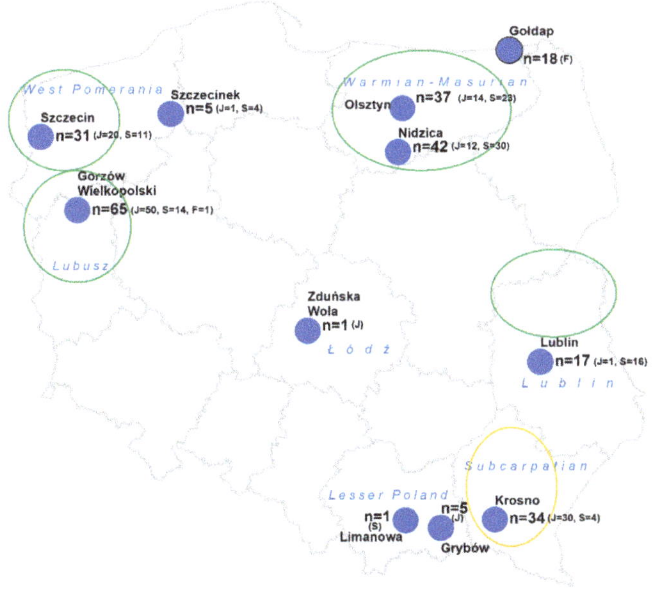

Figure 1. Geographic distribution of samples collected from wild deer in Poland. Blue dots show the areas of the samples collection which correspond to closest cities, n—the number of samples collected in the particular areas. F—no. of fallow deer, J—no. of red deer, S—no. of roe deer; green rings—the major regions of dairy cow production in big farms; orange ring—regions with moderate dairy cow production, mainly in small family farms.

Due to the differences of overall reactivity, scatter plot analyses of the net OD values for Gag and Bet antigens were separately performed for European bison (Figure 2a) and the different deer species (Figure 2b), which showed that the correlation between the seroreactivity to both antigens was strong in the population of bison, while in deer, it was weaker.

Cut-off values were calculated for Gag and Bet separately, using two methods commonly used in serodiagnostics for the different tests and animal populations (see Materials and Methods, grey and red dashed lines) (Figure 2). This approach distinguished between very high reactive sera, as well as those assessed as inconclusive with reactivity in the grey intermediate zone between the two independently calculated cut-off values (Figure 2).

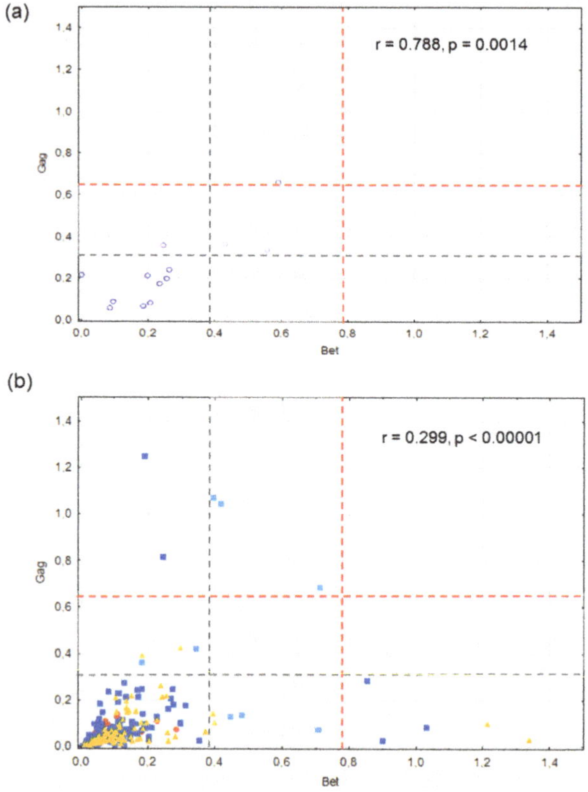

Figure 2. Distribution of Gag and Bet serological reactivity presented as scatter plots: (**a**) serum samples of bison origin, (**b**) serum samples of cervid origin. Each point represents a data pair of an individual serum of the following origins: blue dot—European bison, red dot—fallow deer, blue square—red deer, and yellow triangle—roe deer. Dashed lines, grey and red, indicate the cut-off values calculated in two ways grey—cut-off = 1 × (mean + 3SD), red—cut-off = 2 × (mean + 3SD). The grey boxes between the dashed lines indicate the grey zones of inconclusive ELISA results. The upper right sector shows double-positive, the lower-left double-negative, the lower-right sector displays sera positive for Bet only, and the upper left sector represents sera positive for Gag exclusively. The correlation coefficient (r) and *p*-value (p) are indicated in the graphs.

This analysis indicated that seven samples showed clearly high reactivity in comparison to other samples only in deer populations, while the reactivity of another 16 samples was in the intermediate grey zones. Out of these 23 samples with high or intermediate reactivity, four were from European bison, representing 30% of bison samples tested. The remaining 19 samples represent 7.4% of deer specimens tested, including six from roe deer and 13 from red deer origin. Interestingly, all highly reactive deer samples came from six locations, with seven samples (7/256, 2.7%) from Gorzów Wielkopolski in the western part of Poland, and six samples (6/256, 2.3%) from Nidzica in the north of the country (Figure 1, Table 1). Three samples from bison and three from red deer showed high reactivity to both, Gag and Bet antigens. One bison and six deer samples reacted strongly with Gag only (4 from red deer and 2 from roe deer), while ten samples were reactive to Bet antigen (6 from red deer and 4 from roe deer).

Table 1. Summary of Gag and Bet ELISA, western blotting (WB), and PCR results.

Sample No.	Species	OD Gag	OD Bet	OD Env	WB Gag	WB Bet	PCR	Area of Samples Collection
95/24	red deer	0.083	1.033	0.002	+	+/-	-	Gorzów Wlkp
113/11	red deer	0.13	0.447	0.002	n.t.	n.t.	n.t.	Gorzów Wlkp
113/13	red deer	0.074	0.709	0.008	+/-	+	+	Gorzów Wlkp
113/14	roe deer	0.102	0.399	0.003	n.t.	n.t.	n.t.	Gorzów Wlkp
125/9	red deer	1.07	0.395	0.018	+/-	-	-	Gorzów Wlkp
125/10	red deer	1.047	0.478	0.023	+	-	-	Gorzów Wlkp
95/10	red deer	0.286	0.855	0.001	+	+	-	Gorzów Wlkp.
81/05	red deer	1.246	0.192	n.t.	+	+	-	Krosno
98/04	roe deer	0.391	0.183	0	-	-	-	Lublin
80/05	roe deer	0.141	0.394	n.t.	n.t.	n.t.	-	Nidzica
80/16	roe deer	0.423	0.297	n.t.	n.t.	n.t.	n.t.	Nidzica
80/17	red deer	0.424	0.342	n.t.	n.t.	n.t.	n.t.	Nidzica
80/20	red deer	0.685	0.710	n.t.	+	+	-	Nidzica
80/24	roe deer	0.031	1.339	n.t.	+/-	+/-	-	Nidzica
80/32	red deer	0.36	0.182	n.t.	n.t.	n.t.	n.t.	Nidzica
91/15	red deer	0.138	0.48	n.t.	n.t.	n.t.	-	Olsztyn
130/1	roe deer	0.097	1.214	0.013	+	+/-	-	Olsztyn
127/9	red deer	0.026	0.901	0.028	+	+	-	Szczecin
127/16	red deer	0.915	0.246	0.093	+	+	-	Szczecin
76/01	Bison	0.359	0.245	nt	n.t.	n.t.	n.a.	n.a.
76/02	Bison	0.366	0.432	n.t.	+	-	n.a.	n.a.
87/01	Bison	0.338	0.556	n.t.	+	-	n.a.	n.a.
87/04	Bison	0.660	0.590	n.t.	+	+	n.a.	n.a.

n.t.—not tested, n.a.—not available. Areas of sample collection are indicated according to Figure 1.

To verify the ELISA results, 15 samples with reactivity to at least one BFV antigen were subsequently tested by western blotting assay (WB) with lysates of BFV_{100}-infected Cf2Th cells, used as an antigen. Uninfected Cf2Th cells were used as a control antigen. Specific reactivity against Gag results in the presence of a double band at about 60/58 kDa and, for Bet, a single band at approximately 46 kDa is characteristic (own unpublished study). Out of the 15 samples tested, eleven samples showed strong reactivity to the BFV cellular antigen (Figure 3) including three ELISA-positive samples from bison, while three samples from deer showed only very faint bands in WB, marked by +/-, in Table 1. The pattern of bison sera WB reactivity was very similar to the positive control, which contained pooled sera of naturally BFV-infected cows. In contrast, the pattern of deer reactivity was slightly different, especially for Bet reactivity, which was, in most cases, clearly weaker and even completely missing in animals 125/9 and 125/10. One sample, no. 98/4 showed no reactivity in WB.

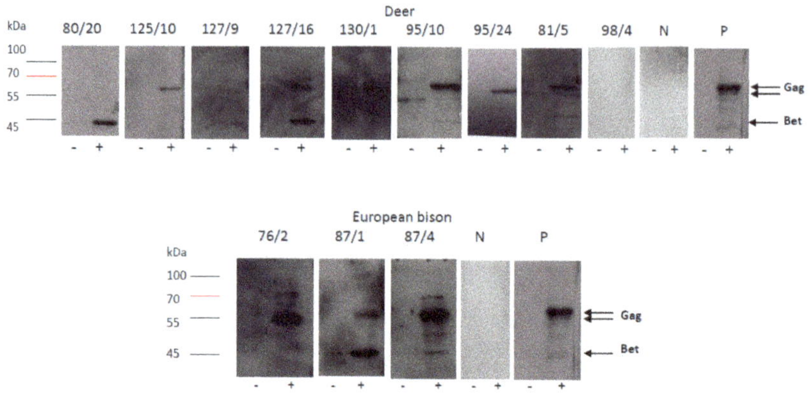

Figure 3. Detection of foamy virus (FV)-specific antibodies by immunoblotting analysis with a cellular antigen in representative serum samples of deer and European bison; (−) lane with uninfected Cf2Th cells lysate as antigen, (+) lane with Cf2Th/BFV100 cells lysate as antigen; P—BFV positive control serum, N—BFV negative serum.

3.2. Detection of FV DNA

We then aimed to detect FV-specific DNA in the total DNA extracted from the blood cells of ruminants with high reactivity towards BFV antigens, as determined by serology. A set of specific PCR primers was designed to match a conserved region of the *pol* gene encoding the BFV, EFV, and FFV reverse transcriptase. DNA extracted from blood cells of animals with serum reactivity towards BFV antigens was used as the template in semi-nested PCRs. Specific amplification was obtained for only one sample collected from red deer no. 113/13 (Figure 4). The 275 bp PCR product was cloned and sequenced. Alignment of sequences of six clones with all sequences of BFV, EFV, and FFV isolates available in GenBank showed the highest homology with the Polish BFV_{100} isolate and German BFV Riems, both representing the European clade of BFV [37] (97% identity for clone 0 and 100% for the other four clones) (Figure 5). Such a high similarity is comparable to the homology of FFV sequences of domestic cat and mountain lion origin.

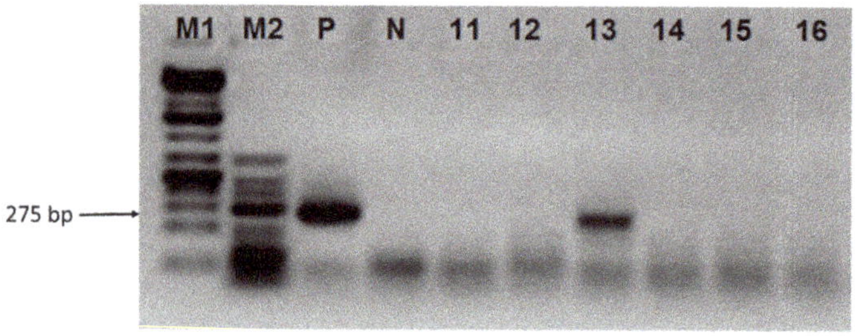

Figure 4. Electrophoretic analysis of semi-nested PCR amplification products. M1, Gene Ruler 1 kb Plus DNA Ladder; M2, GeneRuler Low Range DNA Ladder, Fermentas, **P**, positive control (blood DNA of calf experimentally inoculated with BFV), N, negative reaction control, samples no. 113/11–113-16.

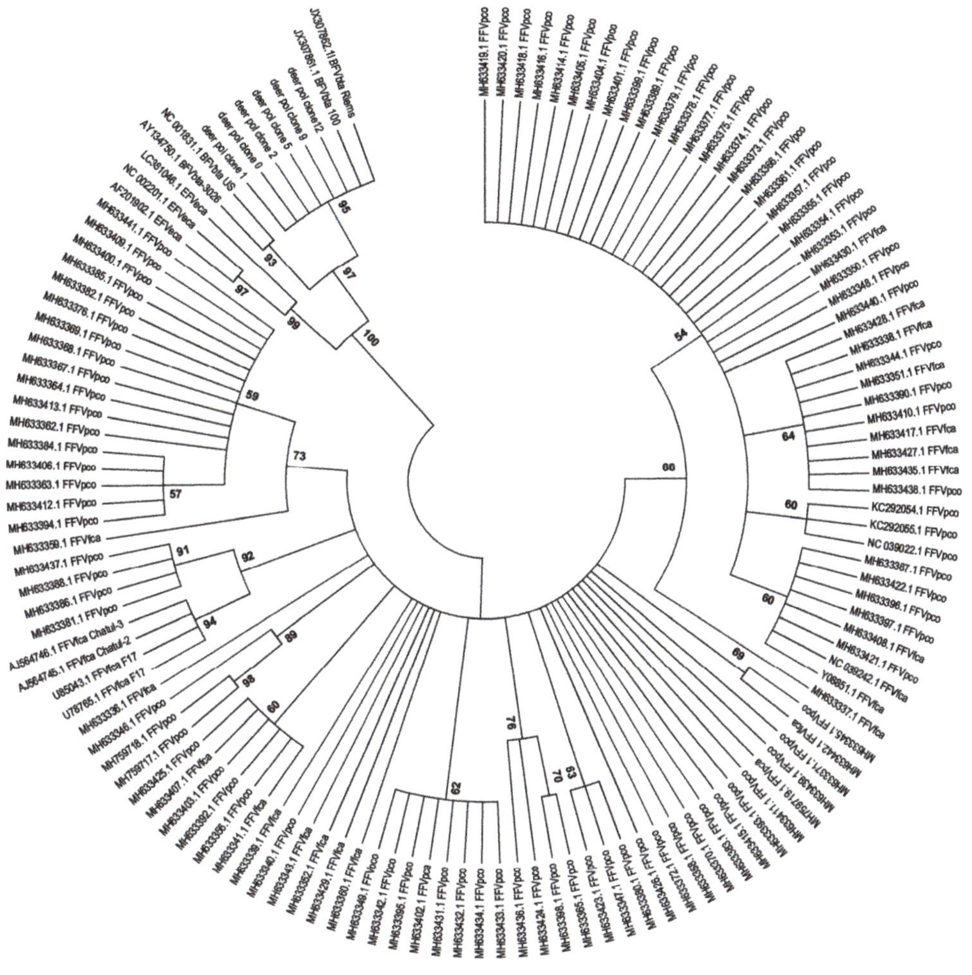

Figure 5. Phylogenetic tree inferred from the 275 bp amplicons of the *pol* region from deer 113/13 and extracted from the sequences of all BFV, EFV, and FFV isolates (the majority of the sequences) available in GenBank. The origin of FV isolates has been indicated as follows: BFVbta, cow (*Bos taurus*); EFVeca, horse (*Equus caballus*); FFVfca, cat (*Felis catus*); FFVpco, mountain lion (*Puma concolor*). All analyzed sequences were devoid of primer sequences. The tree was generated with MEGA 6.0 software by maximum likelihood method and presented with condensed branches.

Furthermore, a set of pan-BFV specific primers was used to amplify part of the LTR sequences from red deer no. 113/13. The LTR PCR amplicons were cloned, sequenced, and aligned to the respective sequences of BFV isolates available in GenBank (Figure 6). Unfortunately, no successful amplification was achieved when primers specific for BFV *gag* were used.

Both phylogenetic analyses (Figures 5 and 7) clearly show that the new sequences from European red deer are most closely related to the European clade of known BFV isolates [37]. In addition, LTR clones showed the highest similarity to the Polish BFV_{100} isolate (99.2% to 99.8% identity for analyzed clones) (Figure 6). The overall similarity for both sequences was very high and most changes were single transitions or transversion. Interestingly a deletion of two nucleotides at the LTR position

803/804 nt, the beginning of the R region of the LTR, was present in all clones from red deer, which is not present in any of the European clade BFV isolates.

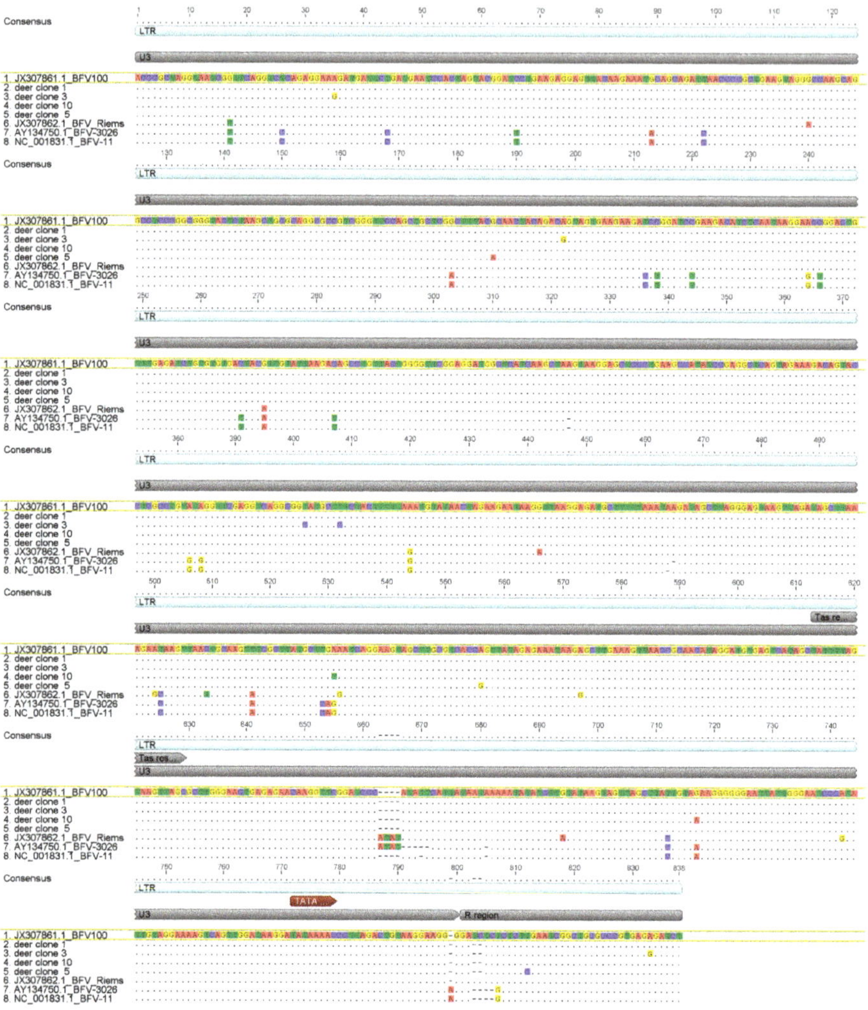

Figure 6. Alignment of the LTR clones sequences derived from red deer no. 113/13 with respective sequences extracted from BFV isolates available in GenBank.

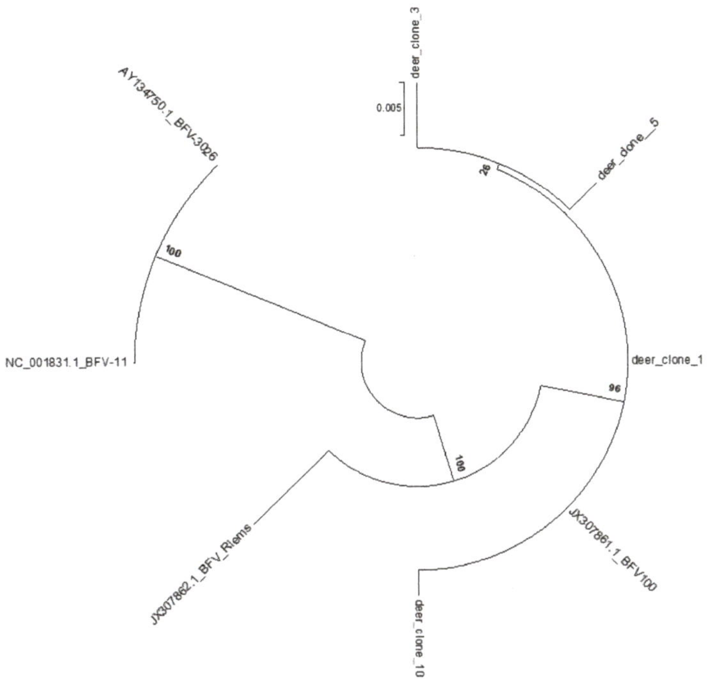

Figure 7. Phylogenetic tree inferred from the 874 bp sequence of the LTR region amplified from deer no. 113/13 and extracted from sequences of all BFV isolates available in GenBank. All analyzed sequences were devoid of primer sequences. The tree was generated with MEGA 6.0 software by maximum likelihood method. Bar—nucleotide substitutions per site.

4. Discussion

Most known FVs are highly prevalent in their hosts. For instance, the prevalence of BFV among cattle ranges between 7% and 50% of cattle worldwide, while in Poland it reaches over 30% (see for summary [10]). Transmission of BFV is suggested to occur through saliva, and, therefore, there is likely to be a risk of its spread through shared grazing areas or direct social or environmental contacts [5,6]. Serological investigation of sera from wild ruminants, presented in this study using BFV Gag and Bet antigens, clearly showed that about 8.5% of the sera reacted with at least one BFV antigen in a generic ELISA system. None of the tested samples reacted with the BFV Env antigen, which has already been shown to be an antigen with low diagnostic value in BFV-infected cattle [7,38]. Interestingly, about one fourth (3/13) of European bison sera analyzed specifically reacted with both BFV Gag and Bet in two independent serological assays. In contrast, only 9.7% of red deer and 5.8% of roe deer serum samples tested with the Gag and Bet ELISA and the WB based on the BFV-infected cells showed reactivity and it was often either against Bet or Gag but rarely (1.1%) against both antigens together. None of the fallow deer serum samples reacted with Gag or Bet antigens, which may be because of the low number of samples tested in comparison to red or roe deer. Highly BFV-related, conserved non-primate FV *pol* and LTR sequences were detected by diagnostic PCR in blood cell samples from one red deer, corresponding analyses could not be performed for bison due to the lack of DNA samples.

If the strongly BFV-related sequences isolated from the BFV-reactive red deer 113/13 are also representative for the other deer scored seropositive, this would indicate that these animals have probably been infected with BFV derived from domestic cattle. Since contact between deer and grazing cattle is possible under the farming conditions in Poland, we assume that inter-species transmission from cattle to red and roe deer and possibly other deer species occurs at a low but consistent level similar to the transmission of SFVs to humans highly exposed to non-human primates [18,39–41]. In simian-to-human transmissions, aggressive behavior, biting, and blood exchange are the major route of infection, this is different in ruminants. In BFV, free and mixed grazing of cattle and deer in rural areas may lead to BFV transmission as has been well documented for small ruminant lentiviruses in France by Erhouma and others [30], where close contact between wild ibex and goats at pastures led to small ruminant lentiviruses infections in wild animals, or for BoHV-1 which was detected in cervid populations in Germany and in Poland [24,42]. BFV transmission through saliva has been described as the most frequent route of transmission in natural conditions [3,10]; however, our own studies showed that the isolation of BFV from saliva is possible only from a small percentage of animals [32]. Unpublished data also showed that, in contrast to SFV or FFV, BFV viral load in the saliva of naturally and experimentally infected cows is very variable, from quite high to undetectable in some BFV-positive animals, but the explanation for this phenomenon is still unclear. However, a similar scenario in the wild may limit the possibility of BFV transmission to wildlife animals.

The low correlation of Bet and Gag reactivity in both deer species can also be taken as an indication for individual inter-species transmission events. These interspecies transmissions may result in attenuated or abortive replication, which could lead to incomplete or variable immune recognition of BFV antigens and thus a deviant pattern of immune responses compared to BFV in productively infected cattle [43]. In addition, the abrogation of the immune response after the transgression of the species barrier and adaptation to the new host has been reported for some viruses [43,44] and may explain the immune response pattern seen here in deer. Alternatively, wild-ranging red, roe, and fallow deer may be also exposed to currently unknown BFV-like viruses from other ruminants leading to unexpected and variant patterns of immune reactivity. This point may also explain the high number of PCR negative deer samples in contrast to the results of serological tests. The genetic differences of BFV-like viruses from different species could affect primer binding, leading to a lack of amplification, but, on the other hand, a very low number of BFV copies (below the sensitivity of PCR reaction reaching 10 copies) in peripheral blood of infected animals or the presence of any PCR inhibitors could also lead to negative PCR results. However, such discordance between the presence of BFV-specific antibodies and viral DNA may also result from the natural clearance of the productive BFV infection in heterologous hosts as was observed by Morin and co-workers [44] in experimental infection of calves with caprine arthritis-encephalitis virus.

The high prevalence (3 out of 13 animals tested) and overall tight correlation of reactivity against BFV Gag and Bet in European bison (see ELISA and WB data, Figures 2 and 3) may indicate that a currently unknown BFV-like virus is endemic in bison. This may be similar to the isolation of a retrovirus similar to the bovine foamy virus from American bison, reported years ago by Amborski and co-workers [12]. While such a bison-specific FV is serologically related but distinct (comparably low signal intensities in the Gag and Bet ELISAs, [7,38]), it may also be genetically distinct from the BFV of cattle. In contrast to deer, the habitats of bison and domestic cattle do not overlap frequently since bison are kept in nature reserves, clearly reducing the chance of exposure to BFV from cattle.

European bison are an endangered large European animal that was close to extinction at the beginning of the 20th century. Tight protection programs, especially in Poland and other countries [45], have led to the recovery of this iconic species at the price of severe inbreeding. Loss of genetic diversity within a species increases the susceptibility to infection with many pathogens, including bacteria, viruses, and parasites [23,46,47]. Under such conditions, even innocuous infectious agents like BFV may gain pathogenic potential, either on their own or as part of the microbiome/virome. This indicates a strong rationale for further investigations into old and emerging ruminant FVs. In addition, since only low numbers of bison have been studied here, further research that includes higher numbers of samples is warranted. These new studies should also go beyond serology and PCR-mediated DNA detection and should include the analysis of oral samples and milk for virus detection and isolation and maybe even encompass novel DNA detection methods based on deep sequencing.

In summary, we demonstrate clear evidence that free-ranging ruminants are exposed to and infected by FVs closely related to BFV. However, more studies are required to know whether the highly endangered, inbred, and iconic bison and the different deer species are infected by species-specific, novel FVs or by BFV of cattle origin crossing species barriers.

Author Contributions: M.M.-K. was involved in the study design, performed research and data analysis, and wrote the manuscript; M.L. was involved in the study design and wrote the manuscript; J.K. designed and supervised the study and wrote the manuscript; J.R. was involved in samples collection and preparation. All authors have read and agreed to the published version of the manuscript.

Funding: This research received no external funding.

Acknowledgments: The authors would like to thank Martha Krumbach (DKFZ, Heidelberg) for critically reading the manuscript and the veterinarians and hunters for their assistance in the sample collection.

Conflicts of Interest: The authors declare no conflict of interest.

References

1. Khan, A.S.; Bodem, J.; Buseyne, F.; Gessain, A.; Johnson, W.; Kuhn, J.H.; Kuzmak, J.; Lindemann, D.; Linial, M.L.; Löchelt, M.; et al. Spumaretroviruses: Updated taxonomy and nomenclature. *Virology* **2018**, *516*, 158–164. [CrossRef]
2. Rethwilm, A.; Bodem, J. Evolution of Foamy Viruses: The Most Ancient of All Retroviruses. *Viruses* **2013**, *5*, 2349–2374. [CrossRef]
3. Kehl, T.; Tan, J.; Materniak, M.; Kehl, T.; Tan, J.; Materniak, M. Non-Simian Foamy Viruses: Molecular Virology, Tropism and Prevalence and Zoonotic/Interspecies Transmission. *Viruses* **2013**, *5*, 2169–2209. [CrossRef]
4. Materniak, M.; Bicka, L.; Kuźmak, J. Isolation and partial characterization of bovine foamy virus from Polish cattle. *Pol. J. Vet. Sci.* **2006**, *9*, 207–211.
5. Johnson, R.H.; de la Rosa, J.; Abher, I.; Kertayadnya, I.G.; Entwistle, K.W.; Fordyce, G.; Holroyd, R.G. Epidemiological studies of bovine spumavirus. *Vet. Microbiol.* **1988**, *16*, 25–33. [CrossRef]
6. Kertayadnya, I.G.; Johnson, R.H.; Abher, I.; Burgess, G.W. Detection of immunological tolerance to bovine spumavirus (BSV) with evidence for salivary excretion and spread of BSV from the tolerant animal. *Vet. Microbiol.* **1988**, *16*, 35–39. [CrossRef]
7. Romen, F.; Backes, P.; Materniak, M.; Sting, R.; Vahlenkamp, T.W.; Riebe, R.; Pawlita, M.; Kuzmak, J.; Löchelt, M. Serological detection systems for identification of cows shedding bovine foamy virus via milk. *Virology* **2007**, *364*, 123–131. [CrossRef] [PubMed]
8. Murray, S.M.; Linial, M.L. Simian Foamy Virus Co-Infections. *Viruses* **2019**, *11*, 902. [CrossRef] [PubMed]
9. Malmquist, W.A.; Van der Maaten, M.J.; Boothe, A.D. Isolation, immunodiffusion, immunofluorescence, and electron microscopy of a syncytial virus of lymphosarcomatous and apparently normal cattle. *Cancer Res.* **1969**, *29*, 188–200.
10. Materniak-Kornas, M.; Tan, J.; Heit-Mondrzyk, A.; Hotz-Wagenblatt, A.; Löchelt, M. Bovine Foamy Virus: Shared and Unique Molecular Features In Vitro and In Vivo. *Viruses* **2019**, *11*, 1084. [CrossRef]
11. Tobaly-Tapiero, J.; Bittoun, P.; Neves, M.; Guillemin, M.C.; Lecellier, C.H.; Puvion-Dutilleul, F.; Gicquel, B.; Zientara, S.; Giron, M.L.; de Thé, H.; et al. Isolation and characterization of an equine foamy virus. *J. Virol.* **2000**, *74*, 4064–4073. [CrossRef] [PubMed]
12. Amborski, G.F.; Storz, J.; Keney, D.; Lo, J.; McChesney, A.E. Isolation of a retrovirus from the American bison and its relation to bovine retroviruses. *J. Wildl. Dis.* **1987**, *23*, 7–11. [CrossRef] [PubMed]
13. Flanagan, M. Isolation of a spumavirus from a sheep. *Aust. Vet. J.* **1992**, *69*, 112–113. [CrossRef] [PubMed]
14. Nakamura, K.; Miyazawa, T.; Ikeda, Y.; Sato, E.; Nishimura, Y. Contrastive Prevalence of Feline Retrovirus Infections between Northern and. *Vet. Med. Sci.* **2000**, *62*, 921–923. [CrossRef] [PubMed]
15. Kechejian, S.R.; Dannemiller, N.; Kraberger, S.; Ledesma-Feliciano, C.; Malmberg, J.; Roelke Parker, M.; Cunningham, M.; McBride, R.; Riley, S.P.D.; Vickers, W.T.; et al. Feline Foamy Virus is Highly Prevalent in Free-Ranging Puma concolor from Colorado, Florida and Southern California. *Viruses* **2019**, *11*, 359. [CrossRef]

16. Hruska, J.F.; Takemoto, K.K. Biochemical properties of a hamster syncytium-forming virus. *J. Natl. Cancer Inst.* **1975**, *54*, 601–605.
17. Delelis, O.; Lehmann-Che, J.; Saïb, A. Foamy viruses—A world apart. *Curr. Opin. Microbiol.* **2004**, *7*, 400–406. [CrossRef]
18. Pinto-Santini, D.M.; Stenbak, C.R.; Linial, M.L. Foamy virus zoonotic infections. *Retrovirology* **2017**, *14*, 55. [CrossRef]
19. Meiering, C.D.; Linial, M.L. Historical perspective of foamy virus epidemiology and infection. *Clin. Microbiol. Rev.* **2001**, *14*, 165–176. [CrossRef]
20. Materniak-Kornas, M.; Osiński, Z.; Rudzki, M.; Kuźmak, J. Development of a recombinant protein-based ELISA for detection of antibodies against bovine foamy virus. *J. Vet. Res.* **2017**, *61*, 247–252. [CrossRef]
21. Gortazar, C.; Diez-Delgado, I.; Barasona, J.A.; Vicente, J.; De La Fuente, J.; Boadella, M. The Wild Side of Disease Control at the Wildlife-Livestock-Human Interface: A Review. *Front. Vet. Sci.* **2014**, *1*, 27. [CrossRef] [PubMed]
22. Yon, L.; Duff, J.P.; Ågren, E.O.; Erdélyi, K.; Ferroglio, E.; Godfroid, J.; Hars, J.; Hestvik, G.; Horton, D.; Kuiken, T.; et al. Recent changes in infectious diseases in European wildlife. *J. Wildl. Dis.* **2019**, *55*, 3. [CrossRef] [PubMed]
23. Krzysiak, M.K.; Jabłoński, A.; Iwaniak, W.; Krajewska, M.; Kęsik-Maliszewska, J.; Larska, M. Seroprevalence and risk factors for selected respiratory and reproductive tract pathogen exposure in European bison (Bison bonasus) in Poland. *Vet. Microbiol.* **2018**, *215*, 57–65. [CrossRef] [PubMed]
24. Rola, J.; Larska, M.; Socha, W.; Rola, J.G.; Materniak, M.; Urban-Chmiel, R.; Thiry, E.; Żmudziński, J.F. Seroprevalence of bovine herpesvirus 1 related alphaherpesvirus infections in free-living and captive cervids in Poland. *Vet. Microbiol.* **2017**, *204*, 77–83. [CrossRef] [PubMed]
25. Kita, J.; Anusz, K. Serologic survey for bovine pathogens in free-ranging European bison from Poland. *J. Wildl. Dis.* **1991**, *27*, 16–20. [CrossRef] [PubMed]
26. Lee, L.C.; Scarratt, W.K.; Buehring, G.C.; Saunders, G.K. Bovine leukemia virus infection in a juvenile alpaca with multicentric lymphoma. *Can. Vet. J.* **2012**, *53*, 283–286.
27. Patton, K.M.; Bildfell, R.J.; Anderson, M.L.; Cebra, C.K.; Valentine, B.A. Fatal Caprine arthritis encephalitis virus–like infection in 4 Rocky Mountain goats (Oreamnos americanus). *J. Vet. Diagn. Investig.* **2012**, *24*, 392–396. [CrossRef]
28. Gufler, H.; Moroni, P.; Casu, S.; Pisoni, G. Seroprevalence, clinical incidence, and molecular and epidemiological characterisation of small ruminant lentivirus in the indigenous Passirian goat in northern Italy. *Arch. Virol.* **2008**, *153*, 1581–1585. [CrossRef]
29. Sanjosé, L.; Crespo, H.; Blatti-Cardinaux, L.; Glaria, I.; Martínez-Carrasco, C.; Berriatua, E.; Amorena, B.; De Andrés, D.; Bertoni, G.; Reina, R. Post-entry blockade of small ruminant lentiviruses by wild ruminants. *Vet. Res.* **2016**, *47*, 1. [CrossRef]
30. Erhouma, E.; Guiguen, F.; Chebloune, Y.; Gauthier, D.; Lakhal, L.M.; Greenland, T.; Mornex, J.F.; Leroux, C.; Alogninouwa, T. Small ruminant lentivirus proviral sequences from wild ibexes in contact with domestic goats. *J. Gen. Virol.* **2008**, *89*, 1478–1484. [CrossRef]
31. Kramsky, J.A.; Manning, E.J.B.; Collins, M.T. Protein G binding to enriched serum immunoglobulin from nondomestic hoofstock species. *J. Vet. Diagn. Investig.* **2003**, *15*, 253–261. [CrossRef] [PubMed]
32. Materniak, M.; Sieradzki, Z.; Kuźmak, J. Detection of bovine foamy virus in milk and saliva of BFV seropositive cattle. *Bull. Vet. Inst. Pulawy* **2010**, *54*, 461–465.
33. Romen, F.; Pawlita, M.; Sehr, P.; Bachmann, S.; Schröder, J.; Lutz, H.; Löchelt, M. Antibodies against Gag are diagnostic markers for feline foamy virus infections while Env and Bet reactivity is undetectable in a substantial fraction of infected cats. *Virology* **2006**, *345*, 502–508. [CrossRef] [PubMed]
34. Pamba, R.; Jeronimo, C.; Archambault, D. Detection of bovine retrospumavirus by the polymerase chain reaction. *J. Virol. Methods* **1999**, *78*, 199–208. [CrossRef]
35. Sanger, F.; Nicklen, S.; Coulson, R. DNA sequencing with chain-terminating. *Proc. Natl. Acad. Sci. USA* **1977**, *74*, 5463–5467. [CrossRef]
36. Tamura, K.; Stecher, G.; Peterson, D.; Filipski, A.; Kumar, S. MEGA6: Molecular Evolutionary Genetics Analysis Version 6.0. *Mol. Biol. Evol.* **2013**, *30*, 2725–2729. [CrossRef]
37. Hechler, T.; Materniak, M.; Kehl, T.; Kuzmak, J.; Lochelt, M. Complete Genome Sequences of Two Novel European Clade Bovine Foamy Viruses from Germany and Poland. *J. Virol.* **2012**, *86*, 10905–10906. [CrossRef]

38. Materniak, M.; Hechler, T.; Lochelt, M.; Kuzmak, J.; Löchelt, M.; Kuźmak, J. Similar Patterns of Infection with Bovine Foamy Virus in Experimentally Inoculated Calves and Sheep. *J. Virol.* **2013**, *87*, 3516–3525. [CrossRef]
39. Wolfe, N.D.; Switzer, W.M.; Carr, J.K.; Bhullar, V.B.; Shanmugam, V.; Tamoufe, U.; Prosser, A.T.; Torimiro, J.N.; Wright, A.; Mpoudi-Ngole, E.; et al. Naturally acquired simian retrovirus infections in central African hunters. *Lancet* **2004**, *363*, 932–937. [CrossRef]
40. Calattini, S.; Betsem, E.B.A.; Froment, A.; Mauclère, P.; Tortevoye, P.; Schmitt, C.; Njouom, R.; Saib, A.; Gessain, A. Simian foamy virus transmission from apes to humans, rural Cameroon. *Emerg. Infect. Dis.* **2007**, *13*, 1314–1320. [CrossRef]
41. Betsem, E.; Rua, R.; Tortevoye, P.; Froment, A.; Gessain, A. Frequent and recent human acquisition of simian foamy viruses through apes' bites in central africa. *PLoS Pathog.* **2011**, *7*, e1002306. [CrossRef] [PubMed]
42. Frölich, K.; Hamblin, C.; Parida, S.; Tuppurainen, E.; Schettler, E. Serological Survey for Potential Disease Agents of Free-ranging Cervids in Six Selected National Parks from Germany. *J. Wildl. Dis.* **2006**, *42*, 836–843. [CrossRef] [PubMed]
43. Solórzano, A.; Foni, E.; Córdoba, L.; Baratelli, M.; Razzuoli, E.; Bilato, D.; Martín del Burgo, M.Á.; Perlin, D.S.; Martínez, J.; Martínez-Orellana, P.; et al. Cross-Species Infectivity of H3N8 Influenza Virus in an Experimental Infection in Swine. *J. Virol.* **2015**, *89*, 11190–11202. [CrossRef] [PubMed]
44. Morin, T.; Guiguen, F.; Bouzar, B.A.; Villet, S.; Greenland, T.; Grezel, D.; Gounel, F.; Gallay, K.; Garnier, C.; Durand, J.; et al. Clearance of a productive lentivirus infection in calves experimentally inoculated with caprine arthritis-encephalitis virus. *J. Virol.* **2003**, *77*, 6430–6437. [CrossRef] [PubMed]
45. Miller, M.L. The Remarkable Story of How the Bison Returned to Europe. Available online: https://blog.nature.org/science/2017/08/22/remarkable-story-how-bison-returned-europe/ (accessed on 9 October 2019).
46. Kita, J.; Anusz, K.; Zaleska, M.; Malicka, E.; Bielecki, W.; Osińska, B.; Kowalski, B.; Krasiński, Z.; Demiaszkiewicz, A.; Rhyan, J.; et al. Relationships among ecology, demography and diseases of European bison (Bison bonasus). *Pol. J. Vet. Sci.* **2003**, *6*, 261–266.
47. Krzysiak, M.K.; Iwaniak, W.; Kęsik-Maliszewska, J.; Olech, W.; Larska, M. Serological Study of Exposure to Selected Arthropod-Borne Pathogens in European Bison (Bison bonasus) in Poland. *Transbound. Emerg. Dis.* **2017**, *64*, 1411–1423. [CrossRef]

viruses

MDPI

Article

Isolation of an Equine Foamy Virus and Sero-Epidemiology of the Viral Infection in Horses in Japan

Rikio Kirisawa [1,*], Yuko Toishi [2], Hiromitsu Hashimoto [3] and Nobuo Tsunoda [2]

1 Laboratory of Veterinary Virology, Department of Pathobiology, School of Veterinary Medicine, Rakuno Gakuen University, Ebetsu, Hokkaido 069-8501, Japan
2 Shadai Stallion Station, Abira-cho, Hokkaido 059-1432, Japan
3 Shiraoi Farm, Shiraoi-cho, Hokkaido 059-0901, Japan
* Correspondence: r-kirisa@rakuno.ac.jp; Tel.: +81-11-388-4748; Fax: +81-11-387-5890

Received: 10 June 2019; Accepted: 3 July 2019; Published: 5 July 2019

Abstract: An equine foamy virus (EFV) was isolated for the first time in Japan from peripheral blood mononuclear cells of a broodmare that showed wobbler syndrome after surgery for intestinal volvulus and the isolate was designated as EFVeca_LM. Complete nucleotide sequences of EFVeca_LM were determined. Nucleotide sequence analysis of the long terminal repeat (LTR) region, *gag*, *pol*, *env*, *tas*, and *bel2* genes revealed that EFVeca_LM and the EFV reference strain had 97.2% to 99.1% identities. For a sero-epidemiological survey, indirect immunofluorescent antibody tests were carried out using EFVeca_LM-infected cells as an antigen against 166 sera of horses in five farms collected in 2001 to 2002 and 293 sera of horses in eight farms collected in 2014 to 2016 in Hokkaido, Japan. All of the farms had EFV antibody-positive horses, and average positive rates were 24.6% in sera obtained in 2001 to 2002 and 25.6% in sera obtained in 2014 to 2016 from broodmare farms. The positive rate in a stallion farm (Farm A) in 2002 was 10.7%, and the positive rates in two stallion farms, Farms A and B, in 2015 were 40.9% and 13.3%, respectively. The results suggested that EFV infection is maintained widely in horses in Japan.

Keywords: equine foamy virus; isolation; Japan; sero-epidemiology; spumaretrovirus

1. Introduction

Foamy viruses (FVs) belong to the subfamily *Spumaretrovirinae* within the family *Retroviridae* [1]. FVs have been isolated from a wide range of mammals, including nonhuman primates [2–5], cats [6], cows [7], horses [8] and bats [9], and it has been shown that they establish lifelong infection [10,11]. FV infections have not been shown to be associated with any defined disease [1,12]. The non-pathogenicity of FVs is an essential factor for the development of a foamy viral vector in gene therapy [13]. The FV genome consists of genes encoding canonical retroviral Gag, Pol and Env proteins and a regulatory protein Tas and an accessory protein Bet [1].

The prevalence of simian FVs has been studied in detail, but there have been few studies on the prevalence of other animal FVs [14]. The prevalence of feline FV (FFV) in domestic cats and wild cats was reported to range from about 30% to 100% depending on sex, age, and the geographical region [14–22]. The prevalence of bovine FV (BFV) infection in cattle was reported to range from 7% to 45% [23–26]. The prevalence of equine FV (EFV) in horses has not been reported.

In 2000, equine foamy virus was isolated for the first time from blood samples of naturally infected healthy horses after co-cultivation of phytohemagglutinin (PHA)-activated lymphocytes derived from sero-positive horses with permissive human U373-MG cells and hamster BHK21 cells [8]. Nucleotide sequence analysis revealed that EFV is phylogenetically close to non-primate FVs, especially BFV. There has been no further isolation of EFV since the first isolation in 2000.

In this report, the first isolation of EFV in Japan (the second isolation of EFV in the world) in primary horse kidney cells co-cultured with fresh peripheral blood mononuclear cells (PBMC) from a broodmare showing wobbler syndrome after surgery for intestinal volvulus and the molecular characterization of the isolated virus are described. The results of a serological survey using the Japanese EFV isolate in thoroughbred horses in Japan are also described.

2. Materials and Methods

2.1. Cell Cultures and Virus Isolation

Primary horse fetal kidney (HFK) cells were prepared according to the standard method from a fetal kidney that was obtained from a euthanized pregnant mare due to the judgment of a poor prognosis for a forelimb fracture, and the cells were cultured in MEM supplemented with 10% fetal calf serum (FCS) as the growth medium at 37 °C. A blood sample from a horse (Horse A) that exhibited wobbler syndrome the day after a surgical operation for intestinal volvulus in an equine hospital, not in our medical center of Rakuno Gakuen University, as veterinary medicine was collected in heparin-containing tubes on October 1, 2001, and peripheral blood mononuclear cells (PBMC) were isolated by Ficoll-Paque gradients (density of 1.077 g/mL). The PBMC were co-cultured with HFK cells in culture dishes (35 mm in diameter) in the growth medium for virus isolation at 37 °C under a 5% CO_2 atmosphere. The culture medium was removed the next day, fresh MEM supplemented with 4% FCS as a maintenance medium was added, and the cells were cultured at 37 °C. The cultured cells were observed daily and the maintenance medium was changed at 4-day intervals until the appearance of a cytopathic effect (CPE). A CPE was observed 10 days after the start of cultivation and the HFK cells showing a CPE were detached by trypsin-EDTA solution and harvested as virus-infected single cells 4 days after the appearance of a CPE. The infected cells were stored at −80 °C using CELLBANKER I (Takara Bio Inc., Kusatsu, Shiga, Japan) as the cryopreservation medium. Serum of Horse A was collected on October 1, 2001. Horse A was euthanized due to the judgment of a poor prognosis about 1 week after the operation. We also used conserved sera of Horse A that had been stocked monthly in our laboratory from January 2000.

2.2. DNA Extraction

Total DNA was extracted from HFK cells showing a CPE (about 80% of the cells) as described previously [27].

2.3. Polymerase Chain Reaction (PCR) for Detection of the Equine Foamy Virus Genome

To detect EFV DNA in cells showing a CPE, PCR assays targeting LTR were carried out using the Expand High Fidelity PCR system (Roche Diagnostic GmbH, Mannheim, Germany) and primers listed in Table 1, which were designed on the basis of the complete EFV sequence (GenBank AF201902) by using DNASIS Pro (Hitachi Software Engineering Co., Ltd., Tokyo, Japan). PCR amplification was carried out as described previously [28] under the following conditions: an initial denaturation step of 94 °C for 5 min, 35 cycles of 94 °C for 30 s, 55 °C for 30 s, 72 °C for 1 min and 30 s, and a final extension step of 72 °C for 5 min. The PCR products were purified and sequenced as described below.

Table 1. Primers used in PCR amplification.

Primer	Sequence (5′–3′)	Location [1]
LTR-F	TGTCATGGAATGAGGATCCAG	1–21 10587–10607
LTR-R	ATTGTCGCGGTATCTCCTTAA	1449–1429 12035–12015

Table 1. *Cont.*

Primer	Sequence (5′–3′)	Location [1]
Gag-F	AGATACCGCGACAATTGGCG	1435–1454
Gag-R3	CCATTGTCCCGAGGTAAATC	1637–1618
Gag-F3	AAGAAGAGGCCCTGGAAGAA	3071–3090
Gag-R	AGGGACACAAGTTATTTCAGCTC	3246–3224
Pol-F	GGCGTTATTGAAGGCATTTG	4670–4690
Pol-R	CCCATACCTGCTGAATGTTG	4997–4978
Env-F	ATGACACCTCCAATGACTCTAC	6536–6557
Env-R3	CAGGTATGGCCTCTCTGAT	6617–6599
Env-R	TTATTCTCCTTTGTCCTCTC	9496–9477
Env-F2	TTTGGGTAAAGTACCAGCCTC	8113–8133
Env-R2	GGATAAGTCCACTTCCCAGAG	9528–9508
TAS-F	AGGATATTATCATGGCTAGCA	9431–9451
TAS-R	ATGGTTCTCGAATAAAGCGGT	11885–11865
		1299–1279

[1] Location at the complete nucleotide sequence of EFV (Genbank AF201902).

2.4. Restriction Enzyme Digestion and Southern Blot Hybridization

The DNA extracted from cells showing a CPE was digested to completion with restriction endonuclease *Bam*HI under conditions recommended by the manufacturer (Takara Bio Inc., Tokyo, Japan). The digested fragments were separated by electrophoresis in 0.7% agarose gels in Tris-acetate-EDTA buffer (40 mM Tris-acetate, 1 mM EDTA, pH 8.0) and were transferred to nitrocellulose filters (0.45 μm, Schleicher & Schuell, Dassel, Germany) according to the method by Southern [29]. The filters were pre-hybridized for 2 h and then hybridized for 14 h with a probe of the isolated viral LTR labeled with the non-isotopic reagent digoxigenin-dUTP [27]. An enzyme immunoassay kit (Roche Diagnostics, Basel, Switzerland) was used for detecting hybridized fragments. For a DNA molecular weight marker, *Hin*dIII-digested lambda DNA labeled with digoxigenin-dUTP (Roche Diagnostics) was used.

2.5. Sequence and Phylogenetic Analyses

Regions coding for Gag, Pol, Env, Tas and Bet were amplified by PCR with the Expand High Fidelity PCR system (Roche Diagnostics) and each of the specific primers listed in Tables 1 and 2. The PCR products were purified by Chroma spin columns (Clontech Laboratories, Inc., Mountain View, CA, USA) or a High Pure PCR Product Purification kit (Roche Diagnostic) and used for sequencing. Sequencing was conducted in Hokkaido System Science Co. Ltd. (Sapporo, Japan) using specific primers and walking primers. Sequence analyses were conducted by DNASIS Pro (Hitachi Software Engineering Co., Ltd., Tokyo, Japan). Phylogenetic analysis of the nucleotide sequences was conducted by using MEGA7 software with 1000 bootstrap replicates of the neighbor-joining method [30]. Evolutionary distances were estimated according to the Kimura 2-parameter method [31]. The DDBJ accession number assigned to the complete sequence of the analyzed isolate is LC381046.

Table 2. PCR-amplified regions.

Primer Pair	Amplified Region [1]	PCR Product Size (bp)
LTR-F & LTR-R	1–1429, 10587–12035	1429
LTR-F & Gag-R3	1–1637	1637
Gag-F & Gag-R	1435–3246	1812
Gag-F3 & Pol-R	3071–4997	1927
Pol-F & Env-R3	4670–6617	1948
Env-F & Env-R	6536–9496	2961

Table 2. *Cont.*

Primer Pair	Amplified Region [1]	PCR Product Size (bp)
Env-F2 & Env-R2	8113–9528	1416
TAS-F & TAS-R	9431–11885	2454

[1] Region at the complete nucleotide sequence of EFV (Genbank AF201902).

2.6. Serum Samples

Sera obtained from horses in 10 farms (Farms A to J) in Hokkaido in Japan were used for a sero-epidemiological survey. Farms A and B were stud farms, and the others were breeding farms. In 2001 to 2002, sera were collected from 28 stallions in Farm A on June 7, 2002; 72 mares in Farm C on June 13, 2002; 25 mares in Farm D on April 17, 2001; and 29 mares in Farm E and 12 mares in Farm F on June 30, 2002. In 2014 to 2016, sera were collected from 44 stallions in Farm A on June 30, 2015; 15 stallions in Farm B on May 15, 2015; 107 mares in Farm C on June 30, 2015; 25 mares in Farm D on January 26, 2015; 30 mares in Farm G on March 11, 2015; 39 mares in Farm H on January 17, 2014; 22 mares in Farm I on January 28, 2016; and 11 mares in Farm J on October 31, 2016. For the broodmare from which EFV was isolated (Horse A, Farm C), serum collected on October 1, 2001 (date of onset of wobbler syndrome) and sera collected on February 14, 2001; October 11, 2000; and January 26, 2000 were used. All of the serum samples were initially sent to our laboratory to test for equine herpesvirus 1 (EHV-1) infection. The serum separation procedure was as follows. A blood sample from each horse was collected in a plain tube and was allowed to clot by leaving it at room temperature. The clot was removed by centrifugation at 1000× g for 10 min and the resulting supernatant, designated as a serum, was transferred to a clean polypropylene micro tube. After inactivation of the complement at 56 °C for 30 min, the serum was used for a serological test of EHV-1 infection. After the test, the serum was stored at −20 °C.

2.7. Indirect Immunofluorescence Assay (IFA) for Detection of Antibodies to EFV

EFV-infected HFK cells were detached by trypsin-EDTA solution and washed three times with phosphate-buffered saline (PBS, pH 7.4) by centrifugation at 200× *g* for 5 min. The cells were re-suspended in a small volume in PBS and smeared on a 15-well multitest slide glass (MP Biomedicals, LLC, Solon, OH, USA) and then fixed in 100% acetone on ice for 30 min. Equine sera were diluted serially from 1:20 to 320 and incubated with the fixed cells at 37 °C for 30 min in an incubation chamber. The cells were washed three times with PBS. After drying the cells at room temperature, the cells were incubated with 1:80 diluted fluorescein isothiocyanate conjugated goat-anti horse IgG (Jackson Immuno Research Inc., West Grove, PA, USA) at 37 °C for 30 min. After a final wash, infected cells were visualized under a fluorescence microscope (Olympus, Tokyo, Japan). An IFA titer of 20 or greater was regarded as positive. Uninfected HFK cells were used as control cells.

3. Results

3.1. Virus Isolation and Identification

Initially, we suspected a neurological type of equine herpesvirus 1 infection in a horse showing clinical symptoms of wobbler syndrome. However, co-cultivation of PBMC from the affected horse and HFK cells did not show any herpes viral-like CPE after incubation for 1 week. At 10 days after cultivation, small syncytia were observed and they gradually increased in size, and many vacuoles were observed in the syncytia. These morphological changes resembled the foamy CPE in response to FV infection [1]. The isolate was designated as EFVeca_LM. EFVeca_LM was highly cell-associated in HFK cells, and cell-free virus was not released in culture supernatants. Cell-free virus was also not obtained after three cycles of freeze-and-thawing of EFVeca_LM-infected HFK cells. By PCR amplification using primers for the LTR region of EFV, identical products with the same estimated size, approximately 1450 bp, were observed in agarose gel electrophoresis. The nucleotide sequence identity of the amplified products without primer sequences was 98.2% (1381/1407) against that of EFV (Figure 1). In Southern blot analysis, the LTR probe detected a 12-kbp fragment in DNAs from virus-infected cells without restriction enzyme digestion and 7.1-kbp and 1.4-kbp fragments in *Bam*HI-digested DNAs (Figure 2A). By analogy to the EFV genome, the 12-kbp fragment represents unintegrated linear viral genomic DNA and the 7.1-kbp and 1.4-kbp fragments correspond to about 60% of the region of the genome from the 5′ end and the LTR region located at the 3′ end, respectively (Figure 2B,C). We could not detect the integrated viral DNA in host chromosomal DNA in Figure 2A. Possible reasons were that copy numbers of the integrated DNA were extremely low compared to those of unintegrated viral DNA and that sensitivity of our Southern blot analysis was insufficient for detecting the integrated viral DNA. The same results were obtained by Tobaly-Tapiero et al. [8].

```
EFV (AF201902)   22 AGACTAAGAATATAGCTATT TTTTTCCAGTACTGAAGTAC AAGAATGGTTCCAGATGGAG GATGTAGATGATAGAGCAAG 101
LM (LC381046)    22 ....C............... .................... .................... ..............A....A 101

EFV (AF201902)  102 AGAACCACTAGATGGCAGTG AAACACATCAAGAAATAGCA GAATTTGCTTGTGCTATGCT GCCCCCTGGTTGGTGTATAG 181
LM (LC381046)   102 .................... .................A.. ...........C........ .................... 181

EFV (AF201902)  182 TCAGACCCGAAGGAAGAACT TATATATCCACTGGGCCTGA TACTTCAGATGAGGAAGAAG ATAAAGCCTTAGCTCCTAAG 261
LM (LC381046)   182 .........G.......... .................... ...C................ .................... 261

EFV (AF201902)  262 ATTCTAAAGACACATCCTAG CATATGTCCAAAACACCCTC GCCACCATAAAATAGGAGGA CGCTTTGTCTCTGACCTTTT 341
LM (LC381046)   262 .................... .................... ..........G......... ........T........... 341

EFV (AF201902)  342 AGATAGTCCCAGCAGTTCAG ACGATGAGGAGGAGGCTCGC CAGAACTTGGCTCGTGTCCT TGAGGCGGCGCTTCCTCACC 421
LM (LC381046)   342 .................... .T.................T ..A................. .................... 421

EFV (AF201902)  422 CTGGCGAAGATTCCTCTGAT GACGATCCTCTTTATCTAGG AGAACCAGAAAGGGATTAAA GGATTATGGGGCTAGCTCAG 501
LM (LC381046)   422 .................... .................... .................... .................... 501

EFV (AF201902)  502 CTCGCTAATGCATAATAGCA TTCAACTGACAGCAACCCCA TAGTCTGGTGCTCATGACAG TGTGAGAGTTCAATACTCAC 581
LM (LC381046)   502 .................... .................... .................... ..............A..... 581

EFV (AF201902)  582 CTCTCCACTGTCGTGAGGAC CCTTATGTTAACCACAAACC TTATATTTTTAGGAGCCGGG AGGATAGCTCAACCTGTTAA 661
LM (LC381046)   582 .................... .................... .................... ...........C........ 661

EFV (AF201902)  662 GAACTCAGAAGGTTATGTAT ATTCTTCCTTGCTCCCGGTG GTTCGATCCCTGTTTAGCCT GATACGATAGCCGCTAACCT 741
LM (LC381046)   662 .................... .................... .................... .................... 741

EFV (AF201902)  742 GGGACGAACTCCCCTTTTAG TTTCGGTTTTAAGATGCTTC CGCATACGCATATAGATAGA AGTAGGAAGTAGTTAATCCC 821
LM (LC381046)   742 .................... .................... .................... .................... 821

EFV (AF201902)  822 AGTCTGAGGGATGGCTCGTA CAACAAAACACACATCGAGG AATGTAATACCTGTCCTCTC TCAGATCAGTGGACGGACAG 901
LM (LC381046)   822 .................... .................... .................... .................... 901

EFV (AF201902)  902 GATGAACGTACATATATAAG TTCATCCAGCCAGTTCACTT TTTAGGAATTTATATTAGTC AATATGAAATACATAAGTTA 981
LM (LC381046)   902 .................... .................... .................... .................... 981

EFV (AF201902)  982 ATAAACGAATATGAAATACA ATTAGGAAGTGAAACCAAGC GTGACGCATTCTGTGTTCGA GTACACTGACAGAACTCTGA 1061
LM (LC381046)   982 ....TA...A...G...... .................... .................... .............G...... 1061

EFV (AF201902) 1062 TTCGAATCAATGGACAAAAT AAGTTTTTCCAACCAAATTA AAATATAAATAAGATCAGAT TGTGAGGGCCACTCACTCAC 1141
LM (LC381046)  1062 .................... .................... .............G...... .................... 1141

EFV (AF201902) 1142 ATATTCGGCTGCGTCCGGAG TGAGTCGAGCAGGCCACAGA CTGGGTAAGAATATATTTTA TGATTATTTGGAGTTTGATG 1221
LM (LC381046)  1142 .................... .................... .................... .A..............A... 1221

EFV (AF201902) 1222 ATGCACTTAATTTGCTCTGC ATAAAATAATATAAATGTGT GATTGCTTATACAATAAACC GCTTTATTCGAGAACCATAA 1301
LM (LC381046)  1222 .................... ...G................ .................... .................... 1301

EFV (AF201902) 1302 AATAAATTTATTGTTGCTTT CTTATCACTCTTAAGTGAGA AACATCTCCTTAAAGGAAAT AAATACCTGGGCTACTTAAG 1381
LM (LC381046)  1302 .................... .................G.. ..T................. .................... 1381

EFV (AF201902) 1382 AGAGTTTTATACTCATACTT AATATAGGCCTTAGAGTATT CCCTATT 1428
LM (LC381046)  1382 .................... ......A............. ....... 1428
```

Figure 1. Comparison of the nucleotide sequences of LTR regions in the Japanese isolate EFVeca_LM and reference EFV. Identical nucleotides are indicated by dots. Numbers on the left and right sides are the nucleotide positions of EFV complete genome sequence (AF201902).

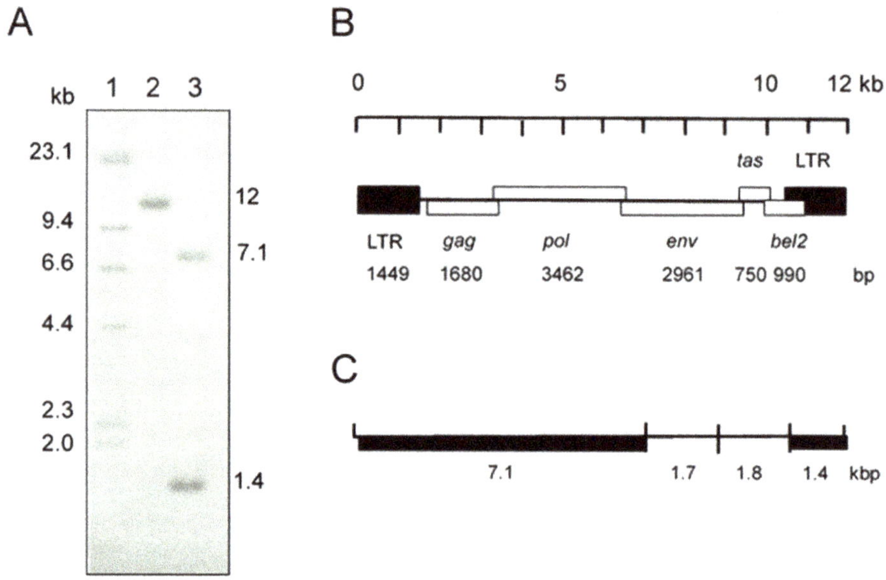

Figure 2. (**A**) Southern blot analysis of total DNA from HFK cells infected with the isolate. The LTR region was used as a probe. Lane 1: molecular weight marker, lambda DNA *Hind*III digest labeled with digoxigenin-dUTP, Lane 2: uncut DNA, Lane 3: *Bam*HI-digested DNA. (**B**) EFV genomic structure. (**C**) *Bam*HI restriction map of the EFV genome. Fragments of thick lines were detected by the LTR probe in lane 3 in (**A**).

Altogether, the isolated virus, EFVeca_LM, was identified as equine foamy virus belonging to the *Spumaretrovirinae* subfamily.

EFV IFA titers of Horse A are shown in Table 3. EFV antibody already existed in the serum collected at the time of onset of wobbler syndrome. In three conserved sera, EFV antibodies were also detected and showed almost the same IFA titers as that in serum collected at the time of onset of wobbler syndrome. The titers of all of the tested sera against uninfected control HFK cells were less than 20.

Table 3. EFV antibody titers determined by IFA tests in Horse A.

	Serum Collection Date			
	26 Jan, 2000	**11 Oct, 2000**	**14 Feb, 2001**	**1 Oct, 2001** [1]
IFA titer	160	160	160	80

[1] Date of onset of wobbler syndrome.

3.2. Sequence Analysis

The provirus DNA of EFVeca_LM was completely sequenced and found to be 12,034 bp. The complete provirus genomic sequence of EFVeca_LM was submitted to DDBJ under the accession number LC381046. The complete genomic sequences of EFVeca_LM were compared to those of EFV (GenBank AF201902) (Table 4). The LTR nucleotide sequences of EFVeca_LM and EFV showed 98.2% identity. The nucleotide sequence and amino acid sequence of the *gag* gene showed 98.6% and 99.1% identities, respectively. The nucleotide sequence and amino acid sequence of the *pol* gene showed 98.6% and 99.1% identities, respectively. The nucleotide sequence and amino acid sequence of the *env* gene showed 98.3% and 98.5% identities, respectively. The nucleotide sequence and amino acid sequence of the *tas* gene showed 99.1% and 100.0% identities, respectively. The nucleotide sequence and amino acid sequence of the *bel2* gene showed 97.2% and 97.3% identities, respectively.

Table 4. Identities of nucleotide sequences and amino acid sequences of an isolated virus and EFV.

	Identity (%)	
Region	**Nucleotide Sequence**	**Amino Acid Sequence**
LTR	98.2 (1449) [1]	
gag	98.6 (1680)	99.1 (559) [2]
pol	98.6 (3462)	99.1 (1153)
env	98.3 (2961)	98.5 (986)
tas	99.1 (750)	100.0 (249)
bel2	97.2 (990)	97.3 (329)

[1] Number in parenthesis is the size of the nucleotide sequence; [2] Number in parenthesis is the size of the amino acid sequence.

Phylogenetic comparisons of the full-length provirus genome of EFVeca_LM and those of various animal foamy virus isolates revealed that EFVeca_LM belonged to the same clade as EFV (Figure 3).

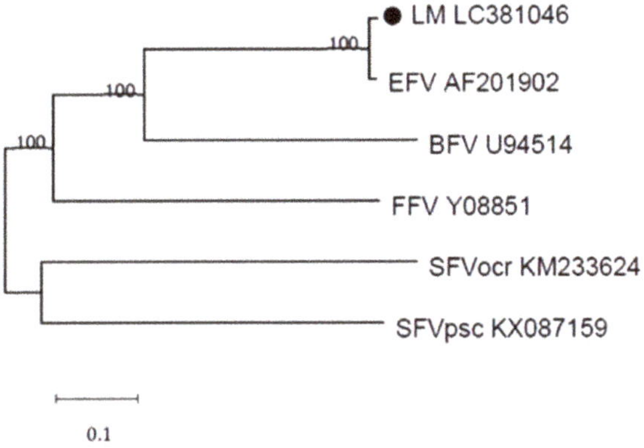

Figure 3. Phylogenetic analysis of the Japanese isolate EFVeca_LM (LM LC301046) and other foamy virus strains. The phylogenetic tree was generated using complete nucleotide genome sequences. EFVeca_LM is indicated by a closed circle. Bootstrap values less than 50% are not shown on the corresponding nodes. BFV: bovine foamy virus, FFV: feline foamy virus, SFVocr: simian foamy virus Otolemur crassicaudatus, SFVpsc: simian foamy virus Pan troglodytes schweinfurthii.

3.3. Sero-Epizootiology

To examine the prevalence of EFV antibodies in Japanese horses, we conducted IFA tests using EFVeca_LM and a total of 166 sera obtained from one stallion farm (Farm A) and four broodmare farms (Farms C to F) in 2001 to 2002 and a total of 293 sera obtained from two stallion farms (Farms A and B) and six broodmare farms (Farms C, D, G to J) in 2014 to 2016 (Table 5). The titers of all of the tested sera against uninfected control HFK cells were less than 20. All of the farms had EFV antibody-positive horses. The positive rates in sera obtained from broodmare farms in 2001 to 2002 ranged from 20.7% to 28.0% (average: 24.6%), and the positive rates in sera obtained from broodmare farms in 2014 to 2016 ranged from 12.8% to 35.5% (average: 25.6%). The positive rate in sera obtained from a stallion farm (Farm A) in 2002 was 10.7% and the positive rates in sera obtained from two stallion farms, Farm A and Farm B, in 2015, were 40.9% and 13.3%, respectively. Average ages of broodmares for which sera were tested and broodmares for which sera were antibody-positive in 2001 to 2002 were

9.8 years and 10.3 years, respectively. The average ages of broodmares for which sera were tested and broodmares for which sera were antibody-positive in 2014 to 2016 were 10.7 years and 12.0 years, respectively. The average ages of stallions in Farm A for which sera were tested in 2002 and in 2015 were 9.1 years and 11.3 years, respectively. The average ages of stallions in Farm A for which sera were antibody-positive in 2002 and in 2015 were 8.0 years and 13.7 years, respectively. Positive rates in sera obtained from Farms A and C in 2015 were higher than those in sera obtained in 2002, and there was a relationship between the positive rate and aging in Farms A and C in 2015 (Table 6). In Farm A, the positive rate in sera obtained in 2015 from stallions aged 15 to 24 years (83.3%) was clearly higher than the positive rates for other age groups (27.3% in stallions aged 4 to 9 years and 20.0% in stallions aged 10 to 14 years). In Farm C, the positive rates in sera obtained in 2015 from broodmares aged 10 to 14 years old (42.0%) and broodmares aged 15 to 24 years (56.3%) were clearly higher than the positive rate for broodmares aged 4 to 9 years (19.5%). In Farm C in 2002, the positive rates in sera were similar for the three age groups. The average ages of horses reared in Farms A and C had increased from 9.1 years to 11.3 years and from 9.4 years to 10.6 years in 2015, respectively. In Farm A, the same four horses were reared both in 2002 and 2015, and two horses were EFV antibody-positive in 2002 (one 4-year-old horse and one 10-year-old horse) and also antibody-positive in 2015 (one 17-year-old horse and one 23-year-old horse). The remaining two horses did not possess EFV antibody in 2002 (one 9-year-old horse and one 10-year-old horse) but possessed EFV antibody in 2015. In Farm C, there was no same horse reared both in 2002 and 2015.

Table 5. Prevalence of EFV antibody in horses in Hokkaido in Japan.

		In 2001 to 2002		In 2014 to 2016	
Farm	**Category**	**Collection Date**	**Positive/Negative/Tested Sera**	**Collection Date**	**Positive/Negative/Tested Sera**
A	Stallion	7 Jun, 2002	3 (8.0y) [1]/ 25 (9.6y)/ 28 (9.1y) [2] (10.7%) [3]	30 Jun, 2015	18 (13.7y)/ 26 (9.7y)/ 44 (11.3y) (40.9%)
B	Stallion			15 May, 2015	2 (10.0y)/ 13 (10.8y)/ 15 (10.7y) (13.3%)
C	Broodmare	13 Jun, 2002	18 (9.6y)/ 54 (9.4y)/ 72 (9.4y) (25.0%)	30 Jun, 2015	38 (12.0y)/ 69 (9.9y)/ 107 (10.6y) (35.5%)
D	Broodmare	17 Apr, 2001	7 (11.0y)/ 18 (8.6y)/ 25 (9.2y) (28.0%)	26 Jan, 2015	7 (11.7y)/ 18 (9.4y)/ 25 (10.0y) (28.0%)
E	Broodmare	30 Jun, 2002	6 (12.7y)/ 23 (10.7y)/ 29 (11.1y) (20.7%)		
F	Broodmare	30 Jun, 2002	3 (8.7y)/ 9 (9.7y)/ 12 (9.4y) (25.0%)		
G	Broodmare			11 Mar, 2015	5 (14.0y)/ 25 (11.0y)/ 30 (11.5y) (16.7%)
H	Broodmare			17 Jan, 2014	5 (11.4y)/ 34 (10.8y)/ 39 (10.9y) (12.8%)
I	Broodmare			28 Jan, 2016	3 (11.3y)/ 19 (9.3y)/ 22 (9.6y) (13.6%)
J	Broodmare			31 Oct, 2016	2 (11.5y)/ 9 (12.2y)/ 11 (12.1y) (18.2%)
Subtotal	Stallion		3 (8.0y)/ 25 (9.6y) 28 (9.1y) (10.7%)		20 (13.3y)/ 39 (10.1y)/ 59 (11.2y) (33.9%)
	Broodmare		34 (10.3y)/ 104 (9.6y) 138 (9.8y) (24.6%)		60 (12.0y)/174 (10.2y)/ 234 (10.7y) (25.6%)
Total			37/166 [4] (22.3%)		80/293 (27.3%)

[1] Number in parenthesis is the average age (years) of antibody-positive horses; [2] Number in parenthesis is the average age of tested horses; [3] Number in parenthesis is antibody-positive rate; [4] Positive sera/ tested sera.

Table 6. Relationship between average ages of EFV antibody-positive horses and EFV antibody-positive rates.

Age (years)	Farm A		Farm C	
	2002	2015	2002	2015
	Positive/Tested	Positive/Tested	Positive/Tested	Positive/Tested
4	1/2 (50.0%) [1]	1/1 (100.0%)	0/2	
5	0/2		0/7	0/3
6	0/1	0/7	2/7 (28.6%)	1/5 (20.0%)
7	0/5	2/5 (40.0%)	4/9 (44.4%)	2/11 (18.2%)
8	0/3	2/6 (33.3%)	1/4 (25.0%)	3/13 (23.1%)
9	0/4	1/3 (33.3%)	2/5 (40.0%)	2/9 (22.2%)
10	2/3 (66.7%)	1/3 (33.3%)	2/10 (20.0%)	6/19 (31.6%)
11	0/2	0/1	2/11 (18.2%)	4/10 (40.0%)
12	0/1	0/1	3/6 (50.0%)	5/9 (55.6%)
13	0/1	1/2 (50.0%)	1/2 (50.0%)	2/4 (50.0%)
14	0/1	0/3	0/4	4/8 (50.0%)
15	0/1	2/2 (100.0%)	1/2 (50.0%)	3/7 (42.9%)
16	0/1	3/3 (100.0%)	0/1	1/2 (50.0%)
17		2/3 [3] (66.7%)	0/2	4/5 [6] (80.0%)
18				1/1 [6] (100.0%)
19				0/1 [6]
20				
21				
22		1/1 [4] (100.0%)		
23	0/1	2/2 [5] (100.0%)		
24		0/1 [6]		
Subtotal 4y to 9y	1/17 (5.9%)	6/22 (27.3%)	9/34 (26.5%)	8/41 (19.5%)
10y to 14y	2/8 (25.0%)	2/10 (20.0%)	8/33 (24.2%)	21/50 (42.0%)
15y to 24y	0/3	10/12 (83.3%)	1/5 (20.0%)	9/16 (56.3%)
total	3/28 (10.7%)	18/44 (40.9%)	18/72 (25.0%)	38/107 (35.5%)
Average age	8.0y/ 9.6y/ 9.1y [2]	13.7y/ 9.7y/ 11.3y	9.6y/ 9.4y/ 9.4y	12.0y/ 9.9y/ 10.6y

[1] Number in parenthesis is antibody-positive rate; [2] Average age of antibody-positive horses/ average age of antibody-negative horses/ average age of total tested horses; [3] One positive horse also had the antibody in 2002 (4-year-old horse). The remaining two horses were not reared in 2002; [4] This horse was reared in 2002 (9 years old) and was antibody-negative in 2002; [5] Both horses were reared in 2002 (10 years old) and one horse was antibody-positive in 2002; [6] These horses were not reared in 2002.

4. Discussion

In this study, we isolated an EFV strain for the first time in Japan from PBMC obtained from a horse that showed symptoms of wobbler syndrome after surgery for intestinal volvulus. In general, spumaretroviruses have no pathogenicity in animals. Although pathogenicity of EFV has not been clearly demonstrated, the EFV we isolated and the symptoms observed in the horse might have no relationship. Concerning EFV isolation from PBMC, Tobaly-Tapiero et al. [8,32] reported that it took 4 weeks to isolate EFV in a highly FV-permissive adherent cell line (either human U373-MG cells or hamster BHK21 cells) after pre-cultivation of PBMC with the mitogenic lectin PHA-P for 2 days. On the other hand, we were able to isolate EFV from mitogen-untreated PBMC in HFK after co-cultivation for 10 days. Recently, we isolated another EFV from PBMC obtained from an EFV antibody-positive horse in HFK after co-cultivation for 10 days. These results suggested that isolation of EFV from PBMC could be conducted by co-cultivation with HFK without pre-cultivation of PBMC with mitogens. However, in our system, cell-free EFV was not released into the supernatant of EFV-infected HFK cell culture. Furthermore, cell-free EFV was not produced after three cycles of freezing and thawing of infected cells in culture medium. BFV is also highly cell-associated and spreads mainly through cell-to-cell transmission [33–36]. Most primate foamy viruses budded from intracellular membranes and cell-free viruses were produced following three cycles of freezing and thawing of infected cells [32]. However, Tobaly-Tapiero et al. [32] obtained cell-free EFV in the culture supernatant of EFV-infected human U373-MG cells without a freezing and thawing procedure. In ref. [32], it was reported that this phenomenon might be due to the lack of a dilysine motif in the C-terminus of the primate Env glycoprotein [37,38]. Our EFV isolate also lacked the dilysine motif. Therefore, the process of EFV replication in cells might be different depending on the cell type. We plan to propagate our EHV isolate in human U373-MG cells to confirm the results obtained by Tobaly-Tapiero et al. [32].

Nucleotide sequence data for EFVeca_LM showed high identities to those for prototype EFV (97.2% to 99.1% in various coding regions). The FFV clade clusters with a sequence identity of about 94% to 99% in partial *gag* and *pol* genes [14,39]. However, in the partial *env* gene, FFVs were divided into two distinct genotypes corresponding to two distinct serotypes [39–42]. In BFVs, phylogenetic analysis of complete genomic sequences revealed two clades, the European clade and non-European clade [39]. A recent Japanese BFV isolate belonged to the non-European clade based on results of phylogenetic analysis of partial *env* gene sequences [36]. Therefore, EFV might also be divided into two or more clades if more EFV isolates are obtained worldwide.

Since sero-prevalence of the EFV antibody in broodmares in Japan was about 25% in both the periods 2001 to 2002 and 2014 and 2016, it is thought that EFV infection might persist in almost a constant percentage of horse populations. This is the first report on sero-epidemiology in horses, though preliminary studies in horses in Poland showed the presence of provirus nucleic acid of EFV in about 15% of the tested animals [43]. In our study, the EFV-positive rate increased in an age-dependent manner, especially in Farms A and C in 2015. Furthermore, the average ages of horses reared in both farms in 2015 were slightly increased compared to those in 2002. In Farm A, two horses were sero-converted between 2002 and 2015. The mechanism of EFV transmission is not known, but it is likely that the longer the time spent in the same farm, the greater is the chance to become sero-positive [23]. A significant interaction between age and sero-positivity to BFV has also been reported and it was suggested that this phenomenon is due to horizontal transmission [23]. Furthermore, since the EFV-antibody positive rate in stallions of Farm A in 2015 was the highest among all farms in both periods, sexual transmission might have occurred in the breeding season. In any case, it is thought that most infections result from horizontal transmission.

Fortunately, we have sera from Farms A and C that have been stocked monthly for about 18 years in our laboratory, and we plan to conduct a detailed serological survey to determine the epidemiology of EFV infection in horses. Furthermore, we plan to isolate other EFVs from sero-positive horses and examine the molecular epidemiology of EFV infection in horses in Japan.

Author Contributions: Conceptualization, R.K.; Methodology, R.K.; Formal Analysis, R.K.; Resources, Y.T., H.H., N.T.; Writing-Original Draft Preparation, R.K.; Writing-Review & Editing, Y.T., N.T.; Supervision, R.K.

Funding: This research received no external funding.

Conflicts of Interest: The authors declare no conflict of interest.

References

1. Rethwilm, A.; Lindemann, D. Foamy viruses. In *Fields Virology*, 6th ed.; Knipe, D.M., Howley, P., Eds.; Lippincott, Willilams & Wilkins: Philadelphia, PA, USA, 2013; pp. 1613–1632.
2. Johnston, P.B. A second immunologic type of simian foamy virus: Monkey throat infections and unmasking by both types. *J. Infect. Dis.* **1961**, *109*, 1–9. [CrossRef] [PubMed]
3. Stiles, G.E.; Bittle, J.L.; Cabasso, V.J. Comparison of simian foamy virus strains including a new serological type. *Nature* **1964**, *201*, 1350–1351. [CrossRef] [PubMed]
4. Rogers, N.G.; Basnight, M.; Gibbs, C.J.; Gajdusek, D.C. Latent viruses in chimpanzees with experimental kuru. *Nature* **1967**, *216*, 446–449. [CrossRef] [PubMed]
5. Achong, B.G.; Mansell, P.W.; Epstein, M.A.; Clifford, P. An unusual virus in cultures from a human nasopharyngeal carcinoma. *J. Natl. Cancer Inst.* **1971**, *46*, 299–307. [PubMed]
6. Riggs, J.L.; Oshirls, L.S.; Taylor, D.O.; Lennette, E.H. Syncytium-forming agent isolated from domestic cats. *Nature* **1969**, *222*, 1190–1191. [CrossRef] [PubMed]

7. Malmquist, W.A.; van der Maaten, M.J.; Boothe, A.D. Isolation, immunodiffusion, immunofluorescence, and electron microscopy of a syncytial virus of lymphosarcomatous and apparently normal cattle. *Cancer Res.* **1969**, *29*, 188–200. [PubMed]
8. Tobaly-Tapiero, J.; Bittoun, P.; Neves, M.; Guillemin, M.C.; Lecellier, C.H.; Puvion-Dutilleul, F.; Gicquel, B.; Zientara, S.; Giron, M.L.; de Thé, H.; et al. Isolation and characterization of an equine foamy virus. *J. Virol.* **2000**, *74*, 4064–4073. [CrossRef]
9. Wu, Z.; Ren, X.; Yang, L.; Hu, Y.; Yang, J.; He, G.; Zhang, J.; Dong, J.; Sun, L.; Du, J.; et al. Virome analysis for identification of novel mammalian viruses in bat species from Chinese provinces. *J. Virol.* **2012**, *86*, 10999–11012. [CrossRef]
10. Meiering, C.D.; Linial, M.L. Historical perspective of foamy virus epidemiology and infection. *Clin. Microbiol. Rev.* **2001**, *14*, 165–176. [CrossRef]
11. Saïb, A. Non-primate foamy viruses. *Curr. Top. Microbiol. Immunol.* **2003**, *277*, 197–211.
12. Linial, M. Why aren't foamy viruses pathogenic? *Trends Microbiol.* **2000**, *8*, 284–289. [CrossRef]
13. Rethwilm, A.; Bodem, J. Evolution of foamy viruses: The most ancient of all retroviruses. *Viruses* **2013**, *5*, 2349–2374. [CrossRef] [PubMed]
14. Kehl, T.; Tan, J.; Materniak, M. Non-simian foamy viruses: Molecular virology, tropism and prevalence and zoonotic/interspecies transmission. *Viruses* **2013**, *5*, 2169–2209. [CrossRef] [PubMed]
15. Nakamura, K.; Miyazawa, T.; Ikeda, Y.; Sato, E.; Nishimura, Y.; Nguyen, N.T.; Takahashi, E.; Mochizuki, M.; Mikami, T. Contrastive prevalence of feline retrovirus infections between northern and southern Vietnam. *J. Vet. Med. Sci.* **2000**, *62*, 921–923. [CrossRef]
16. Bandecchi, P.; Matteucci, D.; Baldinotti, F.; Guidi, G.; Abramo, F.; Tozzini, F.; Bendinelli, M. Prevalence of feline immunodeficiency virus and other retroviral infections in sick cats in Italy. *Vet. Immunol. Immunopathol.* **1992**, *31*, 337–345. [CrossRef]
17. Lin, J.A.; Cheng, M.C.; Inoshima, Y.; Tomonaga, K.; Miyazawa, T.; Tohya, Y.; Toh, K.; Lu, Y.S.; Mikami, T. Seroepidemiological survey of feline retrovirus infections in cats in Taiwan in 1993 and 1994. *J. Vet. Med. Sci.* **1995**, *57*, 161–163. [CrossRef] [PubMed]
18. Daniels, M.J.; Golder, M.C.; Jarrett, O.; MacDonald, D.W. Feline viruses in wildcats from Scotland. *J. Wildl. Dis.* **1999**, *35*, 121–124. [CrossRef] [PubMed]
19. Glaus, T.; Hofmann-Lehmann, R.; Greene, C.; Glaus, B.; Wolfensberger, C.; Lutz, H. Seroprevalence of Bartonella henselae infection and correlation with disease status in cats in Switzerland. *J. Clin. Microbiol.* **1997**, *35*, 2883–2885.
20. Winkler, I.G.; Löchelt, M.; Flower, R.L. Epidemiology of feline foamy virus and feline immunodeficiency virus infections in domestic and feral cats: A seroepidemiological study. *J. Clin. Microbiol.* **1999**, *37*, 2848–2851.
21. Mochizuki, M.; Akuzawa, M.; Nagatomo, H. Serological survey of the Iriomote cat (Felis iriomotensis) in Japan. *J. Wildl. Dis.* **1990**, *26*, 236–245. [CrossRef]
22. Miyazawa, T.; Ikeda, Y.; Maeda, K.; Horimoto, T.; Tohya, Y.; Mochizuki, M.; Vu, D.; Vu, G.D.; Cu, D.X.; Ono, K.; et al. Seroepidemiological survey of feline retrovirus infections in domestic and leopard cats in northern Vietnam in 1997. *J. Vet. Med. Sci.* **1998**, *60*, 1273–1275. [CrossRef] [PubMed]
23. Jacobs, R.M.; Pollari, F.L.; McNab, W.B.; Jefferson, B. A serological survey of bovine syncytial virus in Ontario: Associations with bovine leukemia and immunodeficiency-like viruses, production records, and management practices. *Can. J. Vet. Res.* **1995**, *59*, 271–278. [PubMed]
24. Johnson, R.H.; de la Rosa, J.; Abher, I.; Kertayadnya, I.G.; Entwistle, K.W.; Fordyce, G.; Holroyd, R.G. Epidemiological studies of bovine spumavirus. *Vet. Microbiol.* **1988**, *16*, 25–33. [CrossRef]
25. Romen, F.; Backes, P.; Materniak, M.; Sting, R.; Vahlenkamp, T.W.; Riebe, R.; Pawlita, M.; Kuzmak, J.; Löchelt, M. Serological detection systems for identification of cows shedding bovine foamy virus via milk. *Virology* **2007**, *364*, 123–131. [CrossRef] [PubMed]
26. Materniak-Kornas, M.; Osiński, Z.; Rudzki, M.; Kuźmak, J. Development of a recombinant protein-based ELISA for detection of antibodies against bovine foamy virus. *J. Vet. Res.* **2017**, *61*, 247–252. [CrossRef]
27. Kirisawa, R.; Ohmori, H.; Iwai, H.; Kawakami, Y. The genomic diversity among equine herpesvirus-1 strains isolated in Japan. *Arch. Virol.* **1993**, *129*, 11–22. [CrossRef] [PubMed]
28. Kirisawa, R.; Fukuda, T.; Yamanaka, H.; Hagiwara, K.; Goto, M.; Obata, Y.; Yoshino, T.; Iwai, H. Enzymatic amplification and expression of bovine interleukin-1 receptor antagonist cDNA. *Vet. Immunol. Immunopathol.* **1998**, *62*, 197–208. [CrossRef]

29. Southern, E.M. Detection of specific sequences among DNA fragments separated by gel electrophoresis. *J. Mol. Biol.* **1975**, *98*, 503–517. [CrossRef]
30. Kumar, S.; Stecher, G.; Tamura, K. MEGA7: Molecular evolutionary genetics analysis version 7.0 for bigger datasets. *Mol. Biol. Evol.* **2016**, *33*, 1870–1874. [CrossRef]
31. Kimura, M. A simple method for estimating evolutionary rates of base substitutions through comparative studies of nucleotide sequences. *J. Mol. Evol.* **1980**, *16*, 111–120. [CrossRef]
32. Tobaly-Tapiero, J.; Bittoun, P.; Saïb, A. Isolation of foamy viruses from peripheral blood lymphocytes. *Methods Mol. Biol.* **2005**, *304*, 125–137. [PubMed]
33. Liebermann, H.; Riebe, R. Isolation of bovine syncytial virus in East Germany. *Arch. Exp. Veterinarmed.* **1981**, *35*, 917–919. [PubMed]
34. Bao, Q.; Hipp, M.; Hugo, A.; Lei, J.; Liu, Y.; Kehl, T.; Hechler, T.; Löchelt, M. In vitro evolution of bovine foamy virus variants with enhanced cell-free virus titers and transmission. *Viruses* **2015**, *7*, 5855–5874. [CrossRef] [PubMed]
35. Zhang, S.; Liu, X.; Liang, Z.; Bing, T.; Qiao, W.; Tan, J. The influence of envelope C-terminus amino acid composition on the ratio of cell-free to cell-cell transmission for bovine foamy virus. *Viruses* **2019**, *11*, 130. [CrossRef] [PubMed]
36. Hachiya, Y.; Kimura, K.; Oguma, K.; Ono, M.; Horikita, T.; Sentsui, H. Isolation of bovine foamy virus in Japan. *J. Vet. Med. Sci.* **2018**, *80*, 1604–1609. [CrossRef] [PubMed]
37. Goepfert, P.A.; Shaw, K.L.; Ritter, G.D., Jr.; Mulligan, M.J. A sorting motif localizes the foamy virus glycoprotein to the endoplasmic reticulum. *J. Virol.* **1997**, *71*, 778–784. [PubMed]
38. Goepfert, P.A.; Shaw, K.; Wang, G.; Bansal, A.; Edwards, B.H.; Mulligan, M.J. An endoplasmic reticulum retrieval signal partitions human foamy virus maturation to intracytoplasmic membranes. *J. Virol.* **1999**, *73*, 7210–7217.
39. Phung, H.T.; Ikeda, Y.; Miyazawa, T.; Nakamura, K.; Mochizuki, M.; Izumiya, Y.; Sato, E.; Nishimura, Y.; Tohya, Y.; Takahashi, E.; et al. Genetic analyses of feline foamy virus isolates from domestic and wild feline species in geographically distinct areas. *Virus Res.* **2001**, *76*, 171–181. [CrossRef]
40. Flower, R.L.; Wilcox, G.E.; Cook, R.D.; Ellis, T.M. Detection and prevalence of serotypes of feline syncytial spumaviruses. *Arch. Virol.* **1985**, *83*, 53–63. [CrossRef]
41. Winkler, I.G.; Flügel, R.M.; Löchelt, M.; Flower, R.L. Detection and molecular characterisation of feline foamy virus serotypes in naturally infected cats. *Virology* **1998**, *247*, 144–151. [CrossRef]
42. Hechler, T.; Materniak, M.; Kehl, T.; Kuzmak, J.; Löchelt, M. Complete genome sequences of two novel European clade bovine foamy viruses from Germany and Poland. *J. Virol.* **2012**, *86*, 10905–10906. [CrossRef] [PubMed]
43. Materniak, M.; Kuzmak, J. Occurrence of equine foamy virus infection in horses from Poland. In Proceedings of the 9th International Foamy Conference, Bethesda, MD, USA, 29–30 May 2012.

viruses

MDPI

Article

Feline Foamy Virus is Highly Prevalent in Free-Ranging *Puma concolor* from Colorado, Florida and Southern California

Sarah R. Kechejian [1], Nick Dannemiller [1], Simona Kraberger [2], Carmen Ledesma-Feliciano [3], Jennifer Malmberg [4], Melody Roelke Parker [5], Mark Cunningham [6], Roy McBride [7], Seth P. D. Riley [8], Winston T. Vickers [9], Ken Logan [10], Mat Alldredge [11], Kevin Crooks [12], Martin Löchelt [13], Scott Carver [14] and Sue VandeWoude [1,*]

1 Department of Microbiology, Immunology, and Pathology, College of Veterinary Medicine and Biomedical Sciences, Colorado State University, Fort Collins, CO 80523, USA; skecheji@colostate.edu (S.R.K.); dannemillern@gmail.com (N.D.)
2 Biodesign Institute, Arizona State University, Tempe, AZ 85281, USA; simona.kraberger@gmail.com
3 Division of Infectious Diseases, University of Colorado Anschutz Medical Campus, 12700 E 19th Ave, Aurora, CO 80045, USA; Carmen.Ledesma_Feliciano@colostate.edu
4 Wyoming State Vet Lab, University of Wyoming, 1174 Snowy Range Road, Laramie, WY 82072, USA; jennifer.malmberg@uwyo.edu
5 Frederick National Laboratory of Cancer Research, Leidos Biomedical Research, Inc., Frederick, MD 21701, USA; melody.roelke-parker@nih.gov
6 Florida Fish and Wildlife Conservation Commission, 1105 SW Williston Road, Gainesville, FL 32601, USA; mark.cunningham@myfwc.com
7 Rancher's Supply Inc., Alpine, TX 79830, USA; livestockprotection@gmail.com
8 National Park Service, Santa Monica Mountains National Recreation Area, Thousand Oaks, CA 90265, USA; seth_riley@nps.gov
9 Karen C. Drayer Wildlife Health Center, University of California, Davis, CA 95616, USA; twvickers@ucdavis.edu
10 Wildlife Researcher Colorado Parks and Wildlife, 2300 S. Townsend Avenue, Montrose, CO 80203, USA; ken.logan@state.co.us
11 Colorado Division of Wildlife Office, Mammals Research, 317 W. Prospect Rd, For Collins, CO 80526, USA; Mat.alldredge@state.co.us
12 Department of Fish, Wildlife, and Conservation Biology, Colorado State University 115 Wagar, Fort Collins, CO 80523, USA; kevin.crooks@colostate.edu
13 Department of Molecular Diagnostics of Oncogenic Infections, Research Program Infection, Inflammation and Cancer, German Cancer Research Center, (Deutsches Krebsforschungszentrum Heidelberg, DKFZ), Im Neuenheimer Feld 242, 69120 Heidelberg, Germany; m.loechelt@dkfz-heidelberg.de
14 School of Biological Sciences, University of Tasmania, Sandy Bay, Tasmania 7005, Australia; Scott.carver@utas.edu.au
* Correspondence: sue.vandewoude@colostate.edu

Received: 7 March 2019; Accepted: 17 April 2019; Published: 19 April 2019

Abstract: Feline foamy virus (FFV) is a retrovirus that has been detected in multiple feline species, including domestic cats (*Felis catus*) and pumas (*Puma concolor*). FFV results in persistent infection but is generally thought to be apathogenic. Sero-prevalence in domestic cat populations has been documented in several countries, but the extent of viral infections in nondomestic felids has not been reported. In this study, we screened sera from 348 individual pumas from Colorado, Southern California and Florida for FFV exposure by assessing sero-reactivity using an FFV anti-Gag ELISA. We documented a sero-prevalence of 78.6% across all sampled subpopulations, representing 69.1% in Southern California, 77.3% in Colorado, and 83.5% in Florida. Age was a significant risk factor for FFV infection when analyzing the combined populations. This high prevalence in geographically distinct populations reveals widespread exposure of puma to FFV and suggests efficient shedding and transmission in wild populations.

Keywords: feline foamy virus; epidemiology; retrovirus; *Spumaretrovirus*; mountain lion; *Puma concolor*; ELISA

---

1. Introduction

Feline foamy virus (FFV) is a member of the oldest retrovirus family, *Spumaretrovirinae* [1]. The virus is reportedly contact-dependent and causes life-long infections in felines worldwide [2]. FFV was originally identified as a tissue culture contaminant from primary feline cell cultures [3] and named for its characteristic cytopathic effects. In comparison to other feline retroviruses, the relevance of FFV infection to felid behavior and health is not yet well-understood despite its high prevalence in populations worldwide [4]. Existing epidemiological studies on FFV have almost exclusively evaluated domestic cat (*Felis catus*) populations [5,6], with only a handful evaluating prevalence in wild feline species [7–10]. Additionally, published literature has found FFV to be putatively apathogenic in domestic cats [11] but no literature has explored the virus' relationship to pathology in wild felids. Puma (*Puma concolor*) are the largest felid in North America and have frequent contact (e.g. predation) with domestic cats [12], making them a unique subject for this analysis.

In this study we exploited an extensive archive [13] to investigate FFV sero-prevalence and risk factors in pumas in the United States using a serologic assay validated for use in domestic cats [14–16]. Relationships between puma demography (e.g. age and sex) and FFV infection was determined using a Bayesian hierarchical modeling approach. We additionally explored the effect of a regional treatment (sport-hunting ban) on FFV sero-positivity in one Colorado subpopulation in order to investigate the effect of management interventions on the spread of the virus. Our results suggested that FFV sero-prevalence in U.S. puma was high (78.6% overall), risk factors varied by sampling location, and that a ban on hunting did not affect FFV sero-prevalence in Colorado.

2. Materials and Methods

We evaluated FFV sero-prevalence in three states: Colorado ($n = 130$, collected 2005–2011), Florida ($n = 150$, collected 1983–2010), and Southern California ($n = 68$, collected 2001–2011). Puma samples were opportunistically collected by government and local authorities engaged in independent management studies as previously described [13,17]. Sex and age of sampled pumas, if recorded, were determined via manager expertise, categorized as male or female and adult or young. Due to inconsistent location information, each state's sample population was considered a uniform population.

Sera were tested in duplicate on separate 96-well plates at 1:50 dilution using a non-quantitative GST-capture ELISA targeting the FFV Gag antigen, as previously described [14–16]. The ELISA has high sensitivity and specificity for the detection of FFV antibodies in naturally and experimentally infected domestic cats and has been validated against western blot [14–16]. This ELISA utilizes recombinant FFV Gag antigen generated from domestic cat FV sequences, which are 98% similar to the published puma FFV Gag [18,19]. Additional data evaluating more than 50 *gag* sequences from Colorado pumas has determined 95–100% similarity between puma and domestic cat FFVs [20]. A positive ELISA result was defined as having an OD absorbance over [2 × (meanGag + 3 SD)], with "meanGag" being the average negative control absorbance, and "SD" being the standard deviation of the negative control absorbance. This calculation employs very stringent cut off criteria [14–16], and is similar to methods of analytical detection reported by Lardeux et al. (2016) [21]. OD calculation was revised for each run, assuring each analysis was compared to its own negative control. Serum from experimentally infected domestic cats (positive) or specific pathogen free domestic cats (negative) were used as controls [15]. All plates were run in the same laboratory by the same individual over the course of one month.

Reagents were reconstituted on an as-needed basis. ELISA plates were prepared with fresh coating buffer the night prior to use.

Normalization of results was conducted by calculating each sample's absorbance as a percent of average positive control absorbance on the same plate. Each sample was additionally recorded as positive or negative using OD cut off values calculated as described above.

FFV sero-prevalence across the sampling period, stratified by sex (male and female) and age (young and adult) across all locations was compared using a chi-square test. Sex, age, and the interaction between sex and age were evaluated as possible risk factors for FFV infection for each state and across all samples using Bayesian generalized linear models (GLMs, a style of linear regression accounting for response variables with non-normal error distributions). For each coefficient (i.e., variable), we used weakly informative priors and extracted a 95% credible interval from the posterior distribution. Any coefficient whose 95% credible interval did not contain 0 was considered important. GLMs were ranked and compared using Akaike information criterion (AIC, an estimator of the relative quality of a statistical model when compared to other models for a given set of data). The model with the lowest AIC value was considered to better fit the data and subsequently the important variable(s) within that model were considered potential risk factors for puma FFV infection. If a model had an important predictor and was within 2 AIC of the best fit model, it was considered to reveal the most credible risk factor for FFV infection in pumas. Puma with unrecorded sex (n = 10) or age (n = 74) were excluded from risk factor analyses. There were 173 female, 167 male, 190 adult and 86 young pumas used in the analysis.

We additionally evaluated FFV sero-prevalence during and after a management intervention in Colorado. Between 2004 and 2009, Colorado Parks and Wildlife implemented a sport hunting ban in the Western Slope to evaluate management programs [22]. We compared FFV sero-prevalence during (2004–2009) and after (2010–2014) the sport hunting ban using a chi square statistic.

3. Results

3.1. Sero-Prevalence

FFV sero-prevalence is reported in Figure 1 and was high in all three states with an overall sero-prevalence of 78.6% (95% CI: 74, 82.7). There was no significant association of FFV sero-prevalence with location at the state level.

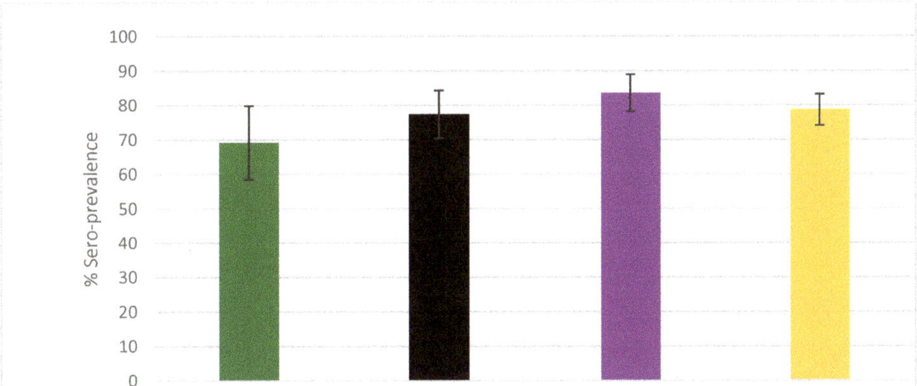

Figure 1. Puma feline foamy virus was found in high sero-prevalence in the U.S. Sero-prevalence by state: Southern California 69.1% (95% CI: 56.7, 79.8%); Colorado 77.3% (95% CI: 69.1, 84.3%); Florida 83.5% (95% CI: 77.0, 88.9%). Sero-prevalence across all sampling locations (overall) was 78.6% (95% CI: 74.0, 82.7%). There was no significant difference between states (p = 0.14).

Figure 2 displays the normalized distribution of all samples used in this analysis, grouped by location, and colored by negative and positive assignment. Colorado samples with normalized absorbance >70% of the positive control values were consistently classified as positive, while samples <70% of the positive control's absorbance were negative. Southern California samples classified as positive had absorbance values >50% of the positive control absorbance except for one sample that was classified 31% of positive control value but still above negative cut off for the plate. All other Southern California samples classified as negative had absorbance <50%. Colorado and Southern California samples classified as positive were clearly distinguished by negative cut off values (Figure 2). While there was less demarcation of clearly negative and positive samples in the Florida population, only two positive samples were <30% absorbance and all negative samples were <30%. Reclassification of all Florida panthers with an absorbance less than 49% ($n = 7$) as negative would have resulted in a sero-positivity of 74% which fell outside of the calculated 95% confidence interval (estimated as 77.0–88.9%); however, exclusion of these samples would have resulted in a sero-positivity of 78%, which remained within the calculated 95% confidence interval (estimated as 77.0–88.9%).

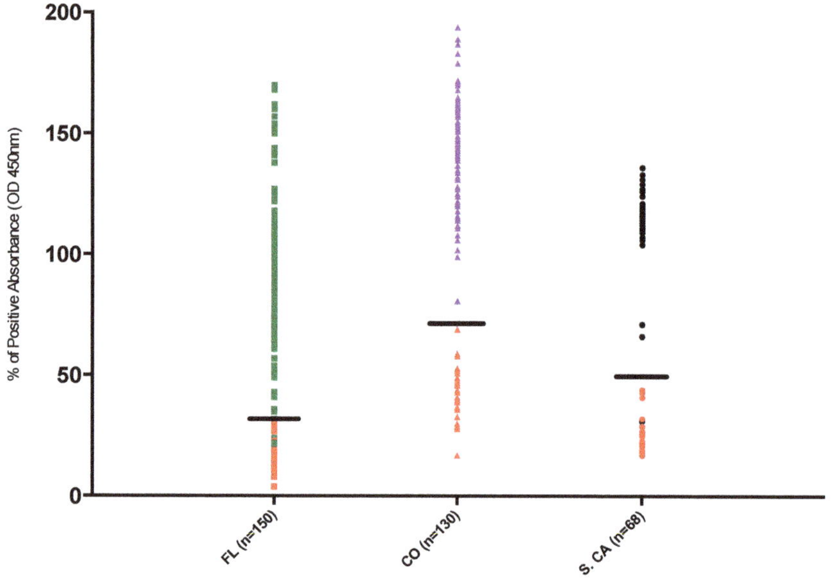

Figure 2. Seropositive OD values were well distinguished from samples classified as seronegative. The sample points in red were negative; the sample points in green, purple or black were classified as positive for their respective locations. All Colorado and all but one Southern California sample fell into positive absorbance ranges that were clearly segregated (noted with black lines) from samples classified as negative (<70% for CO, <50% for S.CA). 112 of 119 Florida samples classified as seropositive were at least 49% of positive control OD values, with only two positive samples <30% (noted with black line).

3.2. Demographic Associations

Results of Bayesian GLMs are reported and graphically portrayed in Table 1 and Figure 3, respectively. Neither sex nor age were predictors of FFV infection in Southern California, but there was a trend for higher FFV exposure in adults relative to younger pumas. Age was a predictor for FFV infection over all sites and also in Colorado and Southern California as individual sites, with adult pumas being at greater risk. In Florida as an individual site, sex, not age, was a predictor of FFV infection, with females being at greater risk.

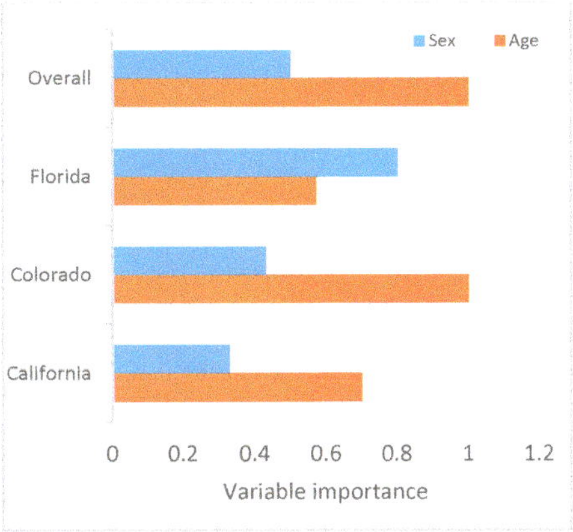

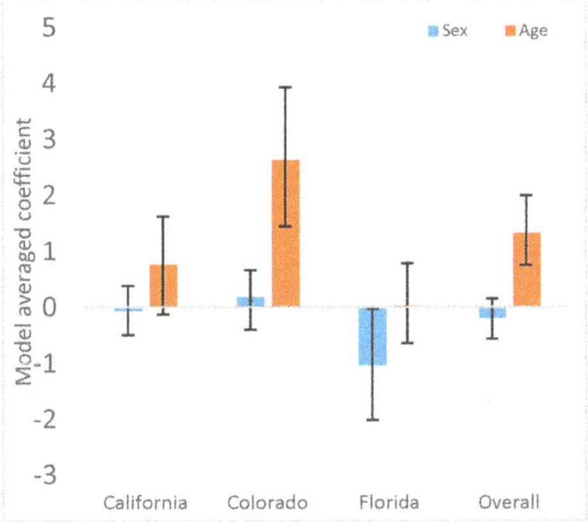

(A) **(B)**

Figure 3. Older pumas and female Florida panthers at higher risk of feline foamy virus (FFV) infection. (**A**) The plot displays variable importance weights for puma sex or age as risk factors for FFV, showing age to be more important in Colorado, Southern California and across the sampling locations (overall). (**B**) The plot displays model averaged coefficients with 95% confidence intervals, with adult and male being >0, and young and female being <0. If the 95% confidence interval did not cross 0, the variable was considered important. Females were weakly associated with infection risk in Florida only.

Table 1. Age alone as a risk factor for feline foamy virus (FFV) infection produced the best fit model in Southern California, Colorado and across all sampling locations (overall), while in Florida sex was the risk factor that produced the best fit model. Models were ranked from most to least supported by the data.

Model	AIC	ΔAIC	Model Weight
SOUTHERN CALIFORNIA			
Age	63.39	0.00	0.46
Null	64.98	1.59	0.21
Sex + Age	65.34	1.94	0.18
Sex	66.7	3.38	0.09
Sex + Age + Sex*Age	67.34	3.94	0.06
COLORADO			
Age	62.09	0.00	0.57
Sex + Age	63.87	1.78	0.23
Sex + Age + Sex*Age	64.20	2.11	0.20
Null	77.69	15.60	0.00
Sex	79.23	17.14	0.00
FLORIDA			
Sex	111.53	0.00	0.32
Sex + Age + Sex*Age	111.77	0.24	0.29
Sex + Age	112.55	1.02	0.19
Null	113.77	2.24	0.11
Age	114.02	2.49	0.09
OVERALL			
Age	240.22	0.00	0.50
Sex + Age	240.84	0.62	0.37
Sex + Age + Sex*Age	242.83	2.61	0.14
Sex	254.40	14.18	0.00
Null	256.12	15.90	0.00

There was no significant difference in FFV sero-prevalence during (n = 40) and after (n = 85) the sport hunting ban implemented on the Western Slope of Colorado (X^2: 2.5, $p > 0.11$).

4. Discussion

This study provides the first broad scale investigation of FFV sero-prevalence in a large, geographically-dispersed sampling of free-ranging pumas. The high overall puma FFV sero-prevalence of 78.6% was higher than what had been recorded in domestic cat populations using similar ELISA assays [5,6]. Reported FFV infection rates in domestic cats have ranged from 30 to 70%, and have varied across locations and analytical methodology [2,5–7,15]. Although the puma sampling locations have marked differences in their landscapes and ecology [13] similarly high infection rates were detected in all populations. This suggests that FFV is readily transmitted across varied landscapes.

While it was not possible to validate this study using sera from known positive and negative individuals, our stringency for negative and positive values was set using strict criteria [21]. Analysis of OD values illustrated distinct clustering of positive and negative sample absorbance (Figure 2), providing confidence that positive values truly reflected actual sero-prevalence. Florida samples were not as clearly distinguished as Colorado and Southern California samples. Samples from Florida were typically older and more likely to have been collected under less-than-ideal conditions from autolyzed animals (i.e., from road kill specimens). While this would typically result in the detection of more false negatives than false positives (due to degradation of circulating antibodies) it was also possible that there was higher nonspecific binding in this cohort. While exclusion of positive samples falling below 50% OD values of positive controls would still result in sero-prevalence estimates within the estimated 95% confidence interval in this population, further confirmatory analysis by PCR or other serologic assay would be warranted.

The significant difference in sero-prevalence between age groups in Colorado and across the sampled locations suggests that adults have higher exposure to FFV. If adult pumas are at increased risk of FFV infection, it is necessary to further investigate FFV transmission and the potential for horizontal transmission between individuals being the dominant mode. The significantly lower sero-prevalence of FFV in kittens suggests that this age group does not have the same exposure to the virus as adults in the same populations, supporting horizontal transmission as the primary mode of transmission in these populations. We recognize the difficult task of sampling family units is needed to fully explore the possibility of vertical transmission of the virus; however, a future study with this goal could help to more clearly determine mother to cub transmission events.

This reported high FFV sero-prevalence in adults exceeded the prevalence of most other infectious agents reported in these populations [13]. Adult pumas are traditionally considered to be solitary animals with rare documented instances of geographic and temporal overlap [23–25] though recent behavioral studies have exposed more social interactions between pumas [26]. In either case, inferred horizontal transmission of FFV resulting in four of five adults being exposed suggests facile transmission among adults. High FFV sero-prevalence could be explained by the virus maybe being able to survive on fomites (e.g., carcasses) long enough to infect other pumas without the need for physical contact between pumas. Further investigation of FFV degradation outside the host is needed to explore this alternative hypothesis. Further investigation of the virus' genetic and biological attributes may provide unique insights into puma behavior and capacity for transmission of other pathogens similar to Fountain-Jones et al. (2018) [27].

The lack of significant difference in sero-prevalence between sex groups in Southern California, Colorado and overall is consistent with what we found in domestic cats [28]. This suggests transmission may be via non-antagonistic intraspecific interactions. Physical contacts during mating or saliva swapping during kill sharing may be the most likely types of primary transmission events, as there is no substantial evidence that prolonged amicable physical contact (e.g., grooming) is common between adults [23,24,26]. A recent report has documented higher FFV loads in saliva versus blood in naturally infected domestic cats [29], which could suggest a mechanism for puma to puma transmission. Further studies of FFV ecology in the endangered and federally protected Florida panther (Puma concolor coryi) are needed to further our understanding of female sex as a risk factor for FFV infection.

FFV has not been documented to cause acute disease or easily recognized clinical signs of disease in domestic cats [2,14,30]. However, simian Foamy Virus (SFV) has been associated with accelerated SIV disease [31] and an association between FFV viral load and exogenous Feline leukemia virus (FeLV) viremia has been noted [31,32]. Therefore, results from this study can be used to compare the prevalence of FFV to other retroviruses of pumas such as feline immunodeficiency virus (FIV) and evaluate possible potentiation of disease. Furthermore, since FFV is a lifelong infection and viral sequences can be isolated from circulating blood cells, genotypic analysis of puma FFV may be useful as a marker of animal movement and pathogen transmission within or between populations [33].

Author Contributions: Conceptualization, S.R.K., S.K., and S.V.; data curation, S.R.K.; formal analysis, S.R.K., N.D. and S.C.; funding acquisition, S.R.K., N.D., S.C. and S.V.; methodology, C.L.F. and M.L.; project administration, S.V.; resources, M.R.P., M.C., R.M., S.P.D.R., W.V., K.L., M.A. and K.C.; supervision, C.L.F., S.C. and S.V.; writing—original draft, S.R.K., N.D. and S.V.; writing—review and editing, S.R.K., N.D., S.K., C.L.F., J.M., M.C., S.P.D.R., W.V., K.L., M.A., K.C., M.L., S.C. and S.V.

Funding: Funding and support were provided by Colorado State University, Colorado Parks and Wildlife (CPW), Boulder County Parks and Open Space, Boulder City Open Space and Mountain Parks, the Bureau of Land Management, U.S. Forest Service, Arizona State University, University of California at Davis, National Park Service, California State Parks, the Calabasas Landfill, The Santa Monica Mountains Fund, German Cancer Research Center, Boehringer Ingelheim, and a grant from the National Science Foundation-Ecology of Infectious Diseases Program (NSF EF-0723676; EF-1413925).

Conflicts of Interest: The authors declare no conflicts of interest. The funders had no role in the design of the study; in the collection, analyses, or interpretation of data; in the writing of the manuscript, or in the decision to publish the results.

References

1. Fields, B.N.; Knipe, D.M.; Howley, P.M.; Griffin, D.E. Foamy Viruses. In *Fields Virology*, 6th ed.; Rethwilm, A., Lindemann, D., Eds.; Lippincott Williams & Wilkins: Philadelphia, PA, USA, 2013; p. 1614.
2. Linial, M. Why aren't foamy viruses pathogenic? *Trends Microbiol.* **2000**, *8*, 284–289. [CrossRef]
3. Riggs, J.L.; Oshiro, L.S.; Taylor, D.O.N.; Lenette, E.H. Syncytium-forming agent isolated from domestic cats. *Nature* **1969**, *11*, 1190–1191. [CrossRef]
4. Linial, M.L. Foamy Viruses are Unconventional Retroviruses. *J. Virol.* **1999**, *73*, 1747–1755. [PubMed]
5. Lin, J.A.; Cheng, M.C.; Inoshima, Y.; Tomonaga, K.; Miyazawa, T.; Tohya, Y.; Toh, K.; Lu, Y.S.; Mikami, T. Seroepidemiological survey of feline retrovirus infections in cats in Taiwan in 1993 and 1994. *J. Vet. Med. Sci.* **1995**, *57*, 161–163. [CrossRef] [PubMed]
6. Winkler, I.G.; Lochelt, M.; Flower, R.L.P. Epidemiology of Feline Foamy virus and Feline Immunodeficiency virus infections in domestic and feral cats: a seroepidemiological study. *J. Clin. Microbiol.* **1999**, *37*, 2848–2851. [PubMed]
7. Mochizuki, M.; Akuzawa, M.; Nagatomo, H. Serological Survey of the Iriomote Cat (Felis-Iriomotensis) in Japan. *J. Wildl. Dis.* **1990**, *26*, 236–245. [CrossRef] [PubMed]
8. Miyazawa, T.; Ikeda, Y.; Maeda, K.; Horimoto, T.; Tohya, Y.; Mochizuki, M.; Vu, D.; Vu, G.D.; Cu, D.X.; Ono, K.; et al. Seroepidemiological survey of feline retrovirus infections in domestic and leopard cats in northern Vietnam in 1997. *J. Vet. Med. Sci.* **1998**, *60*, 1273–1275. [CrossRef]
9. Daniels, M.J.; Golder, M.C.; Jarrett, O.; MacDonald, D.W. Feline viruses in wildcats from Scotland. *J. Wildl. Dis.* **1999**, *35*, 121–124. [CrossRef] [PubMed]
10. Cleaveland, S.; Mlengeya, T.; Kaare, M.; Haydon, D.; Lembo, T.; Luarenson, M.K.; Packer, C. The conservation relevance of epidemiological research into carnivore viral diseases in the Serengeti. *Conservation Biol.* **2007**, *21*, 612–622. [CrossRef] [PubMed]
11. German, A.C.; Harbour, D.A.; Helps, C.R.; Gruffydd-Jones, T.J. Is feline foamy virus really apathogenic? *Vet. Immunol. Immunopathol.* **2008**, *123*, 114–118. [CrossRef] [PubMed]

12. Smith, J.; Wang, Y.; Wilmers, C. Spatial characteristics of residential development shift large carnivore prey habits. *J. Wildl. Manage.* **2016**, *80*, 1040–1048. [CrossRef]
13. Carver, S.; Bevins, S.N.; Lappin, M.R.; Boydston, E.E.; Lyren, L.M.; Alldredge, M.; Logan, K.; Sweanor, L.L.; Riley, S.P.D.; Serieys, L.E.K.; et al. Pathogen exposure varies widely among sympatric populations of wild and domestic felids across the United States. *Ecol. Appl.* **2016**, *26*, 367–381. [CrossRef]
14. Ledesma-Feliciano, C.; Hagen, S.; Troyer, R.; Zheng, X.; Musselman, E.; Slavkovic, L.D.; Franke, A.-M.; Maeda, D.; Zielonka, J.; Munk, C.; et al. Replacement of feline fomay virus bet by feline immunodeficiency virus vif yields replicative virus with novel vaccine candidate potential. *Retrovirology* **2018**, *15*, 38. [CrossRef]
15. Bleiholder, A.; Muhle, M.; Hechler, T.; Bevins, S.; VandeWoude, S.; Denner, J.; Lochelt, M. Pattern of seroreactivity against feline foamy virus proteins in domestic cats from Germany. *Vet. Immunol. Immunop.* **2011**, *143*, 292–300. [CrossRef]
16. Romen, F.; Pawlita, M.; Sehr, P.; Bachmann, S.; Schröder, J.; Lutz, H.; Löchelt, M. Antibodies against Gag are diagnostic markers for feline foamy virus infections while Env and Bet reactivity is undetectable in a substantial fraction of infected cats. *Virology* **2006**, *345*, 502–508. [CrossRef] [PubMed]
17. Bevins, S.N.; Carver, S.; Boydston, E.E.; Lyren, L.M.; Alldredge, M.; Logan, K.A.; Riley, S.P.D.; Fisher, R.N.; Vickers, T.W.; Boyce, W.; et al. Three pathogens in sympatric populations of pumas, bobcats, and domestic cats: implications for infectious disease transmission. *PLoS ONE* **2006**, *7*, 31403. [CrossRef] [PubMed]
18. Winkler, I.; Bodem, J.; Haas, L.; Zemba, M.; Delius, H.; Flower, R.; Flugel, R.M.; Löchelt, M. Characterization of the genome of feline foamy virus virus and its proteins shows distinct features different from those of primate spumaviruses. *J. Virol.* **1997**, *71*, 6727–6741. [PubMed]
19. Kehl, T.; Bleiholder, A.; Roßmann, F.; Rupp, S.; Lei, J.; Lee, J.; Boyce, W.; Vickers, W.; Crooks, K.; VandeWoude, S. Complete Genome Sequences of Two Novel Puma concolor Foamy Viruses from California. *Genome Announc.* **2013**, *1*, e0020112. [CrossRef] [PubMed]
20. Kraberger, S.; Arizona State University, Tempe, AZ, USA. Personal communication, 2019.
21. Lardeux, F.; Torrico, G.; Aliaga, C. Calculation of ELISA's cut-off based on the change-point analysis method for detection of *Trypanosoma cruzi* infection in Bolivian dogs in the absence of controls. *Mem. Inst. Oswaldo Cruz.* **2016**, *111*, 501–504. [CrossRef] [PubMed]
22. Logan, K.A. *Assessing Effects of Hunting on a Puma Population on the Uncompahgre Plateau, Colorado. Wildlife Research Report*; Colorado Parks and Wildlife: Fort Collins, CO, USA, 2015.
23. Seidensticker, J.; Hornocker, M.; Wiles, W.; Messick, J. Mountain Lion Social Organization in the Idaho Primitive Area. *Wildl. Monogr.* **1973**, *35*, 3–60.
24. Hemker, T.; Lindzey, F.; Ackerman, B. Population Characteristics and Movement Patterns of Cougars in Southern Utah. *J. Wildl. Manage.* **1984**, *48*, 1275–1284. [CrossRef]
25. Logan, K.A.; Sweanor, L. Behavior and social organization of a solitary carnivore. In *Cougar: Ecology and Conservation*; Hornocker, M., Negri, S., Eds.; University of Chicago Press: Chicago, IL, USA, 2010; pp. 105–117.
26. Elbroch, M.; Levy, M.; Lubell, M.; Quigley, H.; Caragiulo, A. Adaptive social strategies in a solitary carnivore. *Sci. Adv.* **2017**, *3*, 1701218. [CrossRef] [PubMed]
27. Fountain-Jones, N.M.; Pearse, W.D.; Escobar, L.E.; Alba-Casals, A.; Carver, S.; Davies, T.J.; Kraberger, S.; Papes, M.; Vandegrift, K.; Worsley-Tonks, K.; et al. Towards an eco-phylogenetic framework for infectious disease ecology. *Biol. Reviews.* **2017**, *93*, 950–970. [CrossRef]
28. Kechejian, S.; Dannemiller, N.; Kraberger, S.; Ledesma-Feliciano, C.; Löchelt, M.; Carver, S.; VandeWoude, S. Feline foamy virus sero-prevalence and demographic risk factors in United States stray domestic cat populations. *J. Feline Med. Surg.* **2019**. in revision.
29. Cavalcante, L.T.F.; Muniz, C.P.; Jia, H.; Augusto, A.; Troccoli, F.; Medeiros, S.; Dias, C.; Switzer, W.; Soares, M.; Santos, A. Clinical and Molecular Features of Feline Foamy Virus and Feline Leukemia Virus Co-Infection in Naturally-Infected Cats. *Viruses* **2018**, *10*, 702. [CrossRef] [PubMed]
30. Saib, A. Non-primate foamy viruses. *Curr. Top. Microbiol. Immunol.* **2003**, *277*, 197–211. [PubMed]
31. Choudhary, A.; Galvin, T.A.; Williams, D.K.; Beren, J.; Bryant, M.A.; Khan, A.S. Influence of naturally occurring simian foamy viruses (SFVs) on SIV disease progression in the rhesus macaque (*Macaca mulatta*) model. *Viruses* **2013**, *5*, 1414–1430. [CrossRef]

32. Powers, J.A.; Chiu, E.S.; Kraberger, S.; Roelke-Parker, M.; Lowery, I.; Erbeck, K.; Troyer, R.; Carver, S.; VandeWoude, S. Feline leukemia virus disease outcomes in a domestic cat breeding colony: Relationship to endogenous FeLV and other chronic viral infections. *J. Virol.* **2018**, *92*, e00649-18. [CrossRef]
33. Biek, R.; Real, L.A. The landscape genetics of infectious disease emergence and spread. *Mol. Ecol.* **2010**, *19*, 3515–3531. [CrossRef] [PubMed]

viruses MDPI

Article

Clinical and Molecular Features of Feline Foamy Virus and Feline Leukemia Virus Co-Infection in Naturally-Infected Cats

Liliane T. F. Cavalcante [1], Cláudia P. Muniz [1,2], Hongwei Jia [3], Anderson M. Augusto [4], Fernando Troccoli [4], Sheila de O. Medeiros [1], Carlos G. A. Dias [5], William M. Switzer [3], Marcelo A. Soares [1,2] and André F. Santos [1,*]

1 Departamento de Genética, Universidade Federal do Rio de Janeiro, Rio de Janeiro 21941-590, Brazil; liliane.tavaresdefaria@gmail.com (L.T.F.C.); claudia.muniz16@gmail.com (C.P.M.); sheila.omedeiros@gmail.com (S.d.O.M.); masoares@biologia.ufrj.br (M.A.S.)
2 Programa de Oncovirologia, Instituto Nacional de Câncer, Rio de Janeiro 20231-050, Brazil
3 Laboratory Branch, Division of HIV/AIDS Prevention, National Center for HIV/AIDS, Hepatitis, STD, and TB Prevention, Centers for Disease Control and Prevention, Atlanta, GA 30329-4027, USA; hjia@cdc.gov (H.J.); bis3@cdc.gov (W.M.S.)
4 Fundação Rio-Zoo, Parque da Quinta da Boa Vista, S/N, Rio de Janeiro 20940-040, Brazil; andersonriozoo@gmail.com (A.M.A.); fernando.troccoli@riozoo.com.br (F.T.)
5 CAT (Centro de Atendimento e Terapia) para Gatos, Rua Mariz e Barros, 292, Rio de Janeiro 20270-001, Brazil; cgabrielvet@hotmail.com
* Correspondence: andre20@globo.com

Received: 14 October 2018; Accepted: 7 December 2018; Published: 11 December 2018

Abstract: Feline foamy virus (FFV) and feline leukemia virus (FeLV) belong to the *Retroviridae* family. While disease has not been reported for FFV infection, FeLV infection can cause anemia and immunosuppression (progressive infection). Co-infection with FFV/FeLV allows evaluation of the pathogenic potential and epidemiology of FFV infection in cats with FeLV pathology. Blood and buccal swab samples from 81 cats were collected in Rio de Janeiro. Plasma was serologically tested for FeLV. DNA extracted from peripheral blood mononuclear cells and buccal swabs was used to PCR detect FFV and FeLV. A qPCR was developed to detect and measure FFV proviral loads (pVLs) in cats. FeLV qPCR was performed using previous methods. The median log10 pVL of FFV mono-infected individuals was lower than found in FFV/FeLV co-infected cats in buccal swabs ($p = 0.003$). We found 78% of cats had detectable buccal FFV DNA in FFV mono-infected and FFV co-infected FeLV-progressive cats, while in FeLV-regressive cats (those without signs of disease) 22% of cats had detectable buccal FFV DNA ($p = 0.004$). Our results suggest that regressive FeLV infection may reduce FFV saliva transmission, the main mode of FV transmission. We did not find evidence of differences in pathogenicity in FFV mono- and -dually infected cats. In summary, we show that FVs may interact with FeLV within the same host. Our study supports the utility of cats naturally co-infected with retroviruses as a model to investigate the impact of FV on immunocompromised mammalian hosts.

Keywords: spumavirus; feline illness; proviral load; neglected virus

1. Introduction

Foamy viruses (FV) are complex retroviruses that belong to the *Retroviridae* family and comprise a unique genus within the *Spumaretrovirinae* subfamily that naturally infect many vertebrates, including feline, simian, bovine, and equine [1]. FV infection in humans is invariably associated with zoonotic transmission from other primate species [2,3]. Despite causing a highly cytopathic effect in many cell types in vitro [4], little is known about the pathogenic potential of FV in vivo. A single case-control study reported the presence of hematological abnormalities in humans infected with gorilla simian foamy viruses (SFVs) [5]. Other studies failed to report diseases associated with FV in either natural infection of nonhuman primates or in zoonotic infection of humans with SFVs [6–11]. It has been hypothesized that FVs are not able to cause disease in healthy, naturally-infected individuals due to functional immune systems that control virus infection, but these results may be limited by the small numbers of infected persons followed longitudinally [12]. Similarly, an absence of disease association with FVs may reflect an absence of systematic studies following infected individuals, animals or humans for long periods of time since other retroviruses can take decades for disease appearance and disease is not always found in all infected individuals. For example, persons with SFV infection can also be co-infected with HIV and HTLV but longitudinal studies have not been reported on disease outcomes in these persons [8,13,14]. Other viruses, including cytomegalovirus, varicella-zoster and herpes simplex, only rarely cause disease in healthy individuals, but when in co-infection with the human immunodeficiency virus (HIV), can become be activated with pathogenic consequences [15]. Similarly, rhesus macaques naturally infected with SFV and experimentally infected with simian immunodeficiency virus (SIV) progress more frequently to simian acquired immunodeficiency syndrome (SAIDS) compared to SIV-monoinfected macaques [16]. SIV/SFV co-infection in that study was associated with higher SIV viral loads (VLs), lower $CD4^+$ T-cell counts and lower survival.

Domestic cats (*Felis catus*) can be persistently infected with feline spumaretrovirus (the updated name for feline foamy virus—FFV). FFV elicits anti-FFV host immune responses. FFV prevalence in these animals ranges between 30–100% depending on sex, age and geographical region analyzed [17–21]. Upon experimental inoculation, FFV is found in oral mucosa cells 2–3 weeks after infection [22], and is initially detected by qPCR in the blood within the first two weeks of infection [23]. In this same study, two peaks of viremia were observed, at days 20 (80–170 FFU/mL blood) and 155 (332–415 FFU/mL blood). Furthermore, domestic cats are naturally infected by two other retroviruses which cause severe immunodeficiency: the feline immunodeficiency virus (FIV), another complex retrovirus, and feline leukemia virus (FeLV), a simple retrovirus characterized by the absence of accessory genes. Infection of cats with FIV or FeLV allows an evaluation of FFV co-infection in hosts with a compromised immune system and determination of FFV pathogenic potential.

FeLV was discovered decades ago in a group of cats with lymphoma [24], is more pathogenic than FIV, and for many years was responsible for more clinical manifestations than any other etiological agent in cats [25]. FeLV prevalence ranges between 1–3.6% in healthy individuals but between 7.3–12.2% in sick cats [26–29]. The main transmission route of FeLV is oropharyngeal exposure to mucosal secretions containing the virus [30]. Different infection outcomes have been identified in experimentally infected cats over the years. Regressive infection is defined as a transient antigenemia followed by the establishment of low to moderate proviral loads (pVLs) [31,32]. In contrast, viremic cats are considered to have a progressive infection, with high proviral and plasma RNA VLs [32]. Cats with progressive FeLV infection can develop tumors, anemia and immunosuppression and FeLV has also been associated with hematological disorders, immune-mediated diseases, and other syndromes, including neuropathy and reproductive disorders [25].

FIV was first identified in 1986 [33] in domestic cats in the United States (US). FIV prevalence ranges between 0.9–4.3% in healthy cats and between 7.9–31.3% in sick cats [26,27]. FIV is a feline lentivirus with structure, genome and pathogenesis that parallel those of HIV. Infection occurs primarily through biting [34], but can also occur through vertical transmission [35,36]. Experimentally infected cats undergo an initial acute phase, followed by a chronic or clinically asymptomatic phase, which may persist for over eight years, and a final symptomatic phase, also called feline acquired immunodeficiency syndrome (FAIDS) [37]. In this phase, opportunistic diseases are observed more frequently, such as neoplasia, myelosuppression, glomerulonephritis, neurological diseases and stomatitis. The risk of developing lymphoid malignancy is estimated to be 5 to 6-fold greater in FIV-infected only cats compared with uninfected cats [38].

Several studies have investigated co-infection in domestic cats [29,39,40]. Other studies have investigated the virologic factors involved in retrovirus co-infection [41]. But they mostly focused on FIV/FeLV co-infections. A study by Yamamoto et al. showed that a pre-existent FeLV infection enhanced the expression of FIV in the body and increased the severity of transient primary and chronic secondary stages of FIV infection [42]. Only a single study has evaluated the presence of all three retroviruses in cats [17], but was limited only to prevalence estimates and not their possible interactions or associations with disease. In another study, FeLV and FIV co-infection was examined and showed a greater risk for lymphoid cancers in dually infected cats [38]. The combination of susceptibility to multiple retroviral infections and varied possible disease outcomes makes domestic cats an attractive animal model to study the epidemiology and pathogenesis of co-infection by distinct retroviruses. We examined blood and buccal swab specimens of domestic cats in Brazil for detection and quantification of each feline virus to evaluate their potential association with disease and transmissibility in animals with single or multiple retroviral infections.

2. Materials and Methods

2.1. Specimen Collection

This project was approved by the Ethics Committee on Animal Use of the Center for Health Sciences at Federal University of Rio de Janeiro (CEUA-CCS) (protocol IBO08-07/16). Blood and buccal swab samples from 81 domestic cats were collected between 2013 and 2014 from three different veterinary clinics in Rio de Janeiro (n = 54) or captured within the grounds of Fundação Jardim Zoológico da Cidade do Rio de Janeiro (RIOZOO, n = 27), an urban area in the north zone of the city. Cats coming from veterinary clinics were selected for this study once they were suspected of FeLV infection, while cats from RIOZOO were selected randomly, independently whether they looked sick or not.

The cats from clinics were not previously vaccinated for FeLV, while for captured animals we are not sure about their vaccination status although the chances they have been vaccinated are minimal, since Brazilian public policies do not include FeLV vaccination. Upon presentation at the clinics or after capture, the cats were weighed and anesthetized with the administration of 10 g of ketamine or 0.5 μg of xylazine per kilogram of body weight. After anesthesia, 1–3 mL of whole blood was collected from the jugular vein by experienced veterinarians and placed into an EDTA blood tube and stored at room temperature until processing. Buccal swabs were collected from 68 cats by rubbing the upper, bottom and side of the oral cavity with a sterile cotton swab.

Hemogram tests displaying blood cell counts of 35 animals were performed by a veterinarian diagnostic laboratory. Hemogram results were kindly provided by Dr. Carlos Gabriel Dias. Cats with low erythrocytes (below 5 milions/μL), hemoglobin (below 8 g/dL) or hematocrit (below 24%) levels were considered anemic.

Twenty-eight cats were followed three years after the initial collection to determine their life status (alive or dead). For FeLV-infected cats, the time elapsed from infection was estimated based on the diagnosis date at the veterinary clinics. For cats whose infection status was unknown before sampling, the time elapsed from infection was considered using the sampling date.

2.2. Demographic and Clinical Variable Description

Cats were classified according to gender, age, outdoor access, household type, neuter status and health status. For age, cats were classified as: (a) kitten, up to 6 months old; (b) young, between 6–12 months of age and (c) adult, above one year of age. For feral cats without a known birthdate, age was estimated by veterinarian evaluation. Household status was classified as: (a) single, cats living alone at home; (b) multicat, cats living with up to 10 cats in the same house; (c) shelter, cats living in a shelter or house with more than 10 cats; and (d) feral, cats that live or have lived in the streets before. Cats classified as single, multicat and shelter were also categorized for outdoor access. Cats were considered sick when any clinical signs, including respiratory tract disease (RTD), progressive weight loss (PWL), ocular secretion (OS), anemia, cachexia, ulcers, hair loss, presence of ectoparasites, tooth loss, prolapses, scabies, pemphigus foliaceous, pyometra, sporotrichosis, diarrhea, neurological symptoms, abortion, kidney disease, stomatitis and neoplasia, or hematological changes were reported. Healthy cats were those without any reported clinical signs at the time of specimen collection.

2.3. Specimen Processing and Genomic DNA Extraction

Blood samples were centrifuged at 568× *g* for 10 min to separate plasma from cells. Plasma aliquots were stored at −80 °C for FIV/FeLV serologic testing. Peripheral blood mononuclear cells (PBMCs) were obtained from the cellular fraction by Ficoll-Paque PLUS (GE Healthcare, Waukesha, WI, USA) centrifugation and were stored at −80 °C until genomic DNA (gDNA) extraction. gDNA from PBMC and buccal swabs was extracted using the PureLink® Genomic DNA Mini Kit (Invitrogen, Carlsbad, CA, USA) and was quantified using a NanoVue Plus™ Nanodrop (GE Healthcare). PCR amplification of cytochrome b oxidase gene (*cytB*) sequences was used to verify DNA integrity of the extracted material as previously described [10].

2.4. Serological Screening of FIV and FeLV

Plasma from domestic cats was tested for FIV/FeLV by two commercial immunochromatographic tests: the FIV ac/FeLV Ag Test Alere® (Bionote Inc., Gyeonggi-do, Korea) or QuickVET FIV/FeLV Ubio (Biotechnology Systems, Kerala, India) kits at a veterinary clinic and UFRJ, respectively. These tests simultaneously detect an FeLV antigen and an FIV antibody. Assay sensitivity of 100% and 96.7% for FeLV and 96% and 97.6% for FIV, and specificity of 100% and 98.5% for FeLV and 98% and 99.3% for FIV were established by Alere® and Ubio, respectively.

2.5. Detection of FFV, FIV and FeLV Using Nested PCR

Nested or semi-nested PCR was performed to diagnose FFV infection by detection of four different FFV genome sequences, including the long terminal repeat (LTR, 215-bp) [43], integrase (*int*, 140-bp) [10], *gag*/polymerase (*pol*) (497-bp) [44] and envelope (*env*, 640-bp) [45]. Three new PCR primers for this study (FFV LTR out, FFV_F1 and FFV_R1) were designed using an alignment of the four available complete FFV genomes from domestic cats (Genbank accession numbers AJ564745, AJ564746, NC001871 and Y08851). Primer sequences are provided in Table 1. Primers used for detection of the FIV reverse transcriptase (RT) portion (603-bp) of the *pol* gene and of FeLV *env* sequences (1689-bp) (Table 1) were published previously ([46]), respectively.

For all published primers, the PCR conditions were followed according to those previous studies [10,43–47]. PCR conditions using newly designed primers were performed using 10× PCR buffer, 25 mM $MgCl_2$, 25 mM dNTPs, 25 pmol forward and reverse primers, 1 unit of Taq platinum polymerase (Invitrogen) and 50–200 nanograms of DNA in a total reaction volume of 50 µL. Amplicons from PCR-positive samples were purified using the PCR DNA Mini Kit (Real Genomics RBC, Banqiao, Taiwan) following the manufacturer's protocol and were sequenced in an ABI 3130xl platform (Thermo Scientific, Waltham, MA, USA).

Table 1. Primers used for PCR amplification of feline retrovirus (FFV, FIV and FeLV) genome sequences.

Virus	Genomic Region	Name	Sense	Primer Sequence (5′-3′)	Reference
FFV	LTR	FFV LTR out	1st forward	TGCACAGGAAGCTCCTTTAGGGTA	Designed herein
		789(rev)	1st and 2nd reverse	TCCCCACGTGTAGAGAAACACCACTC	[43]
		788(fow)	2nd forward	TGTACGGGAGCTCTTCTCACAGACTTGGC	[43]
	glycoprotein/ polymerase (*gag/pol*)	FFV_F1	1st forward	CCTCGGGTCCAAACACAGCC	Designed herein
		FFV_R1	1st reverse	CCAAGGTACATCTCCAGG	Designed herein
		FUV2610s	2nd forward	AACAGCAACACTCTGATGTTCCCG	[44]
		FUV3107a	2nd reverse	ATATACATCTCCTTCCTGCGTTCC	[44]
	integrase (*int*)	SIF5N_mod [a]	1st forward	TACATGGTTATACCCCACKAAGGCTC	[10]
		SIR1NN	1st and 2nd reverse	GTTTTATYTCCYTGTTTTTCCTYTCCA	[10]
		SIP4N	2nd forward	TGCATTCCGATCAAGGATCAGCATT	[10]
	envelope	env-f2	1st forward	GCTACTTCTACTAGAATAATGTTTTGGATA	[45]
		env-r2	1st reverse	AGCCACAGTAGTAATTGCATTGGCCAGGCC	[45]
		env-f3	2nd forward	GCTTTCAAAAATATGGACATTGTTATGTTA	[45]
		env-r3	2nd reverse	GTTTCTCCAAAATCTGCAAGCATATGGATG	[45]
FIV	reverse transcriptase (RT)	RT out F	1st forward	GGAGTAGGAGGAGGAAAAAGAGGAAC	[46]
		RT out R	1st reverse	GCCCATCCACTTATATGGGGGC	[46]
		RT int F	2nd forward	GGGCCTCAGGTAAAACAGTGGC	[46]
		RT int R	2nd reverse	GTCTTCCGGGGTTTCAAATCCCCAC	[46]
FeLV	envelope	Env Fow (1689 bp)	Forward	TCTATGTTAGGAACCTTAACCGATG	[47]
		Env Rev (1689 bp)	Reverse	CAGAATATCTGTGGTAC AAGCCTTAA	[47]
		Env Fow (437 bp)	Forward sequencing	GCYTGGTGGGTCTTAGGAA	[47]
		Env Rev (437 bp)	Reverse sequencing	AACARAAGTAAAGACTGTTGG	[47]

[a] The last four bases were removed from the original primer sequence (TACATGGTTATACCCCACKAAGGCTCCTCC).

2.6. FFV Quantitative PCR (qPCR)

A new quantitative PCR assay was developed to simultaneously detect and measure FFV proviral loads in infected cats. Generic *pol* primers and probe were designed using an alignment of complete FFV genomes at GenBank. The forward and reverse primers FFVPF1 5′-CAT GTT GTC AGC ACC AAG TAT AC-3′ and FFVPR1 5′-TGC AAG AGA GCA AGT TCT TCT TC-3′, respectively, and probe FFVPFP1 5′-FAM-TTG GAA TTG ATT GTA ATT TAC CAT TTGC- BHQ1–3′ were used to detect a 120-bp *pol* sequence.

Cycling conditions included an initial step of 95 °C for 10 min, followed by 55 cycles of 15 s at 95 °C and 30 s at 60 °C with a final hold step at 4 °C using a Bio-Rad iCycler CFX96 (Bio-Rad Laboratories, Hercules, CA, USA). For assay validation, 20 human blood donor PBMC DNAs and five different human cell lines (MCF-7, CEMx174, Jurkat, LNCaP and HeLa) were used as negative controls to assess assay specificity. Specificity and sensitivity were also determined using PBMC lysates from 39 US domestic cats previously found to be FFV-negative (n = 18) or positive (n = 21) by Western blot analysis. These cat specimens were available from a previous study investigating the zoonotic potential of feline retroviruses [48]. The limit of detection (LOD) of the assay was determined by testing of 60–140 replicates (depending on the copy number) ten and fivefold serial dilutions of plasmids containing a cloned fragment of the FFV *int* sequence ranging from 100 to a single copy diluted in 1 µg of negative human gDNA. Once the potential LOD was determined using 10 replicates of the 10-fold dilutions, we used a larger number of five-fold plasmid dilution replicates to further refine the LOD. We tested 60 ten copy replicates, 90 five copy replicates and 140 single copy replicates. Standard curves were constructed using 10^0–10^7 copies of plasmid DNA. The number of provirus copies/cell was estimated using the formula:

$$\text{number of copies detected}/(\text{DNA quantification in picograms}/6\text{ pgs cell})$$

where the mass for each domestic cat cell genome was considered as six picograms DNA per cell [49]. The amount of DNA in nanograms was measured by spectrophotometry.

2.7. FeLV qPCR

The FeLV qPCR test was performed as previously described [49] using a unique region within the U3 of the FeLV LTR with a reported detection limit of 1000 copies per reaction. Specificity of the assay was 100% by obtaining negative results for PBMC DNA from 80 pathogen-free, FeLV-negative cats. Assay sensitivity was also 100% by confirmation of infection in 30 FeLV p27-positive cats. Cats that were experimentally infected and that became persistently antigenaemic as determined by p27 ELISA were considered positive.

The primers and probe FeLV-U3-exo-f 5′-AAC AGC AGA AGT TTC AAG GCC-3′ (forward), FeLV-U3-exo-r 5′-TTA TAG CAG AAA GCG CGC G-3′ (reverse) and FeLV-U3-probe 5′-FAM-CCA GCA GTC TCC AGG CTC CCC A-TAMRA-3′ were used to detect a 131-bp LTR sequence. Standard curves were performed with a plasmid containing the target region in a serial dilution range of 10^3–10^9 copies. The cycling conditions consisted of an initial step of GoTaq (Promega, Madison, WI, USA) activation at 95 °C for 2 min followed by 40 cycles of 15 s at 95 °C and 1 min at 60 °C using an ABI 7500 real-time cycler (Applied Biosystems, Foster City, CA, USA). The number of pVL copies/cell was calculated similarly to the FFV pVL, except the pVL was divided by two to compensate for the presence of two LTR copies per integrated provirus.

2.8. Classification of FFV and FeLV Infections

We classified FFV-infected cats that were tested for both oral swab and PBMC tissues by nested PCR and/or qPCR. FFV-positive cats without virus detected in saliva were considered as latent infections, and were classified as non-transmissible. FFV-positive cats with virus detected in oral swabs were considered as potential FFV transmitters to other cats and were classified as transmissible.

Cats testing qPCR positive for FeLV were classified into two groups based on VL and serostatus: progressives (those with high pVL, most seropositive) and regressives (those with low VL, most seronegative).

2.9. Statistical Analyses

The Mann-Whitney test was used for statistical comparisons of pVL between groups. Kaplan-Meier survival curves were generated for survival analysis. Linear regression was used to evaluate a correlation between the FFV and FeLV VLs. Odds ratios (OR), 95% confidence intervals (95% CI) and *p*-values were determined to analyze risk factors for FeLV and FFV co-infection, including sex, age, whether neutered, and household status. A multivariate analysis was conducted by adjusting the model for variables that showed significant associations with FFV/FeLV co-infection, i.e., that showed *p*-values below 0.10. To test the different proportion of non- and transmissible cats, probabilities (p) were calculated using the Chi-square test. All statistics were performed using MedCalc v.11.3.0.0 or in the *R* environment and *p*-values ≤ 0.05 were considered significant.

3. Results

3.1. Population Profile

All 81 domestic cats sampled in this study were from Fundação Jardim Zoológico da Cidade do Rio de Janeiro (RIOZOO) and from veterinary clinics throughout the city of Rio de Janeiro. Cats were classified according to gender, age, outdoor access, sexual sterilization, household type, and health status (Table 2). We found an approximately equal proportion of male and female cats and a higher number of adult individuals (57%). Twenty of 36 male cats (56%) were neutered, while 15 of 30 females (50%) were spayed.

Table 2. Socio-demographic data and FFV and FeLV prevalence [a] of domestic cats from Brazil in the present study.

Category	Number (%)	FFV Mono-Infected (%)	FeLV Mono-Infected (%)	FFV/FeLV Co-Infected (%)
Total	81 (100)	26 (32)	8 (10)	38 (47)
Gender (n = 81)				
Female	40 (49)	11 (28)	3 (8)	22 (55)
Male	41 (51)	15 (37)	5 (12)	16 (39)
Age group (n = 79)				
Kitten	18 (23)	8 (44)	0 (0)	7 (38)
Young	16 (20)	5 (31)	0 (0)	8 (50)
Adult	45 (57)	13 (29)	7 (16)	22 (49)
Neutered status (n = 66)				
Neutered/spayed	35 (53)	8 (23)	3 (8)	20 (57)
Intact	31 (47)	13 (42)	3 (10)	11 (31)
Household status (n = 78)				
Single	2 (2.6)	1 (50)	0 (0)	1 (50)
Multi-cat	21 (27)	2 (10)	3 (14)	11 (52)
Shelter	12 (15)	1 (8)	2 (17)	9 (75)
Feral	43 (55)	21 (49)	2 (5)	16 (37)
Outdoor Access (n = 29)				
Yes	9 (31)	0 (0)	3 (33)	5 (56)
No	20 (69)	4 (20)	1 (5)	12 (60)
Health status (n = 81)				
Healthy	27 (34)	8 (30)	2 (7)	11 (41)
Sick	52 (66)	18 (35)	5 (10)	26 (50)

[a] Prevalence was calculated with number of infected individuals per total number of animals based on nested PCR/real-time PCR (FFV) or on serology/nested PCR/real-time PCR (FeLV) results. FFV, Feline Foamy Virus; FeLV, Feline Leukemia Virus. Feline immunodeficiency virus (FIV)-infected cats were not reported because only three FIV-positive cats were found (one coinfected with FFV and two multiply infected with FeLV and FFV).

Most cats (55%) were classified as feral and of the 35 cats residing in any household (21 multicats, 12 shelters and 2 singles), the majority (69%) had no outdoor access. The majority of cats (66%) were also sick at the time of sample collection.

3.2. FIV and FeLV Infection of Domestic Cats

Blood DNA specimens from all 81 cats were tested by nested PCR and serology for diagnosis of FIV and FeLV infection. Buccal swab genomic DNA (gDNA) specimens available from 68 cats were also analyzed using PCR testing. Animals were considered PCR-positive when at least one viral sequence was detected in PBMCs and/or buccal swab samples. We found three FIV-positive animals, of which 2/81 (2.5%) were positive only by serology and 1/81 (1.2%) was PCR-positive only. Of two serologically FIV-positive animals, one was a house cat and the other was a feral cat. The FIV PCR-positive only cat was feral (Table 3). We found 22/81 (27%) animals reactive in the FeLV p27 antigen test in plasma and an equal number of PCR-positive animals but cats did not always have concordant p27 and PCR results. Specimens from five cats were PCR-positive only and five different cats were FeLV p27-reactive only.

Table 3. Detection of feline leukemia virus (FeLV) and feline immunodeficiency virus (FIV) in household and feral cats.

Virus	Category	Household (n = 35)	Feral (n = 43)	Total
FeLV	Seropositive only	3/35 (9%)	2/43 (5%)	5/81* (6%)
	PCR-positive only	4/35 (11%)	1/43 (2%)	5/81* (6%)
	PCR-negative and seropositive	9/35 (26%)	8/43 (19%)	17/81* (21%)
	PCR-negative and seronegative	19/35 (54%)	32/43 (74%)	51/81*(63%)
	Total FeLV infections	16/35 (46%)	11/43 (26%)	27/81* (33%)
FIV	PCR-positive	0/35	1/43 (2%)	1/81* (1%)
	Seropositive	1/35 (3%)	1/43 (2%)	2/81* (2%)
	Total FIV infections	1/35 (3%)	2/43 (4.7%)	3/81* (3.7%)

* The total number includes 35 household cats, 43 feral cats and three cats with no information.

Cats positive using at least one assay (serology or PCR) were classified as infected. Among the household cats (single, multi-cat and shelter) and feral cats, FeLV-positive results in both PCR and serological tests tended to be higher in households, 48% (16/35) compared to feral cats 26% (11/43) (p = 0.063; Fisher´s exact test; Table 3). Two cats were dually infected with both FIV and FeLV.

3.3. PCR Detection and Quantification of FFV

The 81 PBMC and 68 buccal swab gDNA samples were screened by nested PCR for amplification of four different FFV genomic sequences (Table 4). Overall, we found a FFV PCR prevalence of 46% (37/81). We found more cats with *gag/pol* PCR-positive results (27/33, 82% in PBMCs and 13/19, 68% in buccal swab gDNA) compared to other viral targets. Of the 37 FFV-positive animals, 33 had both PBMC and buccal swab gDNA specimens available for nested FFV PCR testing. Twenty-nine animals were PCR-positive (88%) in the PBMC compartment, while only 19 (58%) were positive in the buccal swab (p = 0.006). Comparing both tissue compartments, 15 animals were positive in both PBMC and buccal swab, while 14 cats were positive only in PBMC and four were positive only in the buccal swab. No significant differences were found when comparing feral to household cats that were FFV PCR-positive in either the PBMC or the buccal swab compartments (p = 0.788 and p = 0.247, respectively).

Table 4. Nested FFV PCR detection in peripheral blood mononuclear cells (PBMC) and buccal swabs.

Fragment	PBMC (%)	Buccal (%)
long terminal repeat (LTR)	15/79 [b] (19)	0/67 [b] (0)
gag/polymerase (*pol*)	27/81 (33)	13/68 (19)
Integrase	14/81 (17)	9/68 (13)
Envelope	19/81 (23)	1/43 [b] (2)
Nested FFV PCR-positive cats [a]	33/81 (41)	19/68 (28)
FFV qPCR-positive cats	53/73 (73)	19/64 (30)
Total FFV-positive cats	62/81 (77)	31/68 (46)

[a] Cats with at least one virus fragment detected. [b] In three cases, a limited number of samples were tested due to material availability.

We also developed a new quantitative real-time PCR (qPCR) assay to simultaneously detect and measure FFV proviral load (pVL) in cats. Testing of replicates containing serial dilutions of FFV integrase (*int*)-containing plasmids showed that 90/94 replicates (96%) containing five copies/ug DNA tested positive, whereas 96/141 (68%) replicates containing a single FFV copy were qPCR positive. Hence, we set detection limit of the FFV qPCR assay at five FFV copies/ug gDNA or about 8.33×10^{-1} copies/10^6 cells. FFV *int* sequences were not detected in PBMC gDNA from 20 US human blood donors or in five different human cell lines. The sensitivity of the qPCR assay was also evaluated using PBMC lysates from 39 US domestic cats for which the infection status was previously determined by WB testing [48]. Detection of FFV correlated with the WB and/or nested PCR results in 79.5% (31/39) of the samples. The average and median FFV pVLs were 3.49×10^4 and 1.18×10^4 copies/10^6 cells, respectively. Two WB-positive but qPCR-negative samples also tested negative for β-actin, indicating possible DNA degradation or PCR inhibitors in those samples. Five of the 16 FFV WB-negative animals had low pVLs (577–1209 copies/10^6 cells), indicating possible infection during the seroconversion window period or latent infection with a revertant antibody response. One cat with an indeterminate WB result (seroreactivity to a single Gag protein) also tested qPCR negative, suggesting possible nonspecific seroreactivity in this animal.

PBMC gDNA was further available from 34 of 37 Brazilian cats testing positive using the nested PCR assays. Of these 34 cats, 26 were qPCR-positive with a median pVL of −1.74 log10 copies/cell (18,546 copies/10^6 cells) and an average of −1.75 log10 copies/cell (175,154 copies/10^6 cells) (Figure 1A). Of 31 cats with available buccal swab gDNA for qPCR testing, 12 were positive with a median pVL of −0.67 log10 copies/cell (303,671 copies/10^6 cells). Of the 44 cats testing negative by nested PCR, 39 had PBMC gDNA available for qPCR testing. Of these 39 cats, 27 were qPCR-positive with a median pVL of −1.60 log10 copies/cell (24,900 copies/10^6 cells). Buccal swab gDNA from 33 nested PCR-negative animals identified seven qPCR positive cats with a median pVL of −0.7 log10 copies/cell (201,363 copies/10^6 cells). There was no pVL differences between animals that were previously positive or negative for FFV using the nested assays ($p > 0.05$ for both tissues). Interestingly, the pVL was higher in buccal swab than in PBMC specimens ($p = 0.006$). Fifty-three of the 73 PBMC samples tested (73%) were qPCR-positive *versus* 30% (19/64) of buccal swab samples. For FFV-monoinfected cats, we did not find differences between pVL in PBMCs (median pVL of −1.17 log10 copies/cell; $n = 9$) and in buccal swabs (median pVL of −0.98 log10 copies/cell; $n = 4$) ($p = 1$).

By using qPCR, the total number of FFV-positive cats increased from 37 (46%) to 67 (83%). Of these 67 qPCR-positive cats, 26 (38.8%) were monoinfected with FFV. Analysis of cats classified as potentially transmissible and non-transmissible found no statistical difference between FFV pVLs.

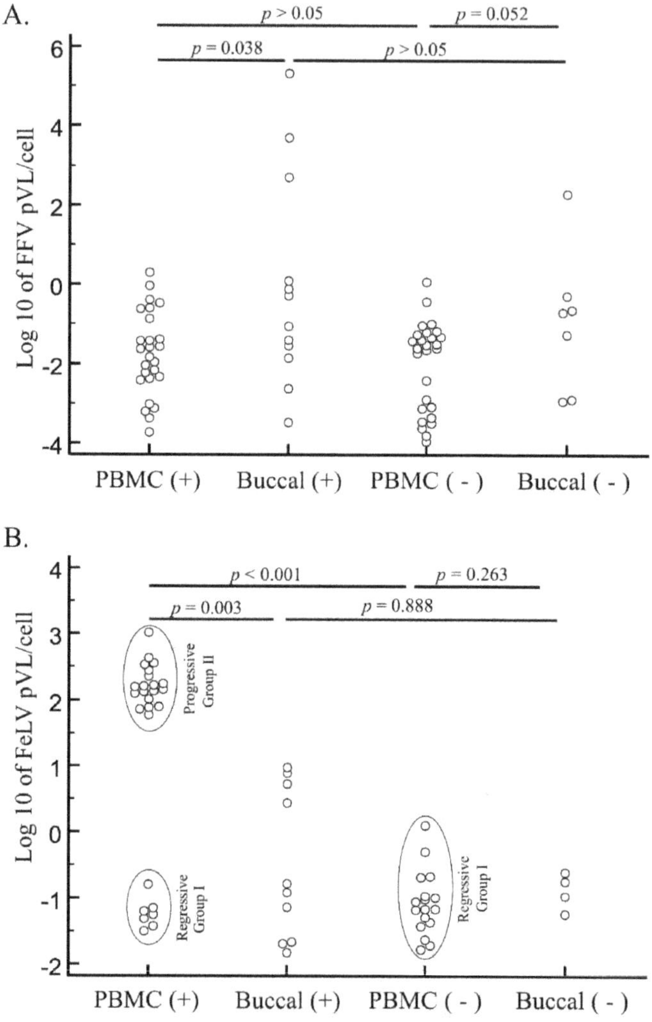

Figure 1. Distribution of feline foamy virus (FFV) and feline leukemia virus (FeLV) log10 proviral loads (pVLs) in blood and oral specimens. FFV (**A**) and FeLV (B) pVLs were measured by quantitative PCR of specimens with nested PCR-positive and -negative test results from domestic cats from Brazil. PCR-positive and -negative cat samples in peripheral blood mononuclear cell (PBMC) or buccal specimens are presented on the *x*-axis. Horizontal lines above each graph depict statistical comparisons between the pVL of specific animal groups or specimen types (Student's *t* tests) with associated probability (*p*) values shown. Ellipses in (**B**) represent different cat groups of FeLV infection outcomes (regressive or progressive).

3.4. FeLV Viral Load Quantification

Of 27 FeLV-positive cats diagnosed by serological and/or molecular assays, 26 with available PBMC gDNA were FeLV qPCR-positive with a median pVL of 2.11 log10 copies/cell (1.29×10^8 copies/10^6 cells) (Figure 1B). Buccal swab gDNA was available for 13 cats, of which 10 were FeLV qPCR-positive with a median pVL of −0.55 log10 copies/cell (2.88×10^5 copies/10^6 cells). The FeLV pVL was approximately 1000× higher in PBMC than in buccal specimens (p = 0.0081). Our pVL data are correlated with FeLV outcome (progressives of Group I, those cats with high VL, mostly seropositive) and regressives (Group II, those with low VL, mostly seronegative). Group I ($n = 19$) had a higher pVL with an average of 2.23 log10 FeLV copies/cell (2.25×10^8 copies/10^6 cells) and median pVL of 2.20 FeLV log10 copies/cell (1.59×10^8 copies/10^6 cells) whereas Group II ($n = 7$) cats had a lower median pVL of −1.25 FeLV log10 copies/cell (5.59×10^4 copies/10^6 cells) ($p < 0.001$). In this case, there was no difference between serological status of the two groups: in group I, 16% ($n = 3$) were FeLV-seronegatives while in group II, 28% ($n = 2$) had that status ($p = 0.588$).

We also tested the 52 of the 54 cats with negative FeLV serology and/or molecular assays with available PBMC gDNA. We found 17 FeLV-positive cats by qPCR with a median of −1.05 log10 copies/cell (8.9×10^4 copies/10^6 cells). This median pVL is almost 2000× lower than the median PBMC pVL in FeLV-seropositive cats ($p < 0.001$). pVLs of FeLV-seronegative cats were similar to those measured in the group II FeLV-positive cats ($p = 0.193$), indicating that the FeLV-seronegative cats with low pVLs likely had a regressive infection. Testing of 35 buccal swab gDNA samples identified four qPCR-positive cats with a median FeLV pVL of −0.55 log10 copies/cell (2.91×10^5 copies/10^6 cells). However, there was no difference between buccal swab pVLs in FeLV-seronegative and seropositive cats ($p = 0.945$). Cats with progressive and regressive infections differed in the qPCR detection of FeLV in buccal tissues. Of 21 regressive animals, only five (24%) had detectable pVL in buccal cells, while all 8 (100%) of animals with progressive infection had detectable pVL in that compartment ($p < 0.001$). Nonetheless, buccal swab pVLs of progressive and regressive animals were similar ($p = 0.608$).

By using qPCR, the total number of FeLV-positive cats increased from 27 (33%) to 48 (59%). Of the 48 qPCR-positive cats, eight (17%) were monoinfected with FeLV, while 38 (79%) were co-infected with both FFV and FeLV and two (4%) were infected with all three feline retroviruses.

3.5. Characteristics of Cats with Feline Retrovirus Co-Infection

We found 32% (26/81) of the cats in our study to be FFV-monoinfected, 10% (8/81) with FeLV monoinfection, 47% (38/81) with dual FFV/FeLV co-infection, 1% (1/81) with dual FFV/FIV co-infection, 2% (2/81) with triple FFV/FeLV/FIV co-infection and 7% (6/81) with no evidence of any feline retrovirus. No FIV monoinfections or dual FeLV/FIV co-infections were identified. Therefore, subsequent statistical analyses were based on the three groups consisting of FFV and FeLV monoinfections and FFV/FeLV dual infections, since these infections were more common in our population.

We found an approximate 1:1 ratio between females and males in all three FFV and FeLV infection groups (Table 2). Kittens, young, and adult cats were present in all three groups, except for the FeLV-monoinfected group which only contained adults. The majority of cats living in multi-cat homes or shelters were FFV/FeLV-co-infected (52% and 75%, respectively). The majority of cats with outdoor access and poor health were also co-infected with FFV and FeLV (Table 2), but these differences were not statistically significant. In captive animals, monoinfection of FFV was 11.4% (4/35) while in feral animals the prevalence was 49% (21/43) ($p < 0.001$). However, the total prevalence of FFV (mono and dual-infection with FeLV) was 86% in captive animals and 71% in feral animals ($p = 0.111$). FeLV monoinfection prevalence was lower in feral (5%) compared to captive (14%) cats, and similarly the total prevalence of FeLV was lower in feral cats (42%) than in the captive cats (74%) ($p = 0.004$).

Odds ratios were determined to evaluate whether FFV infection was a risk factor for FeLV infection. Infection with FFV did not increase the chances of having FeLV infection (OR = 1.09, $p = 0.878$). Among FFV-infected cats, odds ratios were also calculated to evaluate risk factors involved with FeLV co-infection (Table 5). Neutered FFV-infected cats were more likely to be co-infected than non-neutered counterparts. Cats living in shelters showed higher rates of co-infection than those cats in other housing types. Non-feral cats living alone, in a shelter or multicat household had a higher risk of co-infection than feral cats (OR = 6.89, $p = 0.003$). No associations of co-infection were found with either age or sex. We also evaluated risk factors for FFV co-infection of FeLV-infected cats.

No significant differences were observed when considering the same factors analyzed for FFV-infected cats (OR = 0.9, p = 0.878).

Table 5. Univariate analysis of the prevalence and risk factors for FeLV and FFV co-infection in domestic cats.

Factor	Category	FeLV Co-Infection Prevalence	Odds Ratio	95%CI	p Value
Sex	Female	0.67 (22/33)	1.87	0.683–5.148	0.223
	Male	0.52 (16/31)	Reference	-	-
Age	Adult	0.63 (22/35)	1.47	0.534–4.03	0.458
	Non-adult	0.53 (15/28)	Reference	-	-
	Young	0.61 (8/13)	1.1586	0.332–4.046	0.817
	Non-young	0.58 (29/50)	Reference	-	-
	Kitten	0.47 (7/15)	0.5250	0.1628–1.6927	0.281
	Non-kitten	0.62 (30/48)	Reference	-	-
Neuter Status	Neutered	0.71 (20/28)	2.954	0.9378–9.3088	0.064
	Intact	0.46 (11/24)	Reference		
Household	Multicat	0.73 (11/15)	2.221	0.6171–7.9947	0.222
	Non-multicat	0.55 (26/47)	Reference	-	-
	Shelter	1 (9/9)	ND [a]	ND	ND
	Non-shelter	0.47 (28/53)	ND	ND	ND
	Street	0.43 (16/37)	Reference	-	-
	Non-street	0.84 (21/25)	6.89	1.971–24.088	0.0025
	Single	1 (1/1)	ND	ND	ND
	Non-single	0.59 (36/61)	ND	ND	ND

[a] ND = not done. There were no individuals for all comparison groups.

Since the street and neuter variables showed significance at the univariate level, a multivariate analysis was performed with adjustment for those two variables. While the effect of neutering was lost (OR = 2.43; p = 0.161), street cats remained significantly less prone for co-infection with FFV and FeLV than non-street cats (OR = 0.22; p = 0.026).

When we compared median log10 pVLs of FFV mono- and FFV/FeLV co-infected individuals (Figure 2) we found higher FFV pVLs in buccal swab specimens in co-infected cats ($p < 0.003$; Figure 2A). In contrast, differences in PBMC pVLs between mono- and co-infected cats were not significant (p = 0.378). However, pVLs in the buccal specimens were significantly higher than those in PBMC of co-infected cats ($p < 0.001$). No differences were found in FeLV pVLs between buccal swabs and PBMCs or between FeLV mono- and co-infected cats (p = 1 and p = 0.912, respectively; Figure 2B).

We also evaluated pVLs of cat samples that were tested for both FFV and FeLV, but did not observe a correlation between FeLV and FFV pVLs in PBMCs among cats with progressive or regressive infection (Figure 3A). Similarly, there was no correlation between the FFV and FeLV pVLs in buccal specimens (Figure 3B) except for FeLV-regressive individuals (r^2 = 0.998; p = 0.028; Figure 3B), which showed a negative association.

The percentage of potentially transmissible FFV with detectable pVLs in buccal swabs in monoinfected cats (72.7%) was very similar to that in FeLV progressive cats (76.9%) (Figure 4). The opposite was found when comparing FFV-monoinfected cats and FeLV regressives (p = 0.004).

For cats with FFV and FeLV positive results for both buccal swab and PBMC specimens, we compared the FFV pVLs between FFV-monoinfected and FFV/FeLV-co-infected animals and also the pVLs between FeLV progressive and regressive animals. However, we did not observe a correlation between pVLs in buccal swab or PBMC in either situation (data not shown).

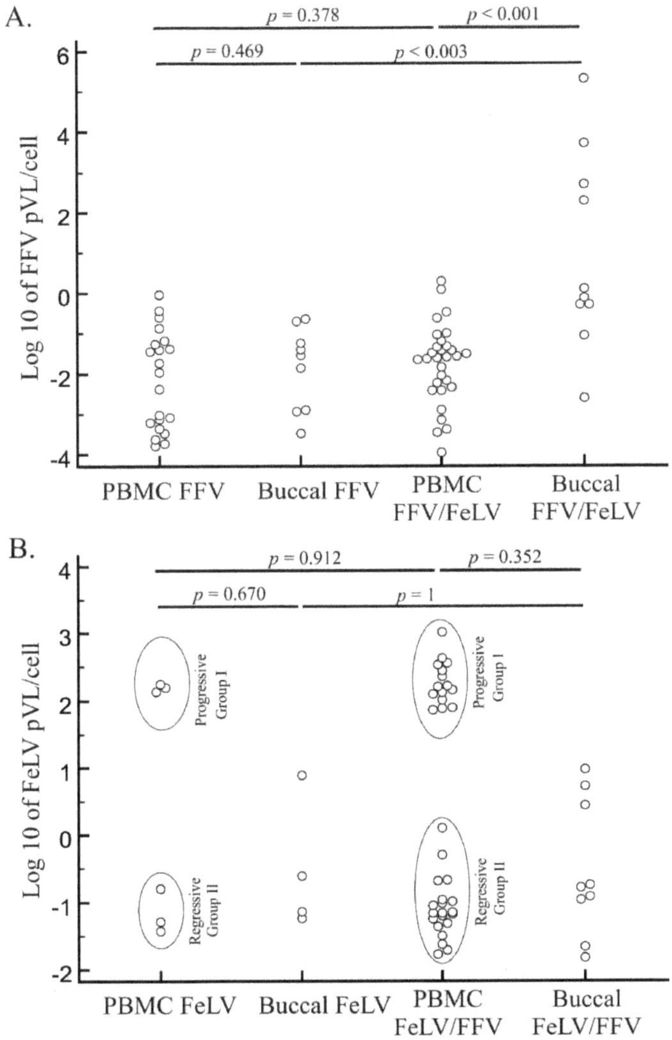

Figure 2. Distribution of feline foamy virus (FFV) and feline leukemia virus (FeLV) log10 proviral loads (pVLs) in blood and oral specimens from singly or dually infected cats. FFV (**A**) and FeLV (**B**) pVLs were measured by quantitative PCR of mono- and co-infected domestic cats from Brazil. Mono- and co-infected cat samples for each retrovirus and in peripheral blood mononuclear cell (PBMC) or buccal specimens are presented. Horizontal lines above each graph depict statistical comparisons between the pVL of specific animal groups or specimen types (Student's *t* tests), with associated probability (*p*) values shown. Ellipses in (**B**) represent different groups of FeLV infection outcome (regressive or progressive).

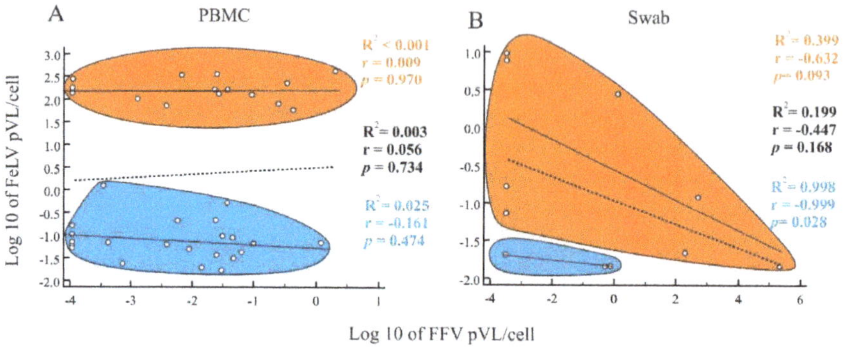

Figure 3. Spearman correlation analysis between feline leukemia virus (FeLV) and feline foamy virus (FFV) log10 proviral loads (pVLs) on blood and oral specimens. Correlations were tested in both peripheral blood mononuclear cells (PBMCs) (**A**) and buccal swab specimens (**B**). Vertical and horizontal axes represent FeLV and FFV pVLs, respectively. Each open circle represents a sample for which pVL was measured for both viruses. Orange and blue ellipsoids represent FeLV progressive and regressive individuals, respectively. Correlation coefficients (R^2) and probabilities (*p*-values) are provided for each group (progressive and regressive) and for all samples together. They are represented in the graph by lines. Dotted lines represent the correlation among all samples, both progressive and regressive. For PBMCs, progressive and regressive cats had FFV and FeLV pVLs with weak correlation ($R^2 < 0.001$, $p = 0.970$ and $R^2 = 0.025$, $p = 0.474$, respectively). pVLs in buccal swab samples of progressive and regressive cats were inversely correlated ($R^2 = 0.399$, $p = 0.093$ and $R^2 = 0.998$, $p = 0.028$, respectively).

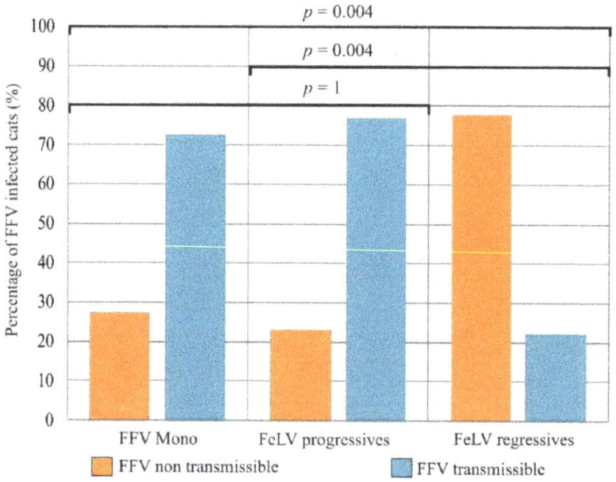

Figure 4. Proportion of potentially transmissible and nontransmisible cats based on proviral loads (pVLs) in different groups of feline foamy virus (FFV). The groups compared include monoinfected cats (FFV Mono), feline leukemia virus (FeLV) progressive (FeLV progressives) and regressive (FeLV regressives) cats in dual infection. In orange, the potentially FFV non-transmissible cats (undetectable buccal swab DNA). In blue, the FFV potentially transmissible cats (detectable DNA). Probabilities (*p*) were calculated using the Chi-square test.

3.6. Association of FFV and FeLV Infection with Clinical Signs

To investigate possible disease associations in cats with mono or dual FFV and FeLV infection we analyzed clinical signs reported in these animals at the time of sampling. We did not detect any differences among the proportions of major clinical signs (RTD, PWL and OS) in FFV-monoinfected, or FeLV-monoinfected regressive or progressive cats (Table 6). Five of seven (71%) cats with FFV/FeLV-progressive infection were anemic at the time of data collection by hemogram testing while none of the FFV/FeLV-regressive cats were anemic (0/2; $p = 0.026$). Less common clinical signs detected were cachexia (2/81), ulcers (2/81), hair loss (3/81), presence of ectoparasites (1/81), tooth loss (1/81), prolapses (1/81), scabies (1/81), pemphigus foliaceous (1/81), pyometra (1/81), sporotrichosis (4/81), diarrhea (1/81), neurological (1/81), abortion (1/81), kidney disease (1/81), stomatitis (3/81) and neoplasia (1/81). However, the low frequency of these clinical signs did not permit an analysis of their association with retrovirus infection of these cats.

Table 6. Proportion of major clinical symptoms by feline retrovirus infection status.

Infection Status (*n*)	Respiratory Tract Disease (%)	Progressive Weight Loss (%)	Ocular Secretion (%)	Anemia (%)
FFV-monoinfected ($n = 26$)	6 (23.1%)	4 (15.4%)	5 (19.2%)	0/1 (0%)
FeLV regressives ($n = 23$)	11 (47.8%)	6 (26.1%)	2 (8.7%)	0/2 (0%)
FeLV progressives ($n = 19$)	6 (31.6%)	5 (26.3%)	0 (0%)	6/8 (75%)
FFV negative/FeLV negative ($n = 5$)	1 (20%)	0 (0%)	0 (0%)	N/A [a]

[a] N/A = not available.

We analyzed FFV pVLs in cats with or without each reported major clinical signs, but did not observe differences between pVLs in cats with or without PWL ($p = 0.456$), RTD ($p = 0.629$) or OS ($p = 0.174$). We also did not find any FFV pVL differences in cats with or without any clinical signs ($p = 0.941$), including anemia and death ($p = 0.885$ and $p = 0.558$, respectively).

For FeLV-positive cats (either by serology or PCR), anemia at the time of sampling was correlated with higher PBMC pVL, with a median of 2.29 log10 FeLV copies/cell (197,784,339 copies/10^6 cells) compared to −1.31 log10 FeLV copies/cell (48,977 copies/10^6 cells) in cats without anemia ($p = 0.045$, Mann-Whitney *U* test). Death was also correlated with higher PBMC pVL, with a median of 2.20 log10 FeLV copies/cell (161,171,526 copies/10^6 cells) among cats who died during follow-up compared to a median of −1 log10 FeLV copies/cell (100,000 copies/10^6 cells) at sampling time among those who were still alive at the end of follow-up ($p = 0.022$, Mann-Whitney *U* test).

We followed 21 cats from entry into the study until 35 months later. Among those, three were FFV-monoinfected, and 13 were FeLV progressives and five were FeLV regressives, irrespective of their FFV infection status. After 25 months of follow-up, all three FFV monoinfected cats were alive. After 35 months, 92.3% (12/13) of cats with progressive infection had died (Figure 5), of which three were feral (25%) and nine were captive (75%), 11 were adults (92%) and one was young (8%) whereas the 13th cat was lost to follow-up at 24 months. In contrast, all regressive cats were alive after 35 months ($p = 0.0008$). Among regressive cats, two were feral (40%) and three were captive (60%), while four were adults (80%) and one was a kitten (20%). There was no difference in age or household status in these cat groups. Similar rates of FFV infection were found in both groups; 10/13 (76.9%) in the first group and 5/7 (71.4%) in the second.

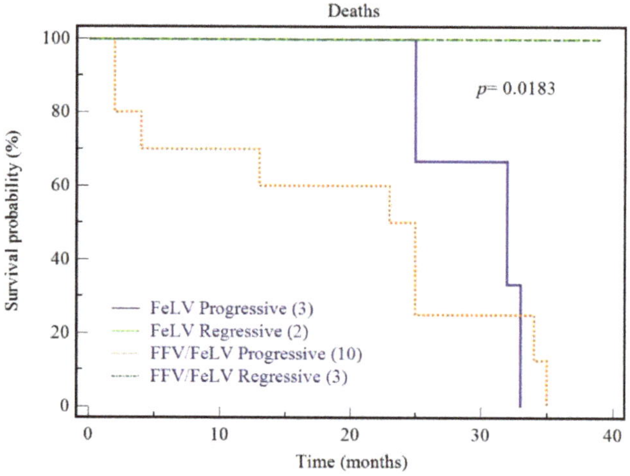

Figure 5. Survival analysis of cats with feline leukemia virus (FeLV) progressive and regressive infections irrespective of their FFV infection status. Kaplan-Meier survival analysis was conducted for cats that were followed-up over 35 months during the study. *p*-value of the comparison (*p*) is shown. Cats with regressive infections were more likely to survive during this period compared to cats with progressive infection ($p = 0.008$).

4. Discussion

In this study, we evaluated FV infection in cats co-infected with other retroviruses known to impair the feline host immune system with pathologic consequences. Retroviral infection of domestic cats was used as a model to investigate possible outcomes associated with mono or dual infections because biological materials such as blood and buccal swabs are usually collected from domestic cats at veterinary clinics for periodic clinical examination and pets can also be easily followed. Moreover, domestic cats can be infected with FeLV, a retrovirus historically considered to be the causative agent of more clinical syndromes than any other single microbial agent in cats, affording an assessment of dual retroviral infections on disease outcomes in cats [25]. Unfortunately, the low FIV prevalence in our study population did not permit an evaluation of dual or triple infection with that retrovirus.

In this study we found that both FFV and FeLV qPCR testing were more sensitive than their respective nested PCR assays for detecting FFV and FeLV, respectively. Even though the FeLV and FFV nested PCR assays in our study targeted multiple viral regions, none were able to detect 100% of the qPCR-positive samples. These results likely reflect viral sequence variation at the primer locations and the target viral genomic fragment size for which detection of smaller amplicon sizes, as those in the qPCR tests, is typically more sensitive. We have obtained similar results when comparing nested PCR and qPCR testing of New World primates (NWP) [9].

In this study, about one fourth of FFV-infected cats were PCR-positive in only the PBMC compartment. These animals may represent recent infections, in which the virus has not yet disseminated to the oral tissues. This hypothesis is supported by a previous report showing a delay in the appearance of SFV in the saliva of cynomolgus macaques (*Macaca fascicularis*) infected through blood transfusion from an SFV-infected animal [50]. Epstein-Barr virus (EBV) shares some features with FV, including a high incidence of infection, a salivary mode of transmission and replication in the oropharyngeal tissues. As it is well established for EBV, it is possible that migratory cells, such as macrophages and other leukocytes initially infected by FV, eventually traffic to the oropharyngeal tissues and spread infection to less differentiated epithelial cells [51].

A recent study with NWP showed an average of −3.1 log10 SFV copies/cell in PBMC [52] whereas in Old World Primates (OWP) the pVL average was −3.08 log10 SFV copies/cell among rhesus macaques [53]. We found a 10× higher FFV pVL (−2.15 log10 copies/cell) in the same tissue compartment in cats. At oral sites, the average NWP SFV pVL was −1.3 log10 copies/cell [52] while in OWPs the pVL ranged from −3.3 to −1 log10 SFV DNA copies/cell [54]. We found similar FFV pVLs in the cat oral cavity (−1.86 log10 copies/cell). Unlike the previous work with primates [52], we did not find significant differences between the pVL in PBMC and in oral tissues of cats. These data suggest that FV pVL distribution at distinct anatomical sites can vary in different natural hosts. We also showed that buccal swabs can be useful as non-invasive biological materials for FFV diagnosis, as recently shown for SFV [52].

Non-feral cats were almost five times more likely to be co-infected with FFV/FeLV than feral cats. We hypothesize that being confined in a household or shelter environment increases the risk of co-infection since these cats may have more intimate contact during grooming or sharing feeding bowls. We also considered possible recruitment bias since clinic cats were suspected to be ill as explained in Methods. These cat behaviors are reported as the most likely routes of FeLV transmission [55], as opposed to biting, which has been more strongly associated with SFV transmission [56]. In our study the FFV prevalence was not different between captive and feral adult cats, while in SFV studies of OWPs the prevalence is higher in adult captive (~70%) [57] than in wild-born primates (~44%) [58], whereas the SFV prevalence in NWP were found very similar in captive and wild animals (14–30%) [10]. These differences can likely be explained by some captive cats having outdoor access and in shelters it is not uncommon for the introduction of new individuals from the street, both increasing the likelihood of exposures to potentially infected cats.

Using qPCR, we identified two distinct cat groups based on FeLV pVL; a regressive group with low pVLs (−1.77 to 0.10 log10 copies/cell) and a progressive group with higher pVLs (1.77 to 3.02 log10 copies/cell). Our results support previous studies showing that pVLs measured by qPCR can be used to identify a regressive infection outcome in which plasma viremia has been cleared [59]. Moreover, the FeLV pVL we detected is within the range reported by others for experimentally and naturally infected cats [60]. However, we show for the first time that naturally-infected cats with progressive FeLV infection can result in death after 35 months of follow-up, although the cause of death cannot be exclusively attributed to FeLV infection. Other studies showed the same outcomes only for experimentally infected cats [60,61]. In one of those studies, progressive and regressive cats were followed for 149 weeks post transfusion and the authors found that 50% (4/8) of regressive cats remained healthy while 100% (2/2) of progressive cats developed non-regenerative anemia and multicentric T-cell lymphoma [61].

To the best of our knowledge, our study is the first to observe the influence of another retrovirus on FV pVL in buccal swabs. A previous co-infection study conducted in the rhesus macaque model has shown that a pre-existing SFV infection can influence the biology and the outcomes of an SIV infection, including higher plasma SIV VL, a decreasing trend in the $CD4^+$ T-cell counts and a greater number of animal deaths [16]. However, SFV pVLs were not assessed in that study. Herein, with the determination of pVLs of two feline retroviruses (FFV and FeLV), it was possible to observe that FeLV progressive or regressive infections were not able to reactivate FFV from latency in PBMC. However, a recent study showed that FFV pVL in blood was positive correlated in cats with status of FeLV progressive, presence of FeLV-B subtype and positive status for feline coronavirus (FeCoV), demonstrating a mechanism of complex interaction that need to be clarified [62]. Furthermore, co-infected cats with progressive FeLV infection are likely more prone to become FFV-transmissible and *vice-versa* as evidenced by the higher pVLs in these oral compartments. As the proportion of potential-transmissible FFV infections was similar between FFV monoinfections and in cats with progressive FeLV infections, but lower in regressive FeLV co-infections, we postulate that the latency mechanism in regressive FeLV could also contribute to reduction of the establishment of FFV colonization of the oral cavity. These findings may also be a consequence of an altered disease susceptibility caused by the cats' virome composition. The virome influences the phenotype of the host in a combinatorial manner by interacting with other components of the microbiome and by interacting with individual variations in host genetics. Together these interactions may influence a range of phenotypes as we observed in the distinct behavior of FeLV progressive and regressive infections as also in the FeLV regressive correlation with reduced FFV saliva transmission [63]. The microbiome composition may also allow the stimulation of specific immune cell subsets, which may carry the FFV proviral DNA, thus indirectly increasing the FFV pVL due to the increased number of cells. We also found that FFV pVL was higher in buccal tissues of FFV/FeLV co-infected cats than among FFV monoinfections. However, we identified a negative correlation between the pVLs of both viruses circulating in this tissue. A previous study has reported FeLV as a cofactor for FIV infection by enhancing the expression and spread of FIV in the host and by increasing the severity of immunodeficiency caused by FIV by an unknown mechanism [42]. Another study evaluated FIV/FeLV interactions in in vitro and in vivo experiments, but did not find evidence of direct viral interactions [63]. Since FeLV is mainly transmitted through saliva [30] and superficial differentiated epithelial cells of the oral mucosa are the major cell types in which FFV replicates [51], we hypothesize that both viruses can infect the same compartment. Just like the Tax protein of HTLV-1 can activate HIV expression in vitro via the LTR [64], FeLV may enhance FFV replication in the oral cavity by a similar mechanism, or related to regulatory protein synergism, or some other means. A simplified model of this hypothesis is presented in Figure 6. Any potential interaction mechanism between these two viruses, and their infectiousness, remains to be determined and any contributions of infectious DNA-containing viral particles compared to integrated proviral DNA sequences was not measured in our study due to the small volumes of materials obtained for analysis.

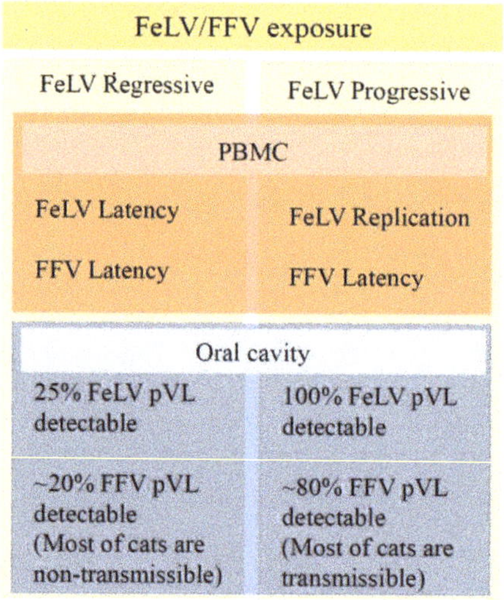

Figure 6. Hypothetical pathway to progressive or regressive outcomes via dual infection with feline foamy virus (FFV) and feline leukaemia virus (FeLV) and potentially active viral replication measured by proviral load (pVL). FeLV progressive and regressive outcome determined by PBMC tissue (blood) pVLs were correlated to different FFV and FeLV pVL patterns of detection in the oral cavity.

Although we found evidence for increased buccal FFV pVLs in cats co-infected with FeLV with the potential for increased transmissibility, we did not observe significant disease associations in these cats. A small number of dually infected cats with FeLV-progressive infection had anemia but this trend was not highly significant. We also did not find large numbers of FIV-infected cats to evaluate the effect of FV co-infection on disease outcomes. Additional studies with larger numbers of naturally or experimentally infected cats and longer periods of follow-up may be needed to determine these potential associations.

Our study also reinforces the importance of FeLV qPCR testing to define FeLV infection outcomes, enabling differential clinical treatment of cats that were negative by serological methods. For example, blood transfusion from regressive cats containing latent feline leukemia provirus caused infection and disease in naïve recipient cats [61]. Moreover, FeLV regressive cats with undetectable antigenemia, but that are immune to vaccination, are often equivocally vaccinated [59].

In summary, we provide evidence that FVs may interact with other retroviruses infecting cats. Our study supports that domestic cats naturally infected by FFV and FeLV can be used as a model to investigate the potential impact of FV on immunocompromised mammalian hosts. The results of these animal model studies may help inform the design of clinical and research investigations into the potential for SFV to cause disease in infected humans. The tools developed in our study will be useful to further explore consequences and interactions of multiple feline retrovirus infections of cats.

Author Contributions: Conceptualization, W.M.S., M.A.S. and A.F.S.; Methodology & Formal Analysis, L.T.F.C., C.P.M., H.J., A.M.A., F.T., S.d.O.M. and C.G.A.D.; Writing-Original Draft Preparation, L.T.F.C.; Writing-Review & Editing, L.T.F.C., W.M.S., M.A.S. and A.F.S.; Supervision & Project Administration, A.F.S.; Funding Acquisition, W.M.S., M.A.S. and A.F.S.

Funding: This research was funded by the Brazilian Science Council (CNPq) grant 480529/2013-2 to AFS, by the Rio de Janeiro State Science Foundation (FAPERJ) grant #E-26/103.059/2011 to MAS and by Centers for Disease Control and Prevention (CDC) intramural funding. LTFC was recipient of a Ph.D. fellowship by the Brazilian Ministry of Education (CAPES) and another by FAPERJ.

Acknowledgments: We thank the veterinary clinicians who collected cat specimens and associated clinical data over the study period. This work is part of the requirements for the PhD Thesis of L.T.F.C. at the Department of Genetics, Universidade Federal do Rio de Janeiro, Brazil. Use of trade names is for identification only and does not imply endorsement by the U.S. Department of Health and Human Services, the Public Health Service, or the CDC. The findings and conclusions in this report are those of the authors and do not necessarily represent the views of the CDC, or any of the authors' affiliated institutions.

Conflicts of Interest: The authors declare no conflict of interest.

References

1. Linial, M.F.H.; Hahn, B.; Löwer, R.; Neil, J.; Quackenbusch, S.; Rethwilm, A.; Sonigo, P.; Stoye, J.; Tristem, M. Retroviridae. In *Virus Taxonomy*; Fauquet, C.M.M.M., Manilo, V.J., Desselberger, U., Ball, L.A., Eds.; Elsevier: San Diego, CA, USA, 2005.
2. Heneine, W.; Switzer, W.M.; Sandstrom, P.; Brown, J.; Vedapuri, S.; Schable, C.A.; Khan, A.S.; Lerche, N.W.; Schweizer, M.; Neumann-Haefelin, D.; et al. Identification of a human population infected with simian foamy viruses. *Nat. Med.* **1998**, *4*, 403–407. [CrossRef] [PubMed]
3. Switzer, W.M.; Bhullar, V.; Shanmugam, V.; Cong, M.E.; Parekh, B.; Lerche, N.W.; Yee, J.L.; Ely, J.J.; Boneva, R.; Chapman, L.E.; et al. Frequent simian foamy virus infection in persons occupationally exposed to nonhuman primates. *J. Virol.* **2004**, *78*, 2780–2789. [CrossRef] [PubMed]
4. Hooks, J.J.; Gibbs, C.J., Jr. The foamy viruses. *Bacteriol. Rev.* **1975**, *39*, 169–185. [PubMed]
5. Buseyne, F.; Betsem, E.; Montange, T.; Njouom, R.; Bilounga Ndongo, C.; Hermine, O.; Gessain, A. Clinical signs and blood test results among humans infected with zoonotic simian foamy virus: A. case-control study. *J. Infect. Dis.* **2018**, *218*, 144–151. [CrossRef] [PubMed]
6. Wolfe, N.D.; Switzer, W.M.; Carr, J.K.; Bhullar, V.B.; Shanmugam, V.; Tamoufe, U.; Prosser, A.T.; Torimiro, J.N.; Wright, A.; Mpoudi-Ngole, E.; et al. Naturally acquired simian retrovirus infections in central african hunters. *Lancet* **2004**, *363*, 932–937. [CrossRef]
7. Calattini, S.; Betsem, E.B.; Froment, A.; Mauclere, P.; Tortevoye, P.; Schmitt, C.; Njouom, R.; Saib, A.; Gessain, A. Simian foamy virus transmission from apes to humans, rural cameroon. *Emerg. Infect. Dis.* **2007**, *13*, 1314–1320. [CrossRef] [PubMed]
8. Filippone, C.; Betsem, E.; Tortevoye, P.; Cassar, O.; Bassot, S.; Froment, A.; Fontanet, A.; Gessain, A. A severe bite from a nonhuman primate is a major risk factor for HTLV-1 infection in hunters from central africa. *Clin. Infect. Dis.* **2015**, *60*, 1667–1676. [CrossRef]

9. Muniz, C.P.; Cavalcante, L.T.F.; Jia, H.; Zheng, H.; Tang, S.; Augusto, A.M.; Pissinatti, A.; Fedullo, L.P.; Santos, A.F.; Soares, M.A.; et al. Zoonotic infection of brazilian primate workers with new world simian foamy virus. *PLoS ONE* **2017**, *12*, e0184502. [CrossRef]
10. Muniz, C.P.; Troncoso, L.L.; Moreira, M.A.; Soares, E.A.; Pissinatti, A.; Bonvicino, C.R.; Seuanez, H.N.; Sharma, B.; Jia, H.; Shankar, A.; et al. Identification and characterization of highly divergent simian foamy viruses in a wide range of new world primates from brazil. *PLoS ONE* **2013**, *8*, e67568. [CrossRef]
11. Huang, F.; Wang, H.; Jing, S.; Zeng, W. Simian foamy virus prevalence in macaca mulatta and zookeepers. *AIDS Res. Hum. Retroviruses* **2012**, *28*, 591–593. [CrossRef]
12. Rua, R.; Gessain, A. Origin, evolution and innate immune control of simian foamy viruses in humans. *Curr. Opin. Virol.* **2015**, *10*, 47–55. [CrossRef] [PubMed]
13. Switzer, W.M.; Tang, S.; Zheng, H.; Shankar, A.; Sprinkle, P.S.; Sullivan, V.; Granade, T.C.; Heneine, W. Dual simian foamy virus/human immunodeficiency virus type 1 infections in persons from cote d'ivoire. *PLoS ONE* **2016**, *11*, e0157709. [CrossRef] [PubMed]
14. Switzer, W.M.; Garcia, A.D.; Yang, C.; Wright, A.; Kalish, M.L.; Folks, T.M.; Heneine, W. Coinfection with hiv-1 and simian foamy virus in west central africans. *J. Infect. Dis* **2008**, *197*, 1389–1393. [CrossRef] [PubMed]
15. Tsigrelis, C.; Berbari, E.; Temesgen, Z. Viral opportunistic infections in hiv-infected adults. *J. Med. Liban.* **2006**, *54*, 91–96. [PubMed]
16. Choudhary, A.; Galvin, T.A.; Williams, D.K.; Beren, J.; Bryant, M.A.; Khan, A.S. Influence of naturally occurring simian foamy viruses (sfvs) on siv disease progression in the rhesus macaque (macaca mulatta) model. *Viruses* **2013**, *5*, 1414–1430. [CrossRef] [PubMed]
17. Nakamura, K.; Miyazawa, T.; Ikeda, Y.; Sato, E.; Nishimura, Y.; Nguyen, N.T.; Takahashi, E.; Mochizuki, M.; Mikami, T. Contrastive prevalence of feline retrovirus infections between northern and southern vietnam. *J. Vet. Med. Sci.* **2000**, *62*, 921–923. [CrossRef]
18. Winkler, I.G.; Lochelt, M.; Flower, R.L. Epidemiology of feline foamy virus and feline immunodeficiency virus infections in domestic and feral cats: A seroepidemiological study. *J. Clin. Microbiol.* **1999**, *37*, 2848–2851.
19. Daniels, M.J.; Golder, M.C.; Jarrett, O.; MacDonald, D.W. Feline viruses in wildcats from scotland. *J. Wildl. Dis.* **1999**, *35*, 121–124. [CrossRef]
20. Glaus, T.; Hofmann-Lehmann, R.; Greene, C.; Glaus, B.; Wolfensberger, C.; Lutz, H. Seroprevalence of bartonella henselae infection and correlation with disease status in cats in switzerland. *J. Clin. Microbiol.* **1997**, *35*, 2883–2885.
21. Bandecchi, P.; Matteucci, D.; Baldinotti, F.; Guidi, G.; Abramo, F.; Tozzini, F.; Bendinelli, M. Prevalence of feline immunodeficiency virus and other retroviral infections in sick cats in italy. *Vet. Immunol. Immunopathol.* **1992**, *31*, 337–345. [CrossRef]
22. Alke, A.; Schwantes, A.; Zemba, M.; Flugel, R.M.; Lochelt, M. Characterization of the humoral immune response and virus replication in cats experimentally infected with feline foamy virus. *Virology* **2000**, *275*, 170–176. [CrossRef] [PubMed]
23. German, A.C.; Harbour, D.A.; Helps, C.R.; Gruffydd-Jones, T.J. Is feline foamy virus really apathogenic? *Vet. Immunol. Immunopathol.* **2008**, *123*, 114–118. [CrossRef] [PubMed]
24. Jarrett, W.F.; Crawford, E.M.; Martin, W.B.; Davie, F. A virus-like particle associated with leukemia (lymphosarcoma). *Nature* **1964**, *202*, 567–569. [CrossRef] [PubMed]
25. Hartmann, K. Clinical aspects of feline retroviruses: A. review. *Viruses* **2012**, *4*, 2684–2710. [CrossRef] [PubMed]
26. Levy, J.; Crawford, C.; Hartmann, K.; Hofmann-Lehmann, R.; Little, S.; Sundahl, E.; Thayer, V. 2008 american association of feline practitioners' feline retrovirus management guidelines. *J. Feline Med. Surg* **2008**, *10*, 300–316. [CrossRef] [PubMed]
27. Bande, F.; Arshad, S.S.; Hassan, L.; Zakaria, Z.; Sapian, N.A.; Rahman, N.A.; Alazawy, A. Prevalence and risk factors of feline leukaemia virus and feline immunodeficiency virus in peninsular malaysia. *BMC Vet. Res.* **2012**, *8*, 33. [CrossRef] [PubMed]
28. de Almeida, N.R.; Danelli, M.G.; da Silva, L.H.; Hagiwara, M.K.; Mazur, C. Prevalence of feline leukemia virus infection in domestic cats in rio de janeiro. *J. Feline Med. Surg* **2012**, *14*, 583–586. [CrossRef] [PubMed]
29. Sivagurunathan, A.; Atwa, A.M.; Lobetti, R. Prevalence of feline immunodeficiency virus and feline leukaemia virus infection in malaysia: A retrospective study. *JFMS Open Rep.* **2018**, *4*, 2055116917752587. [CrossRef]

30. Francis, D.P.; Essex, M.; Hardy, W.D., Jr. Excretion of feline leukaemia virus by naturally infected pet cats. *Nature* **1977**, *269*, 252–254. [CrossRef]
31. Hofmann-Lehmann, R.; Cattori, V.; Tandon, R.; Boretti, F.S.; Meli, M.L.; Riond, B.; Pepin, A.C.; Willi, B.; Ossent, P.; Lutz, H. Vaccination against the feline leukaemia virus: Outcome and response categories and long-term follow-up. *Vaccine* **2007**, *25*, 5531–5539. [CrossRef]
32. Hofmann-Lehmann, R.; Cattori, V.; Tandon, R.; Boretti, F.S.; Meli, M.L.; Riond, B.; Lutz, H. How molecular methods change our views of FELV infection and vaccination. *Vet. Immunol. Immunopathol.* **2008**, *123*, 119–123. [CrossRef] [PubMed]
33. Pedersen, N.C.; Ho, E.W.; Brown, M.L.; Yamamoto, J.K. Isolation of a T-lymphotropic virus from domestic cats with an immunodeficiency-like syndrome. *Science* **1987**, *235*, 790–793. [CrossRef] [PubMed]
34. Jarrett, O. Strategies of retrovirus survival in the cat. *Vet. Microbiol.* **1999**, *69*, 99–107. [CrossRef]
35. Rogers, A.B.; Hoover, E.A. Maternal-fetal feline immunodeficiency virus transmission: Timing and tissue tropisms. *J. Infect. Dis.* **1998**, *178*, 960–967. [CrossRef] [PubMed]
36. Medeiros Sde, O.; Martins, A.N.; Dias, C.G.; Tanuri, A.; Brindeiro Rde, M. Natural transmission of feline immunodeficiency virus from infected queen to kitten. *Virol. J.* **2012**, *9*, 99. [CrossRef] [PubMed]
37. Kohmoto, M.; Uetsuka, K.; Ikeda, Y.; Inoshima, Y.; Shimojima, M.; Sato, E.; Inada, G.; Toyosaki, T.; Miyazawa, T.; Doi, K.; et al. Eight-year observation and comparative study of specific pathogen-free cats experimentally infected with feline immunodeficiency virus (FIV) subtypes a and b: Terminal acquired immunodeficiency syndrome in a cat infected with fiv petaluma strain. *J. Vet. Med. Sci.* **1998**, *60*, 315–321. [CrossRef] [PubMed]
38. Shelton, G.H.; Grant, C.K.; Cotter, S.M.; Gardner, M.B.; Hardy, W.D., Jr.; DiGiacomo, R.F. Feline immunodeficiency virus and feline leukemia virus infections and their relationships to lymphoid malignancies in cats: A retrospective study (1968–1988). *J. Acquir. Immune Defic. Syndr.* **1990**, *3*, 623–630. [PubMed]
39. Munro, H.J.; Berghuis, L.; Lang, A.S.; Rogers, L.; Whitney, H. Seroprevalence of feline immunodeficiency virus (FIV) and feline leukemia virus (FELV) in shelter cats on the island of newfoundland, Canada. *Can. J. Vet. Res.* **2014**, *78*, 140–144.
40. Stavisky, J.; Dean, R.S.; Molloy, M.H. Prevalence of and risk factors for fiv and felv infection in two shelters in the United Kingdom (2011–2012). *Vet. Rec.* **2017**, *181*, 451. [CrossRef]
41. Zenger, E.; Brown, W.C.; Song, W.; Wolf, A.M.; Pedersen, N.C.; Longnecker, M.; Li, J.; Collisson, E.W. Evaluation of cofactor effect of feline syncytium-forming virus on feline immunodeficiency virus infection. *Am. J. Vet. Res.* **1993**, *54*, 713–718.
42. Pedersen, N.C.; Torten, M.; Rideout, B.; Sparger, E.; Tonachini, T.; Luciw, P.A.; Ackley, C.; Levy, N.; Yamamoto, J. Feline leukemia virus infection as a potentiating cofactor for the primary and secondary stages of experimentally induced feline immunodeficiency virus infection. *J. Virol.* **1990**, *64*, 598–606. [PubMed]
43. Roy, J.; Rudolph, W.; Juretzek, T.; Gartner, K.; Bock, M.; Herchenroder, O.; Lindemann, D.; Heinkelein, M.; Rethwilm, A. Feline foamy virus genome and replication strategy. *J. Virol.* **2003**, *77*, 11324–11331. [CrossRef] [PubMed]
44. Winkler, I.G.; Flugel, R.M.; Lochelt, M.; Flower, R.L. Detection and molecular characterisation of feline foamy virus serotypes in naturally infected cats. *Virology* **1998**, *247*, 144–151. [CrossRef] [PubMed]
45. Phung, H.T.; Ikeda, Y.; Miyazawa, T.; Nakamura, K.; Mochizuki, M.; Izumiya, Y.; Sato, E.; Nishimura, Y.; Tohya, Y.; Takahashi, E.; et al. Genetic analyses of feline foamy virus isolates from domestic and wild feline species in geographically distinct areas. *Virus Res.* **2001**, *76*, 171–181. [CrossRef]
46. Martins, A.N.; Medeiros, S.O.; Simonetti, J.P.; Schatzmayr, H.G.; Tanuri, A.; Brindeiro, R.M. Phylogenetic and genetic analysis of feline immunodeficiency virus gag, pol, and env genes from domestic cats undergoing nucleoside reverse transcriptase inhibitor treatment or treatment-naive cats in rio de janeiro, brazil. *J. Virol.* **2008**, *82*, 7863–7874. [CrossRef] [PubMed]
47. Brown, M.A.; Cunningham, M.W.; Roca, A.L.; Troyer, J.L.; Johnson, W.E.; O'Brien, S.J. Genetic characterization of feline leukemia virus from florida panthers. *Emerg. Infect. Dis.* **2008**, *14*, 252–259. [CrossRef] [PubMed]

48. Butera, S.T.; Brown, J.; Callahan, M.E.; Owen, S.M.; Matthews, A.L.; Weigner, D.D.; Chapman, L.E.; Sandstrom, P.A. Survey of veterinary conference attendees for evidence of zoonotic infection by feline retroviruses. *J. Am. Vet. Med. Assoc.* **2000**, *217*, 1475–1479. [CrossRef] [PubMed]
49. Tandon, R.; Cattori, V.; Gomes-Keller, M.A.; Meli, M.L.; Golder, M.C.; Lutz, H.; Hofmann-Lehmann, R. Quantitation of feline leukaemia virus viral and proviral loads by taqman real-time polymerase chain reaction. *J. Virol. Methods* **2005**, *130*, 124–132. [CrossRef]
50. Brooks, J.I.; Merks, H.W.; Fournier, J.; Boneva, R.S.; Sandstrom, P.A. Characterization of blood-borne transmission of simian foamy virus. *Transfusion* **2007**, *47*, 162–170. [CrossRef] [PubMed]
51. Murray, S.M.; Picker, L.J.; Axthelm, M.K.; Hudkins, K.; Alpers, C.E.; Linial, M.L. Replication in a superficial epithelial cell niche explains the lack of pathogenicity of primate foamy virus infections. *J. Virol.* **2008**, *82*, 5981–5985. [CrossRef] [PubMed]
52. Muniz, C.P.; Zheng, H.; Jia, H.; Cavalcante, L.T.F.; Augusto, A.M.; Fedullo, L.P.; Pissinatti, A.; Soares, M.A.; Switzer, W.M.; Santos, A.F. A non-invasive specimen collection method and a novel simian foamy virus (SFV) DNA quantification assay in new world primates reveal aspects of tissue tropism and improved sfv detection. *PLoS ONE* **2017**, *12*, e0184251. [CrossRef] [PubMed]
53. Soliven, K.; Wang, X.; Small, C.T.; Feeroz, M.M.; Lee, E.G.; Craig, K.L.; Hasan, K.; Engel, G.A.; Jones-Engel, L.; Matsen, F.A.t.; et al. Simian foamy virus infection of rhesus macaques in bangladesh: Relationship of latent proviruses and transcriptionally active viruses. *J. Virol.* **2013**, *87*, 13628–13639. [CrossRef] [PubMed]
54. Murray, S.M.; Picker, L.J.; Axthelm, M.K.; Linial, M.L. Expanded tissue targets for foamy virus replication with simian immunodeficiency virus-induced immunosuppression. *J. Virol.* **2006**, *80*, 663–670. [CrossRef] [PubMed]
55. Willett, B.J.; Hosie, M.J. Feline leukaemia virus: Half a century since its discovery. *Vet. J.* **2013**, *195*, 16–23. [CrossRef] [PubMed]
56. Betsem, E.; Rua, R.; Tortevoye, P.; Froment, A.; Gessain, A. Frequent and recent human acquisition of simian foamy viruses through apes' bites in central Africa. *PLoS Pathog* **2011**, *7*, e1002306. [CrossRef] [PubMed]
57. Broussard, S.R.; Comuzzie, A.G.; Leighton, K.L.; Leland, M.M.; Whitehead, E.M.; Allan, J.S. Characterization of new simian foamy viruses from african nonhuman primates. *Virology* **1997**, *237*, 349–359. [CrossRef]
58. Hussain, A.I.; Shanmugam, V.; Bhullar, V.B.; Beer, B.E.; Vallet, D.; Gautier-Hion, A.; Wolfe, N.D.; Karesh, W.B.; Kilbourn, A.M.; Tooze, Z. Screening for simian foamy virus infection by using a combined antigen western blot assay: Evidence for a wide distribution among old world primates and identification of four new divergent viruses. *Virology* **2003**, *309*, 248–257. [CrossRef]
59. Torres, A.N.; Mathiason, C.K.; Hoover, E.A. Re-examination of feline leukemia virus: Host relationships using real-time PCR. *Virology* **2005**, *332*, 272–283. [CrossRef]
60. Hofmann-Lehmann, R.; Huder, J.B.; Gruber, S.; Boretti, F.; Sigrist, B.; Lutz, H. Feline leukaemia provirus load during the course of experimental infection and in naturally infected cats. *J. Gen. Virol.* **2001**, *82*, 1589–1596. [CrossRef]
61. Nesina, S.; Katrin Helfer-Hungerbuehler, A.; Riond, B.; Boretti, F.S.; Willi, B.; Meli, M.L.; Grest, P.; Hofmann-Lehmann, R. Retroviral DNA–the silent winner: Blood transfusion containing latent feline leukemia provirus causes infection and disease in naive recipient cats. *Retrovirology* **2015**, *12*, 105. [CrossRef]
62. Powers, J.A.; Chiu, E.S.; Kraberger, S.J.; Roelke-Parker, M.; Lowery, I.; Erbeck, K.; Troyer, R.; Carver, S.; VandeWoude, S. Feline leukemia virus (FELV) disease outcomes in a domestic cat breeding colony: Relationship to endogenous felv and other chronic viral infections. *J. Virol.* **2018**, *92*. [CrossRef] [PubMed]
63. Beebe, A.M.; Faith, T.G.; Sparger, E.E.; Torten, M.; Pedersen, N.C.; Dandekar, S. Evaluation of in vivo and in vitro interactions of feline immunodeficiency virus and feline leukemia virus. *Aids* **1994**, *8*, 873–878. [CrossRef] [PubMed]
64. Siekevitz, M.; Josephs, S.F.; Dukovich, M.; Peffer, N.; Wong-Staal, F.; Greene, W.C. Activation of the hiv-1 ltr by t cell mitogens and the trans-activator protein of HTLV-i. *Science* **1987**, *238*, 1575–1578. [CrossRef] [PubMed]

viruses

MDPI

Article

Feline Foamy Virus Infection: Characterization of Experimental Infection and Prevalence of Natural Infection in Domestic Cats with and without Chronic Kidney Disease

Carmen Ledesma-Feliciano [1,2], Ryan M. Troyer [1,3], Xin Zheng [1], Craig Miller [1,4], Rachel Cianciolo [5], Matteo Bordicchia [6], Nicholas Dannemiller [1], Roderick Gagne [1], Julia Beatty [6], Jessica Quimby [7,8], Martin Löchelt [9] and Sue VandeWoude [1,*]

1. Department of Microbiology, Immunology, and Pathology, College of Veterinary Medicine and Biomedical Sciences, Colorado State University, Fort Collins, CO 80523, USA
2. Division of Infectious Diseases, Department of Medicine, School of Medicine, University of Colorado Anschutz Medical Campus, 12700 E. 19th Ave., Aurora, CO 80045, USA
3. Department of Microbiology and Immunology, University of Western Ontario, 1151 Richmond St., London, ON N6A 5C1, Canada
4. Department of Veterinary Pathobiology, Oklahoma State University, Stillwater, OK 74075, USA
5. Department of Veterinary Biosciences, The Ohio State University, Columbus, OH 43210, USA
6. Sydney School of Veterinary Science, Faculty of Science, University of Sydney, NSW 2006, Australia
7. Department of Clinical Sciences, College of Veterinary Medicine and Biomedical Sciences, Colorado State University, Fort Collins, CO 80523, USA
8. Department of Veterinary Clinical Sciences, The Ohio State University Veterinary Medical Center, 601 Vernon Tharpe Street, Columbus, OH 43210, USA
9. Department of Viral Transformation Mechanisms, Research Program Infection, Inflammation and Cancer, German Cancer Research Center (DKFZ), Im Neuenheimer Feld 242, 69120 Heidelberg, Germany

* Correspondence: Sue.Vandewoude@colostate.edu; Tel.: +970-491-7162

Received: 25 June 2019; Accepted: 13 July 2019; Published: 19 July 2019

Abstract: Foamy viruses (FVs) are globally prevalent retroviruses that establish apparently apathogenic lifelong infections. Feline FV (FFV) has been isolated from domestic cats with concurrent diseases, including urinary syndromes. We experimentally infected five cats with FFV to study viral kinetics and tropism, peripheral blood mononuclear cell (PBMC) phenotype, urinary parameters, and histopathology. A persistent infection of primarily lymphoid tropism was detected with no evidence of immunological or hematologic perturbations. One cat with a significant negative correlation between lymphocytes and PBMC proviral load displayed an expanded FFV tissue tropism. Significantly increased blood urea nitrogen and ultrastructural kidney changes were noted in all experimentally infected cats, though chemistry parameters were not outside of normal ranges. Histopathological changes were observed in the brain, large intestine, and other tissues. In order to determine if there is an association of FFV with Chronic Kidney Disease, we additionally screened 125 Australian pet cats with and without CKD for FFV infection and found that FFV is highly prevalent in older cats, particularly in males with CKD, though this difference was not statistically significant compared to controls. Acute FFV infection was clinically silent, and while some measures indicated mild changes, there was no overt association of FFV infection with renal disease.

Keywords: foamy virus; spumavirus; retrovirus; viral tropism; infection; kidney; cats; chronic kidney disease; chronic renal disease

---

1. Introduction

Feline foamy virus (FFV) is a retrovirus belonging to the ancient *Spumaretrovirinae* subfamily that infects domestic cats (*Felis catus*) and was originally discovered following development of cytopathic effects (CPEs) in feline cell lines [1,2]. Foamy viruses (FVs) cause multiple CPEs in vitro including multinucleation, giant cell formation, and vacuolization, leading to cells looking "foamy" (and where the "*spuma*" originates) [1,3–5]. In naturally-occurring and experimental infections of the domestic cat, however, FFV infection does not cause obvious disease, and has not been definitively associated with pathology despite establishing a persistent, life-long infection with a wide tissue tropism [3,6–11]. It is believed the apathogenicity of FVs in general is due to long periods of co-evolution with their hosts that has led to a disease-free or highly-attenuated infection [2,12,13]. FV transmission is thought to primarily occur via salivary shedding and ongoing contact between animals, though alternate routes such as vertical transmission through lactating dams have been reported [7,14]. In cats, biting and amicable prolonged contact, such as grooming, have been suggested as routes of transmission [7,15,16]. Global FFV prevalence in pet and feral domestic cats can be high and varies from 8 to 80% based on geographic location, population sampled, and assay type [16–26]. FFV prevalence studies of cats in the USA have documented infection rates of 10 to 75%, with age and male sex identified as risk factors in some cohorts [7,16,27].

FVs are generally host-specific with the exception of simian foamy virus (SFV) where non-human primates may transmit virus to related species and zoonotically to humans [28–34]. Zoonotic transmission of FFV to humans has not been detected thus far [12,19,35]. Because of the apparent apathogenicity, wide tissue tropism, and large vector cassette packaging capacity, FVs have been used to develop vaccine and gene therapy vectors in multiple species including cats and non-human primates as a model for human therapies [10,13,36–42]. Many aspects about FV biology, including target cells, latency reservoirs, the specific receptor used for cell entry, viral kinetics over time following infection, and peripheral blood mononuclear cell (PBMC) population changes during infection have been poorly documented [6,12,43,44]. Experimental FFV infection studies in disease-free specific-pathogen-free (SPF) domestic cats with age-matched negative controls using modern and specific assays are rare; the majority have been conducted with domestic cats kept as pets or from shelters [3,6–8,11,38,42,45].

While FFV has been detected in apparently disease-free and healthy animals and has historically been considered apathogenic, the virus has been detected in animals suffering from co-infecting pathogens including feline immunodeficiency virus (FIV) [16,17,46,47], feline leukemia virus (FeLV) [45,48,49], feline coronavirus (FCoV) [24,50], and *Bartonella henselae* [18]. German and others reported histopathological changes in kidney and lung following experimental FFV inoculation [6]. A recent study of zoonotic infection with SFV in African hunters found alterations of urinary parameters including blood urea nitrogen (BUN) and serum creatinine, among other hematological changes [30]. These findings in both cats and humans call into question whether chronic infections with FVs are truly apathogenic.

FFV has also been isolated from cats with renal and other urinary tract disease [4,6,24,51–55], polyarthritis [45,47], neoplasia [1,3,24,56], upper respiratory illness [6,24], and myeloproliferative diseases [7]. Chronic kidney disease (CKD) is one of the most commonly diagnosed renal diseases in cats, with prevalence rates reaching up to 85% in geriatric cats [57–59]. CKD is characterized by functional and structural loss of kidney tissue likely resulting from prolonged or repeated renal insults [60–63]. As renal function declines, urine concentrating ability is lost and glomerular filtration rate falls, which eventually manifests as azotemia characterized by elevated BUN and serum creatinine. While the etiologies of CKD are often unknown, a list of comorbidities have been associated with the development of CKD, including retroviral infections [64–67].

Due to the widespread presence of FFV in domestic cat populations and the knowledge gaps that remain about FFV pathogenicity, especially considering its use in vaccine and gene therapy development, biochemical and histopathologic data from an in vivo FFV experimental infection in healthy SPF domestic cats [10] were further analyzed with emphasis on clinical, immunological, and pathological characteristics and changes during early infection. Due to the renal findings in this study and the detection of FFV in cats suffering from urinary disease, we sought to establish if there is an association between FFV and CKD in cats. We compared FFV prevalence rates in pet cats suffering from CKD in Australia (AU) (as measured by increased blood creatinine) and compared findings to age-matched cats without evidence of CKD. We hypothesized that (1) FFV causes subtle perturbations in immunological and hematological parameters in addition to histopathological changes that could potentially lead to disease in domestic cats, and that (2) FFV is associated with chronic kidney disease in cats. We identified mildly altered hematological and biochemical parameters associated with mild histopathological changes in the lung, brain, and other tissues, and ultrastructural changes in the kidney. We additionally found that while FFV is highly prevalent in AU, there was no direct association between FFV infection and CKD pathology in our sampled population.

2. Materials and Methods

2.1. Cells and Virus Generation

Plasmid pCF-7 encoding an FFV genome that is replication-competent in vitro and in vivo was used as virus source [10,38]. Crandell feline kidney (CrFK) cells [21,25,68] were used for transfection, viral propagation, and titer determination as described [10]. A CPE end-point dilution assay was used to determine viral titer (50% tissue culture infectious dose, $TCID_{50}$/mL) for cat inoculations [10,69]. CPEs consistent with FFV infection used in our assay include cytomegaly, vacuolization, and syncytia formation [1,3,70].

2.2. Animals and Study Design for Experimental FFV Inoculation

Cats were infected with pCF-7-derived FFV as a control group for a previous study testing an experimental molecularly modified chimeric FFV vector [10]. Domestic cats used in our study were acquired from the Colorado State University (CSU, Fort Collins, CO, USA) specific-pathogen-free (SPF) colony, which is free of FFV, and housed in an animal facility at CSU accredited by the Association for Assessment and Accreditation of Laboratory Animal Care International. The trial was approved by the Colorado State University Institutional Animal Care and Use Committee (IACUC) on 5 December 2013 and registered under IACUC protocol #: 13-4104A.

Nine cats (male castrated and intact females, aged 6–8 months) were separated into naïve (N) and FFV groups based on inoculum (Figure 1, modified with permission from [10]): cats N1-4 received FFV-negative CrFK culture media and cats FFV1-4 were inoculated with 10^5 FFV particles (derived from a 2.78×10^5 $TCID_{50}$/mL as described previously [10]) in CrFK culture supernatant. Each cat was inoculated with 2 mL, divided into 1 mL intravenously (iv) through the cephalic vein and 1 mL intramuscularly (im) into hindlimb musculature. A fifth cat was inoculated at the start of the study with 10^5 viral particles (5.56×10^5 $TCID_{50}$/mL) of the afore-mentioned chimeric FFV but remained PCR negative. This cat was subsequently inoculated with 1.4×10^6 $TCID_{50}$/mL of the pCF-7-derived FFV on day 53 of the study and subsequently became FFV PCR positive [10]. This animal, referred to as FFV5, was included in our analyses to increase the statistical power of this study. The study timeline and sample collection schedule (blood, saliva, urine, and tissues) are shown in Figure 1.

Cats were monitored daily for any clinical signs of disease, and rectal temperature and body weight were recorded weekly. Peripheral blood was used for flow cytometric PBMC phenotype analysis or processed to collect serum and plasma shortly after collection. Whole blood and sera were submitted to the CSU Veterinary Diagnostic Laboratory (VDL) for complete blood count (CBC) and chemistry analyses (normal blood urea nitrogen concentration: 18–35 mg/dl; normal serum creatinine concentration: 0.8–2.4 mg/dl). Saliva was collected by swabbing oral mucosa with a sterile cotton-tip applicator and freezing at −80 °C. Urine was collected through cystocentesis and submitted to the CSU VDL for urinalysis, urine sediment, and urine protein:creatinine (UPC) ratio determination. Urine was considered appropriately concentrated if it had a urine specific gravity (USG) over (>) 1.035. UPC ratio was considered normal if below (<) 0.2 and borderline proteinuric if between 0.2 and 0.4 [71]. On day 176 post-inoculation (pi), cats were euthanized and necropsied to assess gross pathology and harvest tissues for virus detection, histopathology, and renal-specific assays at the International Veterinary Renal Pathology Service (IVRPS) in The Ohio State University (OSU, Columbus, OH, USA).

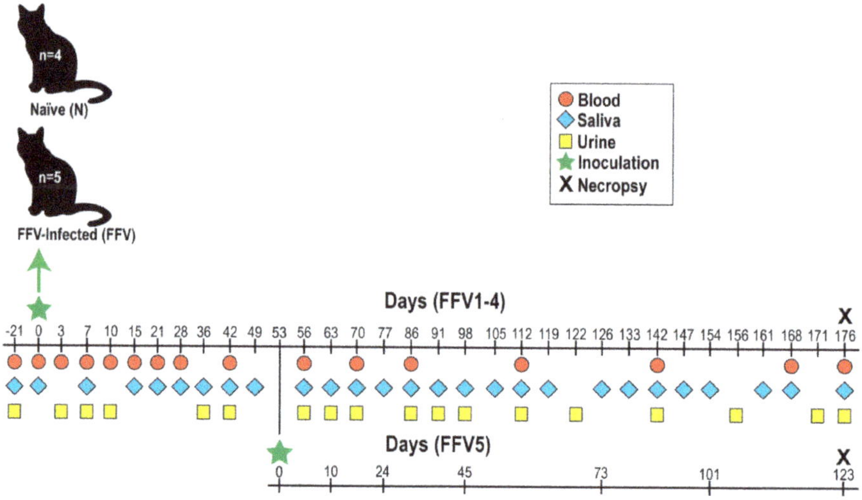

Figure 1. Experimental timeline of feline foamy virus (FFV) (strain pCF-7) inoculation and sample collection in specific-pathogen-free (SPF) domestic cats. Cats were separated into groups based on inoculum type: negative Crandell feline kidney (CrFK) culture media (naïve control cats N1-4) or FFV in CrFK cell culture supernatant (cats FFV1-5). Blood, saliva, urine, and tissues were collected on the dates specified. Sample collection for cat FFV5 was on a different schedule than the rest of the cohort (bottom timeline, adjusted to match rest of FFV cohort). Samples for baseline data were collected on day -21. On day 176 post-inoculation, cats were euthanized to perform necropsy and tissue collection (black **X**). Figure modified with permission from [10].

2.3. *Nested and Real-Time Quantitative PCR for Virus Detection and Quantification*

DNA was purified from whole blood, saliva, and plasma using the DNeasy Blood and Tissue Kit (QIAGEN, Hilden, Germany) and amplified using 0.5 μM forward and reverse primers under conditions described [10,72]. Nested PCR (nPCR) products were electrophoresed in agarose gel and stained to identify the desired PCR product. Real-time quantitative PCR (qPCR) was performed in duplicate to triplicate on purified FFV DNA as described [10,72]. Tissue DNA was purified with the DNeasy Blood and Tissue Kit after homogenizing in Buffer ATL and Proteinase K using the FastPrep®-24 Instrument (MP Biomedicals, Santa Ana, CA, USA). Saliva and plasma RNA was purified using the QIAamp Viral RNA Mini Kit (QIAGEN). RNA was reverse transcribed to cDNA using Superscript II and random hexamer primers (Invitrogen, Carlsbad, CA, USA) and resulting cDNA was used for qPCR as described above.

2.4. *Hematological and Flow Cytometric Analyses for PBMC Phenotyping*

Routine hematology and comprehensive PBMC phenotyping were performed at regular intervals (Figure 1). For flow cytometric PBMC phenotype analysis, EDTA-anticoagulated blood was incubated with fluorescent-labelled antibodies (Table S1) diluted at 4 °C flow buffer (PBS with 5% bovine fetal serum and 0.1% sodium azide) and processed by the IMMUNOPREP whole blood lysis method on a Q-Prep EPICS Immunology Workstation (Beckman Coulter, Fort Collins, CO, USA) to lyse red blood cells. Samples were analyzed with a Gallios Flow Cytometer (Beckman Coulter). Output data were analyzed using FlowJo software (FlowJo, Ashland, OR, USA). Data from the CBC were used to determine absolute neutrophil, lymphocyte, and monocyte cell numbers by multiplying the number of nucleated cells by percentages of each cell population. Absolute cell counts were then multiplied by percentages of each cell subpopulation obtained through flow cytometry for each cat per timepoint. PMBC phenotype analyses were divided into two panels: Panel A assayed T lymphocyte populations while Panel B determined number of B cells, natural killer (NK) cells, and monocytes. Markers for activation (CD134+, CD125+, MHCII+) and apoptosis (Fas+) were also assayed. In total, 24 PBMC phenotypes were measured for each cat per timepoint (Table 1). General white blood cell (WBC) activation and apoptosis were determined by multiplying WBC counts by MHCII+ and Fas+ percentages.

Table 1. White blood cell (WBC) populations assayed for peripheral blood mononuclear cell (PBMC) phenotype analysis.

Assay	Population	Cluster of Differentiation
CBC	WBC	-
	Monocytes	-
	Lymphocytes	-
	Neutrophils	-
Flow Cytometry (Panel A)	Th [1] lymphocytes	CD4+
	Activation	CD4+CD25+
	Activation	CD4+CD134+
	Apoptosis	CD4+Fas+
	Tc [2] lymphocytes	CD8+
	Activation	CD8+CD25+
	Activation	CD8+CD134+
	Apoptosis	CD8+Fas+
	Double-positive T cells	CD4+CD8+
Flow Cytometry (Panel B)	B cells	CD21+
	Activation	CD21+MHCII+
	Apoptosis	CD21+Fas+
	NK cells	CD56+
	Activation	CD56+MHCII+
	Apoptosis	CD56+Fas+
	Monocytes	CD14+
	Activation	CD14+MHCII+
	Apoptosis	CD14+Fas+
	WBC activation	MHCII+
	WBC apoptosis	Fas+

[1] T helper, [2] T cytotoxic.

2.5. Gross Necropsy and Histologic Characterization of Tissues

To evaluate pathologic changes associated with FFV infection, necropsy was performed on cats FFV1-5 and control cat N4 on day 176 pi. The following tissues were collected and stored either frozen at −80 °C for viral tropism determination (qPCR) or in 10% buffered formalin for histopathological evaluation by light microscopy: lymph nodes (submandibular, mesenteric, pre-scapular, retropharyngeal, and ileocecocolic), thyroid, tongue, tonsil, oral mucosa, salivary glands, thymus, heart, lung, spleen, liver, kidney, ovary, testis, mammary tissue, brain (cerebrum, cerebellum, brainstem), small intestine (jejunum, ileum), colon, bone marrow, and hindlimb skeletal muscle. For histopathological assessment, formalin-fixed tissue samples were embedded into paraffin and 5 µm sections were collected onto charged slides (Superfrost; CSU CDL, Fort Collins, CO, USA). One slide of each tissue was stained with hematoxylin and eosin (HE) for microscopic examination.

Tissues were scored using the following scale: 0 = no apparent pathology/change, 1 = minimal change (minimally increased numbers of small lymphocytes, plasma cells, macrophages, and/or mast cells), 2 = mild change (mild inflammation, edema, and/or parafollicular expansion, secondary follicle formation, and presence of tingible body macrophages within lymph nodes), 3 = moderate change (as previously described, but more extensive), 4 = marked changes (as previously described, but with severe inflammation, edema, and/or lymphoid reactivity).

2.6. Renal Tissue Microscopic and Ultrastructural Examination

Renal tissues collected from cats FFV1-5 and N4 during necropsy were submitted to the IVRPS for comprehensive analysis with light microscopy (LM), transmission electron microscopy (TEM), and immunofluorescence (IF). Samples were submitted in 10% buffered formalin for LM, 3% glutaraldehyde for TEM, and Michel's transport media for IF, and were processed as previously described [73]. Briefly, formalin-fixed paraffin embedded samples were sectioned at 3 µm thickness and stained with HE, Periodic Acid Schiff (PAS), Masson's Trichrome (MT), and Jones Methenamine silver method (JMS). Samples for TEM were processed routinely and examined with a JEOL JEM-1400 TEM microscope (JEOL USA, Inc., Peabody, MA, USA) and representative electron micrographs were taken with an Olympus SIS Veleta 2K camera (Olympus Soft Imaging Solutions GmbH, Münster, Germany). For IF, samples were washed to remove residual plasma constituents, embedded in Optimal Cutting Temperature (OCT, Sakura Finetek USA INC, Torrance, CA, USA), and frozen until sectioning. The OCT blocks were sectioned at 5 µm thickness and direct IF performed with FITC-labeled goat anti-feline Immunoglobulin (Ig) G, IgM, and IgA antibodies (Bethyl Laboratories, Montgomery, TX, USA) as well as FITC-labeled rabbit anti-human lambda light chain (LLC), kappa light chain (KLC), and C1q antibodies (Dako-Agilent, Santa Clara, CA). Stained sections were examined using an Olympus BX51 epifluorescence microscope and representative images were taken with a Nikon Digital Sight DS-U2 camera (Nikon, Tokyo, Japan). TEM assessment was not performed on control cat N4.

2.7. Samples from Australian Pet Cats with CKD and Non-Azometic, Age-Matched Controls

To investigate a possible association between FFV infection and naturally-acquired azotemic CKD, biobanked residual samples from pet cats undergoing routine clinical care at the University Veterinary Teaching Hospital Sydney (UVTHS), Sydney School of Veterinary Science, were obtained. Sample collection was approved by the University of Sydney Animal Ethics Committee, approval numbers N00/7-2013/3/6029 (approved 26 August 2013) and 2016/1002 (approved 17 May 2016). Cases were defined as CKD-positive ("CKD") if serum creatinine was elevated above the reference range, USG (measured concurrently) was <1.035, and clinical signs consistent with CKD were present [71]. Age-matched control samples were from non-azotemic clinically healthy cats with USG > 1.050.

A total of 125 samples (53 whole blood and 34 plasma samples in the CKD group and 38 whole blood samples in the control group) were analyzed for FFV infection by either nPCR (whole blood) or specific FFV ELISA against Gag antigen (plasma) as described previously [10]. Detection of FFV antibodies in sera/plasma is more sensitive for detection than FFV PCR [8,10,16,26,72]. Four different laboratories were used for serum creatinine and BUN determination and values were classified as abnormal based upon the references established for each laboratory: BUN: 7.2–10.7 mmol/L (20.16–29.96 mg/dl), 5.7–12.9 mmol/L (15.96–36.12 mg/dl), 5–15 mmol/L (14–42.01 mg/dl), or 3–10 mmol/L (8.4–28 mg/dl) [74]; serum creatinine: 91–180 µmol/L (1.03–2.04 mg/dl), 71–212 µmol/L (0.8–2.4 mg/dl), 40–190 µmol/L (0.45–2.15 mg/dl), or 80–200 µmol/L (0.9–2.26 mg/dl) [75].

2.8. Statistical Analyses

For the experimentally FFV-inoculated cats, two-tailed Student's t test were performed on hematology, flow cytometry, BUN, serum creatinine, and USG data sets. *P*-values < 0.05 were considered statistically significant. For cat FFV5, the timeline following re-inoculation on day 53 with FFV was adjusted so that day 53 equaled day 0 pi. To have consistent timelines with the main FFV group, timepoints after day 53 for cat FFV5 were grouped with either the equivalent day or the nearest date post-inoculation to the cats in the FFV cohort. A Pearson's correlation coefficient was calculated to determine presence of a correlation and its significance between lymphocyte population numbers and FFV proviral load over time. To assess distributions of viral load to lymphocyte counts, we ran a generalized linear mixed model (GLMM) with the individual cat as a random factor and lymphocyte count as a fixed factor. Data were only run through the GLMM if viral load was at detectable levels and the data fit a negative binomial distribution.

For the CKD analyses, risk ratios and chi-square tests were performed to assess the independence of three pairs of categorical variables: (1) sex and FFV infection, (2) sex and CKD, and (3) FFV infection and CKD. For each pair of variables, cats were stratified by sex (M or F), FFV infection status, and CKD status. Given that both nPCR and ELISA were used to determine FFV infection, CKD analyses were performed on both assays' results to see if conclusions differed. If a chi-square test produced a P-value < 0.05, risk ratios and 95% confidence intervals (95% CI) were calculated as an additional post-hoc test. Risk ratios describe the probability of a health outcome occurring in an exposed group to the probability of the event occurring in a comparison, non-exposed group. A Risk ratio >1 suggests an increased risk of that outcome in the exposed group, and a risk ratio <1 suggests a reduced risk in the exposed group. Cats for which sex data were not known (n = 5) were omitted in sex-specific data analyses.

Excel (Microsoft Corporation, Redmond, WA, USA) and Prism (GraphPad, La Jolla, CA, USA) were used to conduct the Student's t tests, calculate the lymphocyte and proviral load Pearson's correlation coefficient, and produce graphs. GLMM and CKD analyses were run using the statistical program R version 3.4.2 [76]. The "fitdistrplus" package [77] was used to determine error distributions of the viral load data and the "glmmTMB" package [78] was used to run the GLMM. Chi-square tests and RRs for CKD were calculated using the 'epitools' package [79].

3. Results

3.1. FFV-Infected Cats Did Not Show Clinical Signs of Infection Despite a Persistent FFV Proviral Load and Specific Humoral Response

As previously reported, all FFV group cats became PBMC FFV DNA positive (PCR), starting at 21 d pi (Figure 2) [10]. One cat (FFV3) was not PCR positive until day 42 but maintained a much higher proviral load than the rest of the cohort from that point on (Figure 5 in [10]). Cat FFV5 was FFV PCR positive by 10 days pi with FFV pCF-7 (Figure 2). FFV DNA was consistently detected in PBMC once the animals showed positivity [10]. Out of 80 FFV saliva samples tested, FFV RNA was detected only once (cat FFV4 on day 133 pi, Table 2); this sample was FFV DNA negative. All plasma samples tested were negative for FFV RNA and DNA (Table 2). Cats in the naïve group remained negative at all times. Additional proviral kinetics and anti-FFV antibody responses were reported previously [10].

Despite evidence of productive infection and specific immune response [10], none of the cats developed a fever, had changes in body weight, or displayed signs of clinical illness related to infection (such as anorexia or lethargy). CBC and chemistry values did not change significantly from the pre-inoculation time point (day -21) or indicate disease [80].

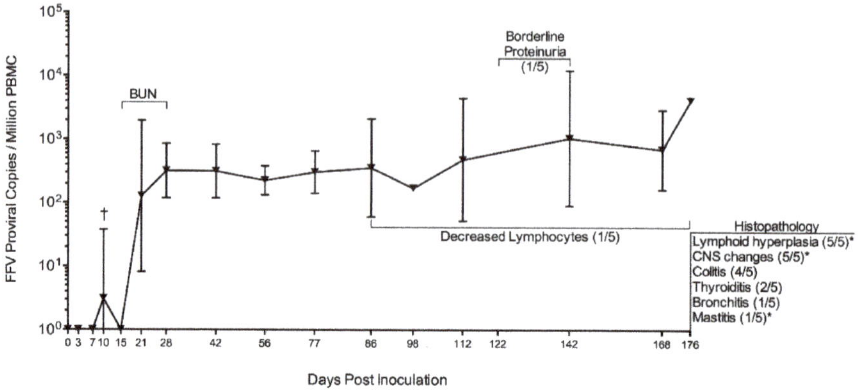

Figure 2. FFV proviral load in PBMC of cats FFV1-5 with summary of significant findings. FFV-infected cats began showing PBMC provirus 21 days pi. Cat FFV5 was re-inoculated and its timeline adjusted to match the rest of the cohort; this cat showed FFV positivity on day 10 post-reinoculation (†) [10]. Blood urea nitrogen (BUN) was significantly increased in infected cats compared to naïve on days 15, 21, and 28. Cat FFV3 had decreased lymphocytes compared to the rest of its cohort, which was negatively correlated to proviral PBMC load (Results Section 3.3). FFV3 also had borderline proteinuria on days 122 and 142 pi. Histopathological changes found after necropsy on day 176 are shown at the right-hand margin. Graph shows mean of FFV group cats' FFV proviral load with bars denoting standard deviation. Numbers in parenthesis indicate number of cats out of the FFV cohort showing findings, with an asterisk (*) indicating findings also observed in control cat N4 to a lesser severity.

Table 2. Summary of findings for diagnostic assays used in the experimental inoculation experiments. Bold font indicates that at least one cat was positive for the measured value, or differences in values between naïve and FFV-infected animals were significant. Cat FFV5 was on a different inoculation and sample collection schedule following re-inoculation on day 53 pi (Figure 1).

Assay	Days Tested	Summary of Findings
Saliva qPCR (RNA)	36, 42, 49, 56, 63, 86, 112, 119, 126, **133**, 142, 147, 154, 161, 168, 176	D133 saliva sample was FFV DNA-negative.
Plasma qPCR (DNA)	42, 86, 142, 176	FFV not detected.
Plasma qPCR (RNA)	15, 56, 112	FFV not detected.
Tissue qPCR (DNA)	176	Virus shows primarily lymphoid tropism. Cat FFV3 had expanded tropism to other lymphoid and non-lymphoid tissues (Table 3). FFV not detected in cat FFV4's tissues.
CBC, Chemistry	−21, 0, 3, 7, 10, 15, 21, 28, 42, 56, 63, 70, 77, 86, 98, 112, 126, 142, 154, 168, 176	Not indicative of disease.
PBMC Phenotype	−21, 0, 3, 7, **10**, **15**, 21, 28, **42**, 56, 70, **86**, **112**, 142, 168	Significantly increased populations in FFV cats included monocytes and CD21+MHCII+, while CD8+CD25+, CD8+CD134+, CD8+FAS+, CD56+, and CD56+MHCII+ cells were decreased.
BUN, Creatinine	−21, 0, 7, **15**, **21**, **28**, 42, 56, 63, 70, 77, 86, 98, 112, 126, 142, 154, 168, 176	While BUN remained within normal limits for all cats, values were significantly increased in FFV group cats compared to naïve on bolded days. Creatinine values were within normal ranges and did not rise above 1.8 mg/dl.
Urinalysis	−21, 3, 7, 10, 42, 56, 63, 70, 86, 91, 98, 112, 122, 142, 156, 171, 176	USG > 1.035 for all cats. Urinalysis and urine sediment were unremarkable.
UPC Ratio	36, 70, 86, 91, 98, **122**, **142**, 156, 171, 176	UPC ratio was 0.1 (normal) for all cats, except cat FFV3 where it increased to 0.2 (borderline proteinuric) on 122 and 142 days pi, during highest PBMC proviral load for this cat [10].

Table 3. FFV provirus has a primarily lymphoid tissue tropism. Viral load was determined through DNA qPCR and is presented as viral copies per million cells. Cat FFV3 had altered PBMC FFV DNA kinetics and expanded tissue tropism compared to the other FFV cats. Cat FFV5 was on a different inoculation schedule than the rest of the FFV cats (Materials and Methods Section 2.2 and Figure 1). Bold text indicates difference in either proviral load or viral detection compared to other cats in the group.

Tissue	N4	FFV1	FFV2	FFV3	FFV4	FFV5	Total Cats
Salivary gland	-	-	-	-	-	-	0
Tongue	-	-	-	-	-	-	0
Oral Mucosa	-	-	-	**2.10×10^2**	-	-	1
Tonsil	-	2.41×10^2	4.03×10^2	-	-	5.10×10^2	3
Prescapular LN	-	**5.89×10^3**	-	-	-	4.96×10^2	2
Submandibular LN	-	3.35×10^2	2.26×10^2	-	-	5.78×10^2	3
Retropharyngeal LN	-	1.86×10^2	1.19×10^2	1.49×10^2	-	2.35×10^2	4
Mesenteric LN	-	-	-	-	-	-	0
Thymus	-	-	-	**3.48×10^2**	-	-	1
Spleen	-	5.93×10^2	3.11×10^2	2.10×10^2	-	3.35×10^2	4
Ileum	-	-	-	-	-	-	0
Bone marrow	-	-	-	**6.10×10^2**	-	-	1
Kidney	-	-	-	-	-	-	0
Muscle	-	-	-	-	-	-	0

3.2. *FFV Provirus Tissue Tropism Is Primarily Lymphoid*

FFV DNA was detected in the tissues of four out of the five FFV-inoculated cats primarily in lymphoid tissue including lymph nodes (submandibular, retropharyngeal, and prescapular, which drain lymph from head, neck, and forelimbs), tonsil, and spleen (Table 3). Cat FFV3 showed an expanded tissue tropism to central lymphoid tissues (thymus and bone marrow) in addition to non-lymphoid tissue (oral mucosa). The prescapular lymph node was the tissue with highest viral load (cat FFV1). Cat FFV5 showed an FFV tissue tropism similar to the rest of the FFV group, with the submandibular lymph node having the highest viral load (Table 3). Control cat N4 and cat FFV4 did not have detectable provirus in any of the tissues tested.

3.3. *Significant PBMC Phenotypic Changes Were Rare though a Negative Correlation Was Found between Lymphocytes and FFV Proviral Load in Cat FFV3*

Out of the 24 cell populations and activation or apoptosis markers assayed for each cat per timepoint (Table 1), there were only 9 instances where significant differences ($P < 0.05$) were found between infected and control animals (Table 2). Significantly increased populations were found between FFV (1–5) and N (1–4) groups in the following instances: (1) absolute monocyte numbers on days 15 ($P = 0.036$) and 42 ($P = 0.025$) pi and (2) CD21+MHCII+ cells on d 86 pi ($P = 0.0076$). FFV-group cats had decreased populations compared to controls in the following instances: (1) CD8+CD25+ cells on d 112 pi ($P = 0.044$), (2) CD8+CD134+ cells on d 10 pi ($P = 0.031$), (3) CD8+FAS+ on d 10 pi ($P = 0.015$), (4) CD56+ cells on d 112 pi ($P = 0.00038$), and (5) CD56+MHCII+ cells on days 15 ($P = 0.049$) and 112 pi ($P = 0.00070$).

We further evaluated WBC populations in cat FFV3 due to the altered PBMC FFV provirus pattern observed [10]. This cat appeared to have lower lymphocytes and a trend for decreasing lymphocyte count over time compared to the rest of the infected and naïve cats (Figure 3A, blue line) as PBMC proviral load increased over time (Figure 3B, black line). A Pearson's correlation coefficient test for this cat showed a significant negative correlation between lymphocyte cell number and viral load over time ($r = -0.653$, $P = 0.006$). There was no correlation found in the rest of the infected cats (data not shown) and there was no significant relationship between viral load and lymphocyte count when we analyzed all cats as a group (GLMM Estimate −0.530, $P = 0.596$).

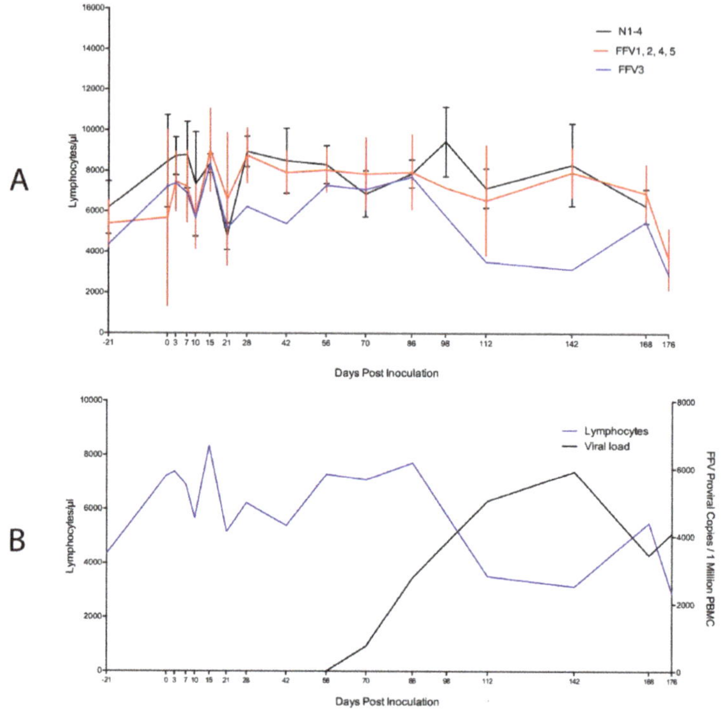

Figure 3. High viral load correlates with decline in circulating lymphocytes in cat FFV3. (**A**) Absolute lymphocyte population numbers determined through complete blood count for cat FFV3 (blue line) appeared to decrease over time compared to all other cats in the study. Naïve cats are grouped on the black line and the rest of the FFV-group cats are displayed on the red line; (**B**) A significant negative correlation ($r = -0.653$, $P = 0.006$) was found between lymphocytes and FFV proviral load [10] in cat FFV3 as lymphocyte population numbers (blue line) decreased and proviral load (determined by qPCR, black line) increased over time. Bars denote standard deviation.

3.4. Subtle Differences in Urine and Hematological Parameters Were Detected between Experimentally Infected and Control Cats

UPC ratios were 0.1 (normal) for all cats throughout the study, with the exception of two timepoints in cat FFV3 (d 122 and 142 pi) where its UPC ratio increased from 0.1 to 0.2 (borderline proteinuric), before decreasing back to normal (0.1) on day 176 pi (Figure 2) [81]. This mild transient increase in UPC coincided with the timepoint when this cat's PBMC FFV proviral load was highest (d 142 pi) (Figure 3B) [10]. BUN concentration remained within normal ranges (18–35 mg/dl) for all cats throughout the study, however values were higher in infected cats compared to naïve controls on three consecutive timepoints: days 15 ($P = 0.012$), 21 ($P = 0.039$), and 28 ($P = 0.025$) (Figures 3 and 4). All cats had USG > 1.035 and urinalyses and urine sediment were unremarkable throughout the study. Serum creatinine concentrations were at or below 1.8 mg/dl at all timepoints, and there were no significant differences in serum creatinine between infected and control cats [82].

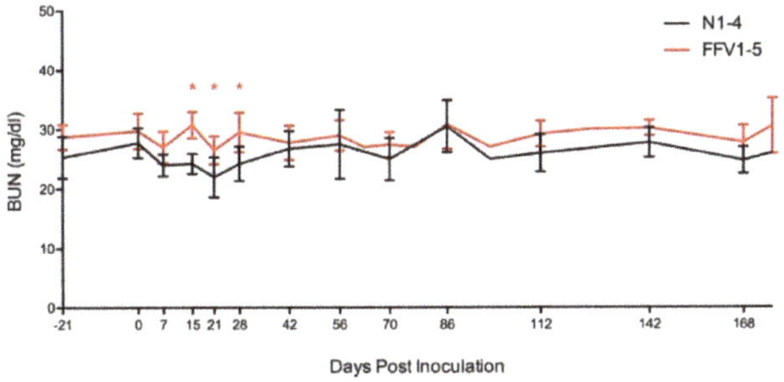

Figure 4. Blood urea nitrogen (BUN) levels are within normal range, but higher in FFV-infected versus naïve control cats. While BUN, one of the biomarkers used to assess renal health, remained within normal range (18–35 mg/dl) for all cats, concentrations tended to be higher in infected cats (red line) compared to naïve cats (black line) on days 15, 21, and 28 pi (red asterisks, $P < 0.05$). Lines represent mean of BUN measurements for the cats in each group. Vertical lines denote the standard deviation for each grouped measurement.

3.5. Mild Lymphoplasmacytic Infiltrates and Lymphoid Hyperplasia of Multiple Tissues Were Associated with FFV Exposure

No significant clinical or pathological findings were grossly observed in control (N4) or FFV-infected cats (FFV1–5) during necropsy. Microscopic evaluation of tissues from FFV-infected cats revealed mild ($n = 3$) to moderate ($n = 2$) lymphoid hyperplasia in retropharyngeal, submandibular, mesenteric, and prescapular lymph nodes, characterized by numerous secondary follicles that contain abundant tingible-body macrophages. The tonsils of infected animals exhibited minimal ($n = 1$), mild ($n = 3$), and moderate ($n = 1$) lymphoid hyperplasia with multifocal infiltration of small numbers of lymphocytes beyond the capsule in one mildly affected animal. Two infected cats exhibited mild thyroiditis characterized by multifocal infiltrates of small lymphocytes, plasma cells, and macrophages within the interstitium and surrounding colloid-filled follicles of varying size. Within the ileum, Peyer's patches were minimally ($n = 1$) to mildly ($n = 4$) hyperplastic, and one animal exhibited multifocal lymphoplasmacytic infiltrates extending deep into the submucosa. Additionally, minimal ($n = 3$) to mild ($n = 1$) lymphoplasmacytic colitis was observed in FFV-infected cats, with lymphoplasmacytic infiltration into the submucosa that caused disruption of the submucosal architecture ($n = 3$), as well as small numbers of degenerate neutrophils scattered within the submucosa ($n = 1$). In the cerebrum of FFV-infected cats, there were minimally ($n = 2$) to mildly ($n = 3$) increased numbers of glial cells (gliosis) and paired astrocytes (astrocytosis) surrounding scattered neurons within the gray matter (satellitosis), a feature that was most prominently noted within the frontal lobe and thalamus (Figure 5B). Cat FFV5 also had small numbers of small lymphocytes within the meninges (lymphocytic meningitis) (Figure 5C). Scattered neurons within these regions were multifocally swollen, rounded, and demonstrated mild central dispersion of Nissl substance (chromatolysis), as well as rare, scattered neurons that exhibited hypereosinophilic and/or fragmented cytoplasm (potentially indicative of neuronal necrosis) ($n = 2$) (Figure 5D). One cat had mild multifocal lymphohistiocytic mastitis. Histologic changes in cat FFV5 were slightly more pronounced when compared to the other infected animals and included moderate lymphoid hyperplasia in the tonsil with moderate numbers of lymphocytes and macrophages within the tonsil medullary sinus, and enlarged germinal centers in the Peyer's patches. Within the lung of this cat, the parabronchial interstitium and alveolar septa were multifocally expanded by small numbers of small lymphocytes, intact neutrophils, and macrophages (interpreted as mild interstitial pneumonia). Alveoli were occasionally filled with small numbers of alveolar macrophages and frequently lined by plump, cuboidal epithelial cells, indicating type 2 pneumocyte hyperplasia, with occasional clubbing of alveolar walls due to mild smooth muscle hypertrophy.

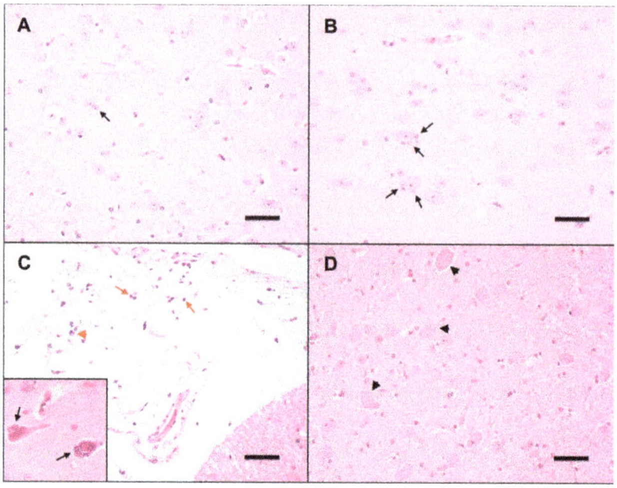

Figure 5. FFV-infected cats exhibit early neurodegenerative changes in the central nervous system. (**A**) Neurons in the CNS of control cat N4 contain uniform, round nuclei, abundant basophilic Nissl substance, and are flanked by few glial cells (black arrow). Frontal lobe, Hematoxylin-eosin (HE) 400×. Scale bar = 100 μm. (**B**) Neurons in the CNS of FFV-infected cat FFV3 exhibit moderate satellitosis, characterized by increased numbers of glial cells (black arrows). Thalamus, HE 400×. Scale bar = 100 μm. (**C**) The meninges of FFV-infected cat FFV5 are expanded by minimal numbers of mature small lymphocytes (red arrows) and plasma cells (red arrowheads). Cerebellum, HE 400×. Scale bar = 100 μm. Neurons in the frontal lobe of this animal (inset) are shrunken, with hypereosinophilic cytoplasm, and exhibit moderate satellitosis (black arrows). Frontal lobe, HE 400×. (**D**) Neurons in the CNS of an FFV-infected cat are swollen and rounded, with an indistinct nucleus and a dispersed Nissl substance (chromatolysis). Thalamus, HE 400×. Scale bar = 100 μm.

Non-specific histologic findings in control cat N4 included mild lymphoid hyperplasia in the mesenteric lymph node, tonsil, and thymus, minimal to mild inflammatory infiltrate in the tongue, and mammary tissue, and minimal chromatolysis in the cerebrum. Findings in this control cat ranged from very subtle to mild, and were less severe than in infected animals.

3.6. Ultrastructural Changes Were Noted in the Kidneys of FFV-Infected Cats

Histopathology of the kidneys from cats FFV1-5 (Table 4) demonstrated a few small foci of tubular degeneration encompassing fewer than 15 tubular cross-sections per focus in cats FFV1 and FFV2; cat FFV1 also had associated atrophy of the tubules. Glomeruli from the remaining cats in the FFV cohort and control cat N4 were within normal limits.

Ultra-structural TEM evaluation of glomeruli from cats FFV1-5 demonstrated minimal to moderate segmental effacement of podocyte foot processes in all infected cats (Figure 6A and Table 4). There were a few small segments of wrinkled glomerular capillary walls in cat FFV5 (Table 4). Electron-dense whorls resembling myelin figures appeared free in the cytoplasm or within cytoplasmic vacuoles in tubular epithelial cells of three of the infected cats (Table 4). Cytoplasmic vacuolization of parietal or tubular epithelial cells was present in two cats (Table 4).

Table 4. Summary of pathological findings in glomeruli and tubulointerstitial compartment of control and FFV-infected cats. Kidney tissue was collected during necropsy on day 176 and submitted to the International Veterinary Renal Pathology Service for analysis. Cat FFV5 was on a different inoculation schedule than the rest of the FFV cats (Materials and Methods Section 2.2 and Figure 1).

Analysis	Finding	N4	FFV1	FFV2	FFV3	FFV4	FFV5	Total Cats
Histology	Tubular degeneration (+/− atrophy)	-	+	+	-	-	-	2
TEM	Podocyte effacement	NT	+/+	++	++	+	+++	5
	Cytoplasmic electron dense figures	NT	-	+	+	+	+	4
	Cytoplasmic myelin figures	NT	+	+	-	+	-	3
	Cytoplasmic vacuolization	NT	-	+	+	-	-	2
	Wrinkled glomerular capillary walls	NT	-	-	-	-	+	1

+ = minimal, +/+ = minimal to mild, ++ = mild, +++ = moderate, NT = not tested.

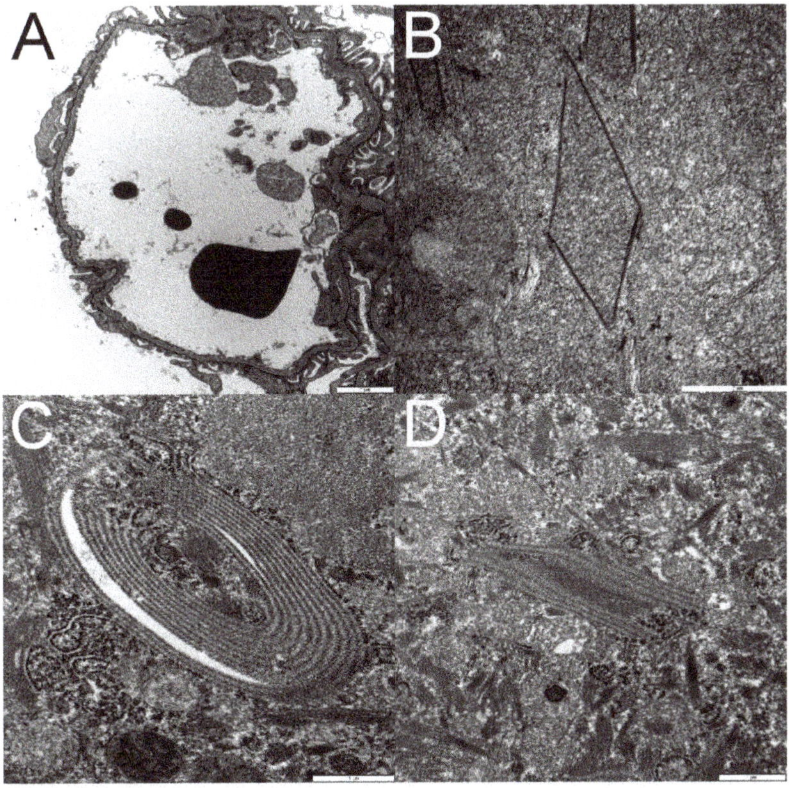

Figure 6. Transmission electron microscopy (TEM) documents podocyte foot process effacement (**A**). Examples of organized linear structures in tubular epithelial cell cytoplasm are depicted in panels **B–D**. These structures ranged from polygonal (**B** and **D**) to ovoid (**C**). Some structures were composed of a single electron dense line (**B**), whereas others were composed of numerous parallel electron dense lines (**C**,**D**) separated by regularly spaced electron lucent lines (**C**,**D**).

Within the cytoplasm of the proximal tubular epithelial cells of four of these cats, there were small electron-dense spirals and linear structures of 10–15 nm in length arranged in pairs, stacks, polygonal shapes, or spirals, and of variable length (Figure 6B–D). Sometimes the linearly shaped ones had a beaded appearance or formed structures resembling a zipper. Mitochondria occasionally wrapped around the structures. In cat FFV5, the structures were similar to the ones found in the other FFV cats but appeared significantly more organized. TEM evaluation was not conducted on cat N4.

Immunofluorescence did not demonstrate definitively positive (granular) labeling for any of the antibodies (IgG, IgM, IgA, LLC, KLC, and C1q). Cat FFV3 had weak blush to linear staining with IgM of the glomerular mesangium and some capillary walls but based on the pattern of staining, it was considered non-specific. Immunofluorescence was negative in tissues from control cat N4.

3.7. FFV Is Highly Prevalent in Australian Domestic Pet Cats

We determined FFV prevalence by either nPCR or ELISA in groups of cats with and without CKD to evaluate associations between FFV infection and the incidence of CKD. Overall FFV prevalence was 67% (Table S2) with no significant difference between CKD and control groups (Figure 7). Overall FFV prevalence was similar between males (68%) and females (69%). Males had a higher FFV prevalence in CKD (73%) versus males without CKD (58%), although this difference was not significant (Figure 7).

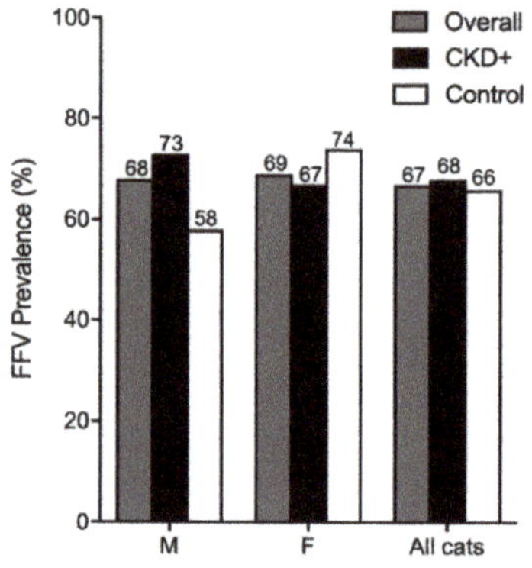

Figure 7. FFV prevalence is high in Australian domestic pet cats. Males with CKD had higher FFV prevalence than male control cats, although not significantly. M = male; F = female.

Chi-square test statistics and P-values are reported in Table S2. Our results suggest there is no significant association between CKD and FFV infection. Chi-square and relative risk ratio results did not differ between nPCR and ELISA indicating that neither assay detected an association between CKD and FFV infection in all groups evaluated.

4. Discussion

This study further characterized early FFV infection and host immune response in healthy SPF domestic cats following experimental FFV inoculation using a well-characterized replicative FFV molecular clone that achieves comparable viral titers, similar gene expression and comparable humoral immune response to wild-type virus in experimentally inoculated cats [42]. Though it is difficult to exactly recapitulate natural exposure route and dose, the FFV experimental exposure protocol used in this study is comparable to inoculation doses others have used in experimental FFV inoculation studies, and resulted in viral loads and antibody responses comparable to those recorded in naturally infected animals [6,8,11,42]. In addition to clinical monitoring, assessing viral kinetics and tropism, determining specific antibody response, and a histopathological assessment of different tissues, we conducted assays to expand infection characterization. This included flow cytometric assessment of specific white blood cell subsets suggested to be involved in FFV infection and renal-specific assays to determine the extent of FFV involvement in renal health or disease. Samples analyzed were obtained from control experimental cats reported in a previous study in which an FFV-based vaccine candidate was tested [10]. Based on microscopic findings from the FFV-infected cohort showing evidence of injury in renal tissues during acute FFV infection (Figure 6A and Table 4), we investigated the potential association of FFV with CKD in Australian client-owned cats following natural FFV infection.

FFV established a detectable, persistent, and clinically apathogenic infection during the relatively acute 6-month time period of our study [6,8,10,38]. Provirus was primarily isolated from lymphoid tissues including PBMC, the retropharyngeal lymph node, and spleen as previously reported (Table 3) [6,11,27]. The expanded tissue tropism found in cat FFV3, with 10-fold higher PBMC proviral load than the other cats, also included the oral mucosa, suggesting that animals with higher viral loads could have dissemination to non-lymphoid sites. We were unable to detect virus in the tissues of one cat (FFV4) which also tended to have lower PBMC proviral load [10]. Viral RNA was detected once in the saliva of cat FFV4 (Table 2), indicating that limited amounts of virus was being shed, and that salivary excretion may not correlate with widespread tissue distribution. A recently published report by Cavalcante and others on FFV-infected cats in Brazil found that pet and feral cats were more likely to be FFV positive in PBMC than in buccal swabs, as tested by PCR [83]. This has also been reported in primates due to a delay in salivary excretion of virus compared to blood [84]. A wide variability of FV positivity has been shown in different nonhuman primate species and even within the same species [85–87]. It is possible that due to the acute time period in our study, viral titer had not yet reached high enough levels in the oral cavity to be detected in the saliva.

A significant negative correlation between lymphocyte numbers and proviral load was found in cat FFV3 (Figure 3B), despite the fact that PBMC phenotype analysis did not indicate increased cell death or lymphocyte population contraction in FFV-infected cats (Table 2). Thus, PBMC phenotyping appears not to be a useful indicator of FFV infection. These findings, however, indicate that a subset of FFV-infected cats may experience higher viral loads with the potential for concurrent lymphocyte decline. Further work analyzing correlates of FFV-infected cats with hematologic indices is warranted to investigate this limited observation.

Necropsy and histologic analysis of experimentally infected cats yielded minimal to moderate changes in the lymphoid compartment, CNS, large intestine, lung, and thyroid. FFV-associated lung lesions have previously been noted in another experimental FFV infection study which reported mixed cellular infiltrates and eosinophilic fluid within alveolar walls [6], similar to findings reported here. Alterations in CNS histopathology of FFV-infected cats suggest viral replication or associated inflammation as is seen in other retroviral infections [88–90]. FFV has previously been isolated from the CNS of cats, and may therefore indicate that FFV is capable of productive CNS infection and subtle neurologic alterations [91]. These findings suggest a potential role for FFV in the development of mild acute inflammation in a variety of parenchymal organs and brain. FFV proviral load did not appear to correlate to the presence or severity of histopathology and histopathological changes were observed in tissues that were not FFV PCR positive and vice-versa. The changes observed were mild and consistent with inflammation due to nonspecific immune stimulation, and cannot be unequivocally associated with FFV infection, which would be ideally confirmed by viral propagation from isolated tissues or immunohistochemistry [11]. Nevertheless, the findings of consistent mild inflammation in multiple tissues of SPF cats exposed to FFV suggest that microscopic alterations occur during acute FFV infection.

FFV has previously been associated with urinary syndrome pathology [4,6,24,51–53]. BUN concentrations remained normal during FFV-infection, but were statistically elevated in FFV-infected compared to naïve groups on days 15, 21, and 28 pi, which coincided with the days when animals were first FFV PCR and ELISA positive [10]. These findings are intriguing given recent reports of chronic zoonotically SFV-infected people with increased BUN compared to un-infected controls [30]. Borderline proteinuria (increased UPC ratio to 0.2 [71]) was also recorded in cat FFV3 on days 122 and 142 pi, which coincided with the timing of the highest viral load measured in the study. While recorded changes in BUN and UPC ratio are interesting, these findings may not specifically indicate renal proteinuria and could be considered a transient systemic response to infection.

Ultrastructural kidney changes (glomerular podocyte foot process effacement, myelin figures, vacuolization, and wrinkled glomerular capillary walls, Figure 6A and Table 4) are non-specific and reversible changes. If enough podocytes are irreversibly injured, then the patient can develop segmental to global glomerulosclerosis, a disease process in humans and small animals that can cause proteinuria, usually with UPC >2. Although a cut-off for the number of irreversibly injured podocytes has not been established in cats, a model of glomerulosclerosis in rats estimated that >40% of the podocytes have to die and detach in order for glomerulosclerosis to develop [92]. Notably, glomerulosclerosis was not identified in any of the cats in the present study. Tubular atrophy noted on histopathology is an irreversible lesion and often seen in cats with clinical evidence of CKD [62,63]. Overall, our findings indicate subtle reversible renal alterations, indicating that FFV does not induce dramatic changes to renal function within 6 months of infection, however it is unknown how the lesions could have progressed in a chronic infection. We did not detect correlations between proviral PBMC load and presence or severity of TEM changes.

Electron-dense structures identified in proximal tubular epithelial cells in the kidney (Figure 6B–D) could represent viral structures at immature stages of assembly before forming the spherical shapes of FFV virions reported in the literature [1,93,94]. Similar structures have been found in the central nervous system in both cats and humans. Cook and others described similar tubular structures as "paramyxovirus nucleocapsid-like" in the cytoplasm of oligodendrocytes taken from demyelinating lesions in the optic nerve of three clinically healthy adult cats [95]. These inclusion-body like structures were of 16–17 nm in diameter and fused into penta- to septa-laminar shapes and 900 nm in length. The authors suggested a possible viral etiology. Wilcox and others (1984) reported similar structures in optic nerves and brains of 24 clinically healthy cats from which FFV was isolated [91]. While also finding 10–18 nm wide and 500 nm long structures, they also reported structures in much smaller shapes, appearing as "short, disorganized fragments," located next to where budding virions were observed, in addition to intranuclearly. These structures were, however, found in the cytoplasm of cells that did not display CPEs and thus these lesions were not attributed to FFV but perhaps a morbillivirus [91].

FFV was highly prevalent in Australian domestic cats as reported previously [16,19], and could be due to the lifestyle of Australian cats which are commonly allowed outside [96,97], allowing more opportunities to interact with other potentially infected cats. The samples analyzed also consisted of sera/plasma assayed by ELISA and whole blood analyzed by PCR. PCR is not as sensitive as ELISA for detection and can yield false negatives [8,10,16,26,72], therefore it is possible that FFV prevalence is even higher in Australia. Similar prevalence rates in males (68%) and females (69%) indicates that there are no sex-related differences in prevalence rates in Australian pet cats [16]. A recent study of feral cats in the USA found an association between FFV infection and male sex [27]. However, our epidemiological results were obtained from client-owned desexed animals. Another epidemiological study of FFV in Australia did not find an association between sex and FFV infection in desexed domestic cats, but did see higher incidences of FFV in female feral cats [16]. Our findings suggest that while overall there appears to be no association between FFV and CKD, CKD in male cats may be associated with FFV infection, though any effect is mild, and evaluation of a much larger cohort is required to assess actual associations. Male sex has not been found to be an overall risk factor for CKD, however males can be overrepresented in certain age groups [98].

5. Conclusions

Collectively, our findings reinforce and expand on the current established notion that FFV is widely prevalent and apathogenic over an acute time period, supporting decades long assumptions that FFV is well adapted to the domestic cat host. Evaluation of a multitude of hematologic and immunological parameters did not reveal significant host responses to infection. However, our detailed analysis of serum chemical and histopathological changes indicates sub-clinical alterations that could contribute to metabolic or degenerative diseases over time, supporting our hypothesis and work conducted by earlier researchers, and recent reports in humans [1,3,4,6,7,24,30,45,47,51–56]. The negative correlation between lymphocyte count and viral load in one cat with higher viral load suggests that a differential susceptibility and potential pathogenicity may exist in some individuals. Studies with larger cohorts of animals with well-characterized disease phenotypes may reveal subtle relationships between FFV and feline health, since the virus is clearly widely distributed in free-ranging cat populations.

Supplementary Materials: The following are available online at http://www.mdpi.com/1999-4915/11/7/662/s1, Table S1: Antibody marker combinations used for PBMC phenotype analysis through flow cytometry. Table S2: FFV prevalence and chi-square analysis data for CKD studies.

Author Contributions: Conceptualization, C.L.-F., R.M.T. and S.V.; Data curation, C.L.-F.; Formal analysis, C.L.-F., N.D., R.G. and S.V.; Funding acquisition, C.L.-F., M.L. and S.V.; Investigation, C.L.-F., R.M.T., X.Z., C.M., R.C. and M.B.; Methodology, C.L.-F., R.M.T., M.L. and S.V.; Project administration, C.L.-F. and S.V.; Resources, C.L.-F., M.B., J.B., M.L. and S.V.; Supervision, S.V.; Validation, C.L.-F. and X.Z.; Visualization, C.L.-F., C.M., R.C. and J.Q.; Writing—original draft, C.L.-F., C.M., R.C., N.D., R.G. and S.V.; Writing—review & editing, C.L.-F., R.M.T., C.M., R.C., N.D., R.G., J.B., J.Q., M.L. and S.V.

Funding: C.L.F. was funded by Morris Animal Foundation (grant number: D16FE-402) and The National Institutes of Health (NIH T32 grant number: 2T32OD010437-16). Funding bodies played no role in the design of the study, collection, analysis, and interpretation of data, or in writing the manuscript.

Acknowledgments: We would like to acknowledge Martha McMillan and Esther Musselman for in vitro FFV training, animal care, and help with regulatory matters (IACUC).

Conflicts of Interest: The authors declare no conflict of interest. The funders had no role in the design of the study; in the collection, analyses, or interpretation of data; in the writing of the manuscript, or in the decision to publish the results.

References

1. Riggs, J.L.; Oshiro, L.S.; Taylor, D.O.; Lennette, E.H. Syncytium-forming agent isolated from domestic cats. *Nature* **1969**, *222*, 1190–1191. [CrossRef] [PubMed]
2. Aiewsakun, P.; Katzourakis, A. Marine origin of retroviruses in the early palaeozoic era. *Nat. Commun.* **2017**, *8*, 13954. [CrossRef] [PubMed]
3. Kasza, L.; Hayward, A.H.; Betts, A.O. Isolation of a virus from a cat sarcoma in an established canine melanoma cell line. *Res. Vet. Sci.* **1969**, *10*, 216–218. [CrossRef]
4. Shroyer, E.L.; Shalaby, M.R. Isolation of feline syncytia-forming virus from oropharyngeal swab samples and buffy coat cells. *Am. J. Vet. Res.* **1978**, *39*, 555–560. [PubMed]
5. Ellis, T.M.; MacKenzie, J.S.; Wilcox, G.E.; Cook, R.D. Isolation of feline syncytia-forming virus from oropharyngeal swabs of cats. *Aust. Vet. J.* **1979**, *55*, 202–203. [CrossRef]
6. German, A.C.; Harbour, D.A.; Helps, C.R.; Gruffydd-Jones, T.J. Is feline foamy virus really apathogenic? *Vet. Immunol. Immunopathol.* **2008**, *123*, 114–118. [CrossRef]
7. Pedersen, N.C. Feline syncytium-forming virus infection. In *Diseases of the Cat*; Holyworth, J., Ed.; The W. B. Saunder Co.: Philadelphia, PA, USA, 1986; pp. 268–272.
8. Alke, A.; Schwantes, A.; Zemba, M.; Flugel, R.M.; Löchelt, M. Characterization of the humoral immune response and virus replication in cats experimentally infected with feline foamy virus. *Virology* **2000**, *275*, 170–176. [CrossRef]
9. Von Laer, D.; Neumann-Haefelin, D.; Heeney, J.L.; Schweizer, M. Lymphocytes are the major reservoir for foamy viruses in peripheral blood. *Virology* **1996**, *221*, 240–244. [CrossRef]
10. Ledesma-Feliciano, C.; Hagen, S.; Troyer, R.; Zheng, X.; Musselman, E.; Slavkovic Lukic, D.; Franke, A.M.; Maeda, D.; Zielonka, J.; Munk, C.; et al. Replacement of feline foamy virus *bet* by feline immunodeficiency virus *vif* yields replicative virus with novel vaccine candidate potential. *Retrovirology* **2018**, *15*, 38. [CrossRef]
11. Weikel, J.; Löchelt, M.; Truyen, U. Demonstration of feline foamy virus in experimentally infected cats by immunohistochemistry. *J. Vet. Med. Physiol. Pathol. Clin. Med.* **2003**, *50*, 415–417. [CrossRef]
12. Kehl, T.; Tan, J.; Materniak, M. Non-simian foamy viruses: Molecular virology, tropism and prevalence and zoonotic/interspecies transmission. *Viruses* **2013**, *5*, 2169–2209. [CrossRef]
13. Liu, W.; Lei, J.; Liu, Y.; Lukic, D.S.; Rathe, A.M.; Bao, Q.; Kehl, T.; Bleiholder, A.; Hechler, T.; Löchelt, M. Feline foamy virus-based vectors: Advantages of an authentic animal model. *Viruses* **2013**, *5*, 1702–1718. [CrossRef]

14. Romen, F.; Backes, P.; Materniak, M.; Sting, R.; Vahlenkamp, T.W.; Riebe, R.; Pawlita, M.; Kuzmak, J.; Löchelt, M. Serological detection systems for identification of cows shedding bovine foamy virus via milk. *Virology* **2007**, *364*, 123–131. [CrossRef]
15. Yamamoto, J.K.; Sparger, E.; Ho, E.W.; Andersen, P.R.; O'connor, T.P.; Mandell, C.P.; Lowenstine, L.; Munn, R.; Pedersen, N.C. Pathogenesis of experimentally induced feline immunodeficiency virus infection in cats. *Am. J. Vet. Res.* **1988**, *49*, 1246–1258.
16. Winkler, I.G.; Löchelt, M.; Flower, R.L.P. Epidemiology of feline foamy virus and feline immunodeficiency virus infections in domestic and feral cats: A seroepidemiological study. *J. Clin. Microbiol.* **1999**, *37*, 2848–2851.
17. Bandecchi, P.; Matteucci, D.; Baldinotti, F.; Guidi, G.; Abramo, F.; Tozzini, F.; Bendinelli, M. Prevalence of feline immunodeficiency virus and other retroviral infections in sick cats in italy. *Vet. Immunol. Immunopathol.* **1992**, *31*, 337–345. [CrossRef]
18. Glaus, T.; Hofmann-Lehmann, R.; Greene, C.; Glaus, B.; Wolfensberger, C.; Lutz, H. Seroprevalence of bartonella henselae infection and correlation with disease status in cats in switzerland. *J. Clin. Microbiol.* **1997**, *35*, 2883–2885.
19. Winkler, I.G.; Lochelt, M.; Levesque, J.P.; Bodem, J.; Flugel, R.M.; Flower, R.L. A rapid streptavidin-capture elisa specific for the detection of antibodies to feline foamy virus. *J. Immunol. Methods* **1997**, *207*, 69–77. [CrossRef]
20. Miyazawa, T.; Ikeda, Y.; Maeda, K.; Horimoto, T.; Tohya, Y.; Mochizuki, M.; Vu, D.; Vu, G.D.; Cu, D.X.; Ono, K.; et al. Seroepidemiological survey of feline retrovirus infections in domestic and leopard cats in northern vietnam in 1997. *J. Vet. Med. Sci.* **1998**, *60*, 1273–1275. [CrossRef]
21. Winkler, I.G.; Flügel, R.M.; Löchelt, M.; Flower, R.L.P. Detection and molecular characterisation of feline foamy virus serotypes in naturally infected cats. *Virology* **1998**, *247*, 144–151. [CrossRef]
22. Nakamura, K.; Miyazawa, T.; Ikeda, Y.; Sato, E.; Nishimura, Y.; Nguyen, N.T.; Takahashi, E.; Mochizuki, M.; Mikami, T. Contrastive prevalence of feline retrovirus infections between northern and southern vietnam. *J. Vet. Med. Sci.* **2000**, *62*, 921–923. [CrossRef]
23. Bleiholder, A.; Mühle, M.; Hechler, T.; Bevins, S.; vandeWoude, S.; Denner, J.; Löchelt, M. Pattern of seroreactivity against feline foamy virus proteins in domestic cats from germany. *Vet. Immunol. Immunopathol.* **2011**, *143*, 292–300. [CrossRef]
24. Mochizuki, M.; Konishi, S. Feline syncytial virus spontaneously detected in feline cell cultures. *Nihon Juigaku Zasshi* **1979**, *41*, 351–362. [CrossRef]
25. Flower, R.L.; Wilcox, G.E.; Cook, R.D.; Ellis, T.M. Detection and prevalence of serotypes of feline syncytial spumaviruses. *Arch. Virol.* **1985**, *83*, 53–63. [CrossRef]
26. Romen, F.; Pawlita, M.; Sehr, P.; Bachmann, S.; Schroder, J.; Lutz, H.; Lochelt, M. Antibodies against Gag are diagnostic markers for feline foamy virus infections while Env and Bet reactivity is undetectable in a substantial fraction of infected cats. *Virology* **2006**, *345*, 502–508. [CrossRef]
27. Kechejian, S.; Dannemiller, N.; Kraberger, S.; Ledesma-Feliciano, C.; Löchelt, M.; Carver, S.; VandeWoude, S. Feline foamy virus sero-prevalence and demographic risk factors in Colorado, Southern California and Florida stray domestic cat populations. *JFMS Open Rep.* **2019**. under review.
28. Switzer, W.M.; Bhullar, V.; Shanmugam, V.; Cong, M.E.; Parekh, B.; Lerche, N.W.; Yee, J.L.; Ely, J.J.; Boneva, R.; Chapman, L.E.; et al. Frequent simian foamy virus infection in persons occupationally exposed to nonhuman primates. *J. Virol.* **2004**, *78*, 2780–2789. [CrossRef]
29. Switzer, W.M.; Garcia, A.D.; Yang, C.; Wright, A.; Kalish, M.L.; Folks, T.M.; Heneine, W. Coinfection with hiv-1 and simian foamy virus in west central africans. *J. Infect. Dis.* **2008**, *197*, 1389–1393. [CrossRef]
30. Buseyne, F.; Betsem, E.; Montange, T.; Njouom, R.; Bilounga Ndongo, C.; Hermine, O.; Gessain, A. Clinical signs and blood test results among humans infected with zoonotic simian foamy virus: A case-control study. *J. Infect. Dis.* **2018**, *218*, 144–151. [CrossRef]
31. Rua, R.; Betsem, E.; Montange, T.; Buseyne, F.; Gessain, A. In vivo cellular tropism of gorilla simian foamy virus in blood of infected humans. *J. Virol.* **2014**, *88*, 13429–13435. [CrossRef]
32. Betsem, E.; Rua, R.; Tortevoye, P.; Froment, A.; Gessain, A. Frequent and recent human acquisition of simian foamy viruses through apes' bites in central africa. *PLoS Pathog* **2011**, *7*, e1002306. [CrossRef]
33. Cummins, J.E., Jr.; Boneva, R.S.; Switzer, W.M.; Christensen, L.L.; Sandstrom, P.; Heneine, W.; Chapman, L.E.; Dezzutti, C.S. Mucosal and systemic antibody responses in humans infected with simian foamy virus. *J. Virol.* **2005**, *79*, 13186–13189. [CrossRef]

34. Boneva, R.S.; Switzer, W.M.; Spira, T.J.; Bhullar, V.B.; Shanmugam, V.; Cong, M.E.; Lam, L.; Heneine, W.; Folks, T.M.; Chapman, L.E. Clinical and virological characterization of persistent human infection with simian foamy viruses. *AIDS Res. Hum. Retrovir.* **2007**, *23*, 1330–1337. [CrossRef]
35. Butera, S.T.; Brown, J.; Callahan, M.E.; Owen, S.M.; Matthews, A.L.; Weigner, D.D.; Chapman, L.E.; Sandstrom, P.A. Survey of veterinary conference attendees for evidence of zoonotic infection by feline retroviruses. *J. Am. Vet. Med. Assoc.* **2000**, *217*, 1475–1479. [CrossRef]
36. Kiem, H.P.; Wu, R.A.; Sun, G.; von Laer, D.; Rossi, J.J.; Trobridge, G.D. Foamy combinatorial anti-hiv vectors with mgmtp140k potently inhibit hiv-1 and shiv replication and mediate selection in vivo. *Gene Ther.* **2010**, *17*, 37–49. [CrossRef]
37. Lei, J.; Osen, W.; Gardyan, A.; Hotz-Wagenblatt, A.; Wei, G.; Gissmann, L.; Eichmuller, S.; Löchelt, M. Replication-competent foamy virus vaccine vectors as novel epitope scaffolds for immunotherapy. *PLoS ONE* **2015**, *10*, e0138458. [CrossRef]
38. Schwantes, A.; Ortlepp, I.; Löchelt, M. Construction and functional characterization of feline foamy virus-based retroviral vectors. *Virology* **2002**, *301*, 53–63. [CrossRef]
39. Trobridge, G.D.; Miller, D.G.; Jacobs, M.A.; Allen, J.M.; Kiem, H.P.; Kaul, R.; Russell, D.W. Foamy virus vector integration sites in normal human cells. *Proc. Natl. Acad. Sci. USA* **2006**, *103*, 1498–1503. [CrossRef]
40. Burtner, C.R.; Beard, B.C.; Kennedy, D.R.; Wohlfahrt, M.E.; Adair, J.E.; Trobridge, G.D.; Scharenberg, A.M.; Torgerson, T.R.; Rawlings, D.J.; Felsburg, P.J.; et al. Intravenous injection of a foamy virus vector to correct canine scid-x1. *Blood* **2014**, *123*, 3578–3584. [CrossRef]
41. Bauer, T.R., Jr.; Allen, J.M.; Hai, M.; Tuschong, L.M.; Khan, I.F.; Olson, E.M.; Adler, R.L.; Burkholder, T.H.; Gu, Y.C.; Russell, D.W.; et al. Successful treatment of canine leukocyte adhesion deficiency by foamy virus vectors. *Nat. Med.* **2008**, *14*, 93–97. [CrossRef]
42. Schwantes, A.; Truyen, U.; Weikel, J.; Weiss, C.; Lochelt, M. Application of chimeric feline foamy virus-based retroviral vectors for the induction of antiviral immunity in cats. *J. Virol.* **2003**, *77*, 7830–7842. [CrossRef]
43. Lindemann, D.; Steffen, I.; Pohlmann, S. Cellular entry of retroviruses. *Adv. Exp. Med. Biol.* **2013**, *790*, 128–149.
44. Plochmann, K.; Horn, A.; Gschmack, E.; Armbruster, N.; Krieg, J.; Wiktorowicz, T.; Weber, C.; Stirnnagel, K.; Lindemann, D.; Rethwilm, A.; et al. Heparan sulfate is an attachment factor for foamy virus entry. *J. Virol.* **2012**, *86*, 10028–10035. [CrossRef]
45. Pedersen, N.C.; Pool, R.R.; O'Brien, T. Feline chronic progressive polyarthritis. *Am. J. Vet. Res.* **1980**, *41*, 522–535.
46. Yamamoto, J.K.; Hansen, H.; Ho, E.W.; Morishita, T.Y.; Okuda, T.; Sawa, T.R.; Nakamura, R.M.; Pedersen, N.C. Epidemiologic and clinical aspects of feline immunodeficiency virus infection in cats from the continental united states and canada and possible mode of transmission. *J. Am. Vet. Med. Assoc.* **1989**, *194*, 213–220.
47. Inkpen, H. Chronic progressive polyarthritis in a domestic shorthair cat. *Can. Vet. J.* **2015**, *56*, 621–623.
48. Whitman, J.E., Jr.; Cockrell, K.O.; Hall, W.T.; Gilmore, C.E. An unusual case of feline leukemia and an associated syncytium-forming virus. *Am. J. Vet. Res.* **1975**, *36*, 873–880.
49. Powers, J.A.; Chiu, E.S.; Kraberger, S.J.; Roelke-Parker, M.; Lowery, I.; Erbeck, K.; Troyer, R.; Carver, S.; VandeWoude, S. Feline Leukemia Virus (FeLV) Disease Outcomes in a Domestic Cat Breeding Colony: Relationship to Endogenous FeLV and Other Chronic Viral. *J. Virol.* **2018**, *92*, e00649-18. [CrossRef]
50. Ward, B.C.; Pederson, N. Infectious peritonitis in cats. *J. Am. Vet. Med. Assoc.* **1969**, *154*, 26–35.
51. Fabricant, C.G.; King, J.M.; Gaskin, J.M.; Gillespie, J.H. Isolation of a virus from a female cat with urolithiasis. *J. Am. Vet. Med. Assoc.* **1971**, *158*, 200–201.
52. Fabricant, C.G.; Rich, L.J.; Gillespie, J.H. Feline viruses. Xi. Isolation of a virus similar to a myxovirus from cats in which urolithiasis was experimentally induced. *Cornell. Vet.* **1969**, *59*, 667–672.
53. Martens, J.G.; McConnell, S.; Swanson, C.L. The role of infectious agents in naturally occurring feline urologic syndrome. *Vet. Clin. North Am. Small Anim. Pract.* **1984**, *14*, 503–511. [CrossRef]
54. Gaskell, R.M.; Gaskell, C.J.; Page, W.; Dennis, P.; Voyle, C.A. Studies on a possible viral aetiology for the feline urological syndrome. *Vet. Rec.* **1979**, *105*, 243–247. [CrossRef]
55. Kruger, J.M.; Osborne, C.A. The role of viruses in feline lower urinary tract disease. *J. Vet. Intern. Med.* **1990**, *4*, 71–78. [CrossRef]
56. McKissick, G.E.; Lamont, P.H. Characteristics of a virus isolated from a feline fibrosarcoma. *J. Virol.* **1970**, *5*, 247–257.

57. Marino, C.L.; Lascelles, B.D.; Vaden, S.L.; Gruen, M.E.; Marks, S.L. Prevalence and classification of chronic kidney disease in cats randomly selected from four age groups and in cats recruited for degenerative joint disease studies. *J. Feline Med. Surg.* **2014**, *16*, 465–472. [CrossRef]
58. Hamilton, J.B.; Hamilton, R.S.; Mestler, G.E. Duration of life and causes of death in domestic cats: Influence of sex, gonadectomy, and inbreeding. *J. Gerontol.* **1969**, *24*, 427–437. [CrossRef]
59. O'Neill, D.G.; Church, D.B.; McGreevy, P.D.; Thomson, P.C.; Brodbelt, D.C. Longevity and mortality of cats attending primary care veterinary practices in england. *J. Feline Med. Surg.* **2015**, *17*, 125–133. [CrossRef]
60. Reynolds, B.S.; Lefebvre, H.P. Feline ckd: Pathophysiology and risk factors–what do we know? *J. Feline Med. Surg.* **2013**, *15*, 3–14. [CrossRef]
61. Bartges, J.W. Chronic kidney disease in dogs and cats. *Vet. Clin. N. Am-Small Anim. Pract.* **2012**, *42*, 669–692. [CrossRef]
62. Brown, C.A.; Elliott, J.; Schmiedt, C.W.; Brown, S.A. Chronic kidney disease in aged cats: Clinical features, morphology, and proposed pathogeneses. *Vet. Pathol.* **2016**, *53*, 309–326. [CrossRef]
63. McLeland, S.M.; Cianciolo, R.E.; Duncan, C.G.; Quimby, J.M. A comparison of biochemical and histopathologic staging in cats with chronic kidney disease. *Vet. Pathol.* **2015**, *52*, 524–534. [CrossRef]
64. Poli, A.; Tozon, N.; Guidi, G.; Pistello, M. Renal alterations in feline immunodeficiency virus (fiv)-infected cats: Anatural model of lentivirus-induced renal disease changes. *Viruses* **2012**, *4*, 1372–1389. [CrossRef]
65. Baxter, K.J.; Levy, J.K.; Edinboro, C.H.; Vaden, S.L.; Tompkins, M.B. Renal disease in cats infected with feline immunodeficiency virus. *J. Vet. Intern. Med.* **2012**, *26*, 238–243. [CrossRef]
66. Poli, A.; Abramo, F.; Taccini, E.; Guidi, G.; Barsotti, P.; Bendinelli, M.; Malvaldi, G. Renal involvement in feline immunodeficiency virus infection: A clinicopathological study. *Nephron* **1993**, *64*, 282–288. [CrossRef]
67. Glick, A.D.; Horn, R.G.; Holscher, M. Characterization of feline glomerulonephritis associated with viral-induced hematopoietic neoplasms. *Am. J. Pathol.* **1978**, *92*, 321–332.
68. Löchelt, M.; Romen, F.; Bastone, P.; Muckenfuss, H.; Kirchner, N.; Kim, Y.B.; Truyen, U.; Rosler, U.; Battenberg, M.; Saib, A.; et al. The antiretroviral activity of APOBEC3 is inhibited by the foamy virus accessory Bet protein. *Proc. Natl. Acad. Sci. USA* **2005**, *102*, 7982–7987. [CrossRef]
69. Reed, L.; Muench, H. A simple method of estimating fifty per cent endpoints. *Am. J. Hyg.* **1938**, *27*, 493–497.
70. Arzi, B.; Kol, A.; Murphy, B.; Walker, N.J.; Wood, J.A.; Clark, K.; Verstraete, F.J.M.; Borjesson, D.L. Feline foamy virus adversely affects feline mesenchymal stem cell culture and expansion: Implications for animal model development. *Stem Cells Dev.* **2014**, *24*, 814–823. [CrossRef]
71. Society, I.R.I. Iris Staging of Ckd. Available online: http://www.iris-kidney.com/guidelines/staging.html (accessed on 28 May 2016).
72. Lee, J.S.; Mackie, R.S.; Harrison, T.; Shariat, B.; Kind, T.; Kehl, T.; Löchelt, M.; Boucher, C.; VandeWoude, S. Targeted enrichment for pathogen detection and characterization in three felid species. *J. Clin. Microbiol.* **2017**, *55*, 1658–1670. [CrossRef]
73. Cianciolo, R.E.; Brown, C.A.; Mohr, F.C.; Spangler, W.L.; Aresu, L.; van der Lugt, J.J.; Jansen, J.H.; James, C.; Clubb, F.J.; Lees, G.E. Pathologic evaluation of canine renal biopsies: Methods for identifying features that differentiate immune-mediated glomerulonephritides from other categories of glomerular diseases. *J. Vet. Intern. Med.* **2013**, *27* (Suppl. S1), S10–S18. [CrossRef]
74. ScyMed. Medicalc: Blood Urea Nitrogen (Unit Conversion). Available online: http://www.scymed.com/en/smnxps/psxff047_c.htm (accessed on 24 June 2019).
75. ScyMed. Medicalc: Creatinine (Unit Conversion). Available online: http://www.scymed.com/en/smnxps/psxdf212_c.htm (accessed on 24 June 2019).
76. Team, R.C. *R: A Language and Environment for Statistical Computing*; R Foundation for Statistical Computing: Vienna, Austria, 2017.
77. Delignette-Muller, M.L.; Dutang, C. fitdistrplus: An R package for fitting distributions. *J. Stat. Softw.* **2015**, *64*, 1–34. [CrossRef]
78. Brooks, M.; Kristensen, K.; van Benthem, K.; Magnusson, A.; Berg, C.; Nielsen, A.; Skaug, H.; Mächler, M.; Bolker, B. Glmmtmb balances speed and flexibility among packages for zero-inflated generalized linear mixed modeling. *R J.* **2017**, *9*, 378–400. [CrossRef]
79. Epitools: Epidemiology Tools. Available online: https://rdrr.io/cran/epitools/ (accessed on 15 July 2019).

80. Ledesma-Feliciano, C.; Department of Microbiology, Immunology, and Pathology, College of Veterinary Medicine and Biomedical Sciences, Colorado State University, Fort Collins, CO, USA. FFV-inoculated and control cat complete blood count and serum chemistry data. 2014.
81. Cowgill, L.D.; Polzin, D.J.; Elliott, J.; Nabity, M.B.; Segev, G.; Grauer, G.F.; Brown, S.; Langston, C.; van Dongen, A.M. Is progressive chronic kidney disease a slow acute kidney injury? *Vet. Clin. Small Anim. Pract.* **2016**, *46*, 995–1013. [CrossRef]
82. Ledesma-Feliciano, C.; Department of Microbiology, Immunology, and Pathology, College of Veterinary Medicine and Biomedical Sciences, Colorado State University, Fort Collins, CO, USA. FFV-inoculated and control cat urinalysis and serum creatinine data. 2014.
83. Cavalcante, L.T.F.; Muniz, C.P.; Jia, H.; Augusto, A.M.; Troccoli, F.; Medeiros, S.O.; Dias, C.G.A.; Switzer, W.M.; Soares, M.A.; Santos, A.F. Clinical and molecular features of feline foamy virus and feline leukemia virus co-infection in naturally-infected cats. *Viruses* **2018**, *10*, 702. [CrossRef]
84. Brooks, J.I.; Merks, H.W.; Fournier, J.; Boneva, R.S.; Sandstrom, P.A. Characterization of blood-borne transmission of simian foamy virus. *Transfusion* **2007**, *47*, 162–170. [CrossRef]
85. Murray, S.M.; Linial, M.L. Foamy virus infection in primates. *J. Med. Primatol.* **2006**, *35*, 225–235. [CrossRef]
86. Soliven, K.; Wang, X.; Small, C.T.; Feeroz, M.M.; Lee, E.-G.; Craig, K.L.; Hasan, K.; Engel, G.a.; Jones-Engel, L.; Matsen, F.a.; et al. Simian foamy virus infection of rhesus macaques in bangladesh: Relationship of latent proviruses and transcriptionally active viruses. *J. Virol.* **2013**, *87*, 13628–13639. [CrossRef]
87. Falcone, V.; Leupold, J.; Clotten, J.; Urbanyi, E.; Herchenroder, O.; Spatz, W.; Volk, B.; Bohm, N.; Toniolo, A.; Neumann-Haefelin, D.; et al. Sites of simian foamy virus persistence in naturally infected african green monkeys: Latent provirus is ubiquitous, whereas viral replication is restricted to the oral mucosa. *Virology* **1999**, *257*, 7–14. [CrossRef]
88. Gray, F.; Lescs, M.C.; Keohane, C.; Paraire, F.; Marc, B.; Durigon, M.; Gherardi, R. Early brain changes in hiv infection: Neuropathological study of 11 hiv seropositive, non-aids cases. *J. Neuropathol. Exp. Neurol.* **1992**, *51*, 177–185. [CrossRef]
89. Bell, J.E. The neuropathology of adult hiv infection. *Rev. Neurol.* **1998**, *154*, 816–829.
90. Torres, L.; Noel, R.J., Jr. Astrocytic expression of hiv-1 viral protein r in the hippocampus causes chromatolysis, synaptic loss and memory impairment. *J. Neuroinflamm.* **2014**, *11*, 53. [CrossRef]
91. Wilcox, G.E.; Flower, R.L.; Cook, R.D. Recovery of viral agents from the central nervous system of cats. *Vet. Microbiol.* **1984**, *9*, 355–366. [CrossRef]
92. Wharram, B.L.; Goyal, M.; Wiggins, J.E.; Sanden, S.K.; Hussain, S.; Filipiak, W.E.; Saunders, T.L.; Dysko, R.C.; Kohno, K.; Holzman, L.B.; et al. Podocyte depletion causes glomerulosclerosis: Diphtheria toxin-induced podocyte depletion in rats expressing human diphtheria toxin receptor transgene. *J. Am. Soc. Nephrol.* **2005**, *16*, 2941–2952. [CrossRef]
93. Chiswell, D.J.; Pringle, C.R. Feline syncytium-forming virus: Identification of a virion associated reverse transcriptase and electron microscopical observations of infected cells. *J. Gen. Virol.* **1979**, *43*, 429–434. [CrossRef]
94. Alke, A.; Schwantes, A.; Kido, K.; Flotenmeyer, M.; Flugel, R.M.; Löchelt, M. The bet gene of feline foamy virus is required for virus replication. *Virology* **2001**, *287*, 310–320. [CrossRef]
95. Cook, R.D. Observations on focal demyelinating lesions in cat optic nerves. *Neuropathol. Appl. Neurobiol.* **1979**, *5*, 395–404. [CrossRef]
96. Toribio, J.A.; Norris, J.M.; White, J.D.; Dhand, N.K.; Hamilton, S.A.; Malik, R. Demographics and husbandry of pet cats living in sydney, australia: Results of cross-sectional survey of pet ownership. *J. Feline Med. Surg.* **2009**, *11*, 449–461. [CrossRef]
97. Johnston, L.; Szczepanski, J.; McDonagh, P. Demographics, lifestyle and veterinary care of cats in australia and new zealand. *J. Feline Med. Surg.* **2017**, *19*, 1199–1205. [CrossRef]
98. White, J.D.; Norris, J.M.; Baral, R.M.; Malik, R. Naturally-occurring chronic renal disease in australian cats: A prospective study of 184 cases. *Aust. Vet. J.* **2006**, *84*, 188–194. [CrossRef]

viruses

MDPI

Article

Insights into Innate Sensing of Prototype Foamy Viruses in Myeloid Cells

Maïwenn Bergez [1,†], Jakob Weber [2,3,†], Maximilian Riess [1], Alexander Erdbeer [2,3], Janna Seifried [1], Nicole Stanke [2,3], Clara Munz [2,3], Veit Hornung [4], Renate König [1,5,6,*] and Dirk Lindemann [2,3,*]

1. Host-Pathogen Interactions, Paul-Ehrlich-Institut, 63225 Langen, Germany; Maiwenn.Bergez@pei.de (M.B.); max.riess@yahoo.de (M.R.); seifriedJ@rki.de (J.S.)
2. Institute of Virology, Medical Faculty "Carl Gustav Carus", Technische Universität Dresden, 01307 Dresden, Germany; j_weber@posteo.de (J.W.); Alexander.Erdbeer@gmx.de (A.E.); nicole.stanke@tu-dresden.de (N.S.); claramarie.munz@gmail.com (C.M.)
3. CRTD/DFG-Center for Regenerative Therapies, Technische Universität Dresden, 01307 Dresden, Germany
4. Gene Center and Department of Biochemistry, Ludwig-Maximilians-Universität München, 81377 München, Germany; hornung@genzentrum.lmu.de
5. German Center for Infection Research (DZIF), 63225 Langen, Germany
6. Immunity and Pathogenesis Program, SBP Medical Discovery Institute, La Jolla, CA 92037, USA

* Correspondence: renate.koenig@pei.de (R.K.); dirk.lindemann@tu-dresden.de (D.L.); Tel.: +49-6103-77-4019 (R.K.); +49-351-458-6210 (D.L.)

† These authors contributed equally to this study.

Received: 30 September 2019; Accepted: 22 November 2019; Published: 26 November 2019

Abstract: Foamy viruses (FVs) belong to the *Spumaretrovirinae* subfamily of retroviruses and are characterized by unique features in their replication strategy. This includes a reverse transcription (RTr) step of the packaged RNA genome late in replication, resulting in the release of particles with a fraction of them already containing an infectious viral DNA (vDNA) genome. Little is known about the immune responses against FVs in their hosts, which control infection and may be responsible for their apparent apathogenic nature. We studied the interaction of FVs with the innate immune system in myeloid cells, and characterized the viral pathogen-associated molecular patterns (PAMPs) and the cellular pattern recognition receptors and sensing pathways involved. Upon cytoplasmic access, full-length but not minimal vector genome containing FVs with active reverse transcriptase, induced an efficient innate immune response in various myeloid cells. It was dependent on cellular cGAS and STING and largely unaffected by RTr inhibition during viral entry. This suggests that RTr products, which are generated during FV morphogenesis in infected cells, and are therefore already present in FV particles taken up by immune cells, are the main PAMPs of FVs with full-length genomes sensed in a cGAS and STING-dependent manner by the innate immune system in host cells of the myeloid lineage.

Keywords: retrovirus; foamy virus; spumavirus; innate sensing; cGAS; STING

1. Introduction

Spuma or foamy viruses (FVs), which constitute several genera in the retrovirus subfamily *Spumaretrovirinae* [1], display a replication strategy with features common to both other retroviruses (*Orthoretrovirinae*) and hepadnaviruses (reviewed in [2,3]). FVs are unique amongst retroviruses, as the initiation of reverse transcription (RTr) of the packaged viral genomic RNA (vgRNA) occurs in a significant fraction of virions (5–10%) during viral assembly [4–7]. Thereby, unlike to orthoretroviruses, both vgRNA and/or viral genomic DNA (vgDNA) containing virions are found in the supernatant of FV infected cells. It is generally accepted that the vgDNA containing virions contribute to the majority of new productive infection events during spreading of FVs in cultures, at least in vitro [5,6]. However, a low level of reverse transcription, probably derived from vgRNA containing virions, has been observed during uptake of FVs at very low multiplicities of infection (MOI) [4,7].

FVs are naturally endemic to most non-human primates (NHPs), including New and Old World monkeys and apes, cats, cows, horses, tree shrews, sea lions, and bats (reviewed in [2,8,9]). In addition, endogenized copies of FV genomes were identified in sloths, the aye-aye, the Cap golden mole [10,11], cod [12], platyfish [12], zebra fish, and the coelacanth. Nowadays, humans are not considered as a natural host, but frequent zoonotic transmissions of NHP simian FVs (SFVs), but not feline FV (FFV) or bovine FV (BFV), have been observed in workers occupationally exposed to NHPs—bush meat hunters in central Africa, and in various contexts of human–NHP interspecies contact in South and Southeast Asia. Cases of spread from human to human have not been reported. The best-studied and characterized isolate to date is the so-called prototype FV (PFV; formerly known as human FV, HFV), which was originally isolated from an African patient who presumably was infected zoonotically by a chimpanzee FV [13–15].

Another characteristic of FVs is their extremely broad tropism. In vitro, only very few species and cell types are known to be non-permissive to FVs or FV Env-mediated entry [16]. FV infection in vitro is highly cytopathic to most cell types, except cell lines or primary cells of myeloid or lymphoid origin, which can become chronically infected [17,18]. The cellular targets of FVs in vivo remain poorly characterized. In infected monkeys, the viral genome is detectable in many tissues but appears to be largely in a latent state, as viral replication is reported to be mainly restricted to the superficial epithelial layer of the oral mucosa [19]. This explains the major transmission mode between monkeys and zoonosis to humans through bites. In the blood, proviral DNA is detected in $CD8^+$- and $CD4^+$ T-cells (memory and naïve) as well as B-cells, and to a lower extent also in monocytes and NK-cells [20–22]. Other types of immune cells that encounter FVs during the course of an infection in vivo have not been characterized.

FVs have co-evolved with their hosts for at least 60 million years and are considered to be non-pathogenic in natural hosts and zoonotically infected humans. The immune system seems to control FV infection very efficiently in natural hosts and zoonotically infected humans, as replication and viral load of FV stays low [20–22]. However, the mechanisms involved are poorly understood (reviewed in [8]). In particular, the interaction of FV with the innate immune system remains to be fully clarified. FVs are known to respond in vitro in a cell type-dependent manner towards IFNs [23]. Furthermore, treatment of cells of different origin with type-I or II IFNs, impairs spreading of FVs or inhibits early steps in FV replication [24–28]. In line with this observation, restriction of FVs by several IFN-induced cellular proteins has been reported, although their relevance for FV replication in vivo has not been tested so far [29–32]. Although FV replication in vitro is impaired by addition of exogenous IFNs, infection of a variety of tissues does not seem to mount an innate immune response [28]. Only recently, stimulation of IFN secretion by human hematopoietic cells, in particular, plasmacytoid dendritic cells (pDCs), upon incubation with SFV virions or SFV infected cells, was demonstrated [23]. pDCs, as the main producer of type-I IFN, detect FV RNA by the TLR7-mediated pathway. However, the contribution of myeloid cells, besides pDCs, to innate sensing and IFN induction has as of yet not been investigated. Above all, conventional dendritic cells (DCs) play a critical role in detecting retroviruses, as shown for the lentivirus HIV-1 [33], and promote, thereby, the activation of adaptive immunity [34]. For HIV-1 and other lentiviruses, it has been demonstrated that the reverse transcribed DNA products generated upon viral entry in DCs mediate the activation of transcription factors, such as IRF3, resulting in ISG expression and IFN synthesis [33,35]. Thereby, the viral reverse transcribed components are sensed by the DNA sensor cyclic GAMP synthase (cGAS) [36] together with polyglutamine binding protein 1 (PQBP1) [37]. Interestingly, and in contrast to lentiviruses, FV infected cells release both vgRNA and vgDNA containing virions, and harbor RTr products late during the assembly steps. Therefore, exposure of DCs and other myeloid cells to

FVs may result in interactions with the innate immune system different to those of other retroviruses. For instance, they could include pathways encountered by hepatitis B virus (HBV), as HBVs, like FVs, reverse transcribe their genome during particle morphogenesis (reviewed in [38]).

The aim of this study was to investigate whether the innate immune system of cells of the human myeloid lineage is capable of sensing FVs. If so, the viral pathogen-associated molecular patterns (PAMPs), the pattern recognition receptors (PRRs), and sensing pathways involved were to be characterized. We found that the innate immune system responds to sensing of RTr products of full-length PFV genomes but not of minimal vector genomes in the cytoplasm of human myeloid cells with an efficient interferon-stimulated gene (ISG) induction within hours of virus exposure. Sensing of PFV RTr products was dependent on cellular cGAS and STING expression and largely insensitive to reverse transcriptase inhibition during viral entry, suggesting that the already viral DNA (vDNA) containing PFV particles are the main stimulator.

2. Materials and Methods

2.1. Cells and Culture Conditions

The human embryonic kidney cell line 293T (ATCC CRL-1573) [39] and a proteoglycan-deficient variant 293T-25A (described elsewhere), the human fibrosarcoma cell line HT1080 (ATCC CCL-121) [40], and the clonal variant HT1080 PLNE containing a PFV LTR driven *EGFP* reporter gene expression cassette [41], were cultivated in Dulbecco's modified Eagle's medium (DMEM) supplemented with 10% (*v*/*v*) heat-inactivated fetal calf serum and antibiotics. The human monocyte cell line THP-1 (ATCC TIB-202) and knockout (KO) variants ΔIFNAR1, ΔSAMHD1 [42], ΔcGAS [43], ΔMAVS [43], ΔMyD88, and ΔSTING [43] were cultivated in Roswell Park Memorial Institute 1640 Medium (RPMI 1640) supplemented with 10% (*v*/*v*) heat-inactivated fetal calf serum, antibiotics, 2.5 g/L glucose, 10 mM Hepes, and 10 mM sodium pyruvate. THP-1 cells were differentiated into macrophage-like cells by the addition of phorbol-12-myristyl-13-acetate (PMA) at 30 to 50 ng/mL final concentrations for 48 h prior to exposure of viral supernatants.

Human buffy coats, of anonymous blood donors, were obtained from German Red Cross Blood Donor Service Baden–Württemberg Hessen. Primary human monocytes were isolated from peripheral blood mononuclear cells (PBMCs) using Ficoll density gradient and subsequent isolation of $CD14^+$ monocytes [44]. Briefly, PBMCs were separated by density gradient centrifugation (30 min, 980× *g*, RT), using Ficoll (Histopaque 1077 Sigma-Aldrich Biochemie GmbH, Hamburg, Germany). The mononuclear layer of the interphase was recovered and washed twice with PBS. PBMCs were subsequently incubated with 0.86% (*w*/*v*) ammonium chloride for erythrocyte lysis (37 °C, 10 min). PBMCs were washed twice and filtered (0.7 µm). $CD14^+$ monocytes were positively selected using CD14-MicroBeads (Miltenyi Biotec, Bergisch Gladbach, Germany) according to the manufacturer's protocol, and separated from unlabeled cells using an AutoMACS device (Miltenyi Biotec). Subsequently, cells were differentiated into monocyte derived dendritic cells (MDDC) or monocyte derived macrophages (MDMs) by cultivating for 5 days in RPMI-1640 medium supplemented with 2 mM L-Glutamine; 10% (*v*/*v*) FCS; 1% (*v*/*v*) HEPES, 1 mM sodium pyruvate; 280 U/mL granulocyte-macrophage colony-stimulating factor (GM-CSF) (Leukine® Sargramostim, Genzyme, Boston, MA, USA); 800 U/mL IL-4 (PeproTech GmbH, Hamburg, Germany) for MDDCs and 560 IU/mL GM-CSF only for type 1 proinflammatory MDMs. The same amounts of medium and cytokines were added on day 3. On day 5 of differentiation, MDMs were detached by a short incubation with PBS-EDTA and MDDCs by gentle resuspension in PBS; they were counted and plated for cell stimulation experiments and simultaneously checked for MDDC and MDM surface markers and their differentiation status.

2.2. Recombinant Plasmid DNAs

A four-component PFV vector system, consisting of the expression-optimized packaging constructs pcoPG4 (PFV Gag), pcoPE (PFV Env), and pcoPP (Pol), and an enhanced green fluorescent protein (EGFP)-expressing PFV transfer vector pMD9 or puc2MD9, has been described previously [16,45,46].

The CMV-driven proviral expression vector pczHSRV2 (wt) and its variants pczHSRV2 M69 (iRT), expressing a Pol protein with enzymatically inactive RT domain (YVDD$_{312–315}$GAAA mutation), pczHSRV2 M73 (iIN), with enzymatically inactive IN domain (D$_{936}$A mutation), and pczHSRV2 EM271 (ΔEnv), with inactivated Env translation start (M1T, ATG to ACG, M5T, ATG to ACG; M16T, ATG to ACG mutation) were described previously [5,47,48]. For this study the variants pczHSRV2 EM284 (ΔGag), with inactivated Gag translation start (M1L, ATG to CTG; S3Stop, TCA to TAA mutation); pczHSRV2 EM270 (ΔPol), with inactivated Pol translation start (M1L, ATG to CTG mutation); pczHSRV2 EM273 (ΔGPE), with simultaneously inactivated Gag, Pol, and Env translation starts; pczHSRV2 EM020 (iFuse), with inactivated Env SU/TM furin cleavage site (R571T mutation); and pczHSRV2 EM010, with inactivated Tas translation start (M1L, ATG to TTG mutation), were generated. All constructs were verified by sequencing analysis. Primer sequences and additional details are available upon request.

For VLP-Vpx production the lentiviral vector pSIV3+, derived from SIVmac251 was used, as previously described [49]. For single-round HIV-1 reporter virus production the plasmid pBR-NL43-Env$^-$-IRES-eGFP-nef$^+$ [50] was used. In both cases the envelope vector pCMV-VSVg was used for pseudotyping.

2.3. Transfection, Virus Production, and Titration

Cell culture supernatants containing recombinant PFV particles and respective mock controls were generated by transfection of the corresponding virus encoding or mock control plasmids (mock A: pUC19; mock B: pczHSRV2 EM273 (ΔGPE)) into 293T cells using polyethyleneimine (PEI) as described previously [41,46], or 293T-25A cells using calcium phosphate (described elsewhere). Cell-free supernatants were generated by passing through a 0.45 µm filter and were either stored in aliquots at −80 °C when used for stimulation experiments or processed further for additional analysis. Viral titers of recombinant, EGFP-expressing PFV vector particles (PFV-SRVs) by fluorescence marker-gene transfer assay on HT1080 cells were determined as described previously [51]. Virus particles generated by use of proviral expression plasmids (PFV-RCPs) were titrated on HT1080 PLNE cells harboring a Tas-inducible nuclear *EGFP* ORF in their genome as described previously [41].

VLP-Vpx and HIV-1 GFP reporter viruses were produced as previously described [52]. Briefly, 2×10^7 HEK293T/17 cells per T175 flask were seeded. The next day, 15.2 µg pSIV3+ and 2.3 µg pCMV-VSVg for VLP-Vpx production and 11.6 µg of pBR-NL43-Env$^-$-IRES-eGFP-nef$^+$ and 5.9 µg pCMV-VSVg, for HIV-1 reporter virus production, per flask, were transfected using 18 mM PEI (Sigma-Aldrich). Medium was changed approximately 16 h later and viral supernatants were harvested 48 and 72 h post-transfection. Supernatants were centrifuged (10 min at 4 °C; 1500 rpm), filtered (0.45 µm), and DNaseI digested (1 U/mL) for one hour. Viral supernatants were purified by ultracentrifugation through 20% (*w*/*v*) sucrose (2 h, at 4 °C; 25,000 rpm); virus pellets from day one and two were resuspended in PBS, pooled, aliquoted and stored at −80 °C. HIV-1 reporter viruses were titrated via serial dilutions on TZM-bl reporter cells using the beta-galactosidase colorimetric assay. VLP-Vpx were titrated according to their ability to target the restriction factor SAMHD1 for degradation, using Western blot.

2.4. Myeloid Cell Stimulation and qPCR Analysis of ISG Induction

For stimulation experiments, THP-1 cells were plated at 2×10^6 cells/well (3×10^4 cells/well) in a total volume of 2 mL (100 µL) in 6-well (96-well) plates and PMA was added to 30 ng/mL (50 ng/mL) final concentration. Forty-eight hours later the medium was replaced by the respective virus supernatant, mock control supernatants (mock A: pUC19, mock B: PFV-RCP ΔGPE mutant) or medium

(medium) as indicated. At different time points post virus exposure, as indicated, viral supernatants were aspirated and cells were snap frozen at −80 °C and stored until subsequent nucleic acid extraction. MDDCs and MDMs were plated at 3×10^4 cells/well in the differentiation medium without cytokines, 24 h prior to infection. Virus supernatants, either PFV or a VSV-G pseudotyped full-length HIV-1 GFP reporter virus, with or without the addition of VLP-Vpx were added. AZT (Sigma) was added during infection in the indicated experiment at a final concentration of 100 µM. MDDC and MDM infections were conducted by spinoculation at 1200 rpm, 32 °C for 1.5 h. Viral supernatants were replaced by fresh medium and cells were cultivated at 37 °C, 5% CO_2. At different time points post infection, cells were either lysed for RNA extraction and subsequent RT-qPCR or stained for FACS analysis.

2.5. Quantitative PCR Analysis

Cellular nucleic acids from cultures in 6-well plates were extracted using the RNeasy Mini kit (QIAGEN, Hilden, Germany) according to the manufacturer's protocol. qPCR analysis of cellular mRNA expression using Maxima Probe qPCR Master Mix including ROX dye (ThermoFisher Scientific, Dreieich, Germany), a StepOnePlus (Applied Biosystems, Foster City, CA, USA) quantitative PCR machine, and plasmid standard curves was performed as previously described [48]. Primers, Taqman probes, and cycling conditions are summarized in Table A1. Cellular nucleic acids from cultures in 96-well plates were extracted using NucleoSpin® RNA Plus Kit (Macherey-Nagel, Düren, Germany) according to the manufacturer's protocol. Relative expression levels of *ISG54* and *RPL13A* were determined using QuantiTect SYBR Green RT-qPCR Kit (QIAGEN) with the respective specific primers on a LightCycler® 480 Instrument (Roche, Basel, Switzerland). Relative mRNA expression levels were normalized to the housekeeping gene *RPL13A* and analyzed using the $2^{(-\Delta\Delta CT)}$ method, finally depicted as fold inductions over mock A, mock B, or medium, as indicated. Primers and cycling conditions are summarized in Table A2. Primer efficiencies have been tested before in 10-fold serial dilutions and were calculated to have >90% efficiency.

2.6. Flow Cytometry Analysis

Purity of MDMs and MDDCs was assessed via flow cytometry analysis. Triple stainings, of 1×10^5 cells with CD14-Pacific blue (BioLegend, San Diego, CA, USA), CD163-PE (BD), CD206-APC (BD) and CD1a-PE (BioLegend), and CD11c-Vio Blue (BioLegend) and CD16-APC (BioLegend) were performed with the matching IgG controls, listed in Table A3. In order to determine CD86 activation, marker expression upon infection with different PFV mutants, 24 h post infection, 6×10^4 cells were stained with CD86-PE (Biolegend) or the corresponding isotype control. Briefly, after 5 days of differentiation, MDMs were detached by a short incubation with PBS-EDTA, MDDCs by gentle resuspension in PBS. Cells were washed twice with FACS staining buffer (PBS containing 10% (*v*/*v*) FCS), FC-Block (1:10, BD) was added to prevent unspecific binding via Fc-receptors (10 min, RT), cells were resuspended in the specific antibody dilutions or corresponding isotype-controls, and they were stained for 20 min on ice. Subsequently, cells were washed twice with FACS staining buffer, fixed with ice-cold 2% (*w*/*v*) Paraformaldehyde, washed twice, and analyzed via flow cytometry using MACSQuant Analyzer 10 (Miltenyi) and FCS Express software (De Novo Software, Glendale, CA, USA). For MDM and MDDC purity, percentages of positive cells of the specific markers are depicted in Figure S1. For CD86 expression of infected MDDCs, mean fluorescent intensities (MFIs) normalized to the IgG controls of each condition are depicted as relative MFIs normalized to the wt treatment. Infection levels by HIV-1 GFP with and without AZT were assessed by determining the percentage of GFP-positive cells (Figure S2). The cut-off was set to 0.1% with the IgG controls or the non-infected controls.

2.7. Analysis of PFV Particle Protein and Nucleic Acid Composition

PFV particles were concentrated from cell-free supernatants by centrifugation at 4 °C and 25,000 rpm for 3 h in a SW32Ti rotor (Beckman Coulter GmbH, Krefeld, Germany) through a 20% (*w*/*v*) sucrose cushion. The particulate material was resuspended in phosphate-buffered saline (PBS) and used immediately for further analysis or stored at −80 °C. Western blot analysis was performed after protein sample buffer addition as described before using PFV Gag and PFV Env leader peptide (LP) specific antisera [48]. DNase digestion of viral particles, extraction of particle-associated nucleic acids, and analysis of nucleic acid composition by qPCR was done using the primer–probe sets listed in Table A1, as described before [46,48,53].

2.8. Analysis of Cellular Protein Expression

For immunoblot analysis of IRF3 phosphorylation and SAMHD1 degradation, 5×10^5 MDDCs/12 wells were seeded and exposed to either PFV-RCP or VLP-Vpx. Six or twenty-four hours post-exposure, cells were harvested by resuspension in ice cold PBS, centrifuged (300× *g*, 6 min, 4 °C), and lysed in 25 µL RIPA-lysis buffer (100 mM NaCl; 10 mM EDTA (pH 7.5), 20 mM Tris (pH 7.5); 1% (*v*/*v*) Triton X-100; 1% (*w*/*v*) sodium deoxycholate) containing protease and phosphatase inhibitor cocktails (Complete Protease Inhibitor Cocktail; PhosSTOP Phosphatase Inhibitor Cocktail, Roche) for 45 min on ice. Lysates were centrifuged (17,000× *g* for 15 min at 4 °C), and protein concentration was determined based on the Bradford assay using the Bio-Rad Protein Assay Dye Reagent Concentrate. Samples containing 20 µg protein were prepared with NuPAGE LDS sample buffer (4×) and NuPAGE Sample Reducing Agent (10×), to a final 1× concentration and denatured at 70 °C for 10 min. Proteins were separated on precasted NuPAGE™ 4–12% Bis-Tris gradient gels (Invitrogen). The gel was run in 1× MOPS buffer (1 M MOPS, 1 M Tris, 69.3 mM SDS, 20.5 mM EDTA Titriplex II) supplemented with 200 µL NuPage Antioxidant 10× (inner chamber) at 200 V for 1 h 10 min. Proteins were transferred to a Hybond P 0.45 PVDF membrane (GE Healthcare, Chicago, IL, USA) using the XCell IITM blotting system with 1× NuPAGE transfer buffer (Invitrogen) at 35 V for 1 h 40 min. Membranes were blocked in 5% (*w*/*v*) BSA (Carl Roth) in 0.01% (*v*/*v*) Tris-buffered saline with Tween 20 (TBST) for 2 h at 4 °C with subsequent incubation in primary antibody dilutions at 4 °C overnight. Horseradish peroxidase (HRP)-linked goat anti-rabbit or horse anti-mouse IgG (heavy and light chain) secondary antibodies (Cell signaling, Danvers, MA, USA) were applied for 2 h at 4 °C. For detection Pierce® ECL Western Blotting Substrate (ThermoFisher Scientific) or ECL Prime (GE Healthcare) were used and the emitted chemiluminescence was detected at different exposure times on autoradiography films (Amersham Hyperfilm ECL, GE Healthcare). The following primary antibodies were used and applied at 4 °C, overnight: Anti-Phospho-IRF-3 (Ser396) (Cell Signaling, number 4947); Anti-IRF3 (Epitomics, number 2241-1); Anti-GAPDH (Cell Signaling, number 2118); and Anti-SAMHD1 (Proteintech; number 12586-1-AP). In order to remove phospho-IRF3 antibody, probed membrane was incubated in stripping buffer (2% (*w*/*v*) SDS, 62.5 mM Tris-HCl (pH 6.8), 100 mM β-mercaptoethanol), rotating for 45 min at 65 °C.

2.9. Statistics

All the statistical analyses were performed using GraphPad Prism 8. The numbers of experimental replicates and information on the statistical methods used for determination of two-tailed *p*-values are described in the individual figure legends. Symbols represent: * $p < 0.05$; ** $p < 0.01$; *** $p < 0.001$; **** $p < 0.0001$; ns: not significant ($p \geq 0.05$).

3. Results

3.1. ISG Induction in Myeloid Cells upon Exposure to Replication-Competent PFV

PMA-differentiated THP-1 monocytic cells represent an in vitro model system recapitulating the functional properties of macrophages and dendritic cells exposed to retroviruses [54]. In order to analyze whether FVs are sensed by cells of the myeloid lineage, replication-competent PFV supernatants derived from full-length, wild type proviral expression constructs (PFV-RCP) (Figure A1) were first used to infect PMA-differentiated THP-1 cells (Figure 1a,b). Relative transcription levels of *ISG54* or

ISG56 were determined as readouts for an IRF-3 dependent stimulation, since the selected ISGs are directly downstream transcriptional targets of IRF3 [55,56].

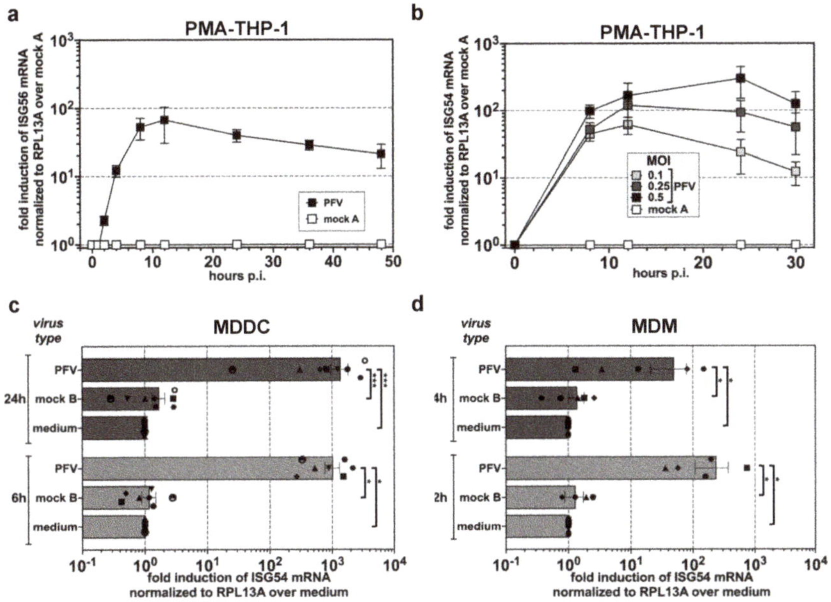

Figure 1. PFV-mediated ISG induction in myeloid cells. (**a**,**b**) Kinetics of *ISG56*/*ISG54* induction in PMA-differentiated THP-1 wild type cells incubated with different amounts of wild type PFV-RCP (a, MOI 0.2) as well as pUC19 (mock A) mock supernatants. ISG mRNA levels normalized for *RPL13A* mRNA levels were determined by qPCR at the indicated time points post exposure. Means ± SDs of *ISG56* ($n = 4$; a) or *ISG54* ($n = 4$; b) induction relative to mock A treatment are shown. (**c**,**d**) Primary human MDDC (**c**) or MDM (**d**) were incubated with wild type PFV-RCP (PFV; MOI 0.25), ΔGPE (mock B) mock supernatant, or medium (medium) for 6, 12, or 24 h, as indicated. Means ± SEMs, plus individual data points, of *ISG54* (n = 5–8) induction normalized to *RPL13A* relative to medium treatment are shown. Mixed-effects analysis with Holm–Sidak's multiple-comparisons test was used to assess significance. * $p < 0.05$; ** $p < 0.01$; *** $p < 0.001$; **** $p < 0.0001$; ns: not significant ($p \geq 0.05$).

Exposure of PMA-differentiated THP-1 cells to PFV-RCPs led to a strong IRF3-dependent ISG induction (Figure 1a,b). Furthermore, a significant, dose-dependent ISG induction was detectable, which peaked at 8 to 12 h and declined slowly thereafter (Figure 1a,b). To corroborate this finding, primary human MDMs and MDDCs were analyzed. As it cannot be ruled out that DCs and macrophages may possess slightly different sets of proteins aiding to sense DNA, we exposed both cell types to wild type PFV-RCP (PFV), mock (mock B) supernatants obtained after 293T transfection of a proviral expression construct with inactivated viral structural protein expression (ΔGPE), or medium (medium). Interestingly, in both MDDCs and MDMs we detected a robust and high ISG induction (Figure 1c,d) after PFV-RCP but not mock supernatant exposure, suggesting that replication-competent PFV derived from full-length proviral expression constructs are efficiently sensed by the innate immune system in different myeloid cell types. In line with this, a strong phosphorylation of IRF3 was detectable in PFV-RCP treated but not in medium treated MDDCs at 6 h post exposure (Figure S3).

3.2. PFV is Sensed by the Cellular cGAS-STING Pathway

To identify the particular innate pathways that are triggered by PFV, we exposed a panel of THP-1 KO cell lines deficient in key molecules of various sensing pathways to wild type PFV-RCP for 8 or

24 h, respectively. Interestingly, PMA-THP-1 cells deficient in cGAS or STING expression, which are key molecules of the DNA-sensing pathway, failed to mount any measurable ISG-response upon PFV exposure (Figure 2). In contrast, cells deficient in MAVS, a key node of the RIG-I/MAVS RNA-sensing pathway, or MyD88 that lies downstream of the endosomal TLR7/9 pathway showed a reduced but clearly detectable ISG induction. These results suggest that FVs are mainly sensed by the cytosolic DNA-sensing pathway in myeloid cells. Furthermore, IFNAR1 deficient PMA-THP-1 cells displayed a similar ISG response as wild type cells indicating that events downstream of IFN production do not influence sensing of FV. Intriguingly, KO of SAMHD1, previously demonstrated to strongly enhance HIV-1 sensing in various myeloid cell types [33,36,37], did not further stimulate the ISG response upon PFV exposure. On the contrary, PFV-mediated ISG induction in SAMHD1 KO cells was moderately reduced, at levels comparable to those observed for MAVS and MyD88 KO cells.

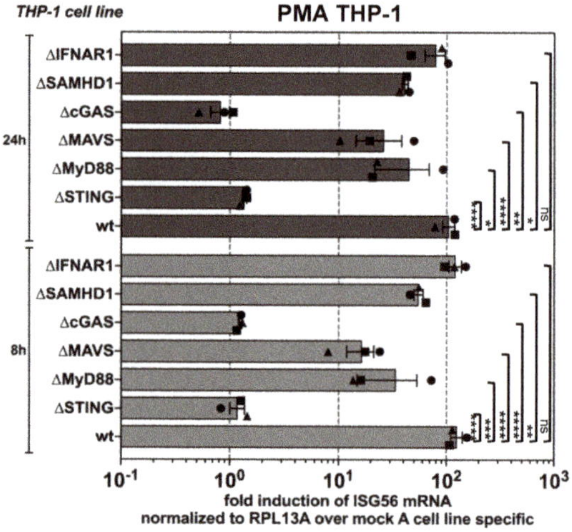

Figure 2. cGAS and STING-mediated sensing of PFV-associated reverse transcription products. PMA-differentiated THP-1 wild type cells and KO variants with deficiencies in components of various innate sensing pathways, as indicated, were incubated with wild type PFV-RCP (MOI 0.2) or pUC19 (mock A) mock supernatants. ISG mRNA levels normalized for *RPL13A* mRNA levels were determined by qPCR at the indicated time points post exposure. Means ± SEM, plus individual data points, of *ISG56* ($n = 3$) induction normalized to *RPL13A* relative to mock A treatment are shown. Two-way ANOVA with Tukey's multiple-comparisons test was used to assess significance. * $p < 0.05$; ** $p < 0.01$; *** $p < 0.001$; **** $p < 0.0001$; ns: not significant ($p \geq 0.05$).

Thus, innate sensing of PFV in host cells of the myeloid lineage occurs mainly in a cGAS and STING dependent manner.

3.3. *Innate Sensing of PFV Requires Cytoplasmic Access and Enzymatically Active Reverse Transcriptase*

Since we determined the cytoplasmic DNA-sensing pathway as the main innate pathway, we aimed at identifying the PAMPs responsible of PFV sensing and at determining the cellular sublocation. For this purpose, myeloid target cells were exposed to viral supernatants derived from various mutant proviral expression constructs, which varied in their nucleic acid compositions and had different blocks in early steps of viral replication (Figure A1, Figure 3a). A significant ISG induction was detectable in PMA-THP-1 and MDDCs not only by wild type PFV-RCP, but also by variants that either failed to express the PFV transactivator Tas and accessory protein Bet (ΔTas-Bet) after proviral integration due to inactivation of the translation start site of the *tas* ORF, or encoded an enzymatically inactive integrase (iIN) and were, therefore, largely integration-deficient (Figure 3b,c). This indicates that FV sensing does not require proviral integration or de novo viral transcription capacity.

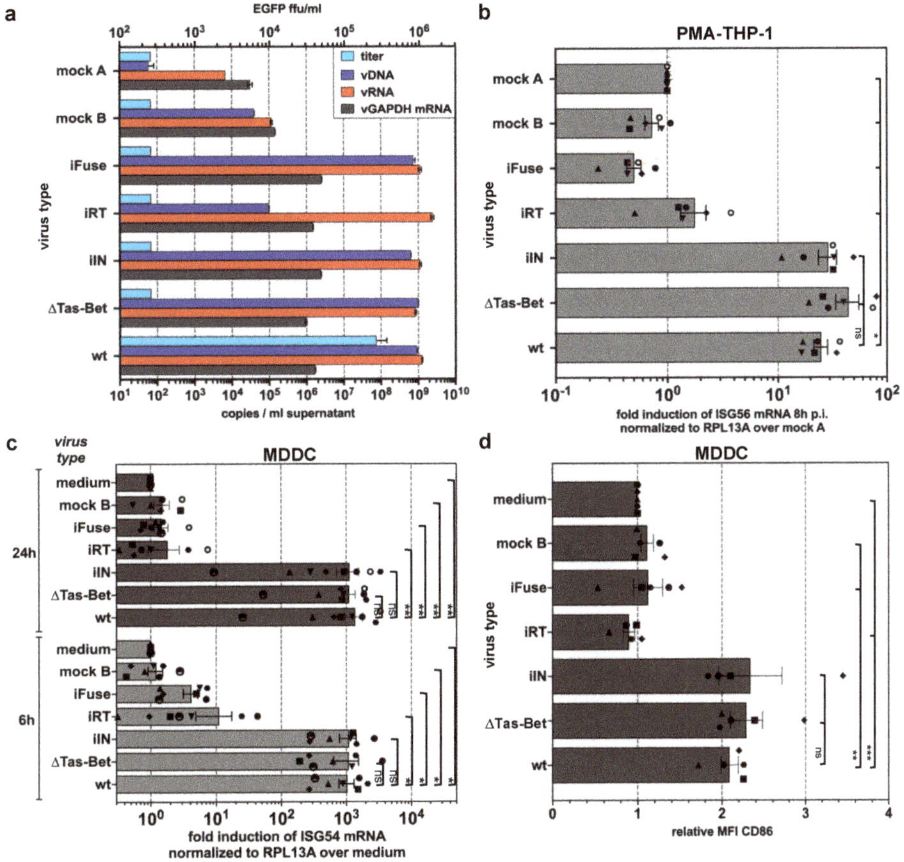

Figure 3. Differential ISG induction profiles of PFV mutants (described in detail in Figure A1 and Material and Methods) varying in their protein and nucleic acid composition. (**a**) Particle-associated nucleic acids extracted from viral particles pelleted by ultracentrifugation of virus supernatants used in (**b–d**) were analyzed by qPCR to quantify the particle-associated viral (vDNA: viral DNA; vRNA: viral RNA) and cellular (vGAPDH mRNA) nucleic acid composition. Mean copy numbers ± SDs per mL supernatant determined from duplicates are shown. (**b**,**c**) ISG induction profile of PMA-differentiated THP-1 wild type cells (**b**) or MDDCs (**c**) incubated with identical amounts of wild type PFV-RCP (MOI 0.1 THP-1; MOI 0.25 MDDCs) supernatants, variants thereof, and pUC19 (mock A) and ΔGPE (mock B) mock supernatants, or medium, as indicated, for 8 h and 24 h. Means ± SEMs, plus individual data points, of *ISG56* ($n = 6$) or *ISG54* ($n = 5$–7) mRNA induction normalized to *RPL13A* mRNA relative to mock A or medium treatment are shown. One-way ANOVA with Tukey's multiple-comparisons test (**b**) or mixed-effects analysis with Tukey's multiple-comparisons test (**c**) was used to assess significance. (**d**) CD86 cell surface expression profile of MDDCs 24 h post exposure to wild type PFV-RCP (MOI 0.25) supernatants and variants thereof as indicated. Means ± SEMs ($n = 5$), plus individual data points, relative to medium treatment are shown. Mixed-effects analysis with Tukey's multiple-comparisons test was used to assess significance. * $p < 0.05$; ** $p < 0.01$; *** $p < 0.001$; **** $p < 0.0001$; ns: not significant ($p \geq 0.05$).

In contrast, ISG induction was strongly reduced or undetectable in cells exposed to supernatants of PFV-RCPs either encoding an enzymatically inactive reverse transcriptase (iRT) or a fusion-deficient envelope glycoprotein (iFuse); and a control supernatant derived from a proviral expression construct with simultaneous inactivation of *gag*, *pol*, and *env* ORF translation start sites (ΔGPE, mock B), which failed to assemble virions (Figure 3b,c). Strikingly, for all individual virus supernatants a perfect correlation between their potentials to induce ISG expression and the upregulation of CD86 cell surface expression in MDDCs was observed (Figure 3d).

Taken together, these results point to the dependence on cytoplasmic access and enzymatically active reverse transcriptase for PFV-mediated ISG induction and activation of MDDCs.

3.4. PFV ISG Induction Does Not Require Reverse Transcription upon Target Cell Entry and Is Not Suppressed by SAMHD1

The above analysis revealed that PFV-RCP mediated induction requires an enzymatically active RT. FVs RTr has been reported to occur both during virus's assembly and upon target cell uptake and entry [4–6]. We therefore aimed to determine whether RTr products already present in PFV-RCP particles or those newly generated during target cell entry, as reported for other retroviruses like HIV-1 [36,37], are the main ISG inductors in myeloid cells. For that purpose, MDDCs were exposed to wild type PFV-RCP and HIV-1 GFP reporter viruses in the presence or absence of AZT, preventing de novo RTr upon target cell entry (Figure S2). Quantification of ISG induction at 24 h p.i. revealed a strong, 5- to 10-fold reduction in *ISG54* induction for HIV-1 GFP exposed samples by AZT treatment (Figure 4a,b). In contrast, AZT treatment diminished the ISG induction potential of PFV-RCP only marginally, a maximum of 2-fold (Figure 4a,b).

Furthermore, we examined whether SIV-Vpx-mediated degradation of endogenous SAMHD1 influences ISG induction mediated by PFV RTr products in MDDCs. MDDCs were exposed to PFV-RCP or HIV-1 GFP supernatants in the presence or absence of SIV-VLPs containing Vpx (Figure S4). Analysis of *ISG54* induction at 6 and 24 h p.i. confirmed the previously reported enhancement of HIV-1 sensing, up to 10-fold at 24 h p.i. (Figure 4c). In contrast, *ISG54* induction levels mediated by PFV-RCPs in MDDCs were not significantly altered by simultaneous Vpx-mediated SAMHD1 inactivation. This is in line with the *ISG56* induction capacity of PFV-RCP in THP-1 SAMHD1 KO cells shown before (Figure 2).

Thus, vDNA or RTr products generated from the encapsidated vRNA genome during virus morphogenesis are the major PFV PAMPs, which are sufficient for efficient sensing of PFV in myeloid cells. Furthermore, unlike HIV, PFV sensing in myeloid cells cannot be enhanced by SIV Vpx pretreatment, arguing against a role of endogenous SAMHD1 in the regulation of PFV sensing.

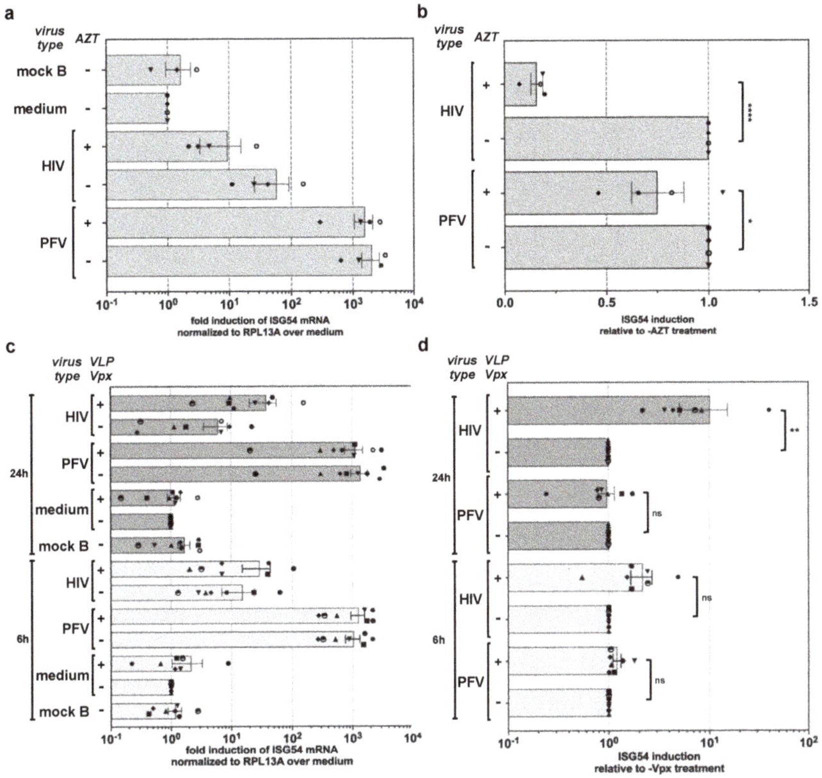

Figure 4. Influence of RTr inhibition and VLP-Vpx treatment on PFV-mediated ISG induction during target-cell entry. (**a**,**b**) MDDCs were incubated with wild type PFV-RCP (MOI 0.25), HIV-1 GFP (MOI 2), and VLP-Vpx or ΔGPE (mock B) mock supernatants in the absence or presence of AZT (100 μM) as indicated. *ISG54* mRNA levels normalized for *RPL13A* mRNA levels were determined by qPCR at 24 h post exposure. (**a**) Mean values ± SEMs, plus individual data points of *ISG54* (n = 3–4) induction relative to medium incubated samples are shown. (**b**) Mean values ± SEMs, plus individual data points of *ISG54* (n = 4) induction relative to the respective sample incubated with the same virus type without AZT addition are shown. One-way ANOVA with Sidak's multiple-comparisons test was used to assess significance. (**c**,**d**) MDDCs were incubated with wild type PFV-RCP (MOI 0.25), HIV-1 GFP (MOI 2) supernatants, or ΔGPE (mock B) mock supernatants in the absence or presence of VLP-Vpx as indicated. *ISG54* mRNA levels normalized for *RPL13A* mRNA levels were determined by qPCR at 6 and 24 h post exposure. (**c**) Mean values ± SEMs, plus individual data points, of *ISG54* (n = 7) induction relative to medium incubated samples are shown. (**d**) Mean values ± SEMs, plus individual data points, of *ISG54* (n = 7) induction relative to the respective sample incubated with the same virus type without VLP-Vpx addition are shown. One-way ANOVA with Sidak's multiple-comparisons test was used to assess significance. * $p < 0.05$; ** $p < 0.01$; *** $p < 0.001$; **** $p < 0.0001$; ns: not significant ($p \geq 0.05$).

3.5. PFV ISG Induction Requires Reverse Transcription of Full-Length Viral Genomes

Reports on level of innate sensing of HIV-1 in various target tissues appear to be strongly influenced by the specific type of HIV-1 viruses (full-length genome replication-competent versus single-round versus minimal vector genome) [57,58]. The characterization of the ISG induction profile of the various PFV-RCP mutants described above and the wild type like ISG profile of IFNAR1 THP-1 KO cells suggested that viral spreading in the culture is not required. This and the time course analysis of ISG induction suggest that the ISG response is induced shortly after cytoplasmic entry. Therefore, we also examined whether single-round PFV vector particles containing minimal viral genomic sequences (PFV-SRV) (Figure A1) induce an ISG response in myeloid cells (Figure 5). Surprisingly, whereas exposure of PMA-THP-1 cells to wild type PFV-RCPs lead to a strong *ISG56* induction, *ISG56* induction levels in cells to PFV-SRVs were strongly reduced (Figure 5a).

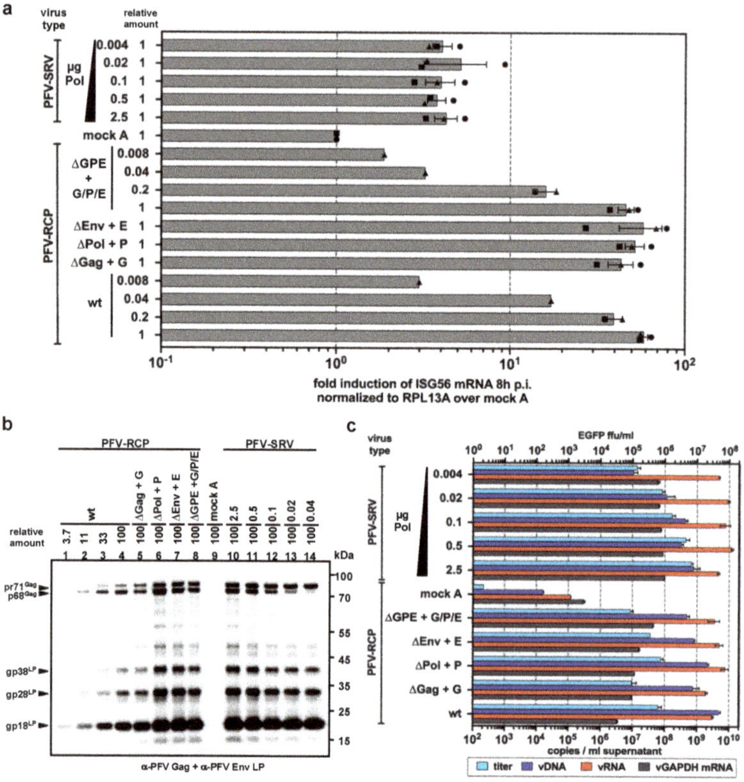

Figure 5. Differential ISG induction profile of single round PFV vector particles harboring full-length or minimal viral genomes. (**a**) PMA-differentiated THP-1 wild type cells were incubated with the indicated relative amounts of wild type PFV-RCP (MOI 0.3) supernatants and variants thereof, or the different PFV-SRV supernatants with variable Pol content (μg Pol packaging plasmid used for supernatant production is indicated; MOI 3 at 2.5 μg Pol) or supernatant from 293T cells transfected with pUC19 (mock A). *ISG56* mRNA levels normalized for *RPL13A* mRNA levels were determined by qPCR at 8 h post exposure. Mean values ± SEMs, plus individual data points of *ISG56* (*n* = 1–3) induction relative to mock A treatment are shown. (**b**,**c**) PFV supernatants characteristics. (**b**) Particle protein composition. Western blot analysis of protein composition of viral particles pelleted by ultracentrifugation of virus supernatants used in panel A employing PFV Gag (α-PFV Gag) and PFV Env LP (α-PFV Env LP) specific polyclonal antisera. The identity of individual protein bands is indicated to the left, the molecular weight to the right. (**c**) Particle nucleic acid composition. Particle-associated nucleic acids extracted from viral particles pelleted by ultracentrifugation of virus supernatants used in panel A were analyzed by qPCR to quantify the particle-associated viral (vDNA: viral DNA; vRNA: viral RNA) and cellular (vGAPDH mRNA) nucleic acid composition. Mean copy numbers ± SDs per mL supernatant determined from duplicates are shown. Viral titers were determined for PFV-SRV supernatants by *EGFP* reporter gene transfer assay on HT1080 cells and for PFV-RCP supernatants by Tas-dependent *EGFP* reporter gene induction assays on HT1080 PLNE cells. Mean titers ± SDs per mL supernatant determined from technical duplicates are shown.

In addition to their replication capacities there are two major differences between PFV-SRV and PFV-RCP. First, PFV-SRVs, unlike PFV-RCP, package Pol also in a vRNA genome independent manner, which leads to higher particle associated RT levels [41]. Second, the packaged and reverse transcribed minimal vRNA genome of PFV-SRVs lacks large genomic regions and does not encode any viral proteins [45].

To examine whether any of these differences are responsible for the differential ISG induction profile, different PFV-SRV and PFV-RCP supernatants were produced. For PFV-SRV, various supernatants were produced, keeping the amounts of vector genome Gag and Env expression vectors constant but using different amounts of Pol packaging plasmid. This resulted in virus supernatants containing similar physical amounts of PFV particles (Figure 5b), which contained similar amounts of viral and cellular RNA, but differed in their vDNA content (Figure 5c) and specific viral infectivity over a 50 to 100-fold range (Figure 5c). When PMA-THP-1 cells were exposed to identical amounts of these different PFV-SRVs, only a very weak ISG response was detectable, which was not influenced by the vDNA content and was at least 10-fold lower than that of PFV-RCP controls (Figure 5a).

Next, PFV-RCPs variants were used in which the translation of individual (ΔGag, ΔPol, ΔEnv) or all (ΔGPE) structural or enzymatic viral ORFs were abolished by point mutagenesis to determine whether the presence of functional ORFs for PFV structural genes in the viral genome is required for efficient innate sensing (Figure A1). Infectious virus supernatants were generated by complementing the individual defective structural functions by using the respective packaging constructs (+G, +P, +E, +G/P/E) also employed for production of PFV-SRVs. RCP virus supernatants contained similar physical amounts of virus particles with similar amounts of vRNA as PFV-SRVs (Figure 5b,c). Mutant PFV-RCP particles contained 2- to 5-fold lower amounts of vDNA and 2- to 8-fold higher amounts of cellular RNA compared to wild type PFV-RCP. Notably, the vDNA of mutant PFV-RCP was similar to that of PFV-SRVs generated with the highest amounts of PFV Pol packaging plasmid (Figure 5c). Strikingly, all mutant PFV-RCP supernatants, including the ΔGPE +G/P/E mutant, did induce an ISG response at wild type level (Figure 5a). When PMA-THP-1 cells were exposed to reducing amounts of PFV-RCP wt and ΔGPE +G/P/E, a dose-dependent decline in the ISG response was observed, with its level correlating well with the amount of vDNA present in the respective supernatants (Figure 5c).

Taken together, these results suggest that the type of PFV RNA genome encapsidated and reverse transcribed is crucial for innate sensing of PFV rather than the amounts of particle-associated Pol and vDNA.

4. Discussion

FV infections of natural hosts and zoonotic transmission to humans appear to be efficiently controlled by the immune system. We have only limited knowledge on the immunological mechanisms involved in this process.

Here, we examined the interaction of PFV with the innate immune system in immune cells of the myeloid lineage. Using an in vitro model cell line, THP-1, and primary human MDDC and MDM cultures, we observed an efficient stimulation of the innate immune system, determined as an IRF3-dependent stimulation of ISG expression and IRF3 phosphorylation, by replication-competent PFV generated from proviral expression constructs (PFV-RCP).

Furthermore, PFV innate sensing was neither dependent on viral transactivator Tas-mediated de novo viral transcription nor on viral integrase enzymatic activity. This indicates that productive infections, late steps of the viral replication cycle and virus spreading are not a prerequisite for PFV innate sensing in myeloid cells.

By use of various PFV-RCP mutants we demonstrated that PFV sensing occurs predominantly in the cytoplasm of myeloid cells as fusion-defective PFV-RCPs failed to stimulate ISG expression.

In contrast, efficient ISG induction required an enzymatically active reverse-transcriptase, indicating that vDNA or RTr products generated during reverse transcription are the major PFV PAMPs sensed by the innate immune system. Since FV RTr is observed both late in the replication cycle after capsid assembly and early during host cell entry [4–6], we investigated whether vDNA and RTr products already being present in PFV particles or those newly generated during uptake are the major PAMPs. Inhibition of RTr during entry by RT inhibitor led only to a minor reduction in PFV-mediated ISG induction, whereas that of HIV-1 was strongly reduced. This indicates that the vDNA and RTr products already present in PFV particles are sufficient for efficient induction of an innate immune response. However, since we are unable to prevent RTr during PFV assembly and at the same time allow subsequent RTr to take place during virus entry, as AZT incorporation leads to dead-end products, we cannot formally exclude that the latter may contribute to a certain extent to the innate immune response.

In line with the ISG induction potentials of the various PFV-RCP mutants, we observed that inactivation of essential key molecules of cellular DNA-sensing pathways, cGAS and STING, in THP-1 cells, abolished PFV-RCP-mediated innate immune stimulation. In accordance with vDNA and RTr products already present in PFV particles before host cell entry, representing the main PFV PAMPs, inactivation of cellular SAMHD1, either by gene KO in THP-1 cells or VLP-Vpx co-delivery in MDDCs, had only minor negative effects on PFV-RCP mediated ISG induction. This is also in agreement with previous reports of SAMHD1, unlike for lentiviruses, not being a restriction factor for PFV [59].

pDCs were shown by Rua and colleagues to mount an innate immune response as a consequence of TLR7-mediated sensing of PFV RNA [23]. Our results suggest that in myeloid cells, the contribution of vRNA sensing to PFV-mediated innate immune stimulation appears to be negligible. This is underlined by clearly detectable, although slightly reduced ISG induction in THP-1 KO cells having key molecules of cellular RNA-sensing pathway, MAVS or MyD88, inactivated. Furthermore, PFV-mediated ISG induction was almost completely abolished when myeloid cells were incubated with PFV-RCP with enzymatically inactive RT, which did not contain vDNA but harbored similar levels of vRNA as wild type virus.

The most striking finding of this study was the requirement of vDNA and/or RTr products to be derived from full-length vRNA genomes (PFV-RCP) instead of RNA genomes with minimal cis-acting viral sequences of PFV single-round vectors (PFV-SRV) for efficient ISG induction in myeloid cells. Interestingly, in contrast to the minimal genome of single-round vectors (PFV-SRV wt), which had a strongly impaired ISG induction capacity, the RTr of single-round vectors encapsidating a full-length genome containing point mutations (PFV-RCP ΔGPE + G/P/E) led to an ISG induction profile similar to replication-competent, wild type PFV particles (PFV-RCP wt). Our results obtained with various kinds of PFV-SRVs and PFV-RCP mutants can rule out differences in the replication capacity, the encoding of structural proteins, and the particle-associated RT levels or vDNA copy numbers as causative for this difference in innate stimulatory capacity. This underscores that most likely the encapsidated and reverse transcribed full-length genome represents the immunostimulatory component. Currently we can envision several potential underlying mechanisms.

A very attractive but perhaps also the most unlikely explanation might be the presence of immunostimulatory determinants in full-length PFV genomes that are absent in minimal PFV vector genomes. A specific **v**iral **s**timulatory **s**equence **e**lement (vSSE), and/or secondary structure thereof, present only in RTr products of full-length PFV genomes, could potentially be sensed.

Alternatively, the size difference between full-length PFV proviral (11,024 nt) and minimal SRV genomes (4348 nt), and not, or not only, a specific vSSE absent in the latter, may be responsible for or contribute to their differential ISG induction potential. This would fit to reports of cGAS activation based on DNA length and based on long DNA pre-structured by host proteins to strongly stimulate DNA sensing [60–62]. HIV-1 minus strand strong stop DNA ((-)sssDNA) was reported to contain short stem-loop structures with flanking unpaired guanosines highly stimulatory for cGAS activity. Notably, full-length PFV-RCP and minimal PFV-SRV genomes are identical up to the translation start of the *gag* ORF, thereby leading to identical PFV (-)sssDNA's (Figure A1). Therefore, even if PFV (-)sssDNA harbors cGAS stimulatory structures analogous to HIV-1 (-)sssDNA, it cannot be the cause for the differential ISG stimulatory capacity of RTr products of full-length PFV-RCP compared to minimal PFV-SRV genomes.

Finally, we cannot rule out that currently unknown differences in stability, structural integrity, or uncoating of the infecting viral cores containing full-length wild type or point mutation-containing genomes in comparison to minimal vector genomes are causing the difference in the innate response.

Further studies, including a detailed bioinformatic analysis of secondary structure prediction of PFV RTr products and their experimental verification, are required to provide experimental evidence for any of the proposed mechanisms, and combinations thereof, or they may reveal a currently unknown way of innate sensing of FV vDNA or RTr products and may identify additional cellular factors involved in this process.

5. Conclusions

To the best of our knowledge, this study is the first to demonstrate that replication-competent FVs can efficiently stimulate an innate immune response in human immune cells of the myeloid lineage. With FV particles known to contain significant amounts of reverse transcribed viral genome, it was not surprising that vDNA and/or RTr intermediates represent the PFV PAMP and cGAS, the main cellular PRR that are responsible for mounting an IRF3-dependent ISG response in this cell type. Elucidation of the underlying mechanism responsible for the differential innate stimulating capacities of full-length and minimal vector genomes in further studies may result in a more detailed characterization of the PFV genomic structures or sequence elements recognized by the host cell's innate immune system.

Supplementary Materials: The following are available online at http://www.mdpi.com/1999-4915/11/12/1095/s1. Figure S1: Characterization of MDDC and MDM differentiation status; Figure S2: AZT-mediated inhibition of MDDC transduction by HIV-1 GFP; Figure S3: PFV-mediated IRF3 phosphorylation in MDDCs; Figure S4: Degradation of endogenous SAMHD1 upon VLP-Vpx transduction.

Author Contributions: Conceptualization, M.B., J.W., R.K., and D.L.; validation, M.B., J.W., R.K., and D.L.; formal analysis, M.B., J.W., R.K., and D.L.; investigation, M.B., J.W., M.R., A.E., J.S., N.S., and C.M.; resources, V.H.; data curation, M.B., J.W., A.E., N.S., R.K., and D.L.; writing—original draft preparation, M.B., R.K., and D.L.; writing—review and editing, M.B., R.K., and D.L.; visualization, M.B. and D.L.; supervision, R.K. and D.L.; project administration, R.K. and D.L.; funding acquisition, R.K. and D.L.

Funding: This research was funded by grants from the Deutsche Forschungsgemeinschaft (DFG: LI 621/10-1; SPP1923 project LI 621/11-1 to D.L. and DFG: SPP1923 project KO4573/1-1 to R.K.). J.W. was supported by a fellowship of the Else Kröner-Promotionskolleg of the Faculty of Medicine of the Technische Universität Dresden.

Acknowledgments: We would like to thank Frank Kirchhoff for providing pBR-NL43-Env^{-}-IRES-eGFP-nef^{+}. We would like to thank Christiane Tondera, Heike Schmitz, Michaela Neuenkirch, and Lavinia Schmitt for technical support. We acknowledge support by the Open Access Publication Funds of the SLUB/TU Dresden.

Conflicts of Interest: The authors declare no conflict of interest. The funders had no role in the design of the study; in the collection, analyses, or interpretation of data; in the writing of the manuscript, or in the decision to publish the results.

Appendix A

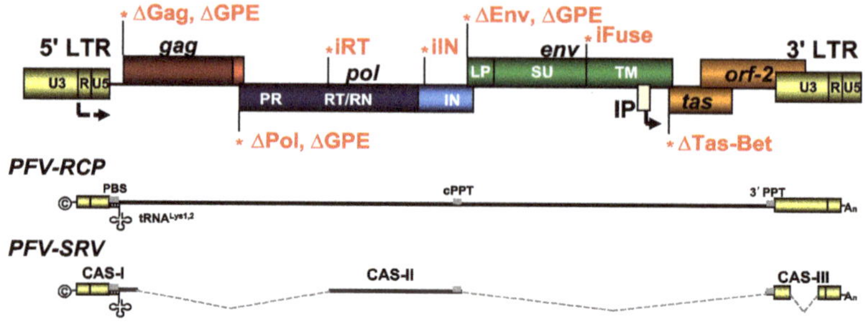

Figure A1. PFV genome organization and viral expression systems used. Schematic outline of the wild type (wt) PFV proviral genome structure with *gag*, *pol*, and *env* ORFs. The locations of the point mutations for the individual proviral mutants resulting in variants with enzymatically inactive integrase (iIN) or reverse transcriptase (iRT); fusion-deficient Env (iFuse); or deficiencies in the translation of, Tas (ΔTas-Bet); Gag (ΔGag); Pol (ΔPol); Env (ΔEnv); or Gag, Pol, and Env (ΔGPE), due to inactivation of the respective translation initiation sites. PFV-RCP supernatants contain full-length viral genomic RNA (vgRNA) whereas PFV-SRV supernatants harbor vgRNA comprising the minimal essential cis-acting viral sequences (CAS). LTR: long terminal repeat; U3: unique 3′ LTR region; U5: unique 5′ LTR region; R: repeat LTR region; PR: protease; RT/RN: reverse transcriptase—RNase H; IN: integrase; LP leader peptide; SU: surface subunit; TM: transmembrane subunit; IP: internal promoter; ©: cap; A_n: poly-A tail; PBS: primer binding site; 3′ PPT: 3′ poly purine tract; cPPT: central PPT.

Table A1. Primer–probe set for Taqman qPCR analysis.

Target	Primer/Probe	Sequence [5′-3′]	Cycle Conditions
PFV RNA/DNA	fwd	TGCAATTCCAAAGGTGATTC	95 °C, 8 min, 1×
	rev	TACCTCTTTCCTTTGCCCAT	95 °C, 30 s, 40×
	probe	TCAAGGTGCAGCATTCACTTCTTCAA	59 °C, 30 s, 40×
			72 °C, 90 s, 40×
hGAPDH	fwd	CATCAATGGAAATCCCATCA	95 °C, 8 min, 1×
	rev	GACTCCACGACGTACTCAGC	95 °C, 30 s, 40×
	probe	TCCAGGAGCGAGATCCCTCCA	59 °C, 30 s, 40×
			72 °C, 90 s, 40×
hISG56	fwd	GAGATCATTCACACCTCATTAT	95 °C, 8 min, 1×
	rev	GGAGTGAGTCTTCTGTTCT	95 °C, 30 s, 40×
	probe	TTCCCTCCCTTGCTAACTGCCATT	58 °C, 30 s, 40×
			72 °C, 90 s, 40×
hRPL13A	fwd	CCACCCTGGAGGAGAAGAGG	95 °C, 8 min, 1×
	rev	GAGTCCGTGGGTCTTGAGGA	95 °C, 30 s, 40×
	probe	TCGGCCTGTTTCCGTAGCCTCA	58 °C, 30 s, 40×
			72 °C, 90 s, 40×

Table A2. Primer–probe set for SYBR Green qPCR analysis.

Target	Primer/Probe	Sequence [5′-3′]	Cycle Conditions
hISG54	fwd rev	GGTGGCAGAAGAGGAAGATT TAGGCCAGTAGGTTGCACAT	50 °C, 30 min, 1× 95 °C, 15 min, 1× 94 °C, 15 s, 40× 56 °C, 45 s, 40× 72 °C, 45 s, 40×
hRPL13A	fwd rev	CCTGGAGGAGAAGAGGAAAGAGA TTGAGGACCTCTGTGTATTTGTCAA	50 °C, 30 min, 1× 95 °C, 15 min, 1× 94 °C, 15 s, 40× 56 °C, 45 s, 40× 72 °C, 45 s, 40×

Table A3. Antibodies used for FACS analysis.

Antibody Specificity	Company	Clone	Volume per Sample in µL	Fluorophore Attached
CD14	BioLegend	M5E2	1	Pacific Blue
CD163	BD Bioscience	GHI/61	2	PE
CD206	BD Bioscience	19.2 (RUO)	2	APC
CD11c	Miltenyi	N418	2	Vio Blue
CD1a	BioLegend	SK9	2	PE
CD16	BioLegend	3G8	2	APC
CD86	BioLegend	IT2.2	1.5	PE
IgG2a, κ; isotype control	BioLegend	MOPC-173	1	Pacific Blue
IgG1, k Isotype control	Beckman Coulter	Clone GHI/61 (RUO)	2	PE
IgG1, k Isotype control	BD Bioscience	MOPC-21	2	APC
IgG2b, isotype control	Miltenyi	IS6-11E5.11	2	Vio Blue
IgG2b, k isotype control	BioLegend	MG2b-57	2 or 1.5	PE

References

1. Khan, A.S.; Bodem, J.; Buseyne, F.; Gessain, A.; Johnson, W.; Kuhn, J.H.; Kuzmak, J.; Lindemann, D.; Linial, M.L.; Lochelt, M.; et al. Spumaretroviruses: Updated taxonomy and nomenclature. *Virology* **2018**, *516*, 158–164. [CrossRef] [PubMed]
2. Rethwilm, A.; Lindemann, D. Foamy viruses. In *Fields Virology*, 6th ed.; Knipe, D.M., Howley, P.M., Eds.; Lippincott Williams & Wilkins, a Wolters Kluwer business: Philadelphia, PA, USA, 2013; Volume 2, pp. 1613–1632.
3. Lindemann, D.; Rethwilm, A. Foamy virus biology and its application for vector development. *Viruses* **2011**, *3*, 561–585. [CrossRef] [PubMed]
4. Delelis, O.; Saib, A.; Sonigo, P. Biphasic DNA synthesis in spumaviruses. *J. Virol.* **2003**, *77*, 8141–8146. [CrossRef] [PubMed]
5. Moebes, A.; Enssle, J.; Bieniasz, P.D.; Heinkelein, M.; Lindemann, D.; Bock, M.; McClure, M.O.; Rethwilm, A. Human foamy virus reverse transcription that occurs late in the viral replication cycle. *J. Virol.* **1997**, *71*, 7305–7311.
6. Yu, S.F.; Baldwin, D.N.; Gwynn, S.R.; Yendapalli, S.; Linial, M.L. Human foamy virus replication: A pathway distinct from that of retroviruses and hepadnaviruses. *Science* **1996**, *271*, 1579–1582. [CrossRef]
7. Zamborlini, A.; Renault, N.; Saib, A.; Delelis, O. Early reverse transcription is essential for productive foamy virus infection. *PLoS ONE* **2010**, *5*, e11023. [CrossRef]

8. Rua, R.; Gessain, A. Origin, evolution and innate immune control of simian foamy viruses in humans. *Curr. Opin. Virol.* **2015**, *10*, 47–55. [CrossRef]
9. Kehl, T.; Tan, J.; Materniak, M. Non-simian foamy viruses: Molecular virology, tropism and prevalence and zoonotic/interspecies transmission. *Viruses* **2013**, *5*, 2169–2209. [CrossRef]
10. Katzourakis, A.; Aiewsakun, P.; Jia, H.; Wolfe, N.D.; LeBreton, M.; Yoder, A.D.; Switzer, W.M. Discovery of prosimian and afrotherian foamy viruses and potential cross species transmissions amidst stable and ancient mammalian co-evolution. *Retrovirology* **2014**, *11*, 61. [CrossRef]
11. Han, G.Z.; Worobey, M. Endogenous viral sequences from the cape golden mole (chrysochloris asiatica) reveal the presence of foamy viruses in all major placental mammal clades. *PLoS ONE* **2014**, *9*, e97931. [CrossRef]
12. Schartl, M.; Walter, R.B.; Shen, Y.; Garcia, T.; Catchen, J.; Amores, A.; Braasch, I.; Chalopin, D.; Volff, J.N.; Lesch, K.P.; et al. The genome of the platyfish, xiphophorus maculatus, provides insights into evolutionary adaptation and several complex traits. *Nat. Genet.* **2013**, *45*, 567–572. [CrossRef] [PubMed]
13. Achong, B.G.; Mansell, P.W.A.; Epstein, M.A.; Clifford, P. An unusual virus in cultures from a human nasopharyngeal carcinoma. *J. Natl. Cancer Inst.* **1971**, *46*, 299–307. [PubMed]
14. Epstein, M.A. Simian retroviral infections in human beings. *Lancet* **2004**, *364*, 138–139, author reply 139–140. [CrossRef]
15. Herchenröder, O.; Turek, R.; Neumann Haefelin, D.; Rethwilm, A.; Schneider, J. Infectious proviral clones of chimpanzee foamy virus (sfvcpz) generated by long pcr reveal close functional relatedness to human foamy virus. *Virology* **1995**, *214*, 685–689. [CrossRef] [PubMed]
16. Stirnnagel, K.; Lüftenegger, D.; Stange, A.; Swiersy, A.; Müllers, E.; Reh, J.; Stanke, N.; Grosse, A.; Chiantia, S.; Keller, H.; et al. Analysis of prototype foamy virus particle-host cell interaction with autofluorescent retroviral particles. *Retrovirology* **2010**, *7*, 45. [CrossRef]
17. Mikovits, J.A.; Hoffman, P.M.; Rethwilm, A.; Ruscetti, F.W. In Vitro infection of primary and retrovirus-infected human leukocytes by human foamy virus. *J. Virol.* **1996**, *70*, 2774–2780.
18. Yu, S.F.; Stone, J.; Linial, M.L. Productive persistent infection of hematopoietic cells by human foamy virus. *J. Virol.* **1996**, *70*, 1250–1254.
19. Murray, S.M.; Picker, L.J.; Axthelm, M.K.; Hudkins, K.; Alpers, C.E.; Linial, M.L. Replication in a superficial epithelial cell niche explains the lack of pathogenicity of primate foamy virus infections. *J. Virol.* **2008**, *82*, 5981–5985. [CrossRef]
20. Callahan, M.E.; Switzer, W.M.; Matthews, A.L.; Roberts, B.D.; Heneine, W.; Folks, T.M.; Sandstrom, P.A. Persistent zoonotic infection of a human with simian foamy virus in the absence of an intact orf-2 accessory gene. *J. Virol.* **1999**, *73*, 9619–9624.
21. von Laer, D.; Neumann Haefelin, D.; Heeney, J.L.; Schweizer, M. Lymphocytes are the major reservoir for foamy viruses in peripheral blood. *Virology* **1996**, *221*, 240–244. [CrossRef]
22. Rua, R.; Betsem, E.; Montange, T.; Buseyne, F.; Gessain, A. In vivo cellular tropism of gorilla simian foamy virus in blood of infected humans. *J. Virol.* **2014**, *88*, 13429–13435. [CrossRef] [PubMed]
23. Rua, R.; Lepelley, A.; Gessain, A.; Schwartz, O. Innate sensing of foamy viruses by human hematopoietic cells. *J. Virol.* **2012**, *86*, 909–918. [CrossRef] [PubMed]
24. Bähr, A.; Singer, A.; Hain, A.; Vasudevan, A.A.; Schilling, M.; Reh, J.; Riess, M.; Panitz, S.; Serrano, V.; Schweizer, M.; et al. Interferon but not mxb inhibits foamy retroviruses. *Virology* **2016**, *488*, 51–60. [CrossRef] [PubMed]
25. Falcone, V.; Schweizer, M.; Toniolo, A.; Neumann-Haefelin, D.; Meyerhans, A. Gamma interferon is a major suppressive factor produced by activated human peripheral blood lymphocytes that is able to inhibit foamy virus-induced cytopathic effects. *J. Virol.* **1999**, *73*, 1724–1728.
26. Matthes, D.; Wiktorowicz, T.; Zahn, J.; Bodem, J.; Stanke, N.; Lindemann, D.; Rethwilm, A. Basic residues in the foamy virus gag protein. *J. Virol.* **2011**, *85*, 3986–3995. [CrossRef]
27. Rhodes Feuillette, A.; Lasneret, J.; Paulien, S.; Ogunkolade, W.; Peries, J.; Canivet, M. Effects of human recombinant alpha and gamma and of highly purified natural beta interferons on simian spumavirinae prototype (simian foamy virus 1) multiplication in human cells. *Res. Virol.* **1990**, *141*, 31–43. [CrossRef]
28. Sabile, A.; Rhodes Feuillette, A.; Jaoui, F.Z.; Tobaly Tapiero, J.; Giron, M.L.; Lasneret, J.; Peries, J.; Canivet, M. In Vitro studies on interferon-inducing capacity and sensitivity to ifn of human foamy virus. *Res. Virol.* **1996**, *147*, 29–37. [CrossRef]

29. Russell, R.A.; Wiegand, H.L.; Moore, M.D.; Schafer, A.; McClure, M.O.; Cullen, B.R. Foamy virus bet proteins function as novel inhibitors of the apobec3 family of innate antiretroviral defense factors. *J. Virol.* **2005**, *79*, 8724–8731. [CrossRef]
30. Löchelt, M.; Romen, F.; Bastone, P.; Muckenfuss, H.; Kirchner, N.; Kim, Y.B.; Truyen, U.; Rösler, U.; Battenberg, M.; Saib, A.; et al. The antiretroviral activity of apobec3 is inhibited by the foamy virus accessory bet protein. *Proc. Natl. Acad. Sci. USA* **2005**, *102*, 7982–7987. [CrossRef]
31. Yap, M.W.; Lindemann, D.; Stanke, N.; Reh, J.; Westphal, D.; Hanenberg, H.; Ohkura, S.; Stoye, J.P. Restriction of foamy viruses by primate trim5alpha. *J. Virol.* **2008**, *82*, 5429–5439. [CrossRef]
32. Jouvenet, N.; Neil, S.J.; Zhadina, M.; Zang, T.; Kratovac, Z.; Lee, Y.; McNatt, M.; Hatziioannou, T.; Bieniasz, P.D. Broad-spectrum inhibition of retroviral and filoviral particle release by tetherin. *J. Virol.* **2009**, *83*, 1837–1844. [CrossRef] [PubMed]
33. Manel, N.; Hogstad, B.; Wang, Y.; Levy, D.E.; Unutmaz, D.; Littman, D.R. A cryptic sensor for hiv-1 activates antiviral innate immunity in dendritic cells. *Nature* **2010**, *467*, 214–217. [CrossRef] [PubMed]
34. Maelfait, J.; Bridgeman, A.; Benlahrech, A.; Cursi, C.; Rehwinkel, J. Restriction by samhd1 limits cgas/sting-dependent innate and adaptive immune responses to hiv-1. *Cell Rep.* **2016**, *16*, 1492–1501. [CrossRef] [PubMed]
35. Luban, J. Innate immune sensing of hiv-1 by dendritic cells. *Cell Host Microbe* **2012**, *12*, 408–418. [CrossRef]
36. Gao, D.; Wu, J.; Wu, Y.T.; Du, F.; Aroh, C.; Yan, N.; Sun, L.; Chen, Z.J. Cyclic gmp-amp synthase is an innate immune sensor of hiv and other retroviruses. *Science* **2013**, *341*, 903–906. [CrossRef]
37. Yoh, S.M.; Schneider, M.; Seifried, J.; Soonthornvacharin, S.; Akleh, R.E.; Olivieri, K.C.; De Jesus, P.D.; Ruan, C.; de Castro, E.; Ruiz, P.A.; et al. Pqbp1 is a proximal sensor of the cgas-dependent innate response to hiv-1. *Cell* **2015**, *161*, 1293–1305. [CrossRef]
38. Leong, C.R.; Oshiumi, H.; Okamoto, M.; Azuma, M.; Takaki, H.; Matsumoto, M.; Chayama, K.; Seya, T. A mavs/ticam-1-independent interferon-inducing pathway contributes to regulation of hepatitis b virus replication in the mouse hydrodynamic injection model. *J. Innate Immun.* **2015**, *7*, 47–58. [CrossRef]
39. DuBridge, R.B.; Tang, P.; Hsia, H.C.; Leong, P.M.; Miller, J.H.; Calos, M.P. Analysis of mutation in human cells by using an epstein-barr virus shuttle system. *Mol. Cell. Biol* **1987**, *7*, 379–387. [CrossRef]
40. Rasheed, S.; Nelson-Rees, W.A.; Toth, E.M.; Arnstein, P.; Gardner, M.B. Characterization of a newly derived human sarcoma cell line (ht-1080). *Cancer* **1974**, *33*, 1027–1033. [CrossRef]
41. Hütter, S.; Müllers, E.; Stanke, N.; Reh, J.; Lindemann, D. Prototype foamy virus protease activity is essential for intraparticle reverse transcription initiation but not absolutely required for uncoating upon host cell entry. *J. Virol.* **2013**, *87*, 3163–3176. [CrossRef]
42. Wittmann, S.; Behrendt, R.; Eissmann, K.; Volkmann, B.; Thomas, D.; Ebert, T.; Cribier, A.; Benkirane, M.; Hornung, V.; Bouzas, N.F.; et al. Phosphorylation of murine samhd1 regulates its antiretroviral activity. *Retrovirology* **2015**, *12*, 103. [CrossRef] [PubMed]
43. Mankan, A.K.; Schmidt, T.; Chauhan, D.; Goldeck, M.; Honing, K.; Gaidt, M.; Kubarenko, A.V.; Andreeva, L.; Hopfner, K.P.; Hornung, V. Cytosolic rna:DNA hybrids activate the cgas-sting axis. *EMBO J.* **2014**, *33*, 2937–2946. [CrossRef] [PubMed]
44. Riess, M.; Fuchs, N.V.; Idica, A.; Hamdorf, M.; Flory, E.; Pedersen, I.M.; Konig, R. Interferons induce expression of samhd1 in monocytes through down-regulation of mir-181a and mir-30a. *J. Biol. Chem.* **2017**, *292*, 264–277. [CrossRef]
45. Heinkelein, M.; Dressler, M.; Jarmy, G.; Rammling, M.; Imrich, H.; Thurow, J.; Lindemann, D.; Rethwilm, A. Improved primate foamy virus vectors and packaging constructs. *J. Virol.* **2002**, *76*, 3774–3783. [CrossRef] [PubMed]
46. Müllers, E.; Uhlig, T.; Stirnnagel, K.; Fiebig, U.; Zentgraf, H.; Lindemann, D. Novel functions of prototype foamy virus gag glycine- arginine-rich boxes in reverse transcription and particle morphogenesis. *J. Virol.* **2011**, *85*, 1452–1463. [CrossRef] [PubMed]
47. Heinkelein, M.; Thurow, J.; Dressler, M.; Imrich, H.; Neumann-Haefelin, D.; McClure, M.O.; Rethwilm, A. Complex effects of deletions in the 5′ untranslated region of primate foamy virus on viral gene expression and rna packaging. *J. Virol.* **2000**, *74*, 3141–3148. [CrossRef]
48. Hamann, M.V.; Müllers, E.; Reh, J.; Stanke, N.; Effantin, G.; Weissenhorn, W.; Lindemann, D. The cooperative function of arginine residues in the prototype foamy virus gag c-terminus mediates viral and cellular rna encapsidation. *Retrovirology* **2014**, *11*, 87. [CrossRef]

49. Negre, D.; Mangeot, P.E.; Duisit, G.; Blanchard, S.; Vidalain, P.O.; Leissner, P.; Winter, A.J.; Rabourdin-Combe, C.; Mehtali, M.; Moullier, P.; et al. Characterization of novel safe lentiviral vectors derived from simian immunodeficiency virus (sivmac251) that efficiently transduce mature human dendritic cells. *Gene Ther.* **2000**, *7*, 1613–1623. [CrossRef]
50. Schindler, M.; Munch, J.; Kirchhoff, F. Human immunodeficiency virus type 1 inhibits DNA damage-triggered apoptosis by a nef-independent mechanism. *J. Virol.* **2005**, *79*, 5489–5498. [CrossRef]
51. Ho, Y.P.; Schnabel, V.; Swiersy, A.; Stirnnagel, K.; Lindemann, D. A small-molecule-controlled system for efficient pseudotyping of prototype foamy virus vectors. *Mol. Ther.* **2012**, *20*, 1167–1176. [CrossRef]
52. Schott, K.; Fuchs, N.V.; Derua, R.; Mahboubi, B.; Schnellbacher, E.; Seifried, J.; Tondera, C.; Schmitz, H.; Shepard, C.; Brandariz-Nunez, A.; et al. Dephosphorylation of the hiv-1 restriction factor samhd1 is mediated by pp2a-b55alpha holoenzymes during mitotic exit. *Nat. Commun.* **2018**, *9*, 2227. [CrossRef] [PubMed]
53. Mannigel, I.; Stange, A.; Zentgraf, H.; Lindemann, D. Correct capsid assembly mediated by a conserved yxxlgl motif in prototype foamy virus gag is essential for infectivity and reverse transcription of the viral genome. *J. Virol.* **2007**, *81*, 3317–3326. [CrossRef] [PubMed]
54. Goujon, C.; Arfi, V.; Pertel, T.; Luban, J.; Lienard, J.; Rigal, D.; Darlix, J.L.; Cimarelli, A. Characterization of simian immunodeficiency virus sivsm/human immunodeficiency virus type 2 vpx function in human myeloid cells. *J. Virol.* **2008**, *82*, 12335–12345. [CrossRef] [PubMed]
55. Nakaya, T.; Sato, M.; Hata, N.; Asagiri, M.; Suemori, H.; Noguchi, S.; Tanaka, N.; Taniguchi, T. Gene induction pathways mediated by distinct irfs during viral infection. *Biochem. Biophys. Res. Commun.* **2001**, *283*, 1150–1156. [CrossRef] [PubMed]
56. Grandvaux, N.; Servant, M.J.; Sen, G.C.; Balachandran, S.; Barber, G.N.; Lin, R.; Hiscott, J. Transcriptional profiling of interferon regulatory factor 3 target genes: Direct involvement in the regulation of interferon-stimulated genes. *J. Virol.* **2002**, *76*, 5532–5539. [CrossRef]
57. McCauley, S.M.; Kim, K.; Nowosielska, A.; Dauphin, A.; Yurkovetskiy, L.; Diehl, W.E.; Luban, J. Intron-containing rna from the hiv-1 provirus activates type i interferon and inflammatory cytokines. *Nat. Commun.* **2018**, *9*, 5305. [CrossRef]
58. Akiyama, H.; Miller, C.M.; Ettinger, C.R.; Belkina, A.C.; Snyder-Cappione, J.E.; Gummuluru, S. Hiv-1 intron-containing rna expression induces innate immune activation and t cell dysfunction. *Nat. Commun.* **2018**, *9*, 3450. [CrossRef]
59. Gramberg, T.; Kahle, T.; Bloch, N.; Wittmann, S.; Müllers, E.; Daddacha, W.; Hofmann, H.; Kim, B.; Lindemann, D.; Landau, N.R. Restriction of Diverse Retroviruses by Samhd1. *Retrovirology* **2013**, *10*, 26. [CrossRef]
60. Herzner, A.M.; Hagmann, C.A.; Goldeck, M.; Wolter, S.; Kubler, K.; Wittmann, S.; Gramberg, T.; Andreeva, L.; Hopfner, K.P.; Mertens, C.; et al. Sequence-specific activation of the DNA sensor cgas by y-form DNA structures as found in primary hiv-1 cdna. *Nat. Immunol.* **2015**, *16*, 1025–1033. [CrossRef]
61. Andreeva, L.; Hiller, B.; Kostrewa, D.; Lassig, C.; de Oliveira Mann, C.C.; Jan Drexler, D.; Maiser, A.; Gaidt, M.; Leonhardt, H.; Hornung, V.; et al. Cgas senses long and hmgb/tfam-bound u-turn DNA by forming protein-DNA ladders. *Nature* **2017**, *549*, 394–398. [CrossRef]
62. Jakobsen, M.R.; Bak, R.O.; Andersen, A.; Berg, R.K.; Jensen, S.B.; Tengchuan, J.; Laustsen, A.; Hansen, K.; Ostergaard, L.; Fitzgerald, K.A.; et al. Ifi16 senses DNA forms of the lentiviral replication cycle and controls hiv-1 replication. *Proc. Natl. Acad. Sci. USA* **2013**, *110*, E4571–E4580. [CrossRef] [PubMed]

viruses

MDPI

Article

Functional Analyses of Bovine Foamy Virus-Encoded miRNAs Reveal the Importance of a Defined miRNA for Virus Replication and Host–Virus Interaction

Wenhu Cao [1], Erik Stricker [1,†], Agnes Hotz-Wagenblatt [2], Anke Heit-Mondrzyk [2], Georgios Pougialis [1], Annette Hugo [1], Jacek Kuźmak [3], Magdalena Materniak-Kornas [3] and Martin Löchelt [1,*]

1 Division Viral Transformation Mechanisms, Research Focus Infection, Inflammation and Cancer, German Cancer Research Center (Deutsches Krebsforschungszentrum, DKFZ), 69120 Heidelberg, Germany; mckf11111@gmail.com (W.C.); stricker@bcm.edu (E.S.); g.pougialis@dkfz.de (G.P.); a.hugo@dkfz.de (A.H.)

2 Core Facility Omics IT and Data Management, German Cancer Research Center (Deutsches Krebsforschungszentrum, DKFZ), 69120 Heidelberg, Germany; hotz-wagenblatt@dkfz.de (A.H.-W.); a.heit@dkfz.de (A.H.-M.)

3 Department of Biochemistry, National Veterinary Research Institute, 24–100 Pulawy, Poland; jkuzmak@piwet.pulawy.pl (J.K.); magdalena.materniak@piwet.pulawy.pl (M.M.-K.)

* Correspondence: m.loechelt@dkfz.de; Tel.: +49-6221-424933

† Current address: Department of Molecular Virology and Microbiology, Baylor College of Medicine, Houston, TX 77030, USA.

Received: 23 September 2020; Accepted: 27 October 2020; Published: 2 November 2020

Abstract: In addition to regulatory or accessory proteins, some complex retroviruses gain a repertoire of micro-RNAs (miRNAs) to regulate and control virus–host interactions for efficient replication and spread. In particular, bovine and simian foamy viruses (BFV and SFV) have recently been shown to express a diverse set of RNA polymerase III-directed miRNAs, some with a unique primary miRNA double-hairpin, dumbbell-shaped structure not known in other viruses or organisms. While the mechanisms of expression and structural requirements have been studied, the functional importance of these miRNAs is still far from understood. Here, we describe the in silico identification of BFV miRNA targets and the subsequent experimental validation of bovine Ankyrin Repeat Domain 17 (ANKRD17) and Bax-interacting factor 1 (Bif1) target genes in vitro and, finally, the suppression of ANKRD17 downstream genes in the affected pathway. Deletion of the entire miRNA cassette in the non-coding part of the U3 region of the long terminal repeats attenuated replication of corresponding BFV mutants in bovine cells. This repression can be almost completely trans-complemented by the most abundant miRNA BF2-5p having the best scores for predicted and validated BFV miRNA target genes. Deletion of the miRNA cassette does not grossly affect particle release and overall particle composition.

Keywords: bovine foamy virus; spumaretrovirus; miRNA expression; virus-host-interaction; miRNA target gene identification; innate immunity; ANKRD17; Bif1 (SH3GLB1); replication in vitro

1. Introduction

In addition to the structural genes, viruses often encode proteins or non-protein regulators of viral replication to modulate the interplay with their hosts. While regulatory proteins are common in many viruses, several DNA viruses additionally encode miRNAs as part of RNA polymerase II or III (RNA Pol II and III) primary transcripts that are common viral factors in the virus–host interaction [1]. On the other side, cellular miRNAs often target essential viral pathways in order to inhibit virus replication, but in rare cases, cellular miRNAs may even fulfill critical functions, for instance, during hepatitis C virus replication [2,3]. By acquisition of counter-acting miRNAs or proteins interfering with host-encoded miRNA expression, maturation, and function, viruses often inhibit this restriction (reviewed in Skalsky et al., 2010; [4]).

In retroviruses, miRNAs are rare compared to regulatory and accessory proteins [1]. There is clear evidence of avian leucosis virus subgroup J (ALV-J) miRNA expression via RNA Pol II [5]. The issue whether HIV expresses miRNAs is controversial: HIV miRNAs are expressed at very low levels and these short RNAs often display deviant features such as their size, as discussed by Balasubramaniam [6]. In clear contrast, canonical miRNAs have been detected at considerable to even very high levels in cells infected with bovine leukemia virus (BLV, [7]), bovine foamy virus (BFV, [8]), and simian foamy virus of African green monkeys (SFV_{agm}, [9]) and Japanese macaques (SFV_{cae}, [10]).

Foamy viruses (FV), or spumaretroviruses, comprise five genera of the Spumaretrovirinae [11]. FVs are characterized by several unique features in their molecular biology and replication strategy compared to the Orthoretrovirinae encompassing the remaining majority of the retrovirus family including the deltaretrovirus BLV [11–15]. Due to their apathogenicity, broad range of susceptible host cells, and other features, FVs are promising candidates for novel virus vectors [16]. In contrast, their capacity to cross species barriers leading to zoonotic infections of humans by simian FVs and their presence in the human food chain are important for human and animal health and may serve as a model for other viruses with similar features [17]. Here, BFV is of particular interest as a co-pathogen in livestock animals, which may or may not modulate the disease potential of other known pathogens [13,18].

Expression of the primary miRNAs (pri-miRNAs) of BLV, BFV, SFV_{agm}, and SFV_{cae} is directed by unique short transcripts generated by RNA Pol III [7–10]. While in BLV the pri-miRNAs consist of individual, single stem-loop structures, the single pri-miRNA species of BFV and some of those from SFV_{agm} and SFV_{cae} consist of two closely spaced stem-loops with an overall dumbbell structure [7–10,13]. In SFV_{agm} and SFV_{cae}, additional pri-miRNAs may be similar to those of BLV consisting of only a single stem-loop [9,10,13]. The single- and double stem-loop RNA Pol III pri-miRNAs of FVs as summarized by Materniak et al., 2019 [13] may be the end-product of complex evolutionary processes that may have been primarily shaped by the limited genetic coding capacity of retro- and spumaviral genomes. In addition, protection of the genomic, full-length RNA from the miRNA processing machinery may have led to the acquisition or emergence of RNA Pol III-directed short pri-miRNAs as discussed by Cullen [2].

To our knowledge, an RNA Pol III-driven dumbbell-shaped pri-miRNA is a unique feature of BFV, SFV_{agm}, and SFV_{cae} with unambiguous experimental data on the expression (abundance), processing, and potential utilization for translational purposes [8–10,13,19]. For both SFVs, target gene prediction has been performed and some of the targets have been validated based on reporter constructs in heterologous cells [9,10]. Since BFV has only a single dumbbell-shaped pri-miRNA and correspondingly only a single expression cassette, it appears to be a comparably simple and easy to engineer model compared to SFV_{agm} and SFV_{cae} with a less defined mix of single- and double-stem-loop structures [8–10,13].

Here, we describe BFV miRNA target gene prediction studies and identification of the importance of the high-abundance BFV BF2-5p miRNA for BFV replication. Bovine ANKRD17 [20–23] and Bif1 [24,25] were shown to be BF2-5p target genes in vitro with respect to moderately decreased RNA and strongly reduced protein steady state levels, similar to the action of most other miRNAs [3,26]. Besides functions in several cellular pathways, ANKRD17 is an upstream regulator of innate immune signaling [20–23] and corresponding changes were detected here. Infectivity of an infectious BFV clone devoid of the miRNA cassette displayed attenuated replication in vitro, which could be trans-complemented by the BF2-5p miRNA. Deletion of the complete miRNA expression cassette had no obvious effects on Gag and Pol expression, processing and particle release and composition.

2. Materials and Methods

2.1. Cell Culture and DNA and miRNA Transfection Techniques

HEK293T human epithelial kidney cell line (ATCC CRL-3216; Manassas, VA, USA), baby hamster kidney cell line 21 (BHK, ATCC CCL-10) and the bovine macrophage cell line BoMac [27] were used for transfection assays. These cells were grown in Dulbecco's modified Eagle medium (DMEM, Sigma, Steinheim, Germany) supplemented with 10% fetal calf serum (Biochrome, Berlin, Germnay) and 1% penicillin–streptomycin (GIBCO, New York, NY, USA). Bovine Madin–Darby bovine kidney (MDBK, ATCC CCL-22) cells and the MDBK-derived BFV Tas reporter MICL cells, carrying an EGFP gene upstream of the BFV LTR promoter were grown in DMEM as above [28]. All cells used were routinely checked for the absence of mycoplasma and cell identity by multiplex analyses (GATC, Konstanz, Germany).

The day before transfection, cells were seeded at a density of 20–30%. The next day, cells were transfected with plasmid DNA by using the lipofectamine LTX reagent (Thermo Fisher Scientific, Darmstadt, Germany) according tothe manufacturer's instruction or polyethylenimine (PEI, Polysciences Inc., Warrington, PA, USA) [8,28]. After incubation for 12 h at 37 °C and 5% CO_2, the medium was replaced by fresh medium and the cells were incubated for an additional 36 h before lysis and luciferase reporter assays.

A molecular mimic and the corresponding scrambled sequence miRNA for BFV BF2-5p miRNA of BFV were purchased from Invitrogen/Thermo Fisher Scientific and transfected using lipofectamine LTX reagent and 25 pmol miRNA per well of a 6-well plate. The miRNA mimic and control are small, chemically modified double-stranded RNAs while the miRNA inhibitor is a small, chemically modified single-stranded RNA designed to specifically bind to and inhibit BF2-5p (for details see: https://www.thermofisher.com/de/de/home/life-science/epigenetics-noncoding-rna-research/mirna-analysis/mirna-mimics-inhibitors/mirvana-mimics-inhibitors.html, accessed on 1.12.2017).

2.2. Molecular Cloning

All BFV miRNA expression plasmids were based on the RNA Pol-II and -III promoter-deficient basal vector pGEM3Z (Promega, Mannheim, Germany) and the different dual reporter constructs have been described previously [19]. To construct additional psiCHECK2-based reporter plasmids for miRNA function, genomic sequences were amplified using the high-fidelity Phusion DNA polymerase (New England Biolabs, Frankfurt, Germany), 0.5 µmol of the primers, and 200 ng target DNA from wt BFV-Riems [29] or bovine MDBK cells under the following conditions: Initial denaturation at 98 °C for 30 s, then 30 cycles of amplification (98 °C for 10 s, 55 °C for 30 s, 72 °C for 1 min), final extension at 72 °C for 10 min as described previously [19]. Reporter constructs for bovine ANKRD17 (NM_001192181.2) and Bif1 (NM_001077993.2) were confirmed by DNA sequencing and each encompassed about 400 nt 3′ UTR sequences.

To conduct reverse genetic experiments, cloned BFV genomes selected for high titer cell-free transmission in bovine MDBK cells [28,30] were further optimized by replacing the U3 region of the 5′LTR by the strong and constitutively active CMV immediate early (IE) promoter using standard cloning strategies as described previously for feline FV [31]. BFV genomes lacking the complete BFV miRNA cassette were obtained by fusion PCR mutagenesis as described [32,33], utilizing the following primer pair 1 (fw-NheI-ENV; 5′-GTTAGTCATCGGAAT- ATTGAGATGGCTAGCGGTG-GGACGCCGG-3′ and rev-AscI-U3; 5′-CAGATCTCAGGCGCGCCGGTTCCTTATTGAGATGTC-TTCG-3′) and primer pair 2 (fw-AscI-AclI-U3, 5′-AATAAGGAACCGGCGCGCCTGAGATCTGTGTGTGACTACATTGAACGTT-GATGTATAACTAGAAGAATAAGATTAAG-3′ and rev-ApaI-U5; 5′-GACTCACTATAGGGCGAATTG-GGCCCTTGTTGTGACCTTCTCC-3′; all from Sigma). The final amplicon was generated in an independent PCR using both initial amplicons and primers fw-NheI-ENV and rev-ApaI-U5 and inserted using the unique NheI and ApaI sites.Mutagenesis resulted in the deletion of a 143 bp region encompassing the BFV miRNA cassette and insertion of unique AscI and AclI restriction sites conserving 5/15 bps. Replacement of the U3 region of the 5′ LTR by CMV-IE promoter sequences avoided recombination between the still intact miRNA cassette in the 5′ LTR and the 3′LTR in which the miRNA cassette sequences had been deleted. In BFV, miRNA deletion mutants carrying the authentic U3 sequence in the 5′LTR such as recombination events were in fact observed and enriched during extended passaging of such clones [34].

2.3. *Dual Luciferase Reporter Assays*

A total of 50 ng of each control or BFV dual-luciferase reporter (DLR) target plasmids was co-transfected with 500 ng of a pGEM3Z-based BFV-miRNA expression vector using Lipofectamine LTX or PEI into 24-well plates containing 10^5 BHK, HEK293T, or MDBK cells per well, which had been plated the previous day as previously described [14]. All transfections for DLR assays were done in duplicate and repeated at least once. At 48 h after transfection, lysates were harvested and renilla and firefly luciferase (Rluc and hluc) activities were measured in triplicate using a dual-luciferase reporter assay system (Promega, Walldorf, Germany) on a TD-20/20 luminometer (Turner Designs, San Jose, CA, USA). The ratio of the activities of RLuc linked to the BFV miRNA target sequences and hluc serving as an internal control was determined for each sample and normalized to the ratio for the parental psiCHECK2 vector.

2.4. *Target Gene Quantification*

Reverse transcription was performed using the QuantiTect Reverse Transcription Kit (Qiagen, Hilden, Germany). In brief, total RNA was extracted by TRIzol reagent as recommended by the supplier (Thermo Fisher Scientific). Then, 1 μL Quantiscript Reverse Transcriptase, 4 μL Quantiscript RT Buffer, and 1 μL RT Primer Mix were combined with 500 ng total RNA and incubated for 15 min at 42 °C. Samples were finally incubated for 3 min at 95 °C to inactivate the reverse transcriptase. Real-time PCR was performed by using the QuantiTect SYBR Green PCR Kit and LightCycler 480 Instrument I, and the reaction conditions were as follows: 95 °C pre-incubation and 40 cycles of 10 s at 95 °C, 40 s at 60 °C, and 1 min at 72 °C. The following primer pairs were used for bovine Ankrd17: fwd, 5′-GCGCGGTACCTATGGAGAAGGCGACGGTTCC-3′; rev, 5′-GCGCGCGGC-CGCTCAGCCAGCTGGTTCATATGCA-3′; bif1: fwd, 5′-TCCTTCCAACCTCAGT-GACCTT-3′; rev, 5′-TCATAGAGAACCCTGGCCTTTC-3′; IFN-beta: fwd, 5′-AAACTCATGAGCAGT-CTGCA-3′; rev, 5′-AAACTCATGAGCAGTCTGCA-3′; NF-kappaB: fwd, 5′-GAAATTCCTGATCCAGA-CAAAAAC-3′; rev, 5′-ATCACTTCAATGGCCTCTGTGTAG-3′; GAPDH: fwd, 5′-CGAGATCCCTCCA-AAATCAA-3′; rev, 5′-TTCACACCCATGACGAACAT-3′. Relative gene abundances were determined using the $\Delta\Delta CT$ method with GAPDH as the reference [35].

2.5. *In Silico Target Gene Prediction and Statistical Analyses*

BFV miRNA sequences were used as inputs for two online target prediction databases: miRanda (http://www.microrna.org/microrna/home.do, accessed on 10 August 2017) and TargetScan (http://www.targetscan.org, accessed on 10.8.2017). In order to increase the identification of meaningful miRNA target candidates, the use of more than one tool is recommended [36,37]. Using the miRanda and TargetScan miRNA prediction algorithms, the bovine *Bos tauris* genome was scanned for complementarity to the three stable BFV miRNAs miR-BF1-5p, miR-BF2-5p, and miR-BF1–3p [8]. TargetScan seems to be a more robust tool, because it enables a more complete search at the isoform level and penalizes the less conserved interactions, and its databases are the most up-to-date. For these reasons, TargetScan can predict the interactions with a higher probability of being biologically validated than the other tools. However, the algorithms used by miRanda (mirSVR score) can complement these prediction studies, as it takes additional biological parameters into consideration that remain interesting to verify. Only those potential target genes that were detected by both algorithms were selected and analyzed further. To reduce the number of hits to biologically meaningful and relevant target genes, the search was restricted to the 3′-untranslated regions (UTR) of the bovine target genes in line with general observation that miRNA target sites are mostly, but not exclusively, located in this region [3,38].

Data are expressed as the means ± standard deviations of the results of at least two independent experiments, in which each assay was performed in triplicate. Statistical analyses were conducted using the Welch's and Student's *T*-test using in-house and online resources (graphpad.com, accessed on 5 February 2018). p values of <0.05 were considered to be statistically significant.

2.6. Virological Methods

High titer cell-free transmitted BFV variants with and without the miRNA expression cassette were transfected into HEK293T cells and supernatants harvested two to four days after transfection as indicated. BFV titrations were done using serially diluted cell-free supernatants under spreading infection conditions with MICL reporter cells seeded at low cell density to allow repeated rounds of virus replication and multiplication. BFV infectivity was determined by quantification of viral foci and is expressed as focus-forming units/mL (FFU/mL) as described [28]. BFV infections with wt and miRNA-deficient BFV for reporter assays and expression studies were at multiplicities of infection (MOI) of 0.1 to 0.05, except otherwise stated. BFV particles released into the cell culture supernatant were enriched by sedimentation through a 20% (*w*/*v*) sucrose cushion in an SW41 rotor at 28,000 rpm for 2 h at 4 °C as described previously [28].

2.7. Protein Analysis by Immunoblotting

Cells and enriched virus particles were lysed in 1% SDS with protease inhibitor, mixed with 5× Reducing Sample Loading Buffer and denatured by heating at 95 °C for 5 min. Samples were loaded onto Novex 4–12% Bis-Tris polyacrylamide gradient gels run in Bolt Mini gel chambers in 1× MOPS buffer (Thermo Fisher Scientific) at 120 V for about 120 min. Proteins were transferred onto nitrocellulose membranes at 15 V for 1 hour in a Bolt Mini blotting chamber. Blots were further processed, and specifically bound antibodies were detected as described [28]. For detection of bovine ANKRD17 and Bif1, cross-reactive antisera PA5-46799 and PA5-15278 (Thermo Fisher Scientific), respectively, were used in addition to a polyclonal rabbit antiserum directed against human ANKRD17 kindly provided by Thomas Kufer, University of Hohenheim, Germany [20]. To detect BFV proteins, a rabbit anti Gag antiserum [28], a cross-reactive rabbit anti PFV integrase (IN) antiserum [39] (kindly provided by Dirk Lindemann, Dresden), and a serum pool from BFV-infected cattle [40] were used. Densitometric analyses were carried out using ImageJ software.

3. Results

3.1. In Silico Target Prediction and Ranking

Using the two online miRNA target site prediction algorithms "miRanda–mirSVR" and "TargetScan", the bovine *Bos tauris* genome was scanned for complementarity to the three stable BFV miRNAs miR-BF1-5p, miR-BF2-5p, and miR-BF1-3p [8]. Using the criteria based on the mean value of both algorithms as defined in Section 2.5, potential target genes for BF2-5p miRNA had scores between 100–95 out of 100 (Table 1). BF1-5p miRNA had combined scores of 80 out of 100 and less (52 out of 100 for hit #20), while scores for the 20 best hits for BF1-3p were even lower.

Table 1. In silico prediction of bovine target gene potentially affected by BFV miRNAs miR-BF1-5p, miR-BF1–3p, and miR-BF2-5p using the miRNA target site prediction tools "miRanda–mirSVR" and "TargetScan".

	miR-BF1-5p		miR-BF1-3p		miR-BF2-5p	
Target Rank	Target Score [1]	Gene Symbol	Target Score [1]	Gene Symbol	Target Score [1]	Gene Symbol
1	80	BCL7A	62	TMEM135	100	ANKRD17
2	73	DUSP4	58	PHF20	99	Bif1 (SH3GLB1)
3	67	BCKDHB	58	BRWD1	99	AFAP
4	64	LYPD1	51	SUN1	98	AK3
5	64	RAD23A	51	DUSP6	96	FLRT3
6	62	ANKRD26	50	PRKCI	96	ARL6IP1
7	62	GAPVD1	41	FAM234B	96	ADAMTSL3
8	59	PPP1R13B	37	PI4K2B	96	PTER
9	59	OOSP2	35	USP38	96	BTBD7
10	58	ZNF701	33	UBE2G1	96	MON2
11	57	ZMYND11	29	ZFP62	96	UTRN
12	56	MKI67	28	COL4A1	96	GABRA1
13	56	GCC2	28	ABL2	96	DGKI
14	55	ATCAY	27	PPP2CA	95	CTDSPL2
15	54	RGPD5	25	STARD13	95	TTC26
16	54	RGPD8	25	CDK19	95	ITPKC
17	54	RGPD6	25	ELOVL4	95	BMP2K
18	52	NCCRP1	25	SEL1L	95	SLC7A1
19	52	HR	23	SNX18	95	DPY19L4
20	52	PAQR8	21	ERMP1	95	ZMYM2

[1] Target scores are expressed as the mean values of the two algorithms used.

3.2. Importance of BFV miRNA Expression for Overall BFV Replication

The parental BFV Riems isolate used here was exclusively grown on primary bovine cells [41]. Recently, molecular clones of the wt BFV Riems and a BFV variant selected in vitro for a high titer (HT) replication and cell-free transmission phenotype in bovine MDBK cells were established and designated as pBFV-Riems34 and pBFV-MDBK-24 [28]. In each of these clones, the U3 promoter in the 5′LTR was replaced here by the highly efficient and constitutively active Cytomegalovirus immediate early (CMV-IE) promoter using standard cloning techniques yielding clones pCMV-BFV-Riems34 and pCMV-BFV-MDBK-24. Next, the complete miRNA cassette [8,19] was deleted by fusion PCR mutagenesis yielding clones pCMV-BFV-Riems-ΔmiRNA and pCMV-BFV-MDBK-ΔmiRNA.

To determine whether the BFV miRNAs have detectable effects on BFV replication in in vitro cultivated bovine cells, all four CMV-IE-based BFV genomes (wt pCMV-BFV-Riems 34, wt pCMV-BFV-Riems 34-ΔmiRNA, high titer pCMV-BFV-MDBK 24, and high titer pCMV-BFV-MDBK 24-ΔmiRNA) were transfected into HEK293T cells since transfection of the approx. 15 kbp large plasmids is highly inefficient using MDBK target cells. Cell-free virus supernatants were harvested two days after transfection and infectious titers were determined by titration in the MDBK cell-based MICL LTR-GFP reporter and titration cells under spreading infection conditions (Figure 1 and ref. [28]). The data clearly show that spreading infection of both miRNA deletion mutants was significantly reduced (10-fold titer downregulation compared to the corresponding intact clones) in bovine MICL/MDBK cells, which are known to be proficient in many innate and intrinsic immunity pathways.

Due to the heterologous CMV-IE promoter that replaces the authentic BFV U3 promoter in all constructs used here (see Section 2.2), even the highly-cell-associated BFV Riems isolate yielded cell-free infectivity [30,42].

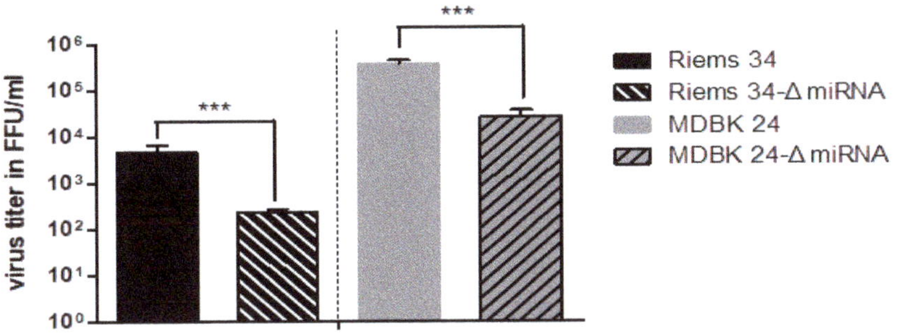

Figure 1. Deletion of the miRNA cassette results in reduced infectivity in bovine MICL reporter cells. Bar diagram of the virus titers (FFU/mL) expressed as number of GFP-positive focus forming units (FFU) from three independent experiments. Low-density MICL cells were infected with serially diluted wt virus (Riem 34 and MDBK 24) and the corresponding miRNA cassette deletion mutants (Riems 34-ΔmiRNA and MDBK 24-ΔmiRNA) originating from transfected HEK293T cells. Five days p.i., viral titers were determined by fluorescence microscopy of GFP-positive cell foci due to the BFV infection-mediated induction of GFP expression. Error bars are given and differences between titers of the wt and the ΔmiRNA mutant virus were analyzed by the Welch's *t*-test and found to be highly significant (***, $p < 0.001$).

3.3. Deletion of the miRNA Cassette Does Not Inhibit Particle Release and Gag and Pol Expression, Processing and Packaging

We next addressed the question whether deletion of the miRNA cassette alters BFV Gag and Pol expression and particle release and composition. For this purpose, each two sub-clones of high titer pCMV-BFV-MDBK 24 and pCMV-BFV-MDBK 24-ΔmiRNA genomes were transfected into HEK293T cells together with an EGFP expression plasmid confirming similar transfection efficacies. After two days, fully permissive MDBK cells were added to enhance virus yield and three days later, cells were harvested for protein analyses. Cell culture supernatants were used to enrich BFV particles by sucrose cushion sedimentation and to infect low-density MICL target cells at a MOI of 0.1. Five days after MICL cell infection and at a comparable degree of infection, cells and supernatants were again harvested for BFV protein analyses. In the transfected and co-cultured cells, HEK293T/MDBK cells, and the corresponding particles (Figure 2), BFV p71 Gag and p127 Pol, precursor protein expression and processing into p68 Gag and the mature p44 IN were comparable between the BFV variants with and without the miRNA cassette. Preparations of released BFV particles contained both cleaved and uncleaved Gag and Pol proteins at comparable concentrations. The BFV-infected MICL cells and the corresponding BFV particle preparations harvested five days p.i. gained results similar to those from the transfected and co-cultured HEK293T and MDBK cells (Figure 2 and Supplementary Figure S1A). However, under the spreading infection conditions in the infected MICL cell cultures, the two independent miRNA-deficient BFV clones showed attenuated replication, which led to slightly lower protein levels in infected cell lysates and released particle preparations. However, Gag and Pol protein processing were comparable. Since FV Gag and Pol protein processing are considered to depend on proper particle formation and Pol protein encapsidation via packaged RNA genomes [43], weconclude that deletion of the BFV miRNA cassette did not detectably affect these processes under either condition. When transfected HEK293T cells were not co-cultivated with MDBK cells, but analyzed four days after transfection, similar data on overall particle release were obtained (Supplementary Figure S1B). All experiments contained duplicates and were done once.

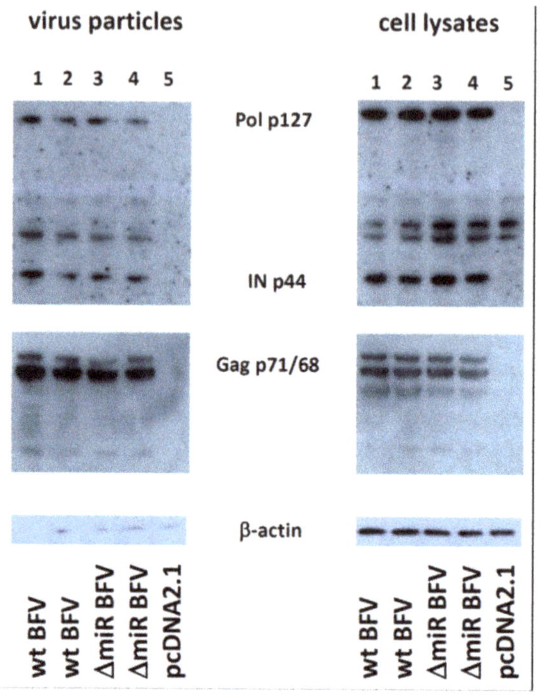

Figure 2. Deletion of the miRNA cassette neither affects BFV Gag and Pol expression and processing nor BFV particle release and composition in transfected and MDBK-co-cultured HEK293T cells. Each two sub-clones of plasmids encoding high titer pCMV-BFV-MDBK 24 (wt BFV) and pCMV-BFV-MDBK 24-ΔmiRNA (ΔmiR BFV) and the pcDNA2.1 control plasmid were transfected into HEK293T cells together with an EGFP expression plasmid using the PEI method. Two days later, MDBK cells were added and three days later, cells were harvested for protein analyses. Cell culture supernatants were used to enrich BFV particles by sucrose cushion sedimentation. Each 15 μg of cell lysates and regular aliquots of enriched particles were subjected to immunoblotting (as given above the panels) using a cross-reactive rabbit anti PFV IN antiserum [39] (top panels) and a serum pool from BFV-infected cattle (middle panels). The BFV-specific proteins detected are labeled between the panels. A directly conjugated antibody against β-actin served as the loading control (bottom panels).

3.4. *Importance of the BF2-5p miRNA for BFV Replication*

Since miR-BF2-5p constitutes the most abundant miRNA in BFV-infected cells [8] and bioinformatics revealed very high target gene identification scores, we propose that this miRNA has a major impact on the BFV life cycle and virus–host interactions. We thus determined whether the differences in titers in bovine MICL target cells were due to the loss of miRNA expression or whether it is a secondary effect unrelated to the miRNAs but due to the unintended deletion of other important functions. For this purpose, miRNA trans-complementation studies using a mimic of the miR-BF2-5p with enhanced stability and identical sequence, together with a scrambled negative control oligonucleotide of the same length, were used in co-transfection studies as described [19] To additionally analyze whether the miRNAs function early or late during BFV infection, MICL cells were first infected with serial dilutions of the cell culture supernatants from pCMV-BFV-Riems 34-ΔmiRNA and high titer cell-free pCMV-BFV-MDBK 24-ΔmiRNA-transfected HEK293T cells. Six h after infection with serially diluted supernatants of the different BFV variants, cells were transfected with the miR-BF2-5p mimic and a negative control miRNA (Figure 3A). Alternatively, MICL cells were first transfected with the miR-BF2-5p mimic and the control miRNA. Approximately 6 h after transfection, the cells were infected with serial dilutions of virus supernatants from pCMV-BFV-Riems 34-ΔmiRNA and high titer cell-free pCMV-BFV-MDBK 24-ΔmiRNA-transfected HEK293T cells (Figure 3B). At four days p.i., the MICL reporter cells were screened for signs of spreading infection as indicated by infection-induced GFP fluorescence. For both BFV miRNA-deficient variants, the co-transfection of the mimic BF2-5p miRNA reproducibly increased the virus titer ten-fold over the control (Figure 3A,B). Furthermore, there was no significant titer difference between the 'infection-first' and 'transfection-first' assays. These data demonstrate that miR-BF2-5p plays an important role in BFV replication, significantly increasing virus spread and infectivity when provided 6 h before and after infection. At the same concentration, an inhibitor of miR-BF2-5p that acts as a sponge to bind and neutralize its target miRNA did not show any effect on the miRNA-containing parental BFV Riems and its high titer variant [44]. This may have been due to the fact that its concentration was too low to neutralize the highly abundant BF2-5p miRNA or that we did not replenish the inhibitor over the incubation period. In addition, the specific expression strategy of the BFV miRNAs and/or the presence of substantial amounts or pri-miRNA in BFV-infected cells (see Figure 4 in reference [8]) may have negatively affected the functions of the inhibitor miRNA.

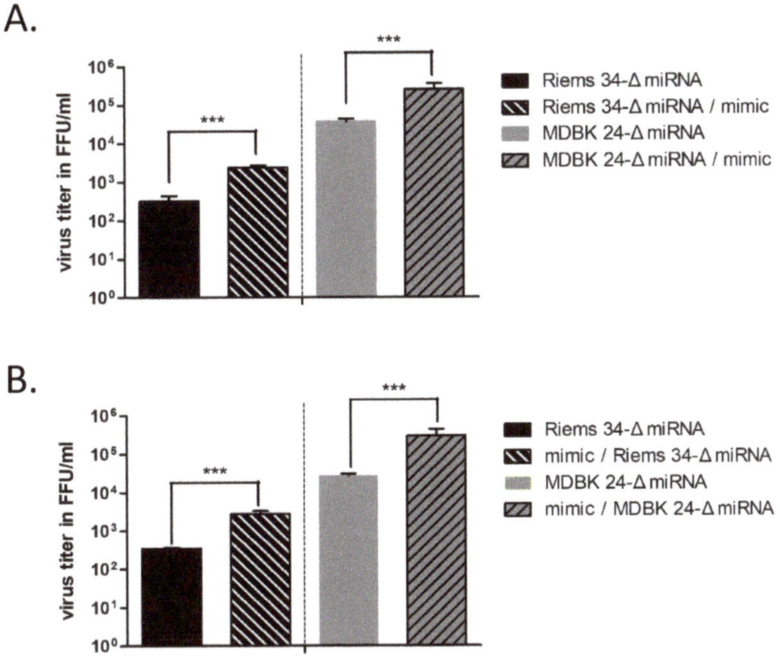

Figure 3. Trans-complementation of miRNA-deficient BFV with miR-BF2-5p restores BFV titers in bovine MICL cells. Bar diagrams of the virus titers (FFU/mL) and the number of GFP-positive focus forming units from three independent experiments. (**A**) MICL cells were infected first with serially diluted miRNA cassette deletion mutants (BFV-Riems 34-ΔmiRNA and BFV-MDBK 24-ΔmiRNA). Six h after infection, the corresponding miR-BF2-5p mimic and negative control were transfected. (**B**) MICL cells were transfected first with the miR-BF2-5p mimic and negative control. Six h after transfection, the cell were infected with serially diluted miRNA cassette deletion mutants (BFV-Riems 34-ΔmiRNA and BFV-MDBK 24-ΔmiRNA). At 4 day p.i., viral titers were determined in both experiments by fluorescence microscopy. Error bars for the titers determined are given and differences between titers of the viruses trans-complemented with the BF2-5p mimic and control miRNA were analyzed by the Welch's *t*-test (***, $p < 0.001$).

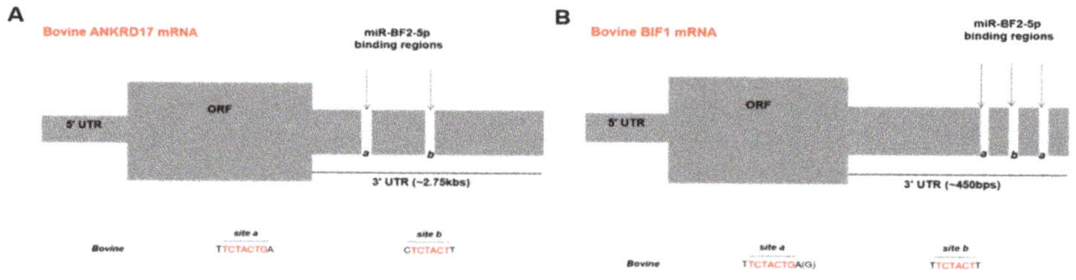

Figure 4. MiR-BF2-5p binding site prediction within ANKRD17 (panel **A**) and Bif1 (panel **B**). The overall bovine ANKRD17 and Bif1 genes consist of 5′UTR, the open reading frame (ORF), and the 3′UTR. Based on sequence complementarity analysis, two possible binding sites (a and b) were identified in the 3′UTR of ANKRD17 starting 85 and 448 nt downstream of the stop codon (**A**), the sequences which are complementary to the seed sequence of miR-BF2-5p, are shown in red. For Bif1 (**B**), three possible binding sites (a-b-a) were found in the 3′UTR, starting 217, 245, and 284 nt downstream of the stop codon, the sequences which are complementary to the seed sequence of miR-BF2-5p are shown in red.

The specificity and absence of significant off-target effects of the BFV miR-BF2-5p mimic, control, and inhibitor (for details see Section 2.1) used throughout the current study were confirmed in one control experiment (with duplicates) using the two high-score target genes encoding for ANKRD17 and Bif1 (Supplementary Figure S2). Importantly, the gene-specific controls presented here do not rule out additional and potentially genome-wide off target effects as known to occur when conducting corresponding functional miRNA analyses [45].

3.5. *In Vitro Validation of ANKRD17 and Bif1 as Direct Targets of miR-BF2-5p*

Data mining of the literature of the high score BF2-5p mRNA targets and potential links to innate immunity and virus replication identified several interesting candidate genes. Among them, the human gene ANKRD17 (ankyrin repeat domain 17) is a regulator of NOD/RLR-mediated inflammatory responses and DNA replication [20], while Bif1 (Bax-interacting factor 1, also designated SH3 domain-containing GRB2-like endophilin B1, SH3GLB1 or ZBTB24) is involved in autophagy and apoptosis-induced virus elimination [24,25]. Since only a few antibodies specifically raised against bovine proteins have been available, we screened several bovine candidate proteins for cross-reactive and commercially available antisera against human or mice counterparts [44]. Based on this survey, target gene validation was performed for bovine ANKRD17 and Bif1.

For validation of ANKRD17 and Bif1 as direct targets of BFV miR-BF2-5p, in silico binding site predictions were performed. The whole mRNA sequences of bovine ANKRD17 (NM_001192181.2, NCBI) and Bif1 (NM_001077993.2, NCBI) were acquired and then the miR-BF2-5p (especially the seed sequences that are important for base-pairing with complementary sequences on the target mRNAs) were aligned with ANKRD17 and Bif1 mRNAs. Using this approach, two potential binding/target sites for miR-BF2-5p were identified inside the 3′UTR region of ANKRD17 (Figure 4A), while three potential binding/target sites for miR-BF2-5p were discovered inside the 3′UTR region of Bif1. Two of the BF2-5p miRNA binding sites inside the 3′UTR region of Bif1 were almost identical (Figure 4B, designated site a with variant flanking sequences).

To verify that miR-BF2-5p can target the predicted binding sites, the subgenomic sequence, which contains the two predicted binding sites in the ANKRD17 3′UTR and the three predicted binding sites in the 3′UTR of Bif1, were amplified via PCR, cloned into the reporter plasmid psiCHECK2, and named psiCHECK2-ANKRD17-original (A.Ori) and psiCHECK2-Bif1-original (B.Ori). The corresponding scrambled target sequence, which is no longer complementary to miR-BF2-5p, were also cloned into the reporter plasmid and named psiCHECK2-ANKRD17-scrambled (A.Scr) and psiCHECK2-Bif1-scrambled (B.Scr).

Then, plasmids pCMV-BFV-MDBK24, pCMV-BFV-MDBK24-ΔmiRNA, and empty plasmid pCR-XL-Topo were transfected into HEK293T cells and 48 h after transfection, BFV, and mock cell culture supernatants were harvested. Each four cultures of MDBK and BoMac cells were infected with normalized amounts of virus supernatants and 2 days p.i., the reporter plasmids A.Ori (Figure 5, panel A) and B.Ori (Figure 5, panel B) were transfected into the infected cells. As the control, two cultures each were mock infected but transfected as above. Twenty-four hours post transfection, the cells were harvested for the dual luciferase reporter (DLR) assay. The normalized DLR readouts showed that in both bovine cell lines, a significant downregulation of Rluc activity in the wt BFV infection group occurred. In contrast, no changes of Rluc activity in the ΔmiRNA BFV infection group and the mock-infected sample were detectable (Figure 5). The data demonstrate that the miR-BF2-5p expressed by the wt BFV virus can target the predicted binding sites within the 3′UTR of ANKRD17 and Bif1.

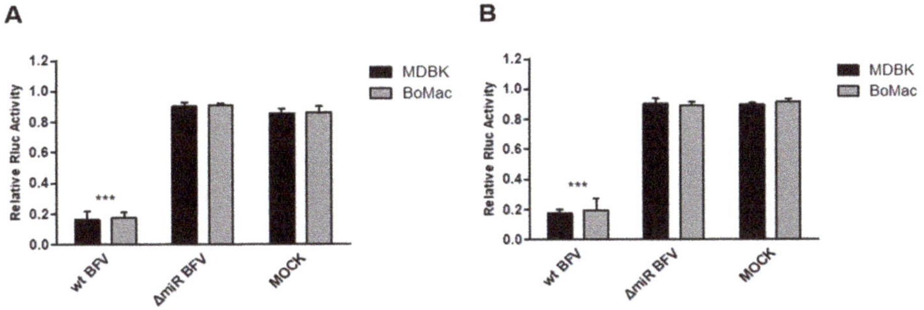

Figure 5. Binding efficacy of miR-BF2-5p and ANKRD17 (**A**) and Bif1 (**B**) target sequences in BFV-infected cells. MDBK and BoMac cells (as given) were infected with high-titer BFV-MDBK24 (wt BFV) and miRNA-deficient BFV-MDBK24 (ΔmiRNA) at a MOI of 0.1 or cell culture medium was added (MOCK). Two days p.i., the reporter plasmids psiCHECK2-ANKRD17-original (A.Ori, panel A) and psiCHECK2-Bif1-original (B.Ori, panel B) were transfected into the cells. At 24 h post-transfection, cell lysates were harvested and analyzed for the suppression of Rluc activity in standard DLR assays as described. Normalized luciferase data (Renilla versus firefly luciferase activity) are presented as bar diagrams of three independent experiments. Differences between treated and control groups (MOCK) were analyzed by the Welch's *t*-test (***, $p < 0.001$).

To confirm that BF2-5p in fact induces suppression of target constructs in BFV-infected cells, a stable mimic of the miR-BF2-5p with enhanced stability and identical sequence together with a scrambled negative control oligonucleotide of the same length were used in co-transfection studies as described [19]. These RNA oligonucleotides together with the two ANKRD17 and Bif1 reporter plasmids (original and scrambled) were co-transfected into HEK293T, MDBK, and BoMac cells in the following four combinations for each target gene (Figure 6A,B): A.Scr/B.Scr reporter plus miR-BF2-5p mimic RNA oligonucleotide; A.Ori/B.Ori reporter plus miR-BF2-5p mimic oligonucleotide; A.Scr/B.Scr reporter plus mimic negative control (mimic NC) oligonucleotide; and A.Ori/B.Ori plus mimic NC. At 24 h post-transfection, cells were harvested for DLR analyses. Transfection of three different cell lines showed significant Rluc activity suppression only for the combination of A.Ori/B.Ori plus miR-BF2-5p mimic, while all other combinations did not result in target gene suppression. These data demonstrate that the miR-BF2-5p mimic specifically targets the predicted binding sites within the 3′UTR of the bovine ANKRD17 and Bif1 genes, leading to their specific suppression (Figure 6).

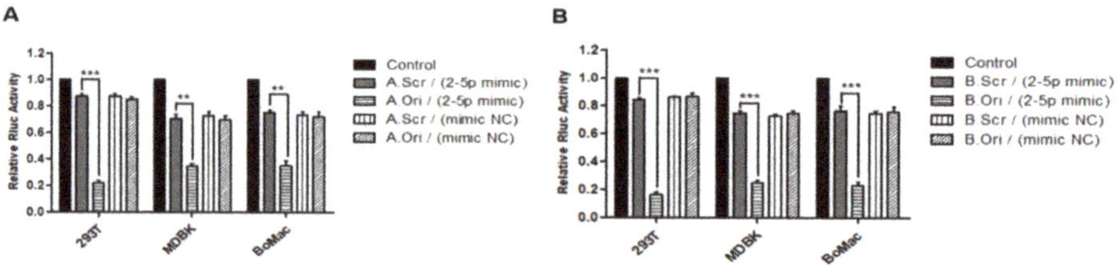

Figure 6. Binding efficacy of miR-BF2-5p mimic and the target sequences in the 3′UTR of bovine ANKRD17 (**A**) and Bif1 (**B**). HEK293T, MDBK, and BoMac cells were transfected with four reporter plasmid/RNA oligonucleotide combinations (letters A and B refer to the ANKRD17 and Bif1 target genes and suffixes Ori and Scr refer to original (wild-type) and scrambled (non-functional control) target sequences, respectively): A.Scr/B.Scr plus miR-BF2-5p mimic (A.Scr/B.Scr (2–5p mimic)); A.Ori/B.Ori plus miR-BF2-5p mimic (A.Ori/B.Ori (2–5p mimic)); A.Scr/B.Scr plus mimic NC (A.Scr/B.Scr (mimic NC)); A.Ori/B.Ori plus mimic NC (A.Ori/B.Ori (mimic NC)). In addition, the empty DLR report plasmid was used as control (black bars). At 24 h post transfection, cell lysates were harvested and analyzed for the suppression of Rluc activity in standard DLR assays as described. Normalized luciferase data (Renilla versus firefly luciferase activity) are presented as bar diagrams of three independent experiments. Differences between treated groups and MOCK or Control groups were analyzed by the Welch's *t*-test (***, $p < 0.001$; **, $p < 0.01$).

To determine whether miR-BF2-5p can suppress the steady state mRNA levels of bovine ANKRD17 (Figure 7A) and Bif1 (Figure 7B), the mimic, the U6 promoter driven BFV miRNA expression vector pBS-U6-BFVmiRNA (4G, [19]) and the corresponding controls were transfected into MDBK cells. In parallel, a second group of MDBK cells was infected with wt BFV-MDBK24 and ΔmiRNA BFV-MDBK24 (MOI of about 0.1). After three days, cells from both experiments (transfection and infections) were harvested and total RNAs extracted for qRT-PCR analyses. The results indicat a moderate but significant suppression of the corresponding bovine mRNA levels for ANKRD17 and Bif1 only in MDBK cells expressing or containing miR-BF2-5p (mimic, U6-cassette, wt BFV infected) (Figure 7). The findings demonstrate that miR-BF2-5p specifically targets ANKRD17 and Bif1 mRNAs and causes moderate but significant suppressions of the steady state mRNA levels. The transfected miRNA species did not lead to gross changes of the transfected cells [44].

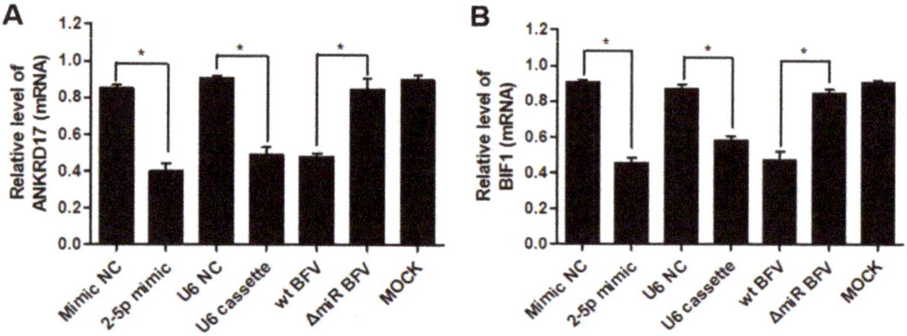

Figure 7. Validation of ANKRD17 (**A**) and Bif1 (**B**) mRNAs as direct targets of miR-BF2-5p. MDBK cells were transfected with miR-BF2-5p mimic and mimic NC (negative control), or U6 promoter driven cassette and U6 promoter empty plasmid (NC), or infected with wt BFV-MDBK24 and ΔmiRNA BFV-MDBK24. After three days, transfected, infected, and untreated cells (MOCK) were harvested and RNA was extracted for qRT-PCR analysis. Expression data normalized relative to GAPDH RNA are shown as bar diagrams of three independent experiments. Differences between treated groups and MOCK or negative control groups were analyzed by the Welch's *t*-test (*, $p < 0.05$).

To analyze whether miR-BF2-5p also suppresses steady-state ANKRD17 (Figure 8A) and Bif1 (Figure 8B) protein levels, the mimic, the U6 promoter driven cassette expression vector pBS-U6-BFVmiRNA (4G), and the corresponding controls were transfected into MDBK cells. In parallel, a second group of MDBK cells was infected with wt BFV-MDBK24 and ΔmiRNA BFV-MDBK24 at a MOI of about 0.1. After three days, total cellular protein lysates were harvested from all samples and identical amounts of protein were subjected to western blot analyses. The results showed, in both experiments (transfections and infections), a strong decrease in the ANKRD17 and Bif1 protein levels (Figure 8A,B) in MDBK cells expressing or containing miR-BF2-5p (mimic, U6-cassette, wt BFV infected). Densitometric analyses revealed about 5-fold decreases of ANKRD17 by co-transfection of the BF2-5p mimic and the U6-based miRNA expression construct and a 20-fold decreases by superinfection with wt BFV compared to the corresponding controls. Bif1 levels were reduced between 12- to 17-fold by the corresponding BFV miRNA treatment while a two-fold decline was seen in this experiment by infection with the miRNA-deficient BFV variant. The experiment demonstrates via different approaches that miR-BF2-5p significantly and specifically targets and decreases steady state protein levels of the 75kD ANKRD17 splice variant and the intact, full-length Bif1 protein. Consistent with the function of miRNAs mainly at the translational level [3,26], target protein levels were much more affected than those of the corresponding mRNAs (see Figure 7).

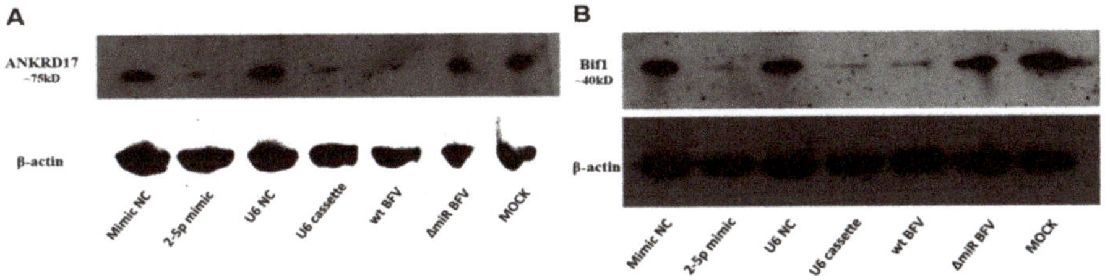

Figure 8. Validation of steady-state protein levels of ANKRD17 (**A**) and Bif1 (**B**) as direct targets of miR-BF2-5p. MDBK cells were transfected with miR-BF2-5p mimic and mimic NC (negative control), or U6 promoter driven cassette and U6 promoter empty plasmid (NC), or infected with wt BFV-MDBK24 and ΔmiRNA BFV-MDBK24. After three days, the transfected and infected cells were harvested and protein was extracted for western blotting. The expression of β-actin was monitored as a control for proper protein loading. In this blot representing one out of two experiments, the 75 kDa splice variant of bovine ANKRD17 and the full-length 40 kDa Bif1 proteins were specifically detected using antibodies as described in Section 2.7.

Overall, the various complementing analyses fully validate bovine ANKRD17 and Bif1 as direct targets of the BFV miR-BF2-5p.

3.6. MiR-BF2-5p Suppresses Expression of Innate Immunity Genes as Predicted Downstream Targets of ANKRD17

Based on the data that ANKRD17 is an upstream regulator in innate immunity [20–23], the role of miR-BF2-5p in host cell innate immunity, specifically in pro-inflammatory signaling via interferon-beta (IFN-β) and nuclear factor kappaB (NF-κB), was evaluated. BoMac cells were infected with wt BFV-MDBK24 and ΔmiRNA BFV-MDBK24 at a MOI of about 0.1 and 2 d p.i., the miR-BF2-5p inhibitor RNA oligonucleotide and negative control (inhibitor NC) were transfected into the cells infected with intact BFV-MDBK24, in parallel, the miR-BF2-5p mimic and negative control (mimic NC) were transfected into the cells infected with miRNA-deficient BFV-MDBK24. Cells were harvested and total RNA was extracted for qRT-PCR analyses 48 h after transfection. The results showed a significant upregulation of IFN-β and NF-κB mRNA levels (Figure 9A,B) for wt and miRNA-deficient BFV-infected and transfected cells compared to mock-treated cells. In wt BFV-infected BoMac cells, the inhibitor of miR-BF2-5p led to a further increase in IFN-β and NF-κB mRNA levels, which was not seen when the corresponding control miRNA was co-transfected. Furthermore, in ΔmiRNA BFV-MDBK24-infected cells, steady state mRNA levels for IFN-β and NF-κB were further enhanced. Co-transfection of the miR-BF2-5p mimic resulted in decreased IFN-β levels while NF-κB levels were not suppressed. Again, transfection of the different miRNAs did not detectably affect cell viability or led to aberrant changes of the analyzed target mRNAs. The results presented here suggest that BFV miR-BF2-5p suppresses cellular pro-inflammatory signaling by IFN-β and NF-κB, which had been increased by BFV infection. The lack of complementarity of the miRNA mimic and inhibitor studies in panel B may be due to different efficacies of the transfected miRNAs or different kinetics of gene activation versus miRNA-induced suppression (see also Section 4).

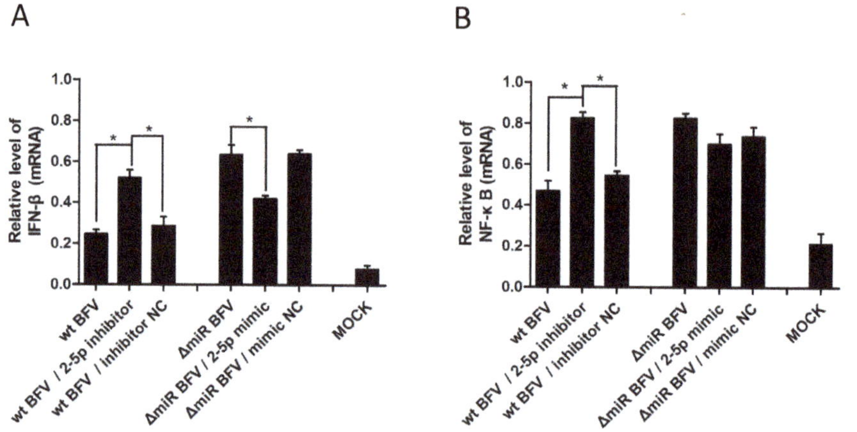

Figure 9. Suppression of pro-inflammatory signaling via IFN-β (**A**) and NF-κB by (**B**) miR-BF2-5p. BoMac cells were infected with wt BFV-MDBK24 and 2 d p.i. transfected with miR-BF2-5p inhibitor and inhibitor negative control (NC) RNA oligonucleotides. In parallel, another group of BoMac cells were infected with ΔmiRNA BFV-MDBK24 and 2 d p.i. transfected with miR-BF2-5p mimic and mimic NC RNA oligonucleotides. At 48 h after transfection, cells were harvested and total RNA was extracted for qRT-PCR analyses, testing the expression level of IFN-β and NF-κB, respectively. Expression data normalized relative to GAPDH RNA are shown as bar diagrams of three independent experiments. For comparison, the relative and GAPDH-normalized expression levels of IFN-β and NF-κB of untreated BoMac cells are given (MOCK). Differences between treated groups and MOCK or negative control groups were analyzed by the Welch's *T*-test (*, $p < 0.05$).

3.7. Kinetics of ANKRD17 and Bif1 Suppression during Productive BFV Infection of MDBK and BoMac Cells

In a final experiment, the kinetics of miR-BF2-5p target gene expression/suppression during low-density BFV infection of BoMac and MDBK cells were analyzed. Cells were infected with wt BFV-MDBK24 (at a MOI of about 0.1) and mock-infected and harvested at 1, 2, 3, and 4 d p.i. for immunoblot analyses (Figure 10). Steady state levels of the BFV miRNA target proteins were determined by densitometry and normalized to β-actin levels. The changes in protein levels in this experiment relative to 1 d after mock- and BFV-infection of bovine BoMac and MDBK cells is shown in the table below the blots.

Importantly, in both bovine target cells, levels of ANKRD17 and, to a lesser degree, Bif1 increased over time in non-infected cells (lanes 1 to 4 and 9 to 12). These increases in steady state levels of both proteins were either strongly or even completely (ANKRD17) or only moderately (Bif1) abrogated in BFV-infected cells. The data indicate a complex relationship between cell growth and BFV infection-induced changes in target protein levels.

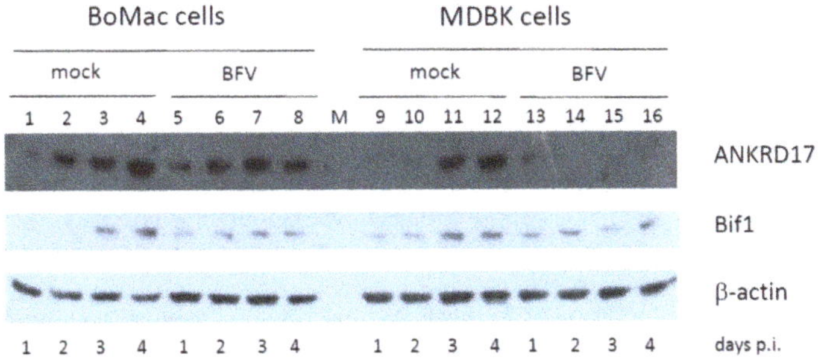

	1 d	2 d	3 d	4 d	1 d p.i.	2 d p.i.	3 d p.i.	4 d p.i.
	mock-infected BoMac cells				BFV-infected BoMac cells			
ANKRD17	1	14.40	14.86	25.82	1	2.07	2.39	2.71
Bif1	1	7.60	51.38	105.94	1	1.50	1.65	1.74
	mock-infected MDBK cells				BFV-infected MDBK cells			
ANKRD17	1	1.16	5.9	10.85	1	0.14	0.23	0.17
Bif1	1	1.21	2.66	2.73	1	1.47	0.67	1.32

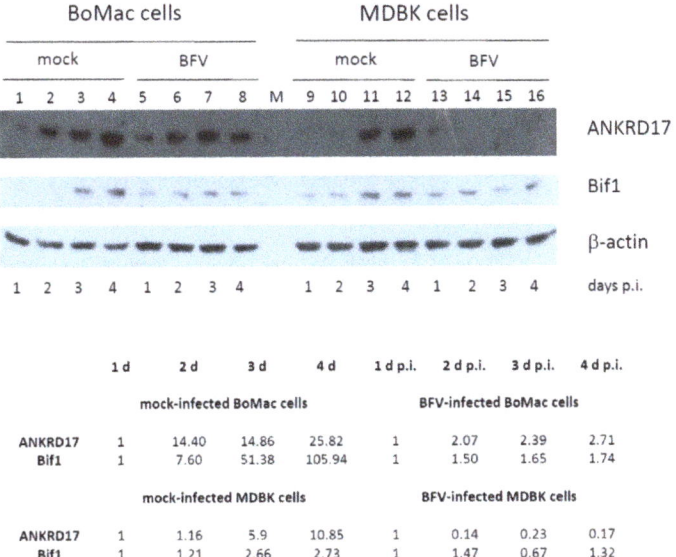

Figure 10. Kinetics of ANKRD17 and Bif1 steady state levels in BFV-infected and mock-infected BoMac (lanes 1 to 8) and MDBK cells (lanes 9 to 16). Sub-confluent BoMac and MDBK cells were either mock-infected (lanes 1 to 4 and 9 to 12) or infected with wt BFV-MDBK24 at a MOI of approximately 0.1 (lanes 5 to 8 and 13 to 16) and harvested 1, 2, 3, and 4 p.i. (as indicated below the blots). Identical amounts of protein were loaded and β-actin expression was monitored for proper protein loading (bottom panel). In this blot, the 75kDa splice variant of bovine ANKRD17 (top panel) was detected using the antiserum provided by T. Kufer and the full-length 40 kDa Bif1 protein was detected using the commercially available antiserum (middle panel). The bands specific for the 75 kDa ANKRD17 form and the 40 kDa Bif and 42 kDa β-actin are shown. Below the blots, the steady state protein levels were determined by densitometry, normalized to β-actin levels, and expression levels are displayed relative to the 1 d mock- and BFV-infected BoMac and MDBK cell values.

4. Discussion

The data presented here show that the miRNA cassette encoded by a distinct region of the U3 sequence of the BFV LTR is important for efficient virus replication in vitro in immortalized bovine cells. The deletion of the about 150 nt-long miRNA cassette in the U3 part of the LTR does not overlap with BFV proteins or BFV Tas response elements or other known cis-acting elements implicated in BFV replication [42,46]. The miRNA deletion can be almost completely complemented in vitro in trans by providing the major BFV miRNA, BF2-5p. This experiment strongly implies that the gross deletion of the miRNA cassette does not affect essential elements at a detectable level and that BF2-5p is of prime importance, at least in vitro, in immortalized bovine cells. This conclusion is also supported by in silico predictions of potential BFV miRNA targets in the bovine genome: for BF2-5p, a high number of high-score target genes was identified while only a few promising targets were found for the second-most abundant miRNA, BF1-5p, whilst the other BFV miRNA yielded no high-score targets.

In addition, the deletion of the complete miRNA cassette from the BFV genome did not detectably impair BFV Gag and Pol expression and processing as detected by analyzing transfected HEK293T and bovine MDBK cells and enriched BFV particles. Proper Gag and Pol processing in particles (and cell lysates) strongly argues for proper genome encapsidation since genome-mediated packaging of Pol into forming FV capsids is considered a necessary prerequisite for Gag and Pol processing by the FV protease [43]. The presence of uncleaved Pol proteins in the particle preparations of the in vitro selected BFV variant with high titer cell-free transmission phenotype may either reflect an impaired adaptation to this novel phenotype in this BFV variant independent of the presence or absence of the miRNA expression cassette. Alternatively, the selected BFV cell-free variants may correspond in this respect to PFV, where unprocessed Pol is also present in purified particle preparations dissimilar to the situation in feline FV (FFV), where unprocessed Pol is undetectable in enriched particle preparations [47,48].

For our proof of concept study on the function and relevance of the potential target genes, we had to focus on those bovine genes where reagents for immune-detection were available. In addition, we intentionally narrowed down to those genes with a known link to virus infection and replication and innate, intrinsic, and adaptive immunity in humans, mice, cattle, and other mammals. For these reasons, bovine Bif1 and ANKRD17 were subjected to in vitro studies on whether they are direct targets of the high-abundant BF2-5p miRNA. The data clearly confirm that both genes are in fact direct targets of this BFV miRNA in immortalized bovine cells. The BF2-5p miRNA effects on the overall levels of the target mRNAs was in both cases modest, but statistically significant. In contrast, Bif1 and ANKRD17 protein levels were substantially suppressed by the miRNA, either expressed from the BFV provirus, an U6 RNA Pol-III expression plasmid, or provided as an miRNA mimic compared to the corresponding controls lacking the miRNA cassette or the control mimic RNA sequence. The quantitatively different effects of the BF2-5p miRNA on target gene mRNA and protein levels are in line with the concept that miRNAs act mostly by suppressing protein translation [3,38].

ANKRD17 is implicated to have an important role in the control and regulation of NOD1 and NOD2 inflammatory immune signaling and thus the restriction and control of virus replication [20–23]. Aside from their function as direct pattern recognition receptors for bacterial peptidoglycans, NOD1 and NOD2 also act as signaling molecules involved in the regulation of inflammation and immunity [49]. ANKRD17 has been shown to physically interact with viral structural and non-structural proteins, however, the functional importance of these interactions is unknown [50,51]. Innate immunity appears to play an important role in controlling FV infections but its role in BFV is almost not understood [52–55]. Thus, potential downstream target genes of ANKRD17 were analyzed for their response toward BF2-5p miRNA expression. Analysis of the effect of BF2-5p on IFN-β and NF-κB RNA levels in vitro showed significant suppression of both potential target mRNAs. Extension of these miRNA studies by inclusion of other downstream targets, the analysis of mRNA and protein steady state levels as well as the effects on immune signaling in vivo and in vitro appears worth doing.

A link between Bif1 and virus replication is suggested by its function in autophagy, which may increase or decrease virus replication [56,57]. In PFV, autophagic flux is increased in infected cells and may result in reduced innate immune signaling [58,59]. However, PFV has suffered severe deletions in the U3 and may thus not or no longer be capable of expressing the authentic repertoire of miRNAs [60]. For time and resource reasons, functional studies have not been done for downstream targets of Bif1, but would be highly desirable in the future.

Due to the basic lack of reagents and a limited understanding of the bovine system compared to the much more intensively studied men or mice, several questions were not easy to study and have therefore not been addressed. For instance, the function(s) of ANKRD17 are currently not fully understood in humans and mice, and details on its function in innate immunity are scant. In addition, validated reporter constructs for immune signaling studies are rare or difficult to obtain. For bovines, no details on alternative splicing and alternative protein forms as described for human ANKRD17 are available. This situation, for instance, prevented trans-complementation studies to elucidate the mechanism of how ANKRD17 interferes with BFV replication. In addition, we do not have detailed information on the kinetics of innate (and adaptive) immune signaling in bovines, and therefore, we may have missed some of the downstream responses since we had simply sampled at the wrong time points. As shown here, the concentrations of ANKRD17 and Bif1 increased during cultivation of mock-treated cells. These increases are suppressed in BFV-infected cells during ongoing virus replication (Figure 10) and thus, steady-state protein levels of both BFV miRNA targets are probably the result of antagonistic effects on their steady-state levels.

Since the RNA Pol III-directed dumbbell-shaped pri-miRNAs cassettes of FVs represent a completely new way of miRNA biogenesis, conventional methods and reagents to study miRNA functions may or may not be appropriate for studying BFV miRNAs. For instance, the very high expression levels of individual BFV miRNAs and the pri-miRNA precursor in persistently infected cells in vitro are not known in other systems [8]. Thus, standard concentrations for transfected miRNA mimics, controls, and/or inhibitors may not be appropriate for BFV. To address this question, we determined whether increased amounts of transfected miRNA inhibitors further recover steady state levels of the identified target proteins in BFV-infected cells. As shown in Supplementary Figure S3, increased amounts of the co-transfected miRNA inhibitor did not further relieve protein suppression, but even appeared to increase suppression.

Finally, experimental inconsistencies and unexpected results related to the use and overexpression of mimic and inhibitor miRNAs may also be due to a "transcriptional override" in complex and currently unresolved regulatory networks [45]. Analyses in other bovine cell types including primary cells or ex vivo analyses would allow better definition of the BFV miRNA functions. The fact that the BFV Riems isolate used in this study was exclusively grown on bovine cells proficient in innate immunity may have, however, contributed to the success of this study. These and other points have to be taken carefully into account before starting future experiments.

Whether BFV miRNAs may have additional functions independent of the posttranscriptional control of cellular gene expression is currently unknown, but taking their high intracellular concentrations in chronically BFV-infected cells into account, this appears possible. The high intracellular concentrations of miR-BF1-5p and miR-BF2-5p [8] may be a prerequisite (or at least an advantage) for extracellular functions (e.g., in the form of free or exosome-associated miRNAs with local or systemic effects) [61]. For instance, it has recently been shown that under conditions of bacterial sepsis, the extracellular form of the murine and human miR-130b-3p is released into the blood and interacts, thereby attenuating the pro-inflammatory function of CIRP (cold-inducible RNA binding protein), a ligand of TLR4-mediated innate inflammatory signaling [62,63].

The data presented here are in line with the miRNA function of oncogenic BLV during in vitro and in vivo infections where deletion of the miRNAs did not abrogate virus replication [64,65]. Unfortunately, the BFV miRNA target genes predicted and validated in this study do not overlap with genes affected by BFV infection of BoMac in vitro, as published recently [55].

In summary, we demonstrate here for the first time that the FV miRNAs play a role during virus replication in vitro, however, more in vitro and especially in vivo studies are required to fully understand their functions for BFV biology and the underlying mechanisms used.

Supplementary Materials: The following are available online at http://www.mdpi.com/1999-4915/12/11/1250/s1, Supplementary Figure S1: Deletion of the miRNA cassette does neither affect BFV Gag and Pol expression and processing nor BFV particle release and composition in infected MICL cells. Supplementary Figure S2: Specificity control for miR-BF2-5p mimic, negative control and inhibitor miRNAs. Supplementary Figure S3: No further increase in protein levels by increased amounts of inhibitor miRNAs in acutely BFV-infected cells.

Author Contributions: W.C. co-designed the study and planned and conducted the in vitro experiments and in silico analyses; A.H.-M. conducted and supported the in silico analyses; A.H.-W. supervised all in silico analyses and data analyses; E.S., G.P., and A.H. supported, finalized, and continued the in vitro work of W.C.; M.M.-K. and J.K. contributed to the design of the study, data evaluation, and interpretation, and reviewed the manuscript; M.L. planned and initiated the study, supervised the in vitro analyses, evaluated data, and wrote the manuscript. Parts of this study have been already been published in the PhD thesis of W.C. and the master's theses of A.H.-M. and E.S. All authors have read and agreed to the published version of the manuscript.

Funding: Work at DKFZ by W.C. E.S. and A.H-M. was supported by the research SID 49 by the Baden-Württemberg Stiftung to M.L. and A.H.-W.

Acknowledgments: We thank Lutz Gissmann and Frank Rösl for continuous and generous support; Rui Cao and Fanny Sanchez-Solis for help in protein quantification; Martha Krumbach for critically reading the manuscript (all DKFZ, Heidelberg, Germany); Dirk Lindemann (Techn. University of Dresden, Germany) for a cross-reactive rabbit anti PFV integrase antiserum; Thomas Kufer, University of Hohenheim, Germany for a cross-reactive ANKRD17 antiserum; and Bryan Cullen (Duke University, Durham, USA) for reagents and scientific support.

Conflicts of Interest: The authors declare no conflict of interest.

References

1. Cullen, B.R. MicroRNA expression by an oncogenic retrovirus. *Proc. Natl. Acad. Sci. USA* **2012**, *109*, 2695–2696. [CrossRef]
2. Cullen, B.R. MicroRNAs as mediators of viral evasion of the immune system. *Nat. Immunol.* **2013**, *14*, 205–210. [CrossRef] [PubMed]
3. Bartel, D.P. Metazoan MicroRNAs. *Cell* **2018**, *173*, 20–51. [CrossRef] [PubMed]
4. Skalsky, R.L.; Cullen, B.R. Viruses, microRNAs, and host interactions. *Annu. Rev. Microbiol.* **2010**, *64*, 123–141. [CrossRef] [PubMed]
5. Yao, Y.; Smith, L.P.; Nair, V.; Watson, M. An avian retrovirus uses canonical expression and processing mechanisms to generate viral microRNA. *J. Virol.* **2014**, *88*, 2–9. [CrossRef] [PubMed]
6. Balasubramaniam, M.; Pandhare, J.; Dash, C. Are microRNAs Important Players in HIV-1 Infection? An Update. *Viruses* **2018**, *10*, 110. [CrossRef] [PubMed]
7. Kincaid, R.P.; Burke, J.M.; Sullivan, C.S. RNA virus microRNA that mimics a B-cell oncomiR. *Proc. Natl. Acad. Sci. USA* **2012**, *109*, 3077–3082. [CrossRef]
8. Whisnant, A.W.; Kehl, T.; Bao, Q.; Materniak, M.; Kuzmak, J.; Löchelt, M.; Cullen, B.R. Identification of novel, highly expressed retroviral microRNAs in cells infected by bovine foamy virus. *J. Virol.* **2014**, *88*, 4679–4686. [CrossRef] [PubMed]
9. Kincaid, R.P.; Chen, Y.; Cox, J.E.; Rethwilm, A.; Sullivan, C.S. Noncanonical microRNA (miRNA) biogenesis gives rise to retroviral mimics of lymphoproliferative and immunosuppressive host miRNAs. *MBio* **2014**, *5*, e00074. [CrossRef] [PubMed]
10. Hashimoto-Gotoh, A.; Kitao, K.; Miyazawa, T. Persistent Infection of Simian Foamy Virus Derived from the Japanese Macaque Leads to the High-Level Expression of microRNA that Resembles the miR-1 microRNA Precursor Family. *Microbes Environ.* **2020**, *35*. [CrossRef]
11. Khan, A.S.; Bodem, J.; Buseyne, F.; Gessain, A.; Johnson, W.; Kuhn, J.H.; Kuzmak, J.; Lindemann, D.; Linial, M.L.; Löchelt, M.; et al. Spumaretroviruses: Updated taxonomy and nomenclature. *Virology* **2018**, *516*, 158–164. [CrossRef] [PubMed]
12. Kehl, T.; Tan, J.; Materniak, M. Non-simian foamy viruses: Molecular virology, tropism and prevalence and zoonotic/interspecies transmission. *Viruses* **2013**, *5*, 2169. [CrossRef]
13. Materniak, M.; Tan, J.; Heit-Mondrzyk, A.; Hotz-Wagenblatt, A.; Löchelt, M. Bovine Foamy Virus: Shared and unique molecular features in vitro and in vivo. *Viruses* **2019**, *11*, 1084. [CrossRef]
14. Lindemann, D.; Rethwilm, A. Foamy virus biology and its application for vector development. *Viruses* **2011**, *3*, 561–585. [CrossRef] [PubMed]
15. Rethwilm, A. Molecular biology of foamy viruses. *Med. Microbiol. Immunol.* **2010**, *199*, 197–207. [CrossRef]
16. Rethwilm, A. Foamy virus vectors: An awaited alternative to gammaretro- and lentiviral vectors. *Curr.Gene Ther.* **2007**, *7*, 261–271. [CrossRef]
17. Pinto-Santini, D.M.; Stenbak, C.R.; Linial, M.L. Foamy virus zoonotic infections. *Retrovirology* **2017**, *14*, 55. [CrossRef]
18. Romen, F.; Backes, P.; Materniak, M.; Sting, R.; Vahlenkamp, T.W.; Riebe, R.; Pawlita, M.; Kuzmak, J.; Löchelt, M. Serological detection systems for identification of cows shedding bovine foamy virus via milk. *Virology* **2007**, *364*, 123–131. [CrossRef]
19. Cao, W.; Heit, A.; Hotz-Wagenblatt, A.; Löchelt, M. Functional characterization of the bovine foamy virus miRNA expression cassette and its dumbbell-shaped pri-miRNA. *Virus Genes* **2018**, *54*, 550–560. [CrossRef]
20. Menning, M.; Kufer, T.A. A role for the Ankyrin repeat containing protein Ankrd17 in Nod1- and Nod2-mediated inflammatory responses. *FEBS Lett.* **2013**, *587*, 2137–2142. [CrossRef]
21. Liu, Y.; Liu, Y.; Wu, J.; Roizman, B.; Zhou, G.G. Innate responses to gene knockouts impact overlapping gene networks and vary with respect to resistance to viral infection. *Proc. Natl. Acad. Sci. USA* **2018**, *115*, E3230–E3237. [CrossRef] [PubMed]
22. Wang, Y.; Tong, X.; Li, G.; Li, J.; Deng, M.; Ye, X. Ankrd17 positively regulates RIG-I-like receptor (RLR)-mediated immune signaling. *Eur. J. Immunol.* **2012**, *42*, 1304–1315. [CrossRef] [PubMed]
23. Piersanti, R.L.; Horlock, A.D.; Block, J.; Santos, J.E.P.; Sheldon, I.M.; Bromfield, J.J. Persistent effects on bovine granulosa cell transcriptome after resolution of uterine disease. *Reproduction* **2019**, *158*, 35–46. [CrossRef]

24. Takahashi, Y.; Meyerkord, C.L.; Hori, T.; Runkle, K.; Fox, T.E.; Kester, M.; Loughran, T.P.; Wang, H.G. Bif-1 regulates Atg9 trafficking by mediating the fission of Golgi membranes during autophagy. *Autophagy* **2011**, *7*, 61–73. [CrossRef]
25. Xu, L.; Wang, Z.; He, S.Y.; Zhang, S.F.; Luo, H.J.; Zhou, K.; Li, X.F.; Qiu, S.P.; Cao, K.Y. Bax-interacting factor-1 inhibits cell proliferation and promotes apoptosis in prostate cancer cells. *Oncol. Rep.* **2016**, *36*, 3513–3521. [CrossRef]
26. Bartel, D.P. MicroRNAs: Genomics, biogenesis, mechanism, and function. *Cell* **2004**, *116*, 281–297. [CrossRef]
27. Stabel, J.R.; Stabel, T.J. Immortalization and characterization of bovine peritoneal macrophages transfected with SV40 plasmid DNA. *Vet. Immunol. Immunopathol.* **1995**, *45*, 211–220. [CrossRef]
28. Bao, Q.; Hipp, M.; Hugo, A.; Lei, J.; Liu, Y.; Kehl, T.; Hechler, T.; Löchelt, M. In Vitro Evolution of Bovine Foamy Virus Variants with Enhanced Cell-Free Virus Titers and Transmission. *Viruses* **2015**, *7*, 5855–5874. [CrossRef]
29. Hechler, T.; Materniak, M.; Kehl, T.; Kuzmak, J.; Löchelt, M. Complete genome sequences of two novel European clade bovine foamy viruses from Germany and Poland. *J. Virol.* **2012**, *86*, 10905–10906. [CrossRef]
30. Bao, Q.; Hotz-Wagenblatt, A.; Betts, M.J.; Hipp, M.; Hugo, A.; Pougialis, G.; Lei-Rossmann, J.; Löchelt, M. Shared and cell type-specific adaptation strategies of Gag and Env yield high titer bovine foamy virus variants. *Infect. Genet. Evol.* **2020**, *82*. [CrossRef]
31. Schwantes, A.; Ortlepp, I.; Löchelt, M. Construction and functional characterization of feline foamy virus-based retroviral vectors. *Virology* **2002**, *301*, 53–63. [CrossRef]
32. Lei, J.; Osen, W.; Gardyan, A.; Hotz-Wagenblatt, A.; Wei, G.; Gissmann, L.; Eichmüller, S.; Löchelt, M. Replication-Competent Foamy Virus Vaccine Vectors as Novel Epitope Scaffolds for Immunotherapy. *PLoS ONE* **2015**, *10*, e0138458. [CrossRef] [PubMed]
33. Gibson, D.G.; Young, L.; Chuang, R.Y.; Venter, J.C.; Hutchison, C.A., 3rd; Smith, H.O. Enzymatic assembly of DNA molecules up to several hundred kilobases. *Nat. Methods* **2009**, *6*, 343–345. [CrossRef] [PubMed]
34. Stricker, E.; Pougialis, G.; Löchelt, M. *Features of Engineered Bovine Foamy Virus Genomes*; German Cancer Research Center (DKFZ): Heidelberg, Germany, 2018.
35. Pfaffl, M.W. A new mathematical model for relative quantification in real-time RT-PCR. *Nucleic Acids Res.* **2001**, *29*, e45. [CrossRef]
36. Lewis, B.P.; Shih, I.H.; Jones-Rhoades, M.W.; Bartel, D.P.; Burge, C.B. Prediction of mammalian microRNA targets. *Cell* **2003**, *115*, 787–798. [CrossRef]
37. John, B.; Enright, A.J.; Aravin, A.; Tuschl, T.; Sander, C.; Marks, D.S. Human MicroRNA targets. *PLoS Biol.* **2004**, *2*, e363. [CrossRef]
38. Gebert, L.F.R.; MacRae, I.J. Regulation of microRNA function in animals. *Nat. Rev. Mol. Cell Biol.* **2019**, *20*, 21–37. [CrossRef]
39. Hutter, S.; Mullers, E.; Stanke, N.; Reh, J.; Lindemann, D. Prototype foamy virus protease activity is essential for intraparticle reverse transcription initiation but not absolutely required for uncoating upon host cell entry. *J. Virol.* **2013**, *87*, 3163–3176. [CrossRef]
40. Materniak, M.; Hechler, T.; Löchelt, M.; Kuzmak, J. Similar patterns of infection with bovine foamy virus in experimentally inoculated calves and sheep. *J. Virol.* **2013**, *87*, 3516–3525. [CrossRef] [PubMed]
41. Liebermann, H.; Riebe, R. Isolation of bovine syncytial virus in East Germany. *Arch. Exp. Vet.* **1981**, *35*, 917–919.
42. Stricker, E. Influence of LTR Variants on Bovine Foamy Virus Replication Kinetics and Gene Expression. Master's Thesis, University of Heidelberg, Heidelberg, Germany, 2017.
43. Wei, G.; Kehl, T.; Bao, Q.; Benner, A.; Lei, J.; Löchelt, M. The chromatin binding domain, including the QPQRYG motif, of feline foamy virus Gag is required for viral DNA integration and nuclear accumulation of Gag and the viral genome. *Virology* **2018**, *524*, 56–68. [CrossRef]
44. Cao, W. Functional Characterization and Target Validation of the Bovine Foamy Virus Encoded miRNAs. Ph.D. Thesis, University of Heidelberg, Heidelberg, Germany, 2018.
45. Hill, C.G.; Matyunina, L.V.; Walker, D.; Benigno, B.B.; McDonald, J.F. Transcriptional override: A regulatory network model of indirect responses to modulations in microRNA expression. *BMC Syst. Biol.* **2014**, *8*, 36. [CrossRef] [PubMed]
46. Tan, J.; Hao, P.; Jia, R.; Yang, W.; Liu, R.; Wang, J.; Xi, Z.; Geng, Y.; Qiao, W. Identification and functional characterization of BTas transactivator as a DNA-binding protein. *Virology* **2010**, *405*, 408–413. [CrossRef] [PubMed]

47. Swiersy, A.; Wiek, C.; Reh, J.; Zentgraf, H.; Lindemann, D. Orthoretroviral-like prototype foamy virus Gag-Pol expression is compatible with viral replication. *Retrovirology* **2011**, *8*, 66. [CrossRef] [PubMed]
48. Wilk, T.; Geiselhart, V.; Frech, M.; Fuller, S.D.; Flugel, R.M.; Löchelt, M. Specific interaction of a novel foamy virus Env leader protein with the N-terminal Gag domain. *J. Virol.* **2001**, *75*, 7995–8007. [CrossRef]
49. Mukherjee, T.; Hovingh, E.S.; Foerster, E.G.; Abdel-Nour, M.; Philpott, D.J.; Girardin, S.E. NOD1 and NOD2 in inflammation, immunity and disease. *Arch. Biochem. Biophys.* **2019**, *670*, 69–81. [CrossRef] [PubMed]
50. Yeo, W.M.; Chow, V.T. The VP1 structural protein of enterovirus 71 interacts with human ornithine decarboxylase and gene trap ankyrin repeat. *Microb. Pathog.* **2007**, *42*, 129–137. [CrossRef]
51. Wang, H.; Liu, X.; Shu, S.; Zhang, J.; Huang, Y.; Fang, F. Murine cytomegalovirus IE3 protein interacts with Ankrd17. *J. Huazhong Univ. Sci. Technol. Med. Sci.* **2011**, *31*, 285–289. [CrossRef]
52. Bergez, M.; Weber, J.; Riess, M.; Erdbeer, A.; Seifried, J.; Stanke, N.; Munz, C.; Hornung, V.; Konig, R.; Lindemann, D. Insights into Innate Sensing of Prototype Foamy Viruses in Myeloid Cells. *Viruses* **2019**, *11*, 1095. [CrossRef]
53. Rua, R.; Lepelley, A.; Gessain, A.; Schwartz, O. Innate sensing of foamy viruses by human hematopoietic cells. *J. Virol.* **2012**, *86*, 909–918. [CrossRef]
54. Bahr, A.; Singer, A.; Hain, A.; Vasudevan, A.A.; Schilling, M.; Reh, J.; Riess, M.; Panitz, S.; Serrano, V.; Schweizer, M.; et al. Interferon but not MxB inhibits foamy retroviruses. *Virology* **2016**, *488*, 51–60. [CrossRef]
55. Rola-Luszczak, M.; Materniak, M.; Pluta, A.; Hulst, M.; Kuzmak, J. Transcriptomic microarray analysis of BoMac cells after infection with bovine foamy virus. *Arch. Virol.* **2014**, *159*, 1515–1519. [CrossRef] [PubMed]
56. Serfass, J.M.; Takahashi, Y.; Zhou, Z.; Kawasawa, Y.I.; Liu, Y.; Tsotakos, N.; Young, M.M.; Tang, Z.; Yang, L.; Atkinson, J.M.; et al. Endophilin B2 facilitates endosome maturation in response to growth factor stimulation, autophagy induction, and influenza A virus infection. *J. Biol. Chem.* **2017**, *292*, 10097–10111. [CrossRef] [PubMed]
57. Santamaria, E.; Mora, M.I.; Potel, C.; Fernandez-Irigoyen, J.; Carro-Roldan, E.; Hernandez-Alcoceba, R.; Prieto, J.; Epstein, A.L.; Corrales, F.J. Identification of replication-competent HSV-1 Cgal+ strain signaling targets in human hepatoma cells by functional organelle proteomics. *Mol. Cell. Proteom.* **2009**, *8*, 805–815. [CrossRef]
58. Yuan, P.; Dong, L.; Cheng, Q.; Wang, S.; Li, Z.; Sun, Y.; Han, S.; Yin, J.; Peng, B.; He, X.; et al. Prototype foamy virus elicits complete autophagy involving the ER stress-related UPR pathway. *Retrovirology* **2017**, *14*, 16. [CrossRef]
59. Zheng, Y.; Zhu, G.; Yan, J.; Tang, Y.; Han, S.; Yin, J.; Peng, B.; He, X.; Liu, W. The Late Domain of Prototype Foamy Virus Gag Facilitates Autophagic Clearance of Stress Granules by Promoting Amphisome Formation. *J. Virol.* **2020**, *94*. [CrossRef]
60. Schmidt, M.; Herchenroder, O.; Heeney, J.; Rethwilm, A. Long terminal repeat U3 length polymorphism of human foamy virus. *Virology* **1997**, *230*, 167–178. [CrossRef]
61. Cai, Q.; He, B.; Weiberg, A.; Buck, A.H.; Jin, H. Small RNAs and extracellular vesicles: New mechanisms of cross-species communication and innovative tools for disease control. *PLoS Pathog.* **2019**, *15*, e1008090. [CrossRef]
62. Gurien, S.D.; Aziz, M.; Jin, H.; Wang, H.; He, M.; Al-Abed, Y.; Nicastro, J.M.; Coppa, G.F.; Wang, P. Extracellular microRNA 130b-3p inhibits eCIRP-induced inflammation. *EMBO Rep.* **2020**, *21*, e48075. [CrossRef]
63. Van Looveren, K.; Van Wyngene, L.; Libert, C. An extracellular microRNA can rescue lives in sepsis. *EMBORep.* **2020**, *21*, e49193. [CrossRef] [PubMed]
64. Safari, R.; Hamaidia, M.; De Brogniez, A.; Gillet, N.; Willems, L. Cis-drivers and trans-drivers of bovine leukemia virus oncogenesis. *Curr. Opin. Virol.* **2017**, *26*, 15–19. [CrossRef] [PubMed]
65. Gillet, N.A.; Hamaidia, M.; De Brogniez, A.; Gutierrez, G.; Renotte, N.; Reichert, M.; Trono, K.; Willems, L. Bovine Leukemia Virus Small Noncoding RNAs Are Functional Elements That Regulate Replication and Contribute to Oncogenesis In Vivo. *PLoS Pathog.* **2016**, *12*, e1005588. [CrossRef] [PubMed]

Publisher's Note: MDPI stays neutral with regard to jurisdictional claims in published maps and institutional affiliations.

viruses

Review

Bovine Foamy Virus: Shared and Unique Molecular Features In Vitro and In Vivo

Magdalena Materniak-Kornas [1], Juan Tan [2], Anke Heit-Mondrzyk [3], Agnes Hotz-Wagenblatt [3] and Martin Löchelt [4,*]

1 Department of Biochemistry, National Veterinary Research Institute, 24-100 Pulawy, Poland; magdalena.materniak@piwet.pulawy.pl
2 Key Laboratory of Molecular Microbiology and Technology, Ministry of Education, College of Life Sciences, Nankai University, Tianjin 300071, China; juantan@nankai.edu.cn
3 German Cancer Research Center DKFZ, Core Facility Omics IT and Data Management, 69120 Heidelberg, Germany; a.heit@dkfz.de (A.H.-M.); hotz-wagenblatt@dkfz.de (A.H.-W.)
4 German Cancer Research Center DKFZ, Program Infection, Inflammation and Cancer, Div. Viral Transformation Mechanisms, 69120 Heidelberg, Germany
* Correspondence: m.loechelt@dkfz.de; Tel.: +49-6221-424933

Received: 27 September 2019; Accepted: 19 November 2019; Published: 21 November 2019

Abstract: The retroviral subfamily of *Spumaretrovirinae* consists of five genera of foamy (spuma) viruses (FVs) that are endemic in some mammalian hosts. Closely related species may be susceptible to the same or highly related FVs. FVs are not known to induce overt disease and thus do not pose medical problems to humans and livestock or companion animals. A robust lab animal model is not available or is a lab animal a natural host of a FV. Due to this, research is limited and often focused on the simian FVs with their well-established zoonotic potential. The authors of this review and their groups have conducted several studies on bovine FV (BFV) in the past with the intention of (i) exploring the risk of zoonotic infection via beef and raw cattle products, (ii) studying a co-factorial role of BFV in different cattle diseases with unclear etiology, (iii) exploring unique features of FV molecular biology and replication strategies in non-simian FVs, and (iv) conducting animal studies and functional virology in BFV-infected calves as a model for corresponding studies in primates or small lab animals. These studies gained new insights into FV-host interactions, mechanisms of gene expression, and transcriptional regulation, including miRNA biology, host-directed restriction of FV replication, spread and distribution in the infected animal, and at the population level. The current review attempts to summarize these findings in BFV and tries to connect them to findings from other FVs.

Keywords: bovine foamy virus; BFV; foamy virus; spuma virus; model system; animal model; animal experiment; miRNA function; gene expression; antiviral host restriction

1. Introduction

The family of *Retroviridae* is divided into two subfamilies: The *Spumaretrovirinae* consist of five genera of different spuma or foamy viruses with shared and unique features that separate them from the canonical *Orthoretrovirinae*, which comprise all other known exogenous retroviruses (Figure 1) [1]. The number of research groups working on FVs is correspondingly small and even further split by their individual research focus or the FV isolate or host species used in their studies but also due to the sheer difference in numbers and an apparent lack of pathogenicity of foamy viruses (FV).

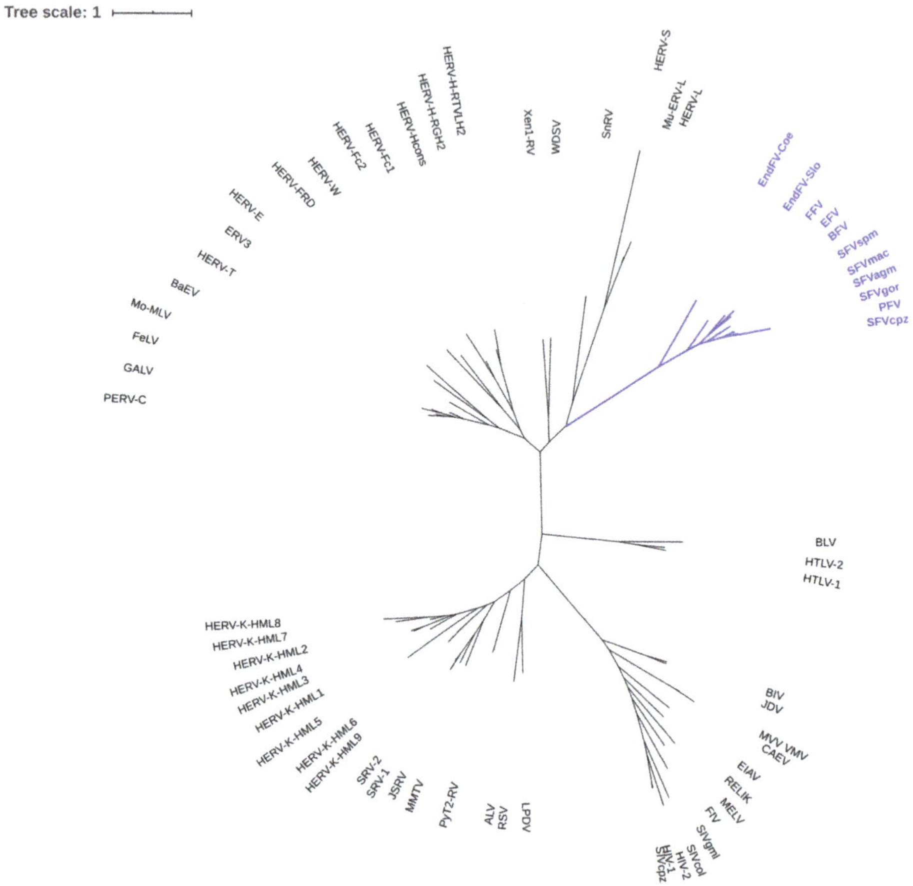

Figure 1. Phylogenetic tree of known exogenous and endogenous foamy viruses (FVs) (blue branches) and members of the *Orthoretrovirinae*. A fasta file with the conserved regions of the Pol proteins (supplement from ref. [2] and prototype FV (PFV, U21247.1) was used for alignment with ClustalW (http://www.clustal.org/). From the alignment, an ML tree was created using fastml (https://fastml.tau.ac.il, default parameters). The resulting newick tree was displayed by Itol (https://itol.embl.de/).

Most molecular analyses have been conducted on the so-called prototype/primate FV isolate, also initially designated human FV, but subsequently shown to be the end-product of the zoonotic transmission of a chimpanzee FV to an East African naso-pharynx cancer patient [3]. Upon subsequent propagation and passaging in diverse human and non-human cell lines and concomitant severe genetic changes [4], this virus became the best-studied FV isolate and it gained the name prototype FV (PFV). However, its prototypic character might be questioned, since research on highly related simian FVs or more distantly related FVs of feline, bovine, and equine origin is lagging behind and has revealed—at least in selected cases—more or less different data (Figure 1 and Table 1) [5]. Simian FVs share substantial relatedness and, despite having a long co-evolutionary history with their cognate hosts, inter-species transmission is frequent and well documented among closely related hosts, like Old World monkeys and apes, including humans, but also between New World monkeys and humans [5–8]. In general—and there are only very few exceptions known—FVs co-speciate with their cognate hosts and more or less closely related species may be susceptible to the same or a highly related FV [5,9–11]. This host range is likely due to the co-evolution of the virus, together with its host with FVs being the most ancient retrovirus according to the presence of endogenous viruses in all of the vertebrate groups [10,12].

Table 1. Special features and novel insights that were gained from past and current work on Bovine Foamy Virus.

Subject/Topic	References
BFV as a well-established infection model in life-stock animals (cattle and sheep)	[13,14]
BFV as the only known FV in the general human food chain (beef and dairy products)	[15,16]
BFV Riems as the only FV passaged exclusively on primary and homologous host cells	[17,18]
Integrase domain: disrupted HH-CC zinc finger and unique sequence insertion into the extreme C-terminus	[19]
Detailed understanding of gene expression and transactivation of a non-simian FV	[20,21]
RNA Pol III miRNAs, unique precursor structure and their functions	[14,22,23]
Extremely tight cell association and identification of residues critical for this phenotype	[24–26]
Detailed understanding of new restriction factors against FVs	[27]
Broad tissue tropism and gene expression in BFV-infected calves	[5,28]

Although a so-called prototype (and/or primate) FV exists in the literature, conserved, prototypic features, besides those basic characteristics that led to the establishment of an independent subfamily of FVs, are currently only partially known. Here, an unbiased comparison of distant FVs and their replication strategies might be worth trying to discriminate basic from deduced, secondary features. In addition, unique data not available for the other FVs have been generated for bovine FV (BFV, see Table 1), and there is the question whether they represent shared or unique features [5]. In this review, we try to use the current data on diverse aspects of the molecular biology of BFV to broaden and complete the overall knowledge of FV biology and indicate avenues of further investigation on BFV biology in vivo and in vitro. In Table 1, the biggest achievements and strengths in the BFV system are summarized and this review will cover some of them in more depth.

2. Specific Topics and Highlights in BFV Biology and Virus-Host Interaction

2.1. Historic View

While the first FV was already described in 1954 [29], the first FV from cattle was isolated 15 years later and designated Bovine Syncytial Virus [30]. The subsequent isolates were also designated Bovine Spuma Virus and Bovine Spumaretrovirus before the name bovine foamy virus (BFV) was coined and finally acknowledged by the ICTV in 1999 (https://talk.ictvonline.org//taxonomy/p/taxonomy-history?taxnode_id=20074661) [1]. Holzschu et al. [19] published the first full-length nucleotide sequence of a BFV isolate from the United States (US) in 1998. These data confirmed the overall genetic structure and coding capacity of BFV as a typical member of the FV genus (Figure 2A).

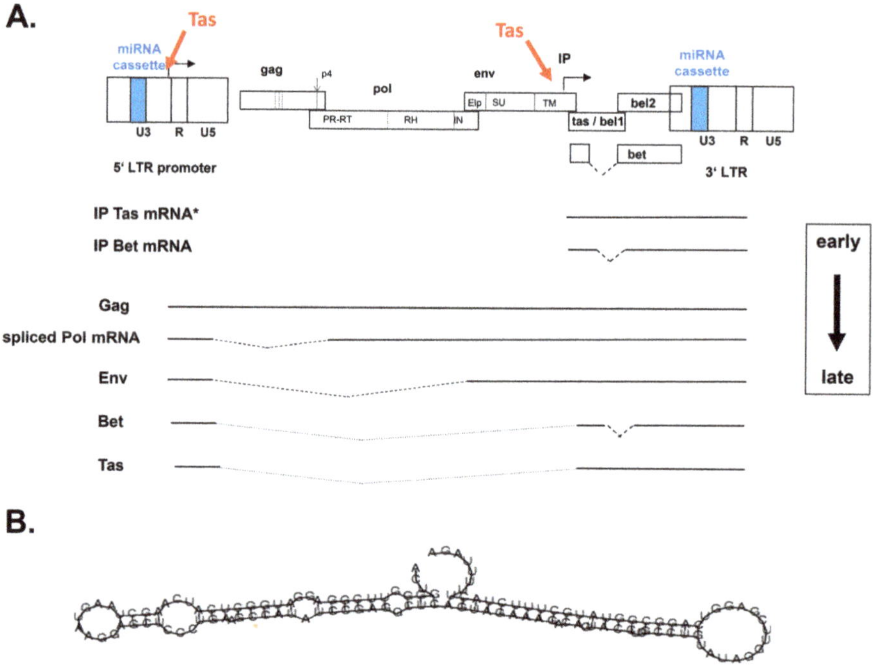

Figure 2. Genetic structure and schematic illustration of bovine foamy virus (BFV) gene expression and the BFV primary miRNA. (**A**) The BFV provirus DNA genome is shown on top schematically and out of scale with the terminal long terminal repeats (LTRs) consisting of the U3, R, and U5 regions. The position of the miRNA cassette in the U3 regions is indicated in color. BFV genes are shown as overlapping open boxes sub-divided into the mature protein domains. Proteolytic processing is marked by dotted lines. The spliced *bet* gene is separately shown below the genome. Broken arrows indicate the transcriptional start sited and direction of LTR- and internal promoter- (IP) directed gene expression and the Tas-mediated transactivation of the 5′LTR and the IP is indicated in red. Below, a selection of the major early and late BFV transcripts starting at the IP and LTR are shown with spliced-out areas indicated by broken lines. Only the major BFV IP-directed Tas mRNA is shown (*). The shift between early and late transcription is marked by a boxed arrow at the right-hand margin. (**B**) The predicted folding and secondary structure of the BFV dumbbell-shaped miRNA precursor (BFV pri-miRNA) is given, for additional information, and the sequence of the mature and stable miRNA, see below and Whisnant et al., 2014 [22].

This opened the way for functional and genetic studies on the molecular biology and replication of BFV in cell cultures and experimentally BFV-infected animals. In addition, it allowed for the establishment of tools for high sensitivity and specificity detection and diagnosis, as described in the subsequent chapters and undertaken in the labs of Jacek Kuzmak and Magdalena Materniak-Kornas, Wentao Qiao, Yunqi Geng and Juan Tan, and Martin Löchelt and co-workers (Figure 3).

Almost unrecognized since exclusively publishing in German, the BFV Riems isolate was established and characterized by Dr. Roland Riebe and co-workers in East Germany (Friedrich Löffler-Institute, Riems, Germany) in the early 80s of the last century [17,18]. The original BFV Riems isolate is, to our knowledge, the only FV that has been exclusively propagated in primary cells of its authentic host species and it thus might have not so much "suffered" genetic changes and co-adaptive imprints due to (repeated) host cell changes and prolonged growth in tumor cells displaying highly selected and aberrant features.

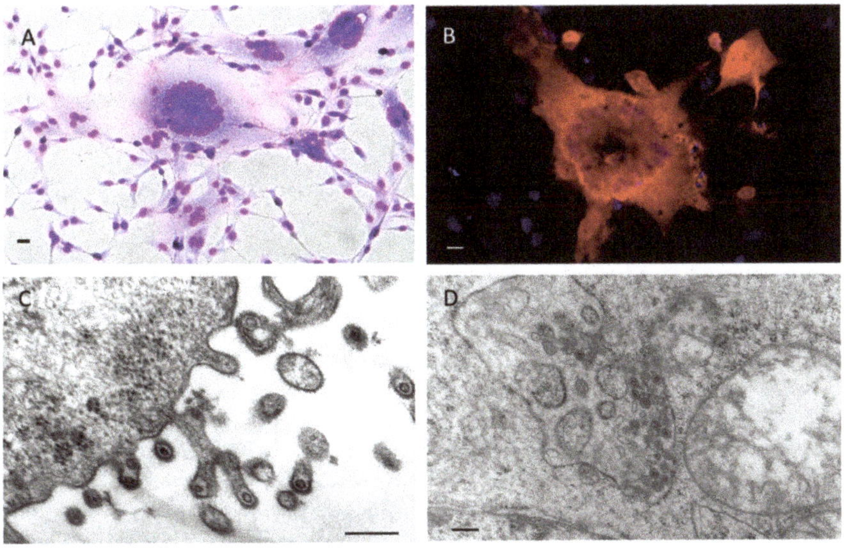

Figure 3. BFV100-infected canine fetal thymus Cf2Th cells: (**A**) Giemsa stained syncytia; (**B**) detection of BFV Gag proteins (red) by indirect immunofluorescence, nuclei were stained in blue; BFV particles budding from the (**C**) plasma membrane (magnification is 60,000-fold) and (**D**) accumulating intracellularly in the endoplasmic reticulum (magnification is 32,000-fold) as visualized by transmission electron microscopy. Scale bars in (**A**,**B**) are 250 μm and in (**C**,**D**) 500 nm.

2.2. Excellent, Well Established Non-Primate FV Model of Transactivation, Gene Expression and Gene Function

Gene expression and transactivation studies have been mainly conducted in the earlier years of PFV and SFV research, in particular between 1990 and 2000. Research regarding the underlying molecular mechanisms of BFV gene expression has only started in 2008 and it is still ongoing in the lab of Wentao Qiao and Juan Tan while using current, state of the art methods and technologies, thus also extending from this perspective our understanding of FV gene expression and replication as reported here by J.T. (Figure 2A). Similarly, BFV Bet and Gag have been additionally studied by this group during the last years and are thus included in this review, allowing for a more comprehensive view on structural and non-structural FV proteins (Figure 2A).

2.2.1. Function of Tas

Unlike PFV Tas, BFV Tas has no classical nuclear localization signal (NLS), but it is mainly present in the nucleus beside some cytoplasmic localization [31–33]. Like most typical DNA-binding transcriptional activators, nuclear localization and multimerization are both required for the transactivation activity of Tas [31,32]. It was reported that PFV Tas has three domains that mediate multimer formation in the nuclei of mammalian cells, but the biological function of PFV Tas multimerization has not been defined [32]. In contrast to PFV Tas, BFV Tas has only one domain that mediates dimer formation. The comparison of the multimerization domains of both proteins does not reveal obvious homologies. Deleting the dimerization region abolishes the Tas-induced transactivation of BFV LTR and internal promoter (IP), which suggests that the active form of BFV Tas is a dimer [31].

There are at least four BFV *tas* mRNAs during BFV infection [34]. These four forms of BFV *tas* mRNA transcripts initiate either at BFV LTR (one) or IP (three), are spliced or unspliced and they have a differential ability to activate the BFV promoters (for clarity, only one representative IP-derived *tas* mRNA is shown in Figure 2A) [34]. According to these findings, we propose the following model of Tas-mediated BFV gene expression. Firstly, activator protein 1 (AP-1) and some other unknown cellular transcriptional genes activate the Tas-mediated transactivation of the BFV IP as the early promoter for BFV gene expression, leading to the transcription of BFV IP *tas* mRNAs [35]. In consequence, BFV Tas quickly accumulates to further enhance BFV IP activity. When a defined threshold level of BFV Tas is reached, the early phase of BFV IP-directed *tas/bet* expression is switched to the late phase of structural gene expression directed by LTR (Figure 2A). The transcription of LTR-spliced BFV *tas* transcripts with low biological activity can ensure modest levels of Tas, which makes it possible to establish persistent viral gene expression to complete the viral life cycle and maintain a balance between the virus and host cells.

Until now, the molecular mechanisms of transcriptional activation by Tas have remained unclear. Past investigations indicate that co-activators p300 and PCAF physically and functionally interact in vivo with PFV Tas, resulting in the enhancement of Tas-dependent transcriptional activation [36]. Subsequently, PCAF acetylation of feline FV (FFV) Tas was shown to augment promoter-binding affinity and virus transcription [37]. Similar to Tas of PFV and FFV, p300 can specifically interact in vivo with BFV Tas, which results in the enhancement of Tas-dependent transcriptional activation [38]. In addition, the p300-mediated acetylation of BFV Tas can increase its DNA binding affinity, and the K66, K109, and K110 residues are critical for the DNA binding ability of BFV Tas; however, they are not conserved among different FVs [38]. The K→R mutations in full-length BFV infectious clones reduce the expression of viral proteins, and the triple mutant completely abrogates viral replication [21]. These findings suggest that acetylation might be an ubiquitous mechanism adopted by FVs as an effective means to regulate gene expression and animal FVs potentially share similarities with PFV in their need for essential host cell factors, e.g., p300 and PACF, etc. In addition to p300, BFV also engages the cellular RelB protein as a co-activator of BFV Tas to enhance its transactivation function [39]. Furthermore, it was found that BFV infection upregulates cellular RelB expression through BFV Tas-induced NF-κB activation [39]. Thus, it is a positive virus-host feedback circuit, in which BFV utilizes the host's NF-κB pathway through the RelB protein for its efficient transcription [39,40]. There are many other unknown factors that are involved in the transactivation of Tas and some advanced techniques, such as tandem affinity purification and proximity labelling, can be used to discover new co-activators of Tas.

2.2.2. Function of Bet

Although the mechanisms of FV Bet expression by splicing-mediated fusion of the N-terminal domain of Tas to the entire *bel2* coding sequence were described almost 25 years ago, its functions are only partly clarified (Figure 2A) [5,41]. FV Bet is highly expressed after infection by different FVs [13,42]. Previously, FFV and PFV Bet were shown to serve as antagonists of apolipoprotein B mRNA-editing, enzyme-catalytic, polypeptide-like 3 (APOBEC3) family antiretroviral proteins for facilitating PFV and FFV replication [43–45]. In addition, Bet might play an important role in the establishment and maintenance of viral persistence in vitro and in vivo [46,47]. Furthermore, Bet has been described as having a negative regulatory effect upon the basal IP activity of PFV and it might limit the expression of the transcriptional transactivator Tas by inhibiting the activation of the IP [48].

BFV Bet consists of 419 aa and it derives from a multiplied spliced mRNA fusing the first N-terminal 35 aa of BFV Tas to the entire Bel2 open reading frame. Although the sequence homology between the Bet proteins of different FVs is very low, some motifs in Bel2 are similar among the different Bet proteins [49]. The Bet proteins of the known BFV isolates [17,19,50–52] are highly conserved. In PFV-infected cells, Bet was shown to fuse with Env and form a glycoprotein of ~170 kDa [53], but a corresponding BFV Env–Bet fusion protein could not be detected while using a BFV Bet antiserum.

BFV3026 Bet is present in both the nucleus and cytoplasm (predominantly in the nucleus) of the infected or transfected cells [54]. Analysis of BFV3026 Bet amino acid sequences did not reveal the apparent structural sequence or functional protein motifs, but a nuclear localization signal (NLS) was predicted at the C-terminal end of BFV3026 Bet (392–396 aa) containing the amino acid sequence RRRRR (PSORT II software, [55]) and NLStradamus model, [56]). PFV Bet was reported to have an effective NLS at the C terminus (between 406 and 459 aa), but it does not contribute to nuclear localization of the protein and PFV Bet is located in both the nucleus and cytoplasm [57]. BFV3026 Bet has a similar subcellular localization as PFV Bet, so it will be interesting to determine whether the predicted NLS of BFV Bet is functional. Nuclear pore complexes are known to allow two modes of transport: the passive diffusion of small molecules (<20–40 kDa) and active transport of larger molecules (50 kDa and more) [58]. As BFV Bet (55 kDa) is slightly too large to freely shuttle between the cytoplasm and nucleus, it might enter the nucleus using the NLS or by a currently unknown mechanism.

The functions of Bet during FV infection and replication are seemingly contradictory. It is required for FFV productive replication, as Bet mutants showed approximately 1,000-fold reduced viral titer in feline kidney cells when compared to the wild-type FFV [59]. This is in contrast to PFV, where different Bet mutations or deletions did not show a defined phenotype or only an approximately 10-fold decreased cell-free viral transmission, which suggests that Bet might play a role in efficient cell-free viral transmission [60]. However, these studies were often conducted in heterologous or genetically altered cells. Similarly, the BFV Bet mutant BFV3026 genome showed a four-fold higher level of replication than the wild-type genome in engineered human 293T cells [50]. In addition, similar to PFV [61], the overexpression of BFV Bet in heterologous canine fetal thymus cells (Cf2Th) reduced BFV3026 replication approximately threefold [50]. Taken together, these data suggest that BFV Bet may serve as a negative regulator for BFV replication; however, analyses in authentic host cells appear to be absolutely mandatory.

In summary, these observations indicate that a biologically relevant FV Bet phenotype might only be detectable in cells expressing the cellular partner or target molecules of the authentic FV Bet protein. This is e.g. exemplified by the controversial finding on the Bet-induced inactivation of APOBEC3-mediated virus restriction: if APOBEC3 is either missing in the host cell used or the FV in question is propagated in different host cells without APOBEC3 expression or expression of heterologous APOBEC3 proteins, the intricate interaction between these partner molecules is lost, resulting in irrelevant phenotypes. Similarly, the repeated shifts of FVs from one to another host cell may have had similar consequences. These different scenarios are a strong case to use in vitro homologous host cells without genetic changes and adaptations often occurring in tumor cells or after extended passages in vitro and/or to conduct animal experiments in the authentic host species.

2.2.3. Function and Localization of Gag

The interaction and subsequent self-multimerization of retro- and foamy virus Gag protein cause capsid formation [62,63]. Unlike Gag proteins from Orthoretroviruses, FVs Gag is not processed into separate matrix (MA), capsid (CA), and nucleocapsid (NC) subunits (see Figure 2). In fact, four processing sites have been identified in the PFV Gag protein, which are divided into the optimal C-terminal cleavage site yielding p68/p3 and three suboptimal cleavage sites yielding p33/p39 or p39/p29 [64,65]. In BFV, four Gag cleavage forms (p71, p68, p33, and p29) were also observed, indicating that both the optimal and suboptimal cleavages of Gag protein also occur in BFV; the Gag p68/p3 cleavage is the most efficiently used cleavage site [66]. In contrast to Orthoretroviruses, the C-terminal domain of PFV Gag (the NC domain equivalent) contains three glycine (G) and arginine (R)-rich motifs (GR boxes) or less-defined RG-rich regions instead of the canonical cysteine-histidine repeat motif [67]. Similar to PFV Gag, BFV Gag also has a nuclear location signal (NLS) in GR box II, which causes the nuclear accumulation of overproduced Gag protein [66,68].

Unlike Orthoretroviruses, but similar to the other FVs, BFV Gag is not myristoylated and it cannot produce cell-free Gag-only virus-like particles [24,25]. Similar to hepatitis B virus (HBV), BFV particle budding and release are instead dependent on the co-expression of the cognate viral envelope (Env) protein [24,25], which suggests that Env provides a critical membrane-targeting function inherently lacking in BFV Gag. In the case of BFV, this occurs at the plasma membrane rather than the endoplasmic reticulum (ER), due to a lack of a functional ER retrieval signal (ERRS) [68]. The addition of a membrane targeting signal to the N-terminus of Gag restores Gag-only budding from the plasma membrane, implying that Myr-membrane targeting substitutes for Env in particle release [24,68].

Unlike PFV, FFV, and SFVs, BFV is highly cell-associated and it can only transmit through cell-to-cell but not via cell-free pathways [17,24]. Interestingly, the Gag protein of BFV-Z1 (an in vitro selected cell-free infectious BFV3026 clone) lost a 14-amino acid sequence as compared to BFV-B (an infectious cell-associated BFV clone). This 14-residue deletion is located in the central and non-conserved region of FV Gag, which strongly contributes to the size differences of simian versus non-simian FVs [69]. This deletion led to a smaller Gag-Z1 that enhanced cell-free infectivity by four- to five-fold [25]. At the same site in Gag in some high titer (HT) cell-free BFV-Riems variants, insertions, and duplications occurred. However, their impact on BFV titers has not been studied [26]. The Gag-Env interaction is very important for the budding and release of FV virions. Yet, the interaction of Gag and Env in BFV-B and BFV-Z1 was almost the same, which suggests that the contribution of Gag-Z1 to enhanced cell-free transmission is not through promoting interaction with Env [25].

Viruses must engage bidirectional cellular transport mechanisms for completing their whole life cycle, and many viruses require microtubules (MTs) during cell entry for efficient nuclear targeting or the cytosolic transport of naked viral particles [70–72]. In BFV, co-localization of MTs and assembling viral particles was clearly observed in BFV infected cells, which implied that BFV particles or assembly intermediates may transport along the cellular MTs to the cellular membrane to ultimately egress from the host cell. In fact, the MTs-depolymerizing assay indicated that MTs are required for the efficient replication of BFV [66]. In conclusion, BFV has evolved this mechanism to hijack the cellular cytoskeleton for its replication. Until now, it is not clear which components of the MTs are involved in a uni- and/or bidirectional cellular transport of BFV particles. Thus, investigations on the direct interaction between the Gag and MT components should be a future research topic.

2.3. BFV-Host Interactions: Restriction Factors, Innate Immunity, miRNAs and Tight Cell Association

2.3.1. Restriction Factors

The innate immune system constitutes a first line of defense against invading viruses. Cellular restriction factors are key players of innate and/or intrinsic immunity, which interferes with defined steps in the viral life cycle, leading to the attenuation or complete suppression of virus replication mainly acting immediately after virus infection [73]. On the other side, viruses have evolved strategies to circumvent this inhibitory activity by co-evolution with host-encoded restriction factors.

Restriction factors are constitutively expressed and their expression can usually be increased by interferons (IFNs) [74–77]. Until now, several restriction factors acting on retroviruses have been characterized in detail: APOBEC3, tripartite motif protein 5α (TRIM5α), bone marrow stromal cell antigen 2 (BST2, also called tetherin), SAMHD1, IFITM, MxB, and SERINC [78–84]. Recently, some restriction factors were found to inhibit the replication of FVs. For instance, TRIM5α is implicated in restricting PFV, SFV, and FFV during viral entry [85,86]; APOBEC3 proteins are known to act during PFV, SFV, and FFV reverse transcription (RT), and introduce lethal mutations in the viral genome [43–45,87]; whereas, human BST2 (hBST2) and bBST2A1 (one isoform of bovine BST2) suppress the release of PFV and BFV [88–90]. Moreover, unlike hBST2, bBST2A1 displays no inhibitory effect on cell-to-cell transmission of PFV and BFV [90]. Other antiviral proteins include promyelocytic leukemia protein (PML), IFN-induced 35-kDa protein (IFP35), N-Myc interactor (Nmi), and p53-induced RING-H2 protein (Pirh2), which have been recently shown to inhibit FV replication through interacting with Tas [27,91–93]. PML directly interacts with PFV Tas and it interferes with its ability to bind the TREs in the PFV LTR and IP [91]. IFP35 might inhibit BFV Tas-induced transactivation by interfering with the interaction of a cellular transcriptional activation factor(s) and BFV Tas [27]. Nmi inhibits the Tas transactivation of the PFV LTR and IP by interacting with Tas and sequestering it in the cytoplasm [92]. Pirh2 negatively influences the Tas-dependent transcriptional activation of the PFV LTR and IP by interacting with the transactivator Tas and down-regulating its expression [93]. These antiviral proteins likely limit or modulate the viral spread in vivo, but other antiviral proteins detected, for instance, in a recent high-throughput screen using PFV might, in addition, lead to FV latency, but are currently mostly unexplored [94].

2.3.2. Innate Immunity

An interesting feature of FVs is their ability to infect a diverse range of cell types and cause a characteristic foam-like cytopathic effect in culture system. However, they appear to be non-pathogenic in either naturally or accidentally infected hosts with a currently "emerging" but still ill-defined capacity to affect blood or kidney parameters without overt clinical consequences [11,95,96]. This suggests that the host immune system controls viral infection and/or FV replication in vivo. Some evidence showed that the innate immune system probably plays an important role in limiting FVs replication to superficial epithelial cells of the oral mucosa [97]. It has been suggested in early studies while using human or primate cell lines that FV does not activate an innate response and cannot induce type I IFNs (IFN-I) [98–100]. However, only in recent years, it was reported that PFV is efficiently sensed by primary human hematopoietic cells via Toll-like receptor (TLR) 7, which leads to the production of high levels of IFN-I [101]. The PFV-induced IFN-I induces the expression of IFN-stimulated genes in line with the finding that factors restricting FV replication are IFN-I-induced (e.g. TRIM5α and APOBEC3, see above). This activation of the innate immune responses might be a prerequisite for controlling viral replication in zoonotically infected humans or natural animal hosts. In line with this finding, previous studies reported that FV replication is sensitive to IFN-I [98,100,102] due to the induction of several IFN-induced cellular proteins with antiviral activity in culture systems [27,43,89–93]. Besides IFN-I, gamma IFN (IFN-γ) that is produced by activated human peripheral blood lymphocytes has also been found to be a major suppressive factor of PFV [103].

Unfortunately, knowledge regarding the host-cell responses (especially innate immune responses) to BFV infection on the level of gene expression is still limited. In a recent study, changes in the transcriptome of the bovine macrophage cell line BoMac after in vitro BFV infection were examined while using bovine long oligo plus microarray (BLOPlus, Michigan State University, US) technology [104]. In total, 124 genes involved in distinct cellular processes were up- or down-regulated. Among the differentially expressed genes, only five are involved in immune response. Three genes (Hsp90b1, hla-drb1, and Cxorf15) were up-regulated while two genes (CXCL2 and SELENBP1) were down-regulated. However, only the results of all three up-regulated genes (Hsp90b1, hla-drb1, and Cxorf15) were confirmed by subsequent RT-qPCR analyses [104].

The Hsp90b1 protein is essential for the broad tropism of vesicular stomatitis virus (VSV) and for the establishment of infection with VSV and activation of innate immunity via TLRs [105]. Therefore, the Hsp90b1 protein might have an effect on the capacity of FVs to infect a variety of tissues from different organisms. In addition, HLA-DRb1 (major histocompatibility complex class II, DR beta 1), an HLA class II antigen, plays central roles in immunity by presenting peptides derived from foreign, non-self proteins. It was found that specific HLA haplotypes, including HLA-DR, may protect against human immunodeficiency virus (HIV) [106], and MHC class II molecules are up-regulated in several lymphoid cell lines following infection with feline immunodeficiency virus (FIV) [107], as well as in T-lymphocytes of FIV-infected cats [108]. Taken together, the increased level of HLA-DRb1 in BFV-infected BoMac cells might be responsible for the sustained elevation of MHC class II antigen levels. Furthermore, Cxorf15 γ-taxilin, together with α- and β-taxilins, is a member of the taxilin family. β- and γ-taxilin may play a role in intracellular vesicle trafficking [109], and the α-taxilin levels are elevated in hepatitis B virus (HBV)-expressing cells and are essential for the release of HBV particles [110]. One can assume that the upregulation of the Cxorf15 gene following BFV infection suggests a possible role of this protein in virion egress while taking similarities in budding strategies for FVs and HBV into consideration [111]. These data offer a basis for further investigation of the immune response of host cells to FV infection, but the above speculation also needs to be further experimentally confirmed.

The effects of BFV infection on immune gene networks were confirmed in a recent study using experimentally infected calves; however, the differentially expressed genes identified one and three days after infection of the animals were different from those reported for the in vitro study while using BoMac cells [14,104].

2.3.3. miRNA Expression as an Additional Layer to Control Host Gene Expression and Innate Immunity

Recently, BFV and simian FV of African green monkey (SFV_{agm}) have been shown to encode miRNAs via RNA polymerase III (RNA Pol III)-directed expression of a complex double-hairpin and, thus, dumbbell-shaped primary miRNA (pri-miRNA) precursor (Figure 2A,B) [22,112]. The identification of such FV miRNA cassettes of about 120 nt length was stimulated and directed by prior findings in bovine leukemia virus (BLV), which is a close relative of human T cell leukemia/lymphotropic viruses (HTLVs) and used as an animal model for its human counterpart [113,114]. The BLV RNA Pol III-driven miRNA cassettes consist of single hairpins structures and they were identified by an algorithm combining the search for RNA Pol III promoters and terminators and the presence of stable RNA hairpin structures that were flanked by these RNA Pol III-specific features [113].

In BFV-Riems, only a single two-hairpin, dumbbell-shaped pri-miRNA with its RNA Pol III promoter and terminator is present in the non-coding part of the LTR U3 region downstream of the *bet/bel2* open reading frame (Figure 2A) [22]. In contrast, in SFV_{agm}, several different miRNAs are encoded by either dumbbell-shaped precursors RNA Pol III cassettes and possibly other pri-miRNAs that have been mapped to corresponding sites in the 3′ end of the SFV_{agm} U3 region [112] (see below and Table 2). In both studies, the miRNAs were identified and characterized by miRNA sequencing. In BFV, two high level expressed miRNAs comprising about 70% of the total miRNA pool and a third one at modest levels were detected, a potential fourth miRNA from the remaining strand of the second hairpin was undetectable [22]. In contrast, and reflecting the complexity of situation in SFV_{agm}, sequencing identified three high-abundant, two intermediate, and at least six low abundant mature miRNAs [112].

The different miRNA expression capacity and underlying mechanisms of BFV versus SFV_{agm} [22,112] encouraged us to conduct bioinformatics while using the online available and further optimized algorithms to study the situation in BFV-Riems, SFV_{agm}, and other FVs. By modifying the original algorithm of Kincaid et al. [112] we especially focused on dumbbell structures of about 130 nucleotides in size in the LTR sequences of 38 FVs (Table 2). Kincaid et al. also analyzed most of them for miRNA structures (Table S1 in [112]). We predicted for 37 of the 38 FV sequences one or more dumbbell miRNA structures while using a fold energy cutoff of −30 kcal/mol and the existence of a terminator together with a TATA- and/or A/B-Box (as overview, see Table 2).

We confirmed the presence of a single miRNA cassette encoding a dumbbell-shaped pri-miRNA [22] in the genome of all known BFV isolates by using the updated algorithm (Table 2). Single dumbbell-shaped pri-miRNAs were also predicted for the closely related EFV and several SFVs from different simian hosts as well PFV derived upon zoonotic transmission into humans. Surprisingly, while a single dumbbell-shaped miRNA cassette was detected in SFV_{gor}, it was absent in another SFV_{gor} sequence that was derived from a zoonotically infected person [115]. Our algorithm found each two independent RNA Pol III dumbbell-type pri-miRNA cassettes in SFV_{agm} (representing S1/S2 and S6/S7 miRNAs in [112]). For other SFVs, two, three, and even five dumbbell-shaped miRNA cassettes were predicted. While the different FFV isolates from domestic cats contained four miRNA cassettes, the highly related FFV variant that was derived from Puma concolor was predicted to only encode three miRNAs.

In general, the predicted dumbbell miRNA cassettes are located in the non-coding region of the U3 LTR sequence, except the first miRNA cassette of all FFV isolates, which partially overlaps the 3′ end of the *bel2/bet* gene. In addition, the fourth miRNA cassette of the domestic cat FFVs is very close to the transcriptional start site of the LTR promoter and it might interfere with RNA Pol II-directed mRNA expression similar to the situation in SFV_{Cni}, where the third miRNA cassette even extends into the R region (Table 2). The size of the predicted dumbbell-shaped pri-miRNA of the different FVs varies between 111 and 128 nt.

Table 2. Results of bioinformatics on dumbbell-type RNA Pol III cassettes in the LTRs of selected FVs flanked by consensus TATA boxes and termination signals.

Virus-Type	Virus Isolate * and Accession Number	Number of Dumbbell-Shaped miRNA Cassettes	Number of AB or BB Boxes
BFV	BFV_Riems [22]; JX307862.1	1	0
	BFV_100; JX307861.1	1	0
	BFV_11; U94514.1	1	0
	BFV_3026; AY134750.1	1	0
EFV	EFV; AF201902.1	1	0
FFV	FFV Chatul-3; AJ564746.1	4	4
	FFV F17; U85043.1	4	4
	FFV FUV; NC_039242.1	4	4
	FFV_{Pco}; KC292054.1	3	3
HFV	HFV; U21247.1	1	0
	HSRV1; Y07723.1	1	0
	HSRV2; Y07724.1	1	0
	PFV; Y07725.1	1	0
SFV	SFV_AG15; JQ867462.1	1	0
	SFV_{agm}; NC_010820.1 [112]	2	1
	SFV_AXX; EU010385.1	5	3
	SFV_BAD327; JQ867463.1	1	0
	SFV_BAD468; JQ867465.1	1	0
	SFV_BAK74; JQ867464.1	0	0
	SFV_CAE_FV2014; MF582544.1	2	1
	SFV_CAE_LK3; M74895.1	2	1
	SFV_CJA; GU356395.1	1	0
	SFV_CNI; JQ867466.1	3	1
	SFV_CPZ; U04327.1	1	0
	SFV_GOR; HM245790.1	1	0
	SFV_MAC; X54482.1	1	0
	SFV_MCY; KF026286.1	1	0
	SFV_MFA; LC094267.1	1	0
	SFV_MFU; AB923518.1	1	0
	SFV_MMU; MF280817.1	1	0
	SFV_OCR; KM233624.1	1	0
	SFV_ORA; NC_039085.1	2	1
	SFV_PPY; AJ544579.1	3	2
	SFV_PSC; KX087159	1	0
	SFV_PVE; NC_001364.1	1	0
	SFV_SSC; GU356394.1	1	0
	SFV_SXA; KP143760.1	1	0
	SFV-6; L25422	1	1

* References are given for those FVs where experimental miRNA data are available.

As experimental miRNA sequencing data are currently only available for SFV_{agm} and BFV-Riems, it is currently an open question as to whether these bioinformatics-based predictions presented here properly reflect the expression capacity and strategy of the different FVs and whether there is a huge variability of miRNAs between different, and even closely related, FVs. Additionally, the experimentally detected central SFV_{agm} miRNA and the corresponding stem-loops 3, 4, and 5 [112] were not detected by our dumbbell-specific miRNA detection tool, so that, in certain FVs, there may be a co-existence of single-hairpin and dumbbell-shaped pri-miRNAs. Alternatively, the central SFV_{agm} stem-loops 3, 4, and 5 may be derived from larger, more complex pri-miRNAs, for instance, with terminal stem-loops but separated by unfolded, single-stranded intervening sequences.

The two independent experimental studies [22,112] and our in silico analyses show that probably all FVs of different origin contain at least one RNA Pol III-directed miRNA cassettes of the dumbbell-shaped type. The miRNA repertoire of in SFV_{agm} is clearly more complex than that of BFV and it is currently unknown as to whether other FVs may or may not encode also SFV_{agm}/BLV-like single hairpin pri-miRNAs. Thus, further wet biology analyses, high throughput sequencing and bioinformatics are needed to allow for full understanding of this highly important regulatory system of FVs.

The importance of cellular miRNA processing factors dicer and drosha was shown for SFV_{agm} [112], while, for BFV, the impact of the overall shape of the dumbbell-shaped pri-miRNA was demonstrated [22]. In BFV, minor modifications of the pri-miRNA sequence are well tolerated, while the replacement of an authentic stem-loop by heterologous shRNA sequences reduced but did not eliminate reporter gene suppression in dual luciferase assays [23]. This finding, together with high-throughput optimization procedures, as done, for instance, for the BLV RNA Pol III miRNA cassettes [116], may open the way to engineer efficient and specific chimeric FV-based pri-miRNA constructs for therapeutic application, as discussed below (see below, Section 2.5).

Similarities to host miRNAs were detected for experimentally validated SFV_{agm} and BFV miRNAs [112,117] (see Table 3). SFV_{agm} miR-S4-3p shares seed identity and functionality with host miR-155, a noted host oncogenic miRNA (oncomiR). SFV_{agm} miR-S6-3p shares seed identity with the host miRNA family miR-132, which suppresses innate immunity. In contrast, the similarities that were detected for BFV miRNAs comprise the miRNAs bta-miR-125a and the human counterpart of this miRNA has been described as stabilizing the suppressive phenotype of R848-stimulated antigen presenting cells on different levels in a hsa-miR-99b/let-7e/miR-125a cluster [118]. Furthermore, miR-125a and miR-125b are both involved in the progression of cervical cancer [119]. MiR-125b inhibits the PI3K/AKT pathway through the down-regulation of mRNA and protein PIK3CD, while miR-125a is anti-oncogenic by the downregulation of TRIB2 and HOXA1 by the family miR-99 clustered in miR-let-7c~99a, miR-125a~let-7e~99b, and miR-100~let-7a-2. The members of these clusters are diminished in cervical cancer [120]. Taking all of this together, the miRNAs coded by FVs seem to interfere with immune and proliferation processes in the cells, but in different ways. The transcription by RNA Pol III makes the expression of miRNAs independent from protein expression, while the location in the LTR avoids the restrictions that are imposed by overlapping coding regions, thus enhancing variability and adaptability.

Table 3. Homology of seed sequences of experimentally identified BFV-Riems and simian FV of African green monkey SFV_{agm}) miRNAs to known miRNAs of other species.

miRNA Name	Human and Bovine miRNA with Seed Identity
SFVagm -S2-5p	hsa-miR-28-5p, hsa-miR-3139, hsa-miR-708-5p
SFVagm -S3-5p	hsa-miR-4739, hsa-miR-4756-5p, hsa-miR-1321
SFVagm -S4-3p	hsa-miR-155-5p
SFVagm -S6-3p	hsa-miR-132-3p, hsa-miR-212-3p
SFVagm -S7-5p	hsa-miR-3154
BFV Riems miR-BF1-3p	bta-miR-125a, bta-miR-125b, bta-miR-670
BFV Riems miR-BF1-5p	bta-miR-3957
BFV Riems miR-BF2-5p	bta-miR-199a-3p

In BFV, three different and closely spaced miRNAs are detectable in chronically or lytically infected cell culture cells and, importantly, also in experimentally BFV-infect calve peripheral blood mononuclear cells (PBMCs), with the latter confirming the relevance of these findings beyond cell culture systems [22]. The three stable miRNAs are generated from both stem-loops of the dumbbell-shaped pri-miRNA [22]. In chronically BFV-infected cells in vitro, two BFV miRNAs make up more than 2/3 of the total cellular miRNA pool pointing to an important role, especially in chronically infected cells [22]. The two high-abundance miRNAs are localized each to the 5'part of the two different stem-loops, while in SFV_{agm}, miRNAs from both strands of the S3 stem-loop are easily detectable [22].

In the BFV system, bovine cells and bovine genomics have been used and the outcomes of bioinformatics-guided target gene prediction as well as wet biology-based experimental validation were mostly conducted in bovine cell cultures and finally in BFV-infected cells and experimentally infected cattle, as described by Cao et al. [14]. In brief, target site predictions for the high abundance BF2-5p miRNA yielded several potential targets with very high scores and two of them with relevance for innate immunity and virus replication, ANKDR17 [121] and Bif-1 (SH3GLB1) [122] were experimentally confirmed in independent assays [14]. In addition, even downstream targets of ANKRD17 showed altered expression in response to BFV miRNA cassette deletion and miRNA co-transfection [14]. A small number of calves were infected with MDBK cells expressing the highly cell-associated BFV Riems isolate and high-titer in vitro-selected BFV variants lacking or carrying the miRNA cassette in order to establish conditions for in depth analyses of the importance of the miRNAs in the authentic host [14]. The data show that all BFV variants are replication-competent in calves; however, the deletion of the miRNA cassette caused a drop of viral infectivity. The deletion of miR-BF2-5p probably reduced the replication competence of the virus, as seen by the lower induction of genes involved in the recognition of viruses by the innate immune system when compared to wt BFV-infected calves. It probably also resulted in the lower level of the humoral response to BFV Gag observed, especially in one of the animal infected with the miR-BF2-5p-deficient BFV variant (for details, see [14]).

2.3.4. Highly Cell-Associated Spread, at Least in Cell Cultures—What Is Behind This Phenotype?

Viruses have two major transmission strategies: cell-free transmission, involving the release of virus particles into the extracellular space, and cell-to-cell transmission [123]. Retroviruses exhibit different degrees of cell-free and cell-to-cell transmission. Unlike most other retroviruses, such as HIV-1, murine leukemia virus (MLV), PFV, FFV, and SFV, which transmit through both cell-to-cell and cell-free pathways, the transmission of BFV is highly cell-associated, with very low to undetectable cell-free transmission [17,24]. This lack, or only low level, of cell-free transmission appears to be independent of whether the BFV isolates have been exclusively propagated in primary bovine cells (the BFV Riems isolate) or whether immortalized bovine (MDBK cells) and hamster and canine cell lines, like BHK-21 and Cf2Th, have been used for virus propagation. BFV is an excellent model for studying virus adaption to cell-free transmission and identifying the principles of viral transmission by in vitro selection and evolution analyses, since the BFV particle budding machinery is similar to that of other FVs [24,25].

In two independent selections screen using established immortal MDBK and BHK-21 cells, BFV Riems was shown to adapt to cell-free transmission within 80 and 130 cell-free passages reaching titers of more than 10^5 and 10^6 FFU/mL, respectively. The resultant HT variants had independently gained the capacity to spread via cell-free particles, but still also use cell-cell transmission [24]. Genetic studies indicate that consistent and cell type-specific, as well as cell-type-independent adaptive changes, occurred in Gag and Env as well as in the LTR regions where larger changes had also been observed [26] (Bao, Stricker, Hotz-Wagenblatt, and Löchelt, to be published). Importantly, cell-free HT BFV-Riems is still neutralized by serum from naturally infected cows [24]. The different selected HT BFV variants will shed light into virus transmission and the potential routes of intervention in the spread of viral infections.

Zhang and colleagues successfully isolated HT cell-free BFV strains from the original cell-to-cell transmissible BFV3026 strain (Chinese isolate) while using in vitro virus evolution and further constructed an infectious cell-free BFV clone, called pBS-BFV-Z1, to independently explore the molecular mechanisms of BFV cell-free transmission [25]. Following sequence comparisons with a cell-associated clone pBS-BFV-B [50], a number of changes in the genome of pBS-BFV-Z1 were identified. Extensive mutagenesis analyses revealed that the C-terminus of Env, especially the K898 residue, controls BFV cell-free transmission by enhancing cell-free virus entry [25]. The authors also claim that virus release of this variant is increased, although this was not experimentally analyzed [25]. It is well-known that lysine (K) can undergo methylation, acetylation, succinylation, ubiquitination, and other modifications, which play an important role in regulating the protein activity and structure adjustment [124]. Interestingly, the equivalent position of the 898 residue in all known BFV isolates (from the United States, NC001831.1. [19], China, AY134750.1 [50], Poland, JX307861 [51,52], and Germany JX307862.1 [17,52], which only spread through cell-to-cell, is not a lysine (K), while the equivalent position is occupied by a lysine in other high titer cell-free FVs, such as SFV, FFV, and PFV. This suggests that the K898 in Env has an important role in FV cell-free transmission. The underlying mechanisms warrant further studies. Interestingly, the Gag protein of BFV-Z1 lost 14 amino acids in the highly divergent sequence between the matrix and capsid regions, which enhanced cell-free infectivity by four- to five-fold [25]. Other changes of the BFV-Z1 genome contributed little to BFV cell-free transmission. Taken together, these data reveal the genetic determinants that regulate cell-to-cell and cell-free transmission of BFV, and suggest the possibility of generating high-titer BFV vectors through engineering viral Env and, in particular, its C-terminal sequence.

2.4. BFV-Host Interactions at the Organismal and Populational Level

2.4.1. BFV Epidemiology and Naturally Occurring Co-Infections

Infections with BFV have been reported worldwide since the first isolation of BFV by Malmquist and co-workers in 1969 [30]; however, sero-epidemiological data are only available from some countries and they show variable rates of BFV infected animals. The highest sero-prevalence was reported in Canada, where it varied between 40 and 50% [125,126]. A slightly lower rate of 39% was observed in Great Britain [127] and Australia [128]. The most recent data come from Germany, where only 7% of tested animals were identified as being BFV positive [15] and from Poland with BFV sero-prevalence of over 30% in dairy cattle [129]. BFV prevalence based on these studies seems to be very diverse. However, these data span a long time-frame; therefore, one of the reasons for these disparities might be the different sensitivity of methods used for serological testing, from agarose gel immuno-diffusion (AGID) and syncytia inhibition assay to ELISA and indirect immuno-fluorescence assays. Additionally, the age of animals tested might be a reason of such diverse BFV prevalence, but, although the age of the animals was not specified in these studies, the importance of this factor was suggested by Jacobs and co-workers, who observed a higher rate of BFV positive status in older animals [126]. This might be due to the persistence of BFV infections and prolonged sero-conversion in animals, but one cannot exclude other factors, like breed and the type of animal rearing. Interestingly, no disease or clear clinical symptoms were ever associated with BFV infection in cows. However a role of BFV as a co-factor of other retroviral infection has been suggested, especially in the context of mixed infections, which are one of the characteristic features of retroviral infections [130]. This has been also suggested for people infected with HIV and HTLV [131], cats infected with FIV, FeLV, and FFV [132], FIV/FeLV [133], and FIV/FFV [134], and monkeys infected with SIV and STLV [135]. Similar studies have been carried out with respect to co-infections with BFV, bovine leukemia virus (BLV), and bovine immunodeficiency virus (BIV) in cattle. Amborski and co-workers published the first report on BFV co-infection with other lymphotropic retroviruses in dairy cows [136]. In the already quoted study by Jacobs and others carried out in Canada, including numerous dairy cattle herds, it was shown that the percentage of animals with antibodies to BIV, BLV, and BFV is 5.5%, 25.7%, and 39.6%, respectively, however with no statistically significant correlation between the individual values [126].

It is assumed that the source of mixed infections might be due to the same route of retroviral transmission, which results in a statistically significant correlation in the occurrence of antibodies, e.g. for BLV and BIV [137] or FIV and FeLV [138,139] and HTLV II and HIV [140]. Mixed infections are particularly important in herds with BLV-infected animals, due to the fact that BLV is the etiological agent of enzootic bovine leukosis and since BFV has been suggested to act as a cofactor in BLV infections [130]. In a recent study, a statistically significant correlation between the occurrence of serologically positive reactions for BLV and BFV at the herd level was shown [141]. Although the results of these studies cannot be related to individual animals, they indicate a certain pattern in the distribution of herds, where BLV and BFV are present. In the study by Jacobs and others, mixed infections of BLV and BFV were recorded in 9.9% of cows [126]. It has been suggested that BFV and BLV co-infections may impair the immune defense capacity of the host [136,142], similarly as proposed for cats co-infected with FIV and FFV [143]. However, it might also be considered that both viruses interact at the molecular level, especially since both of them use the phenomenon of transactivation in the process of viral replication and, even more interesting, they encode miRNAs that interact with genes directly involved in immune defense processes of the host. There is evidence that BLV- and BFV-encoded miRNAs target genes involved in innate and adaptive immunity and, thus, dysregulating their expression levels might facilitate BFV spread, transmission, or persistence. [14,144,145].

BFV is endemic at high prevalence in livestock cattle in different parts of the world, which can be quite easily confirmed by virus isolation in different types of cells (Cf2Th, BoMac, MDBK, KTR, BHK21); however, it is also possible to develop productive infection under experimental in vivo conditions. Only few reports confirmed the possibility of the experimental infection of cattle with BFV [128]. Materniak and co-workers used the experimental BFV inoculation to determine its replication and immunogenicity, not only in its homologous, but also in the heterologous host [13]. Calves and sheep were selected to analyze the infection kinetics in different, but related, species. Although, neither the experimental BFV infection of calves nor sheep resulted in pathology, BFV spread and replicated to similar degrees in both, the homologous and heterologous hosts. Productive BFV infections were established in calves and sheep, as confirmed by virus isolation from leukocytes of all infected animals. BFV was rescued from both infected animal hosts, even in the presence of BFV-specific antibodies, confirming that BFV infection is not cleared by the host immune system [13]. Additional parameters of BFV infection, like humoral immune response to BFV proteins and the presence of BFV DNA in blood cells and organs, also confirmed the persistence of BFV in both hosts [13]. Interestingly, upon long-term replication in sheep, approximately 70% and 40% of the single nucleotide mutations in the sheep-derived BFV *bet* and *env* sequences, respectively, led to changes in the amino acid sequence. As no consistent pattern of adaptive changes was detectable, this proves the utility of sheep as an animal model to study the biology of persistent spumavirus infections [13].

2.4.2. BFV Transmission Route

The transmission of BFV is suggested to occur through close contact. While considering cattle behavior, it is assumed that BFV shedding occurs via saliva through non-aggressive contact, like sneezing or licking and via infected milk [143]. The successful recovery of BFV from saliva and milk of naturally infected cattle tends to confirm this mode of virus shedding and transmission [15,16]. Interestingly, older studies that were reported by Johnson and others, as well as Kertayadnya et al., showed that calves being BFV negative at birth or the beginning of the experiment became infected when placed together with infected adults [128,146]. Additionally, Johnson and others studied different routes of transmission using BFV infected culture fluids containing cell debris. This experiment showed that only throat spray and intravenous application resulted in successful BFV infection in calves, while the swabbing of cell culture-derived BFV into the vagina or onto the prepuce did not lead to infection [128]. Kertayadnya and others also excluded insect or airborne transfer of BFV infection [146].

The authors of both reports state that the most possible source of infection under natural conditions is close contact to a single immunologically tolerant individual, which is productively BFV-infected, but has no or only very low levels of BFV-specific antibodies. However, the source of such BFV tolerance is disputable. One hypothesis is that such animals are characterized by a very early viremic stage of infection before the development of neutralizing antibodies occurs. However, as Kertayadnya and others reported, there are animals that are productively infected with BFV, but do not produce antibodies, even after several months of infection [146]. Another explanation of immunological tolerance towards BFV could be via in utero infection. Such a scenario might be supported by the studies of Bouillant, and Ruckerbauer who recovered BFV from the uterus of BFV infected cows [147]. Finally, perinatal transmission of BFV via colostrum or milk has been proposed. This route of BFV spread is supported by our studies showing that BFV can be reproducibly isolated from the cellular fraction of raw milk [15,16].

2.4.3. Interspecies and Zoonotic Transmission of BFV as Part of the Human Food Chain

It has been clearly demonstrated that SFVs can be zoonotically transmitted to humans in Africa, South America, and Asia upon exposure or contact with SFV-infected monkeys [6,8,148]. The nature of human exposure to BFV is slightly different, but it seems to be constantly present in the human food chain when considering the routes of virus transmission and replication sites of BFV. Additionally, there are many products of cattle origin used in pharmaceutical and cosmetic industry. However, direct contact, which seems to be the most likely mode of zoonotic transmission, is restricted to a limited part of the human population. So far, two serological studies were performed to screen for BFV in humans. One of them focused on dairy cow caretakers, cattle owners, and veterinarians who were tested for BFV-antibodies and showed an overall sero-prevalence of about 7%; however, none of them was PCR positive for BFV DNA in PBMCs [149]. Another study included three groups of humans, who were serologically tested for BFV antibodies [150]. BFV-specific reaction was found in 7% of immunosuppressed patients, 38% of people claiming contact with cattle, and 2% of the general population with no interaction with cows. In each group, a single BFV PCR positive individual was identified and the sequence of short PCR product showed high homology to BFV isolates that are available in GenBank. The data obtained suggest that BFV zoonotic infection may be possible, however it is not common and, in most of the cases, cleared by the host immune system.

2.4.4. BFV Replication in Naturally and Experimentally Infected Animals

In vivo studies play a vital role in virology, since they allow for investigation of the events taking place during the viral infection in the host. Many aspects of infection can be, in fact, only explored by examining naturally infected animals; however, this needs to be done under carefully controlled conditions in the homologous or a heterologous host. In studies on the replication of BFV in vivo, both directions were used; therefore, these data are quite comprehensive. Similar to other FVs, BFV shows a wide tissue tropism. In naturally infected animals, BFV was recovered from peripheral blood leukocytes/lymphocytes, tumors, fetal tissues, placenta, testis, and from fluids used to flush the uterus and oviducts of super-ovulated cows [17,30,51,151–154]. Studies on naturally and experimentally infected animals using PCR-based virus detection showed that BFV DNA is present in most tissues, like lung, salivary glands, liver, spleen, and bone marrow [13]. Interestingly, some reports from SFVs in monkeys previously showed that, although DNA is present in most animal tissues, SFV RNA, indicative of viral gene expression and replication, is mostly if not exclusively detected in oropharyngeal sites [155–157]. In the most recent studies on tissue distribution of BFV DNA and RNA, different organs, as well as blood, bronchoalveolar lavage cells (BALs), and trachea and pharynx epithelium of experimentally infected calves, were analyzed [28]. The highest load of BFV RNA was detected in the lungs, spleen, liver, PBMC, BALs, and trachea epithelium, while in contrast to the previous studies showing BFV isolation from saliva and milk cells of naturally infected cows [15,16], BFV RNA was detected in the saliva of only a single calf. The presence of BFV RNA in such diverse organs seems to be strong proof that active replication of BFV might be not limited to the oral cavity, in contrast to the findings for SFV gene expression in monkeys.

In a recent study, HT BFV Riems, the cell free variant of BFV, and wild type BFV Riems isolate were used for the experimental inoculation of calves [14,24]. The infection pattern was very similar in both groups of calves. The humoral response was comparable in both groups, but BFV viral load measured in PBMCs of infected animals during 16 weeks p.i. was slightly lower in calves that were infected with HT-BFV Riems. However, at the end of experiment, BFV was rescued from PBLs of all, parental and HT BFV-infected, animals. Interestingly, when changes in the expression of selected genes involved in innate immunity were analyzed at day 1 and 3 p.i., the level of induction was clearly lower in the HT-BFV Riems infected calves as compared to wt BFV Riems inoculated animals, which suggests a slightly impaired detection of HT BFV.

Importantly, and confirming the concept that interspecies transmission of FVs is possible to genetically related hosts, sheep have been shown to be permissive to experimental BFV infection while using intravenous inoculation of BFV100-infected Cf2Th cells [13]. Successful inoculation of sheep with BFV as well as its transmission via saliva may support the risk of cross-species infections in mixed farms, where cattle and sheep are kept in close contact. Previous work, in fact, reported the presence of an FV-like virus in sheep [158], but two scenarios are possible since no further characterization of the isolate was performed. One is that the infection was a result of a cross-species transmission of BFV from cattle; alternatively, the isolate was, in fact, a sheep specific foamy virus. Over 500 German sheep serum samples were tested to try to answer this question and 35 sheep sera showed reactivity to BFV Gag antigen in GST ELISA [149]. Unfortunately, further diagnostics of these BFV-cross-reactive animals by virus isolation or PCR amplification were unsuccessful [159]. Recent studies regarding wild ruminants revealed a similar scenario: some sera also reacted with BFV antigens in ELISA test, but PCR mostly failed to identify genetic material of BFV [160]. In fact, the lack of amplification with BFV-specific primers might suggest the infection with novel, species-specific FVs, which generate antibodies that cross-react with BFV-specific antigen. Therefore, the existence of BFV-related FVs in other ruminants still remains open.

2.5. Utilization of BFV as Viral Vector for Translational Applications

As with other retroviruses, different viral vectors for the expression of therapeutic genes or the delivery of vaccine antigens have been constructed for PFV, few SFVs, and FFV, as review see [161]. These vectors mostly include replication-deficient gene transfer vectors generated in producer cells, but they also include replication-competent engineered viruses, which are mostly intended for life vaccine applications. Some of these vectors have been tested beyond cell cultures in small lab animals (mostly mice), but also in outbred hosts like dog (ex vivo PFV-based gene transfer vectors to treat canine leukocyte adhesion deficiency [162]) and cats (FFV-based replication-competent vaccine vectors [163,164]). The recent cloning of full-length BFV genomes that allows for cell-free transmission [14,25,26] is an important prerequisite for conducting and extending corresponding studies also for BFV.

Cattle are important livestock animals and vector-based approaches are likely to meet the costs imposed by bovine infectious disease or the need to engineer defined traits in the future. Such vector-directed gene transfer and vaccination might be an interesting option with a corresponding market to explore and use BFV as a suited viral vector for treatment of cattle. The availability of CMV-IE-driven BFV genomes and recent data that HT cell-free BFV variants replicate in cattle are important prerequisites for such studies [14]. Furthermore, even an engineered HT cell-free BFV variant lacking the entire miRNA cassette replicated in experimentally infected animals and induced immunity against BFV Gag and Bet [14]. Together with the data on the function and core features of the BFV miRNA cassette and the chimerization of the BFV pri-miRNA [23], the insertion of therapeutic or prophylactic miRNAs into replication-competent BFV vectors or the construction of BFV-based miRNA expression tools appear to be new and interesting future developments [161].

3. Conclusions and Outlook

As shown here, research regarding diverse aspects of BFV replication and biology in vitro and in vivo has significantly expanded our understanding of the complexity and diversity of FVs. These new findings are in line with the concept that each of the known exogenous FVs has been shaped by a long history of co-adaptation and co-evolution [10]. It remains to be seen whether, for instance, the host dictates the major pathway of FV transmission: Here, strong differences between herbivorous cattle that do not display aggressive intra-species behavior and carni- and omnivorous simians or felines with a substantial amount of aggressive behavior within and between groups and individual animals can be anticipated. Whether such differences in the host's biology not only affect transmission, but also the repertoire of antiviral restriction, remains to be seen, but appears to be possible.

Additional avenues of high-impact research in BFV may be related to development of vaccine vectors based on the BFV genome or genetic elements thereof. The possibility of cell-free BFV infections recently achieved offset the limitations of a tight cell-associated transmission from BFV as a therapeutic and prophylactic vector candidate [14,24,25]. Vaccines that are based on bovine virus-based vectors could be a great alternative in veterinary science and practice, especially in the context of economically important infections that, due to the high prevalence in cattle populations, cannot be eradicated by culling. Furthermore, extending the studies on the BFV miRNAs as modulators of the virus-host interface and evolutionary struggle, as well as their translational application within a BFV-based vector or as an independent cassette, appears to be a promising extension of ongoing work. Finally, it is of high priority to explore the "requirements" of BFV—as part of the human food chain and present in several raw cattle products—to enter the human population. Such studies may be pretty challenging and also—to a certain degree—unpredictable, but of high medical and epidemiological importance. Here, in vitro selection and evolution screens employing either fresh animal-derived BFV or "native" BFV isolates and primary human cells of different tissue/organ origin will be of special value.

Author Contributions: M.M.-K., J.T., A.H.-W. and M.L. wrote, corrected and approved the article, A.H.-M. provided valuable information and conducted bioinformatics analyses together with A.H.-W., the initial layout and final editing were done by M.L.

Funding: Work by M.M.-K. was supported by Polish Ministry of Science and Higher Education and DAAD, gants no. 5 PO6K 043 27, 484/N-DAAD/2009/2010 and KNOW (Leading National Research Centre) scientific Consortium, "Healthy Animal—Safe Food", decision of Ministry of Science and Higher Education 05-/KNOW2/2015. J.T. was funded by the National Natural Science Foundation of China, grant number 31670151 and A.H.-M., A.H.-W and M.L. were supported by the Baden-Württemberg Stiftung, research grant SID 49 and PPP Polish-German DAAD travel grants.

Acknowledgments: M.M.-K. would like to thank Jacek Kuźmak for introduction into the foamy virus field and his continuous support. M.L. thanks his partners and supporters on BFV research, in particular Roland Riebe, Frank Rösl, Jacek Kuźmak, Timo Kehl, Torsten Hechler, Wentao Qiao, Bryan Cullen, Thomas Vahlenkamp, Lutz Gissmann and M.M.-K. The authors thank Martha Krumbach (DKFZ) for critically reading the manuscript.

Conflicts of Interest: The authors declare no conflict of interest.

References

1. Khan, A.S.; Bodem, J.; Buseyne, F.; Gessain, A.; Johnson, W.; Kuhn, J.H.; Kuzmak, J.; Lindemann, D.; Linial, M.L.; Löchelt, M.; et al. Spumaretroviruses: Updated taxonomy and nomenclature. *Virology* **2018**, *516*, 158–164. [CrossRef] [PubMed]
2. Han, G.Z.; Worobey, M. An endogenous foamy-like viral element in the coelacanth genome. *PLoS Pathog.* **2012**, *8*, e1002790. [CrossRef] [PubMed]
3. Achong, B.G.; Mansell, P.W.; Epstein, M.A.; Clifford, P. An unusual virus in cultures from a human nasopharyngeal carcinoma. *J. Natl. Cancer Inst.* **1971**, *46*, 299–307. [PubMed]
4. Herchenröder, O.; Renne, R.; Loncar, D.; Cobb, E.K.; Murthy, K.K.; Schneider, J.; Mergia, A.; Luciw, P.A. Isolation, cloning, and sequencing of simian foamy viruses from chimpanzees (sfvcpz): High homology to human foamy virus (hfv). *Virology* **1994**, *201*, 187–199. [CrossRef]

5. Kehl, T.; Tan, J.; Materniak, M. Non-simian foamy viruses: Molecular virology, tropism and prevalence and zoonotic/interspecies transmission. *Viruses* **2013**, *5*, 2169–2209. [CrossRef]
6. Wolfe, N.D.; Switzer, W.M.; Carr, J.K.; Bhullar, V.B.; Shanmugam, V.; Tamoufe, U.; Prosser, A.T.; Torimiro, J.N.; Wright, A.; Mpoudi-Ngole, E.; et al. Naturally acquired simian retrovirus infections in central african hunters. *Lancet* **2004**, *363*, 932–937. [CrossRef]
7. Pinto-Santini, D.M.; Stenbak, C.R.; Linial, M.L. Foamy virus zoonotic infections. *Retrovirology* **2017**, *14*, 55. [CrossRef]
8. Muniz, C.P.; Cavalcante, L.T.F.; Jia, H.; Zheng, H.; Tang, S.; Augusto, A.M.; Pissinatti, A.; Fedullo, L.P.; Santos, A.F.; Soares, M.A.; et al. Zoonotic infection of brazilian primate workers with new world simian foamy virus. *PLoS ONE* **2017**, *12*, e0184502. [CrossRef]
9. Chen, Y.; Wei, X.; Zhang, G.; Holmes, E.C.; Cui, J. Identification and evolution of avian endogenous foamy viruses. *Virus Evol.* **2019**, in press. [CrossRef]
10. Katzourakis, A.; Gifford, R.J.; Tristem, M.; Gilbert, M.T.; Pybus, O.G. Macroevolution of complex retroviruses. *Science* **2009**, *325*, 1512. [CrossRef]
11. Linial, M. Why aren't foamy viruses pathogenic? *Trends Microbiol.* **2000**, *8*, 284–289. [CrossRef]
12. Aiewsakun, P.; Simmonds, P.; Katzourakis, A. The first co-opted endogenous foamy viruses and the evolutionary history of reptilian foamy viruses. *Viruses* **2019**, *11*, 641. [CrossRef] [PubMed]
13. Materniak, M.; Hechler, T.; Löchelt, M.; Kuzmak, J. Similar patterns of infection with bovine foamy virus in experimentally inoculated calves and sheep. *J. Virol.* **2013**, *87*, 3516–3525. [CrossRef] [PubMed]
14. Cao, W.; Materniak-Kornas, M.; Stricker, E.; Heit-Mondrzyk, A.; Pougialis, G.; Hugo, A.; Kubis, P.; Sell, B.; Hotz-Wagenblatt, A.; Kuzmak, J.; et al. Functional analysis of bovine foamy virus-encoded mirnas reveals the prime importance of defined mirna for virus replication and host-virus interaction. *Viruses* **2019**, under review.
15. Romen, F.; Backes, P.; Materniak, M.; Sting, R.; Vahlenkamp, T.W.; Riebe, R.; Pawlita, M.; Kuzmak, J.; Löchelt, M. Serological detection systems for identification of cows shedding bovine foamy virus via milk. *Virology* **2007**, *364*, 123–131. [CrossRef]
16. Materniak, M.; Sieradzki, Z.; Kuzmak, J. Detection of bovine foamy virus in milk and saliva of bfv seropositive cattle. *Bull. Vet. Inst. Pulawy* **2010**, *54*, 461–465.
17. Liebermann, H.; Riebe, R. Isolation of bovine syncytial virus in east germany. *Arch. Exp. Vet.* **1981**, *35*, 917–919.
18. Liebermann, H.; Riebe, R. Cellular spectrum of bovine syncytial virus. *Arch. Exp. Vet.* **1981**, *35*, 945–953.
19. Holzschu, D.L.; Delaney, M.A.; Renshaw, R.W.; Casey, J.W. The nucleotide sequence and spliced pol mrna levels of the nonprimate spumavirus bovine foamy virus. *J. Virol.* **1998**, *72*, 2177–2182.
20. Rethwilm, A.; Bodem, J. Evolution of foamy viruses: The most ancient of all retroviruses. *Viruses* **2013**, *5*, 2349–2374. [CrossRef]
21. Zhang, S.; Cui, X.; Li, J.; Liang, Z.; Qiao, W.; Tan, J. Lysine residues k66, k109, and k110 in the bovine foamy virus transactivator protein are required for transactivation and viral replication. *Virol. Sin.* **2016**, *31*, 142–149. [CrossRef] [PubMed]
22. Whisnant, A.W.; Kehl, T.; Bao, Q.; Materniak, M.; Kuzmak, J.; Löchelt, M.; Cullen, B.R. Identification of novel, highly expressed retroviral micrornas in cells infected by bovine foamy virus. *J. Virol.* **2014**, *88*, 4679–4686. [CrossRef] [PubMed]
23. Cao, W.; Heit, A.; Hotz-Wagenblatt, A.; Löchelt, M. Functional characterization of the bovine foamy virus mirna expression cassette and its dumbbell-shaped pri-mirna. *Virus Genes* **2018**, *54*, 550–560. [CrossRef] [PubMed]
24. Bao, Q.; Hipp, M.; Hugo, A.; Lei, J.; Liu, Y.; Kehl, T.; Hechler, T.; Löchelt, M. In vitro evolution of bovine foamy virus variants with enhanced cell-free virus titers and transmission. *Viruses* **2015**, *7*, 5855–5874. [CrossRef]
25. Zhang, S.; Liu, X.; Liang, Z.; Bing, T.; Qiao, W.; Tan, J. The influence of envelope c-terminus amino acid composition on the ratio of cell-free to cell-cell transmission for bovine foamy virus. *Viruses* **2019**, *11*, 130. [CrossRef]
26. Bao, Q.; Hotz-Wagenblatt, A.; Betts, M.J.; Hipp, M.; Hugo, A.; Pougialis, G.; Lei-Rossmann, J.; Löchelt, M. Distinct cell and isolate-specific adaptation strategies of gag and env yield high titer bovine foamy virus variants. *Infect. Genet. Evol.* **2019**, under review.

27. Tan, J.; Qiao, W.; Wang, J.; Xu, F.; Li, Y.; Zhou, J.; Chen, Q.; Geng, Y. Ifp35 is involved in the antiviral function of interferon by association with the viral tas transactivator of bovine foamy virus. *J. Virol.* **2008**, *82*, 4275–4283. [CrossRef]
28. Materniak-Kornas, M.; Kubis, P.; Kuzmak, J. Investigation of active replication sites of BFV in different tissues of experimentally inoculated calves. In Proceedings of the 12th International Foamy Virus Conference, Paris, France, 9–10 June 2016.
29. Enders, J.F.; Peebles, T.C. Propagation in tissue cultures of cytopathogenic agents from patients with measles. *Proc. Soc. Exp. Biol. Med.* **1954**, *86*, 277–286. [CrossRef]
30. Malmquist, W.A.; Van der Maaten, M.J.; Boothe, A.D. Isolation, immunodiffusion, immunofluorescence, and electron microscopy of a syncytial virus of lymphosarcomatous and apparently normal cattle. *Cancer Res.* **1969**, *29*, 188–200.
31. Tan, J.; Qiao, W.; Xu, F.; Han, H.; Chen, Q.; Geng, Y. Dimerization of btas is required for the transactivational activity of bovine foamy virus. *Virology* **2008**, *376*, 236–241. [CrossRef]
32. Chang, J.; Lee, K.J.; Jang, K.L.; Lee, E.K.; Baek, G.H.; Sung, Y.C. Human foamy virus bel1 transactivator contains a bipartite nuclear localization determinant which is sensitive to protein context and triple multimerization domains. *J. Virol.* **1995**, *69*, 801–808. [PubMed]
33. Ma, Q.; Tan, J.; Cui, X.; Luo, D.; Yu, M.; Liang, C.; Qiao, W. Residues r(199)h(200) of prototype foamy virus transactivator bel1 contribute to its binding with ltr and ip promoters but not its nuclear localization. *Virology* **2014**, *449*, 215–223. [CrossRef] [PubMed]
34. Wang, W.; Tan, J.; Wang, J.; Chen, Q.; Geng, Y.; Qiao, W. Analysis of bovine foamy virus btas mrna transcripts during persistent infection. *Virus Genes* **2010**, *40*, 84–93. [CrossRef] [PubMed]
35. Wu, Y.; Tan, J.; Su, Y.; Qiao, W.; Geng, Y.; Chen, Q. Transcription factor ap1 modulates the internal promoter activity of bovine foamy virus. *Virus Res.* **2010**, *147*, 139–144. [CrossRef]
36. Bannert, H.; Muranyi, W.; Ogryzko, V.V.; Nakatani, Y.; Flugel, R.M. Coactivators p300 and pcaf physically and functionally interact with the foamy viral trans-activator. *BMC Mol. Biol.* **2004**, *5*, 16. [CrossRef] [PubMed]
37. Bodem, J.; Krausslich, H.G.; Rethwilm, A. Acetylation of the foamy virus transactivator tas by pcaf augments promoter-binding affinity and virus transcription. *J. Gen. Virol.* **2007**, *88*, 259–263. [CrossRef]
38. Chang, R.; Tan, J.; Xu, F.; Han, H.; Geng, Y.; Li, Y.; Qiao, W. Lysine acetylation sites in bovine foamy virus transactivator btas are important for its DNA binding activity. *Virology* **2011**, *418*, 21–26. [CrossRef]
39. Wang, J.; Tan, J.; Guo, H.; Zhang, Q.; Jia, R.; Xu, X.; Geng, Y.; Qiao, W. Bovine foamy virus transactivator btas interacts with cellular relb to enhance viral transcription. *J. Virol.* **2010**, *84*, 11888–11897. [CrossRef]
40. Wang, J.; Tan, J.; Zhang, X.; Guo, H.; Zhang, Q.; Guo, T.; Geng, Y.; Qiao, W. Bfv activates the nf-kappab pathway through its transactivator (btas) to enhance viral transcription. *Virology* **2010**, *400*, 215–223. [CrossRef]
41. Löchelt, M. Foamy virus transactivation and gene expression. *Curr. Top. Microbiol. Immunol.* **2003**, *277*, 27–61.
42. Hahn, H.; Baunach, G.; Brautigam, S.; Mergia, A.; Neumann-Haefelin, D.; Daniel, M.D.; McClure, M.O.; Rethwilm, A. Reactivity of primate sera to foamy virus gag and bet proteins. *J. Gen. Virol.* **1994**, *75*, 2635–2644. [CrossRef] [PubMed]
43. Löchelt, M.; Romen, F.; Bastone, P.; Muckenfuss, H.; Kirchner, N.; Kim, Y.B.; Truyen, U.; Rosler, U.; Battenberg, M.; Saib, A.; et al. The antiretroviral activity of apobec3 is inhibited by the foamy virus accessory bet protein. *Proc. Natl. Acad. Sci. USA* **2005**, *102*, 7982–7987. [CrossRef] [PubMed]
44. Russell, R.A.; Wiegand, H.L.; Moore, M.D.; Schafer, A.; McClure, M.O.; Cullen, B.R. Foamy virus bet proteins function as novel inhibitors of the apobec3 family of innate antiretroviral defense factors. *J. Virol.* **2005**, *79*, 8724–8731. [CrossRef] [PubMed]
45. Perkovic, M.; Schmidt, S.; Marino, D.; Russell, R.A.; Stauch, B.; Hofmann, H.; Kopietz, F.; Kloke, B.P.; Zielonka, J.; Strover, H.; et al. Species-specific inhibition of apobec3c by the prototype foamy virus protein bet. *J. Biol. Chem.* **2009**, *284*, 5819–5826. [CrossRef]
46. Saib, A.; Koken, M.H.; van der Spek, P.; Peries, J.; de Thé, H. Involvement of a spliced and defective human foamy virus in the establishment of chronic infection. *J. Virol.* **1995**, *69*, 5261–5268.
47. Callahan, M.E.; Switzer, W.M.; Matthews, A.L.; Roberts, B.D.; Heneine, W.; Folks, T.M.; Sandstrom, P.A. Persistent zoonotic infection of a human with simian foamy virus in the absence of an intact orf-2 accessory gene. *J. Virol.* **1999**, *73*, 9619–9624.

48. Meiering, C.D.; Linial, M.L. Reactivation of a complex retrovirus is controlled by a molecular switch and is inhibited by a viral protein. *Proc. Natl. Acad. Sci. USA* **2002**, *99*, 15130–15135. [CrossRef]
49. Lukic, D.S.; Hotz-Wagenblatt, A.; Lei, J.; Räthe, A.M.; Muhle, M.; Denner, J.; Münk, C.; Löchelt, M. Identification of the feline foamy virus bet domain essential for apobec3 counteraction. *Retrovirology* **2013**, *10*, 76. [CrossRef]
50. Bing, T.; Yu, H.; Li, Y.; Sun, L.; Tan, J.; Geng, Y.; Qiao, W. Characterization of a full-length infectious clone of bovine foamy virus 3026. *Virol. Sin.* **2014**, *29*, 94–102. [CrossRef]
51. Materniak, M.; Bicka, L.; Kuzmak, J. Isolation and partial characterization of bovine foamy virus from polish cattle. *Pol. J. Vet. Sci.* **2006**, *9*, 207–211.
52. Hechler, T.; Materniak, M.; Kehl, T.; Kuzmak, J.; Löchelt, M. Complete genome sequences of two novel european clade bovine foamy viruses from germany and poland. *J. Virol.* **2012**, *86*, 10905–10906. [CrossRef] [PubMed]
53. Lindemann, D.; Rethwilm, A. Characterization of a human foamy virus 170-kilodalton env-bet fusion protein generated by alternative splicing. *J. Virol.* **1998**, *72*, 4088–4094.
54. Bing, T.; Wu, K.; Cui, X.; Shao, P.; Zhang, Q.; Bai, X.; Tan, J.; Qiao, W. Identification and functional characterization of bet protein as a negative regulator of bfv3026 replication. *Virus Genes* **2014**, *48*, 464–473. [CrossRef] [PubMed]
55. Horton, P.; Park, K.J.; Obayashi, T.; Fujita, N.; Harada, H.; Adams-Collier, C.J.; Nakai, K. Wolf psort: Protein localization predictor. *Nucleic Acids Res.* **2007**, *35*, W585–W587. [CrossRef] [PubMed]
56. Nguyen Ba, A.N.; Pogoutse, A.; Provart, N.; Moses, A.M. Nlstradamus: A simple hidden markov model for nuclear localization signal prediction. *BMC Bioinform.* **2009**, *10*, 202. [CrossRef] [PubMed]
57. Lecellier, C.H.; Vermeulen, W.; Bachelerie, F.; Giron, M.L.; Saib, A. Intra- and intercellular trafficking of the foamy virus auxiliary bet protein. *J. Virol.* **2002**, *76*, 3388–3394. [CrossRef]
58. Corbett, A.H.; Silver, P.A. Nucleocytoplasmic transport of macromolecules. *Microbiol. Mol. Biol. Rev.* **1997**, *61*, 193–211.
59. Alke, A.; Schwantes, A.; Kido, K.; Flötenmeyer, M.; Flügel, R.M.; Löchelt, M. The bet gene of feline foamy virus is required for virus replication. *Virology* **2001**, *287*, 310–320. [CrossRef]
60. Yu, S.F.; Linial, M.L. Analysis of the role of the bel and bet open reading frames of human foamy virus by using a new quantitative assay. *J. Virol.* **1993**, *67*, 6618–6624.
61. Bock, M.; Heinkelein, M.; Lindemann, D.; Rethwilm, A. Cells expressing the human foamy virus (hfv) accessory bet protein are resistant to productive hfv superinfection. *Virology* **1998**, *250*, 194–204. [CrossRef]
62. Mullers, E. The foamy virus gag proteins: What makes them different? *Viruses* **2013**, *5*, 1023–1041. [CrossRef] [PubMed]
63. Eastman, S.W.; Linial, M.L. Identification of a conserved residue of foamy virus gag required for intracellular capsid assembly. *J. Virol.* **2001**, *75*, 6857–6864. [CrossRef] [PubMed]
64. Pfrepper, K.I.; Löchelt, M.; Rackwitz, H.R.; Schnölzer, M.; Heid, H.; Flügel, R.M. Molecular characterization of proteolytic processing of the gag proteins of human spumavirus. *J. Virol.* **1999**, *73*, 7907–7911. [PubMed]
65. Pfrepper, K.I.; Rackwitz, H.R.; Schnölzer, M.; Heid, H.; Löchelt, M.; Flügel, R.M. Molecular characterization of proteolytic processing of the pol proteins of human foamy virus reveals novel features of the viral protease. *J. Virol.* **1998**, *72*, 7648–7652.
66. Wang, J.; Guo, H.Y.; Jia, R.; Xu, X.; Tan, J.; Geng, Y.Q.; Qiao, W.T. Preparation of bfv gag antiserum and preliminary study on cellular distribution of bfv. *Virol. Sin.* **2010**, *25*, 115–122. [CrossRef]
67. Yu, S.F.; Edelmann, K.; Strong, R.K.; Moebes, A.; Rethwilm, A.; Linial, M.L. The carboxyl terminus of the human foamy virus gag protein contains separable nucleic acid binding and nuclear transport domains. *J. Virol.* **1996**, *70*, 8255–8262.
68. Kong, X.H.; Yu, H.; Xuan, C.H.; Wang, J.Z.; Chen, Q.M.; Geng, Y.Q. The requirements and mechanism for capsid assembly and budding of bovine foamy virus. *Arch. Virol.* **2005**, *150*, 1677–1684. [CrossRef]
69. Winkler, I.; Bodem, J.; Haas, L.; Zemba, M.; Delius, H.; Flower, R.; Flügel, R.M.; Löchelt, M. Characterization of the genome of feline foamy virus and its proteins shows distinct features different from those of primate spumaviruses. *J. Virol.* **1997**, *71*, 6727–6741.
70. Wang, I.H.; Burckhardt, C.J.; Yakimovich, A.; Greber, U.F. Imaging, tracking and computational analyses of virus entry and egress with the cytoskeleton. *Viruses* **2018**, *10*, 166. [CrossRef]

71. Naghavi, M.H.; Walsh, D. Microtubule regulation and function during virus infection. *J. Virol.* **2017**, *91*, e00538-17. [CrossRef]
72. Arriagada, G. Retroviruses and microtubule-associated motor proteins. *Cell Microbiol* **2017**, *19*. [CrossRef] [PubMed]
73. Harris, R.S.; Hultquist, J.F.; Evans, D.T. The restriction factors of human immunodeficiency virus. *J. Biol. Chem.* **2012**, *287*, 40875–40883. [CrossRef] [PubMed]
74. Peng, G.; Lei, K.J.; Jin, W.; Greenwell-Wild, T.; Wahl, S.M. Induction of apobec3 family proteins, a defensive maneuver underlying interferon-induced anti-hiv-1 activity. *J. Exp. Med.* **2006**, *203*, 41–46. [CrossRef] [PubMed]
75. Stopak, K.S.; Chiu, Y.L.; Kropp, J.; Grant, R.M.; Greene, W.C. Distinct patterns of cytokine regulation of apobec3g expression and activity in primary lymphocytes, macrophages, and dendritic cells. *J. Biol. Chem.* **2007**, *282*, 3539–3546. [CrossRef]
76. Carthagena, L.; Bergamaschi, A.; Luna, J.M.; David, A.; Uchil, P.D.; Margottin-Goguet, F.; Mothes, W.; Hazan, U.; Transy, C.; Pancino, G.; et al. Human trim gene expression in response to interferons. *PLoS ONE* **2009**, *4*, e4894. [CrossRef]
77. Liberatore, R.A.; Bieniasz, P.D. Tetherin is a key effector of the antiretroviral activity of type i interferon in vitro and In Vivo. *Proc. Natl. Acad. Sci. USA* **2011**, *108*, 18097–18101. [CrossRef]
78. Sheehy, A.M.; Gaddis, N.C.; Choi, J.D.; Malim, M.H. Isolation of a human gene that inhibits hiv-1 infection and is suppressed by the viral vif protein. *Nature* **2002**, *418*, 646–650. [CrossRef]
79. Stremlau, M.; Owens, C.M.; Perron, M.J.; Kiessling, M.; Autissier, P.; Sodroski, J. The cytoplasmic body component trim5alpha restricts hiv-1 infection in old world monkeys. *Nature* **2004**, *427*, 848–853. [CrossRef]
80. Neil, S.J.; Zang, T.; Bieniasz, P.D. Tetherin inhibits retrovirus release and is antagonized by hiv-1 vpu. *Nature* **2008**, *451*, 425–430. [CrossRef]
81. Laguette, N.; Sobhian, B.; Casartelli, N.; Ringeard, M.; Chable-Bessia, C.; Segeral, E.; Yatim, A.; Emiliani, S.; Schwartz, O.; Benkirane, M. Samhd1 is the dendritic- and myeloid-cell-specific hiv-1 restriction factor counteracted by vpx. *Nature* **2011**, *474*, 654–657. [CrossRef]
82. Lu, J.; Pan, Q.; Rong, L.; He, W.; Liu, S.L.; Liang, C. The ifitm proteins inhibit hiv-1 infection. *J. Virol.* **2011**, *85*, 2126–2137. [CrossRef] [PubMed]
83. Liu, Z.; Pan, Q.; Ding, S.; Qian, J.; Xu, F.; Zhou, J.; Cen, S.; Guo, F.; Liang, C. The interferon-inducible mxb protein inhibits hiv-1 infection. *Cell Host Microbe* **2013**, *14*, 398–410. [CrossRef] [PubMed]
84. Usami, Y.; Wu, Y.; Gottlinger, H.G. Serinc3 and serinc5 restrict hiv-1 infectivity and are counteracted by nef. *Nature* **2015**, *526*, 218–223. [CrossRef] [PubMed]
85. Yap, M.W.; Lindemann, D.; Stanke, N.; Reh, J.; Westphal, D.; Hanenberg, H.; Ohkura, S.; Stoye, J.P. Restriction of foamy viruses by primate trim5alpha. *J. Virol.* **2008**, *82*, 5429–5439. [CrossRef]
86. Pacheco, B.; Finzi, A.; McGee-Estrada, K.; Sodroski, J. Species-specific inhibition of foamy viruses from south american monkeys by new world monkey trim5{alpha} proteins. *J. Virol.* **2010**, *84*, 4095–4099. [CrossRef]
87. Delebecque, F.; Suspene, R.; Calattini, S.; Casartelli, N.; Saib, A.; Froment, A.; Wain-Hobson, S.; Gessain, A.; Vartanian, J.P.; Schwartz, O. Restriction of foamy viruses by apobec cytidine deaminases. *J. Virol.* **2006**, *80*, 605–614. [CrossRef]
88. Jouvenet, N.; Neil, S.J.; Zhadina, M.; Zang, T.; Kratovac, Z.; Lee, Y.; McNatt, M.; Hatziioannou, T.; Bieniasz, P.D. Broad-spectrum inhibition of retroviral and filoviral particle release by tetherin. *J. Virol.* **2009**, *83*, 1837–1844. [CrossRef]
89. Xu, F.; Tan, J.; Liu, R.; Xu, D.; Li, Y.; Geng, Y.; Liang, C.; Qiao, W. Tetherin inhibits prototypic foamy virus release. *Virol. J.* **2011**, *8*, 198. [CrossRef]
90. Liang, Z.; Zhang, Y.; Song, J.; Zhang, H.; Zhang, S.; Li, Y.; Tan, J.; Qiao, W. The effect of bovine bst2a1 on the release and cell-to-cell transmission of retroviruses. *Virol. J.* **2017**, *14*, 173. [CrossRef]
91. Regad, T.; Saib, A.; Lallemand-Breitenbach, V.; Pandolfi, P.P.; de Thé, H.; Chelbi-Alix, M.K. Pml mediates the interferon-induced antiviral state against a complex retrovirus via its association with the viral transactivator. *EMBO J.* **2001**, *20*, 3495–3505. [CrossRef]
92. Hu, X.; Yang, W.; Liu, R.; Geng, Y.; Qiao, W.; Tan, J. N-myc interactor inhibits prototype foamy virus by sequestering viral tas protein in the cytoplasm. *J. Virol.* **2014**, *88*, 7036–7044. [CrossRef] [PubMed]
93. Dong, L.; Cheng, Q.; Wang, Z.; Yuan, P.; Li, Z.; Sun, Y.; Han, S.; Yin, J.; Peng, B.; He, X.; et al. Human pirh2 is a novel inhibitor of prototype foamy virus replication. *Viruses* **2015**, *7*, 1668–1684. [CrossRef] [PubMed]

94. Kane, M.; Zang, T.M.; Rihn, S.J.; Zhang, F.; Kueck, T.; Alim, M.; Schoggins, J.; Rice, C.M.; Wilson, S.J.; Bieniasz, P.D. Identification of interferon-stimulated genes with antiretroviral activity. *Cell Host Microbe* **2016**, *20*, 392–405. [CrossRef] [PubMed]
95. Herchenröder, O.; Löchelt, M.; Buseyne, F.; Gessain, A.; Soares, M.A.; Khan, A.S.; Lindemann, D. Twelfth international foamy virus conference-meeting report. *Viruses* **2019**, *11*, 134. [CrossRef]
96. Ledesma-Feliciano, C.; Troyer, R.M.; Zheng, X.; Miller, C.; Cianciolo, R.; Bordicchia, M.; Dannemiller, N.; Gagne, R.; Beatty, J.; Quimby, J.; et al. Feline foamy virus infection: Characterization of experimental infection and prevalence of natural infection in domestic cats with and without chronic kidney disease. *Viruses* **2019**, *11*, 662. [CrossRef]
97. Murray, S.M.; Picker, L.J.; Axthelm, M.K.; Hudkins, K.; Alpers, C.E.; Linial, M.L. Replication in a superficial epithelial cell niche explains the lack of pathogenicity of primate foamy virus infections. *J. Virol.* **2008**, *82*, 5981–5985. [CrossRef]
98. Rhodes-Feuillette, A.; Saal, F.; Lasneret, J.; Santillana-Hayat, M.; Peries, J. Studies on in vitro interferon induction capacity and interferon sensitivity of simian foamy viruses. *Arch. Virol.* **1987**, *97*, 77–84. [CrossRef]
99. Colas, S.; Bourge, J.F.; Wybier, J.; Chelbi-Alix, M.K.; Paul, P.; Emanoil-Ravier, R. Human foamy virus infection activates class i major histocompatibility complex antigen expression. *J. Gen. Virol.* **1995**, *76*, 661–667. [CrossRef]
100. Sabile, A.; Rhodes-Feuillette, A.; Jaoui, F.Z.; Tobaly-Tapiero, J.; Giron, M.L.; Lasneret, J.; Peries, J.; Canivet, M. In vitro studies on interferon-inducing capacity and sensitivity to ifn of human foamy virus. *Res. Virol.* **1996**, *147*, 29–37. [CrossRef]
101. Rua, R.; Lepelley, A.; Gessain, A.; Schwartz, O. Innate sensing of foamy viruses by human hematopoietic cells. *J. Virol.* **2012**, *86*, 909–918. [CrossRef]
102. Meiering, C.D.; Linial, M.L. The promyelocytic leukemia protein does not mediate foamy virus latency in vitro. *J. Virol.* **2003**, *77*, 2207–2213. [CrossRef] [PubMed]
103. Falcone, V.; Schweizer, M.; Toniolo, A.; Neumann-Haefelin, D.; Meyerhans, A. Gamma interferon is a major suppressive factor produced by activated human peripheral blood lymphocytes that is able to inhibit foamy virus-induced cytopathic effects. *J. Virol.* **1999**, *73*, 1724–1728. [PubMed]
104. Rola-Luszczak, M.; Materniak, M.; Pluta, A.; Hulst, M.; Kuzmak, J. Transcriptomic microarray analysis of bomac cells after infection with bovine foamy virus. *Arch. Virol.* **2014**, *159*, 1515–1519. [CrossRef] [PubMed]
105. Bloor, S.; Maelfait, J.; Krumbach, R.; Beyaert, R.; Randow, F. Endoplasmic reticulum chaperone gp96 is essential for infection with vesicular stomatitis virus. *Proc. Natl. Acad. Sci. USA* **2010**, *107*, 6970–6975. [CrossRef]
106. Carrington, M.; O'Brien, S.J. The influence of hla genotype on aids. *Annu. Rev. Med.* **2003**, *54*, 535–551. [CrossRef]
107. Lerner, D.L.; Grant, C.K.; de Parseval, A.; Elder, J.H. Fiv infection of il-2-dependent and -independent feline lymphocyte lines: Host cells range distinctions and specific cytokine upregulation. *Vet. Immunol. Immunopathol.* **1998**, *65*, 277–297. [CrossRef]
108. Rideout, B.A.; Moore, P.F.; Pedersen, N.C. Persistent upregulation of mhc class ii antigen expression on t-lymphocytes from cats experimentally infected with feline immunodeficiency virus. *Vet. Immunol. Immunopathol.* **1992**, *35*, 71–81. [CrossRef]
109. Nogami, S.; Satoh, S.; Tanaka-Nakadate, S.; Yoshida, K.; Nakano, M.; Terano, A.; Shirataki, H. Identification and characterization of taxilin isoforms. *Biochem. Biophys. Res. Commun.* **2004**, *319*, 936–943. [CrossRef]
110. Hoffmann, J.; Boehm, C.; Himmelsbach, K.; Donnerhak, C.; Roettger, H.; Weiss, T.S.; Ploen, D.; Hildt, E. Identification of alpha-taxilin as an essential factor for the life cycle of hepatitis b virus. *J. Hepatol.* **2013**, *59*, 934–941. [CrossRef]
111. Hutter, S.; Zurnic, I.; Lindemann, D. Foamy virus budding and release. *Viruses* **2013**, *5*, 1075–1098. [CrossRef]
112. Kincaid, R.P.; Chen, Y.; Cox, J.E.; Rethwilm, A.; Sullivan, C.S. Noncanonical microrna (mirna) biogenesis gives rise to retroviral mimics of lymphoproliferative and immunosuppressive host mirnas. *MBio* **2014**, *5*, e00074. [CrossRef] [PubMed]
113. Kincaid, R.P.; Burke, J.M.; Sullivan, C.S. Rna virus microrna that mimics a b-cell oncomir. *Proc. Natl. Acad. Sci. USA* **2012**, *109*, 3077–3082. [CrossRef] [PubMed]
114. Safari, R.; Hamaidia, M.; de Brogniez, A.; Gillet, N.; Willems, L. Cis-drivers and trans-drivers of bovine leukemia virus oncogenesis. *Curr. Opin. Virol.* **2017**, *26*, 15–19. [CrossRef] [PubMed]
115. Rua, R.; Betsem, E.; Calattini, S.; Saib, A.; Gessain, A. Genetic characterization of simian foamy viruses infecting humans. *J. Virol.* **2012**, *86*, 13350–13359. [CrossRef] [PubMed]

116. Burke, J.M.; Kincaid, R.P.; Aloisio, F.; Welch, N.; Sullivan, C.S. Expression of short hairpin rnas using the compact architecture of retroviral microrna genes. *Nucleic Acids Res.* **2017**, *45*, e154. [CrossRef] [PubMed]
117. Heit, A. In Silico Investigations of Bovine Foamy Virus Micrornas. Master's Thesis, University of Heidelberg, Heidelberg, Germany, 2017.
118. Hildebrand, D.; Eberle, M.E.; Wolfle, S.M.; Egler, F.; Sahin, D.; Sahr, A.; Bode, K.A.; Heeg, K. Hsa-mir-99b/let-7e/mir-125a cluster regulates pathogen recognition receptor-stimulated suppressive antigen-presenting cells. *Front. Immunol.* **2018**, *9*, 1224. [CrossRef]
119. Servin-Gonzalez, L.S.; Granados-Lopez, A.J.; Lopez, J.A. Families of micrornas expressed in clusters regulate cell signaling in cervical cancer. *Int. J. Mol. Sci.* **2015**, *16*, 12773–12790. [CrossRef]
120. Shatseva, T.; Lee, D.Y.; Deng, Z.; Yang, B.B. Microrna mir-199a-3p regulates cell proliferation and survival by targeting caveolin-2. *J. Cell Sci.* **2011**, *124*, 2826–2836. [CrossRef]
121. Menning, M.; Kufer, T.A. A role for the ankyrin repeat containing protein ankrd17 in nod1- and nod2-mediated inflammatory responses. *FEBS Lett.* **2013**, *587*, 2137–2142. [CrossRef]
122. Takahashi, Y.; Meyerkord, C.L.; Hori, T.; Runkle, K.; Fox, T.E.; Kester, M.; Loughran, T.P.; Wang, H.G. Bif-1 regulates atg9 trafficking by mediating the fission of golgi membranes during autophagy. *Autophagy* **2011**, *7*, 61–73. [CrossRef]
123. Zhong, P.; Agosto, L.M.; Munro, J.B.; Mothes, W. Cell-to-cell transmission of viruses. *Curr. Opin. Virol.* **2013**, *3*, 44–50. [CrossRef] [PubMed]
124. Zhang, Z.; Tan, M.; Xie, Z.; Dai, L.; Chen, Y.; Zhao, Y. Identification of lysine succinylation as a new post-translational modification. *Nat. Chem. Biol.* **2011**, *7*, 58–63. [CrossRef] [PubMed]
125. Greig, A.S. A syncytium regression test to detect antibodies to bovine syncytial virus. *Can. J. Comp. Med.* **1979**, *43*, 112–114. [PubMed]
126. Jacobs, R.M.; Pollari, F.L.; McNab, W.B.; Jefferson, B. A serological survey of bovine syncytial virus in ontario: Associations with bovine leukemia and immunodeficiency-like viruses, production records, and management practices. *Can. J. Vet. Res.* **1995**, *59*, 271–278.
127. Appleby, R.C. Antibodies to bovine syncytial virus in dairy cattle. *Vet. Rec.* **1979**, *105*, 80–81. [CrossRef]
128. Johnson, R.H.; de la Rosa, J.; Abher, I.; Kertayadnya, I.G.; Entwistle, K.W.; Fordyce, G.; Holroyd, R.G. Epidemiological studies of bovine spumavirus. *Vet. Microbiol.* **1988**, *16*, 25–33. [CrossRef]
129. Materniak-Kornas, M.; Osinski, Z.; Rudzki, M.; Kuzmak, J. Development of a recombinant protein-based elisa for detection of antibodies against bovine foamy virus. *J. Vet. Res.* **2017**, *61*, 247–252. [CrossRef]
130. Jacobs, R.M.; Smith, H.E.; Gregory, B.; Valli, V.E.; Whetstone, C.A. Detection of multiple retroviral infections in cattle and cross-reactivity of bovine immunodeficiency-like virus and human immunodeficiency virus type 1 proteins using bovine and human sera in a western blot assay. *Can. J. Vet. Res.* **1992**, *56*, 353–359.
131. Adjei, A.A.; Adiku, T.K.; Kumi, P.F.; Domfeh, A.B. Human t-lymphotropic type-1 virus specific antibody detected in sera of hiv/aids patients in ghana. *Jpn. J. Infect. Dis.* **2003**, *56*, 57–59.
132. Bandecchi, P.; Matteucci, D.; Baldinotti, F.; Guidi, G.; Abramo, F.; Tozzini, F.; Bendinelli, M. Prevalence of feline immunodeficiency virus and other retroviral infections in sick cats in italy. *Vet. Immunol. Immunopathol.* **1992**, *31*, 337–345. [CrossRef]
133. Lee, I.T.; Levy, J.K.; Gorman, S.P.; Crawford, P.C.; Slater, M.R. Prevalence of feline leukemia virus infection and serum antibodies against feline immunodeficiency virus in unowned free-roaming cats. *J. Am. Vet. Med. Assoc.* **2002**, *220*, 620–622. [CrossRef] [PubMed]
134. Winkler, I.G.; Löchelt, M.; Flower, R.L. Epidemiology of feline foamy virus and feline immunodeficiency virus infections in domestic and feral cats: A seroepidemiological study. *J. Clin. Microbiol.* **1999**, *37*, 2848–2851. [PubMed]
135. Fultz, P.N.; McGinn, T.; Davis, I.C.; Romano, J.W.; Li, Y. Coinfection of macaques with simian immunodeficiency virus and simian t cell leukemia virus type i: Effects on virus burdens and disease progression. *J. Infect. Dis.* **1999**, *179*, 600–611. [CrossRef] [PubMed]
136. Amborski, G.F.; Lo, J.L.; Seger, C.L. Serological detection of multiple retroviral infections in cattle: Bovine leukemia virus, bovine syncytial virus and bovine visna virus. *Vet. Microbiol.* **1989**, *20*, 247–253. [CrossRef]
137. Rola, M. Development of Elisa Test for the Diagnostics of Biv Infections and Determination of the Biv Influence on the Course of Blv Infection. Ph.D. Thesis, NVRI, Pulawy, Poland, 2003.

138. Cohen, N.D.; Carter, C.N.; Thomas, M.A.; Lester, T.L.; Eugster, A.K. Epizootiologic association between feline immunodeficiency virus infection and feline leukemia virus seropositivity. *J. Am. Vet. Med. Assoc.* **1990**, *197*, 220–225.
139. O'Connor, T.P., Jr.; Tanguay, S.; Steinman, R.; Smith, R.; Barr, M.C.; Yamamoto, J.K.; Pedersen, N.C.; Andersen, P.R.; Tonelli, Q.J. Development and evaluation of immunoassay for detection of antibodies to the feline t-lymphotropic lentivirus (feline immunodeficiency virus). *J. Clin. Microbiol.* **1989**, *27*, 474–479.
140. Briggs, N.C.; Battjes, R.J.; Cantor, K.P.; Blattner, W.A.; Yellin, F.M.; Wilson, S.; Ritz, A.L.; Weiss, S.H.; Goedert, J.J. Seroprevalence of human t cell lymphotropic virus type ii infection, with or without human immunodeficiency virus type 1 coinfection, among us intravenous drug users. *J. Infect. Dis.* **1995**, *172*, 51–58. [CrossRef]
141. Materniak, M. Development of Diagnostic Methods for Bovine Foamy Virus Infections and the Role of Milk and Saliva in Virus Transmission. Ph.D. Thesis, NVRI, Pulawy, Poland, 2008.
142. Jacobs, R.M.; Song, Z.; Poon, H.; Heeney, J.L.; Taylor, J.A.; Jefferson, B.; Vernau, W.; Valli, V.E. Proviral detection and serology in bovine leukemia virus-exposed normal cattle and cattle with lymphoma. *Can. J. Vet. Res.* **1992**, *56*, 339–348.
143. Hooks, J.J.; Gibbs, C.J., Jr. The foamy viruses. *Bacteriol. Rev.* **1975**, *39*, 169–185.
144. Gillet, N.A.; Hamaidia, M.; de Brogniez, A.; Gutierrez, G.; Renotte, N.; Reichert, M.; Trono, K.; Willems, L. Bovine leukemia virus small noncoding rnas are functional elements that regulate replication and contribute to oncogenesis in vivo. *PLoS Pathog.* **2016**, *12*, e1005588. [CrossRef]
145. Frie, M.C.; Droscha, C.J.; Greenlick, A.E.; Coussens, P.M. Micrornas encoded by bovine leukemia virus (blv) are associated with reduced expression of b cell transcriptional regulators in dairy cattle naturally infected with blv. *Front. Vet. Sci.* **2017**, *4*, 245. [CrossRef] [PubMed]
146. Kertayadnya, I.G.; Johnson, R.H.; Abher, I.; Burgess, G.W. Detection of immunological tolerance to bovine spumavirus (bsv) with evidence for salivary excretion and spread of bsv from the tolerant animal. *Vet. Microbiol.* **1988**, *16*, 35–39. [CrossRef]
147. Bouillant, A.M.; Ruckerbauer, G.M. Isolation of bovine syncytial virus from lymphocytes recovered from fluids used to flush uterus and oviducts of superovulated cattle. *Can. J. Comp. Med.* **1984**, *48*, 332–334. [PubMed]
148. Switzer, W.M.; Tang, S.; Zheng, H.; Shankar, A.; Sprinkle, P.S.; Sullivan, V.; Granade, T.C.; Heneine, W. Dual simian foamy virus/human immunodeficiency virus type 1 infections in persons from cote d'ivoire. *PLoS ONE* **2016**, *11*, e0157709. [CrossRef]
149. Materniak, M.; Hechler, T.; Löchelt, M.; Kuzmak, J. Seroreactivity of humans and ruminants to bovine foamy virus—Evidence for zoonotic transmission and existence of new reservoirs for foamy viruses. In Proceedings of the 8th International Foamy Virus Conference, Argos, Greece, 7–8 May 2010.
150. Materniak, M.; Serwacka, A.; Rydzewski, A.; Rudzki, S.; Bocian, L.; Kehl, T.; Löchelt, M.; Kuzmak, J. Seroreactivity to non-primate foamy viruses in patients immunosupressed after kidney transplantation. In Proceedings of the 10th Internationa Foamy Virus Conference, Puławy, Poland, 24–25 June 2014.
151. Ruckerbauer, G.M.; Sugden, E.A.; Bouillant, A.M. A comparison of the bovine leukemia and bovine syncytial virus status in utero-tubal cells recovered from fluids used to flush the uterus and oviducts of blv-infected, superovulated cattle. *Ann. Rech. Vet.* **1988**, *19*, 19–26.
152. Scott, F.W.; Shively, J.N.; Gaskin, J.; Gillespie, J.H. Bovine syncytial virus isolations. *Arch. Gesamte Virusforsch.* **1973**, *43*, 43–52. [CrossRef]
153. Van der Maaten, M.J.; Hubbert, W.T.; Boothe, A.D.; Bryner, J.H.; Estes, P.C. Isolations of bovine syncytial virus from maternal and fetal blood. *Am. J. Vet. Res.* **1973**, *34*, 341–343.
154. Luther, P.D.; Nuttall, P.A.; Gibbons, R.A. Isolation of viruses from cultures of bovine endometrial cells. *J. Infect. Dis.* **1978**, *138*, 660–663. [CrossRef]
155. Falcone, V.; Leupold, J.; Clotten, J.; Urbanyi, E.; Herchenroder, O.; Spatz, W.; Volk, B.; Bohm, N.; Toniolo, A.; Neumann-Haefelin, D.; et al. Sites of simian foamy virus persistence in naturally infected african green monkeys: Latent provirus is ubiquitous, whereas viral replication is restricted to the oral mucosa. *Virology* **1999**, *257*, 7–14. [CrossRef]
156. Murray, S.M.; Linial, M.L. Foamy virus infection in primates. *J. Med. Primatol.* **2006**, *35*, 225–235. [CrossRef]

157. Murray, S.M.; Picker, L.J.; Axthelm, M.K.; Linial, M.L. Expanded tissue targets for foamy virus replication with simian immunodeficiency virus-induced immunosuppression. *J. Virol.* **2006**, *80*, 663–670. [CrossRef] [PubMed]
158. Flanagan, J.R.; Becker, K.G.; Ennist, D.L.; Gleason, S.L.; Driggers, P.H.; Levi, B.Z.; Appella, E.; Ozato, K. Cloning of a negative transcription factor that binds to the upstream conserved region of moloney murine leukemia virus. *Mol. Cell. Biol* **1992**, *12*, 38–44. [CrossRef] [PubMed]
159. Hechler, T.; Khan, A.A.; Löchelt, M.; German Cancer Research Center. Personal communication, 2011.
160. Materniak, M.; Kuzmak, J.; Olech, M. Seroreactivity to bovine foamy virus antigens in wild ruminants—Evidence for new reservoirs of foamy viruses? In Proceedings of the XIII DIAGMOL Conference 2012, SGGW, Warsaw, Poland, 24 November 2012.
161. Liu, W.; Lei, J.; Liu, Y.; Lukic, D.S.; Rathe, A.M.; Bao, Q.; Kehl, T.; Bleiholder, A.; Hechler, T.; Löchelt, M. Feline foamy virus-based vectors: Advantages of an authentic animal model. *Viruses* **2013**, *5*, 1702–1718. [CrossRef] [PubMed]
162. Bauer, T.R., Jr.; Allen, J.M.; Hai, M.; Tuschong, L.M.; Khan, I.F.; Olson, E.M.; Adler, R.L.; Burkholder, T.H.; Gu, Y.C.; Russell, D.W.; et al. Successful treatment of canine leukocyte adhesion deficiency by foamy virus vectors. *Nat. Med.* **2008**, *14*, 93–97. [CrossRef] [PubMed]
163. Ledesma-Feliciano, C.; Hagen, S.; Troyer, R.; Zheng, X.; Musselman, E.; Slavkovic Lukic, D.; Franke, A.M.; Maeda, D.; Zielonka, J.; Münk, C.; et al. Replacement of feline foamy virus bet by feline immunodeficiency virus vif yields replicative virus with novel vaccine candidate potential. *Retrovirology* **2018**, *15*, 38. [CrossRef] [PubMed]
164. Schwantes, A.; Truyen, U.; Weikel, J.; Weiss, C.; Löchelt, M. Application of chimeric feline foamy virus-based retroviral vectors for the induction of antiviral immunity in cats. *J. Virol.* **2003**, *77*, 7830–7842. [CrossRef]

viruses

MDPI

Review

Structural and Functional Aspects of Foamy Virus Protease-Reverse Transcriptase

Birgitta M. Wöhrl

Lehrstuhl Biopolymere, Universität Bayreuth, D-95440 Bayreuth, Germany; birgitta.woehrl@uni-bayreuth.de

Received: 12 June 2019; Accepted: 29 June 2019; Published: 2 July 2019

Abstract: Reverse transcription describes the process of the transformation of single-stranded RNA into double-stranded DNA via an RNA/DNA duplex intermediate, and is catalyzed by the viral enzyme reverse transcriptase (RT). This event is a pivotal step in the life cycle of all retroviruses. In contrast to orthoretroviruses, the domain structure of the mature RT of foamy viruses is different, i.e., it harbors the protease (PR) domain at its N-terminus, thus being a PR-RT. This structural feature has consequences on PR activation, since the enzyme is monomeric in solution and retroviral PRs are only active as dimers. This review focuses on the structural and functional aspects of simian and prototype foamy virus reverse transcription and reverse transcriptase, as well as special features of reverse transcription that deviate from orthoretroviral processes, e.g., PR activation.

Keywords: foamy virus; protease; reverse transcriptase; RNase H; reverse transcription; antiviral drugs; resistance

1. General Features of Foamy Virus Replication

Foamy viruses (FVs) are retroviruses that—based on several differences in their molecular properties—are gathered in the subfamily of *Spumaretrovirinae*, whereas all other retroviruses are members of the subfamily *Orthoretrovirinae* [1]. The latter include well-characterized retroviruses such as human immunodeficiency virus (HIV), murine leukaemia virus (MLV), or Rous sarcoma virus (RSV) [2]. FVs are endemic in various mammalian hosts, including cats, horses and non-human primates, but not humans. The so-called prototype foamy virus (PFV) was first isolated from a human nasopharyngeal cell line [3]. Sequence comparisons with a simian FV revealed that it originally was derived from a chimpanzee [4].

FVs are complex retroviruses, i.e., they contain accessory genes. Similar to orthoretroviruses, their genomes contain the genes *gag*, *pol*, and *env* (Figure 1). However, in contrast to orthoretroviruses such as human immunodeficiency virus (HIV), the Pol protein is expressed from a separate mRNA and translated from its own AUG start codon; thus, no Gag–Pol fusion protein is produced [5–7].

In the proviral genome, the viral genes are flanked by long terminal repeats (LTRs). The 5′ LTR harbors the viral promoter, which controls transcription of the *gag*, *pol*, and *env* mRNAs. However, additionally, FVs possess an internal promoter (IP) near the 3′ end of the *env* gene, which is responsible for transcription of the accessory proteins Bet and Tas [8–11] (Figure 1). Tas activates transcription from the 5′ LTR and enhances transcription from the IP [12]. The Bet protein appears to be important for efficient virus replication [13], and interacts with the cellular proteins of the APOBEC family, which function as antiretroviral restriction factors [14–18].

Another interesting feature of FVs is the processing of the Gag protein. Whereas in orthoretroviruses, Gag is cleaved into matrix (MA), nucleocapsid (NC), and capsid (CA) proteins, the only cleavage in the 71-kDa Gag of FV occurs near the C-terminus, resulting in a 68-kDa Gag and a ca. 3-kDa peptide (Figure 1). The cleavage of Gag by the viral protease (PR) was shown to be essential for infectivity [19–21]. The wild-type virus contains a mixture of Gag p71/p68 proteins at a ratio of ca.

1:4 [22]. Inactivation of the Gag p68/p3 cleavage site inhibits reverse transcription at the first template switch. However, p3 itself is not required for infectivity [20,23–26].

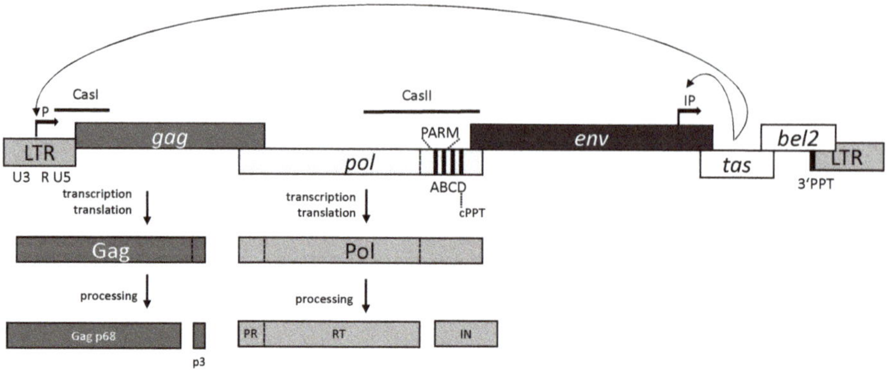

Figure 1. Overview of the foamy virus (FV) genome organisation. The proviral DNA genome is shown. The *gag, pol,* and *env* genes are depicted as boxes. The flanking long terminal repeats (LTRs) comprise the U3, R, and U5 regions, as indicated underneath the 5′ LTR. Transcription starts at the promoter upstream of the R region in the 5′ LTR and at the internal promoter (P and IP, respectively), which are depicted as rectangular arrows. The transactivator protein Tas activates both promoters, as indicated by the arrows. *bel2* encodes the Bet protein. The locations of the Cas sequences, PARM, the purine rich elements A–D, as well as the cPPT and 3′ PPT are illustrated. Only the gene products Gag and Pol, which are processed by the viral PR, are shown.

2. The Pol Protein

Conventional retroviruses express *pol* as a Gag–Pol fusion protein by a rare frameshift event or nonsense codon suppression mechanism. In FVs, Pol is generated from a spliced mRNA independently from Gag [5–7,27–29]. It contains the genes for the PR, polymerase, and RNase H domains, forming the reverse transcriptase (RT) as well as the integrase domain (IN) (Figure 1). The FV Pol protein undergoes only limited proteolysis. A single cleavage between the RNase H and IN domains is carried out, resulting in two mature viral enzymes IN and a PR–RT fusion protein [30,31]. This is in contrast to HIV and other orthoretroviruses, in which Pol is cleaved by the viral PR into three separate proteins, PR, RT and IN (reviewed in [32]).

The existence of a separate Pol poses interesting questions regarding its encapsidation into the FV capsid. It has been suggested that only very few Pol molecules are encapsidated [33,34]. Various studies identified two *cis*-acting sequences (Cas) in the FV pregenomic RNA: CasI and CasII (Figure 1), which are essential and sufficient for the transfer of FV vectors, indicating an important role in virus assembly [35–38]. CasI spans from the 5′ leader sequence into the 5′ *gag* region of the pregenomic RNA of PFV (nucleotides 1–645). CasII is situated in the 3′ region of *pol* (nucleotides 3869–5884) [39]. Within the Cas regions, so-called Pol encapsidation sequences (PES) have been detected that are required to incorporate the full-length Pol protein into the FV capsid. These PES regions range from nucleotides 314 to 354 in CasI and nucleotides 4881 to 5884 in CasII. The deletion of either PES resulted in a significant reduction of Pol uptake into the virus particles [39].

Furthermore, FV Gag binds to pregenomic RNA, and its C-terminus contains determinants that are also important for Pol encapsidation [24,37,39,40]. These results indicate that the pregenomic RNA functions as a bridging molecule between Gag and Pol precursors, and that an interplay of protein–protein as well as protein–RNA interactions is important for correct virus assembly.

3. Reverse Transcription

Reverse transcription—the reverse flow of genetic information from RNA to DNA—is pivotal in the replication cycle of all retroviruses. In the year 1970, the enzyme reverse transcriptase (RT), which catalyses this process, was identified [41,42]. Retroviral RTs exhibit two enzymatic activities that are required to synthesize double-stranded DNA from a single-stranded RNA template: (1) a DNA polymerase activity that can use both DNA and RNA as a template, and (2) an RNase H endonuclease activity that hydrolyzes the RNA strand in an RNA/DNA intermediate. Without the RNase H activity, reverse transcription cannot take place, since RNA degradation is absolutely required for synthesis of the second DNA strand. Misleadingly, the polymerase domain alone is often called the RT domain.

Although the principal order of events is similar in orthoretroviruses and spumaretroviruses, FV reverse transcription takes place late in the replication cycle, i.e., shortly before the virus leaves the cell, whereas conventional retroviruses reverse transcribe their genomic immediately after entering the cell. The pregenomic single-stranded RNA is packaged during virus assembly and reverse transcribed into double-stranded DNA before budding. Thus, the virions of FVs contain mainly double-stranded DNA, which is the functional genome when the virus infects the cell. The packaged pregenomic RNA is diploid. A dimerization signal has been identified at the 5′ end of the RNA [43,44].

Experiments with the RT inhibitor 3′ azido-3′deoxythymidine (AZT) revealed that reverse transcription is largely complete before the infection of new cells [5,45,46]. However, the results of Delelis and Zamborlini suggested a biphasic DNA synthesis with an additional early reverse transcription event, which might optimize genome replication [47,48]. In contrast, in conventional retroviruses such as HIV-1 and MLV, only a very small amount of DNA consisting only of early reverse transcription products—but no full-length DNA—could be detected in virions [49].

In some aspects, FVs resemble hepatitis B virus (HBV). Similar to the FV Gag, the HBV viral structural core protein is not cleaved in virions, and contains Arg-rich regions that interact with RNA in the early stages of reverse transcription and with DNA during encapsidation and in the mature particle [50,51]. In HBV, long reverse transcription products are synthesized by the reverse transcriptase, which is called the P protein. Interactions between the viral pregenomic RNA, the P protein, and the core protein are necessary for particle assembly. In extracellular HBV particles, a partially double-stranded (gapped) circular DNA molecule is present instead of RNA, indicating that reverse transcription takes place during and after particle formation, but before the virus enters a new cell [52,53].

Several groups have investigated the effect of PFV mutants expressing *gag* and *pol* as a Gag–Pol fusion protein [54–57]. The co-expression of Gag with Gag–Pol resulted in a molar ratio of 20:1 in virus particles, which is similar to orthoretroviruses. However, larger variations in the Gag:Pol ratio than in orthoretroviruses are tolerated. Furthermore, virus titers similar to that of the wild type could be achieved as long as a proteolytic cleavage took place between Gag and Pol [54,56]. If the constructs did not allow for removal of the p3 Gag peptide from Pol, particle release resembled that of the wild type, but infectivity was reduced [56]. Reverse transcription with the Gag–Pol mutant virus was also found to be a late event in the replication cycle. However, under AZT treatment, a ca. fivefold drop in virus titer was determined for both wild-type and mutant viruses, implying that early DNA synthesis might also be required [54,57].

Similar to all retroviruses, FV reverse transcription starts at the so-called primer binding site (PBS) close to the 5′ RU5 region of the pregenomic RNA (Figure 1). PFV uses a $tRNA^{Lys1,2}$ primer annealed to the PBS for minus-strand DNA synthesis [30]. Synthesis of the plus-strand DNA is initiated at the 3′ polypurine tract (PPT), which is located upstream of the 3′ U3R region. Additionally, FVs harbor a second so-called central PPT (cPPT), which is located in the CasII region of the *pol* open reading frame. Within CasII, four purine rich sequences (elements A–D) are present. However, only the D element is 100% identical to the 3′ PPT, and thus is likely to constitute the actual cPPT (Figure 1). It is highly conserved in all FV species [58,59]. The C element is required for the regulation of gene expression, and appears to be relevant in *cis* to achieve a sufficient amount of Gag protein. It has been shown recently that it regulates splicing by suppressing the branch point recognition of the strongest *env* splice acceptor. Thus, it plays an essential role in the formation of unspliced *gag* and singly spliced *pol* transcripts [39,58–61]. A and B elements play a role in Pol encapsidation and moreover in PR activation (see below) [59]. Similar to lentiviruses such as HIV, the cPPT of FVs is used as a second initiation site for plus-strand DNA synthesis. In HIV, a so-called central flap region with overlapping single-stranded DNAs is created during reverse transcription. The flap ensures efficient replication in non-dividing cells [62]. However, FVs are not able to establish productive infection in resting cells [63]. Instead of creating a flap, the cPPT is degraded to produce a single-stranded gap region in the double-stranded unintegrated linear PFV DNA [58–60]. The length of the PFV gap varies from 144 to 731 nucleotides with the start and terminal nucleotides being located on either side of the cPPT D element. Mutations in the FV cPPT, which retain the IN amino acid sequence, result in the reduction of the virus titer, indicating the important role of the cPPT in virus replication [59,64]

4. Foamy Virus PR-RT

4.1. Domain organization.

Although the RTs of retroviruses all fulfill the same essential function, i.e., the formation of double-stranded DNA from a single-stranded RNA template, their domain organization is different (Figure 2). HIV RT is a heterodimeric enzyme in which only the larger p66 subunit harbors the polymerase active site and carries the RNase H domain located at the C-terminus. The p51 domain is homologous to the N-terminus of p66, but lacks the RNase H domain, which is cleaved off by the viral PR (Figure 2). Due to the different conformations of p51, no polymerase active site can be formed [65,66]. The RT of RSV is also heterodimeric, consisting of a 63-kDa α subunit and a 95-kDa β subunit, although the respective homodimers can also be isolated from virus particles [67,68]. In addition to the polymerase domain, the connection subdomain and the RNase H domain, the β subunit harbors the IN domain. The active sites of both the polymerase and RNase H are located in the α subunit [69].

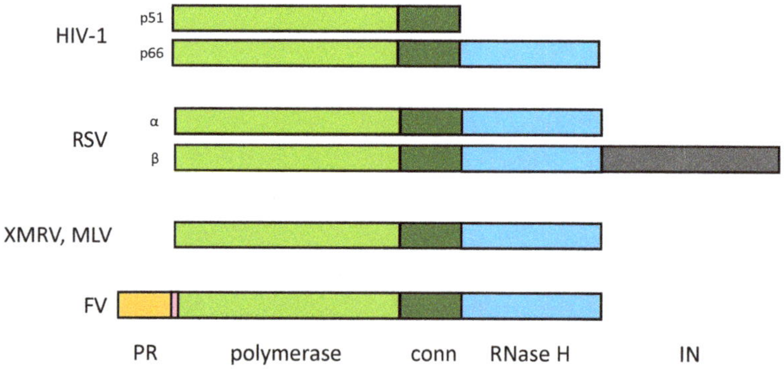

Figure 2. Domain organisation of retroviral RTs. Human immunodeficiency virus (HIV-1) reverse transcriptase (RT) is a heterodimer with a 66-kDa and a 51-kDa subunit. The sequence of the N-terminal region of the two subunits is identical, and comprises the polymerase domain and the connection subdomain, which are highlighted in light and dark green, respectively. The RNase H domain (blue) is located at the C-terminus of the larger subunit. The Rous sarcoma virus (RSV) RT is also heterodimeric. The larger β subunit (95 kDa) carries, in addition to the polymerase, connection, and the RNase H (sub-)domains of the small α subunit (63 kDa), the IN domain (grey). Xenotropic murine leukaemia virus-related virus (XMRV) and murine leukemia virus (MLV) RTs are monomeric enzymes (75 kDa). In addition, the mature monomeric FV enzyme (86 kDa) harbors the PR domain. The stretch ranging from amino acids (aas) 102–143 between the C-terminal end of the PR domain, and the start of the RT domain is highlighted in pink.

The RT of Moloney MLV (MoMLV) and the closely related xenotropic murine leukaemia virus-related virus (XMRV) are monomeric enzymes. The RNase H domain is connected to the polymerase domain via a flexible linker and thus is quite mobile, but becomes ordered in the presence of substrate [70,71]. The mature RT from FVs is actually a PR-RT fusion protein harboring the PR domain at its N-terminus [72,73]. Nevertheless, FV PR-RTs resemble MLV RT in their structural organization and in some biochemical and biophysical properties, but differ from HIV RT. However, since the overall amino acid similarity of FV RTs to MoMLV or XMRV RT is less than 25%, and the PR domain is an integral part of the mature FV enzyme, subdomain assignments cannot be easily obtained from sequence comparisons. Size exclusion chromatography with purified PR-RTs of SFV from macaques (SFVmac) and PFV showed that they are monomers in solution [74,75]. They exhibit polymerase as well as RNase H activities [33,74,76]. Furthermore, similarly to MLV, the isolated RNase H domain is active, but loses specificity (see below) [77–79].

Purified recombinant FV PR-RT monomers do not exhibit PR activity, nor does the separate PR domain. The PR activity of the full-length PR-RT and the separate PR domain can be induced by unphysiological high NaCl concentrations of 3–4 M (see below) [74,80,81]. Unfortunately, no crystal structure of a full-length PR-RT enzyme is available so far. However, the NMR solution structures of isolated FV PR and RNase H domains exist, which give insight into the functions of the FV PR-RT enzyme and its domains [75,77,78,80]. Amino acid sequence comparisons of FV PR-RT with RTs from other retroviruses indicate that the polymerase domain is composed of fingers, palm, and thumb subdomains followed by a connection subdomain and the RNase H. Comparable to HIV RT, the connection subdomain appears to play a role in primer/template binding, protein stability, and polymerization efficiency. The stretch ranging from amino acid (aa) 102 to 143, which is located between the C-terminal end of the PR domain and the start of the RT domain, does not exhibit homology to retroviral PRs or any other RT, but appears to be an intrinsic part of the RT domain that is necessary for solubility and the integrity of the protein [82].

4.2. Polymerization Activities.

The YXDD motif of the polymerase catalytic site is localized in the palm subdomain and is highly conserved among retroviruses. The Asp residues are involved in metal binding. A general model for the catalysis of the polymerase suggests the coordination of two Mg^{2+} ions in which one of them supports the nucleophilic attack of the 3′ OH group of the DNA primer onto the α-phosphate of the incoming dNTP, while the second metal ion is important for pyrophosphate release [83,84].

In most RTs, including the HIV-1 RT, the second site of the motif is a Met (YMDD). However, MLV and FVs contain a Val as the second residue. In HIV-1, mutation of the polymerase active site from YMDD to YVDD causes high level resistance to the inhibitor 3′ thiacytidine (3TC) [85]. Changing YVDD to YMDD in PFV severely impairs virus replication, since reverse transcription cannot be completed. In vitro polymerization assays further indicate that the wild-type YVDD PFV PR-RT is a highly processive DNA polymerase, whereas the YMDD mutant exhibits significantly reduced processivity [34], which is defined as the length of polymerization products synthesized during one round of binding and polymerization before dissociation and reassociation occur. These results indicate that FVs require a highly processive RT for efficient replication. This is probably because in contrast to HIV, only a few Pol molecules are taken up into the virus particle via the direct interaction of Pol with Gag and the viral RNA [33,34]. Interestingly, although the mutant YMDD PFV enzyme resembles the wild-type HIV-1 RT, it still is resistant to 3TC, indicating that probably additional determinants other than the Val in the YXDD motif are involved in the 3TC resistance of FVs [34].

Investigation of the fidelity of PFV PR-RT revealed that it is similar to that of HIV-1 RT for base substitutions; however, it generates more insertions and deletions [33]. Nevertheless, the genetic variation of FV genomes is limited. This might be because although FV genomes can be found in many tissues, high levels of viral RNA were only detected in oral tissues [86]. Compared to

HIV, the replication activities of FVs are restricted to certain tissues, which probably supports the conservation of the genome.

Comparison of the K_M and k_{cat}-values for polymerization on homopolymeric and heteropolymeric substrates indicated similar results for purified SFVmac and PFV PR-RT. The K_M values for both substrate types are also comparable [74,76]. However, the K_M values for FV PR-RTs are about five to 30-fold higher than published values for HIV-1 RT [87–89]. In addition, K_D values for DNA/DNA (PFV 44.4 nM; SFV 36.4 nM) or DNA/RNA (PFV 9.9 nM; SFV 32.4 nM) substrates are much higher than those determined for HIV-1 RT, for which the K_D values for both substrates of ca. 2 nM have been determined [90,91]. Comparison of the pre-steady state kinetics of dNTP incorporation of PFV PR-RT with HIV-1 and MLV showed a severely reduced primer extension capacity of PFV PR-RT at low dNTP concentrations. This behavior is similar to MLV RT, but in strong contrast to HIV-1 RT [92]. For example, k_{pol}/K_D values for dATP incorporation for PFV PR-RT and MLV RT reach values of 2.9 and 2.1, respectively, whereas a value of 55.3 was achieved for HIV-1 RT [92,93]. The authors suggest that the different polymerization properties might have evolved, because HIV and FVs as well as MLV replicate in different cell types. Whereas HIV is able to efficiently propagate in non-dividing cells that have low dNTP concentrations, MLV and FVs replicate in dividing cells. Since these cells contain high dNTP concentrations, FVs did not need to evolve an RT enzyme with high dNTP binding affinities.

5. RNase H Activity and Structure

The catalytic activity of the RNase H domain of retroviral RTs is essential during reverse transcription. Mutations that inactivate the RNase H prevent virus propagation [94,95]. Retroviral RNases H are partially processive endonucleases, which in general do not cleave sequence-specifically. Cleavage of the RNA strand of an RNA/DNA hybrid takes place in the presence of Mg^{2+} ions and results in 5′phosphate and 3′ OH termini. RNase H also exhibits a 3′ to 5′ exonuclease activity during DNA polymerization [96–98]. In addition, during reverse transcription, two specific cleavages are required to remove the extended tRNA and PPT primers, which are used to start minus-strand and plus-strand DNA synthesis. RNase H cleaves specifically between the RNA–DNA junctions [99–103].

To investigate cleavage at the FV PPT-U3 region, DNA/RNA substrates were designed using 5′ end-labeled RNA that contained the entire PPT and part of the U3 region of FV. During reverse transcription, FV PR-RT progressively degrades the RNA until it encounters the PPT. It was shown that FV PR-RT recognizes its own PPT, and cleaves specifically at the U3/PPT boundary. However, it did not properly cleave a similar substrate containing the HIV-1 U3–PPT junction, and vice versa HIV-1 RT did not cleave the FV substrate correctly, suggesting that the two enzymes bind the substrate differently [33]. Gel filtration and NMR data showed that the separate PFV RNase H is a monomer [77,78]. Although the presence of Mg^{2+} ions in the RNase H catalytic center is not required for substrate binding by RTs, NMR spectroscopy indicated that the metal ions are important for stabilization of the overall structure of PFV RNase H [77]. In addition, it has been shown for other RNases that RNA cleavage is achieved by a mechanism that involves two Mg^{2+} ions bound in the catalytic center [104,105].

The K_M values for the RNase H activity of the full-length SFVmac (18.1 nM) and PFV (17.1 nM) enzymes are similar to that of HIV-1 RT (25 nM). This is somewhat surprising, since the amount of RT molecules is much higher in HIV-1 than FV virions [33,34,74].

The isolated RNase H domain of HIV-1 RT is inactive, but activity can be restored by N-terminal extensions, which stabilize the protein [106]. Independent MoMLV and PFV RNase H retain cleavage activity; however, it is remarkably lower than that of the full-length RT enzymes [77,79,107,108]. The RNase H cleavage patterns of the independent PFV RNase H domain and the full-length PR-RT differ, and the K_D value of 23 µM for DNA/RNA substrate binding for the free RNase H is about 4000-fold higher, indicating a substantial role of the polymerase domain for nucleic acid affinity and specificity [74,78].

Moreover, analysis of the RNase H cleavages performed by full-length FV PR-RT and HIV-1 RT on non-specific RNA/DNA substrates revealed different cleavage sites, which also suggests differences in nucleic acid binding [33]. Time-course experiments with PFV and SFVmac PR-RTs indicate that both enzymes cleave endonucleolytically at around −17 to −19 in the RNA. This is followed by a 3′ > 5′ directed processing of the RNA [33,74]. Amino acid sequence comparisons of the RNases H from various retroviruses as well as the human and the *Escherichia coli* RNases H showed that in contrast to the inactive free HIV-1 RNase H, they all contain an additional helix-loop structure, the basic protrusion, which consists of the so-called C-helix and a downstream basic loop element [78]. The basic protrusion of RNases H has been suggested to be important for substrate binding and activity. In HIV-1 RT, this function is probably fulfilled by positively charged residues located in the connection subdomain [109–111].

The structure of the PFV RNase H exhibits the typical fold of an RNase H, which consists of a five-stranded mixed β-sheet flanked by five α-helices (Figure 3). The PFV RNase H structure most closely resembles those of XMRV and HIV-1, even though HIV-1 lacks the basic protrusion [78,112,113]. The catalytic core consists of the highly conserved residues D599, E646, D669, and D740. Helix C precedes the basic loop, which contains four Lys (KKKPLK). On the contrary, in XMRV RNase H, the consecutive basic residues are three Arg, which are part of helix C [78,112]. The structural similarity of the HIV-1 and PFV RNase H was used to examine whether PFV RNase H can serve as a model enzyme for HIV-1 RNase H inhibitors. Indeed, several HIV-1 RNase H inhibitors were identified that also bind and inhibit PFV RNase H at low μmolar concentrations, which are similar to those of the HIV-1 RNase H. Based on NMR binding experiments with PFV, RNase H and the HIV-1 RNase H inhibitor RDS1643 structural overlays with both enzymes, and in silico docking experiments were performed to propose the inhibitor binding site in HIV-1 RNase H [114].

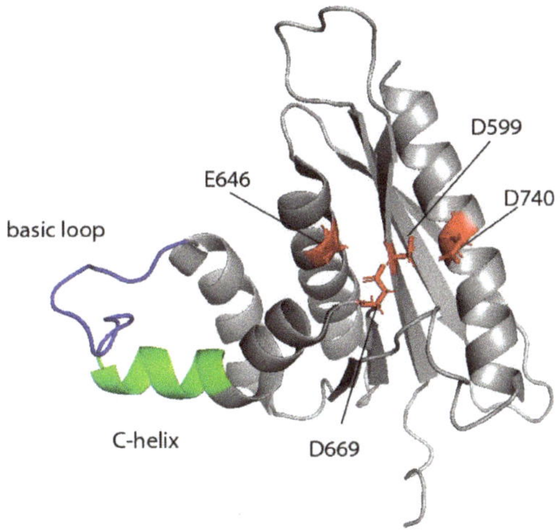

Figure 3. Ribbon diagram of the prototype foamy virus (PFV) RNase H structure. The C-helix is highlighted in green; the basic loop in blue. The active site residues D599, E646, D669, and D740 are depicted in red as sticks (pdb: 2LSN).

NMR titration experiments were performed to identify the residues involved in RNA/DNA substrate binding. ^{1}H-^{15}N heteronuclear single quantum coherence (HSQC) spectra of purified ^{15}N-labeled PFV RNase H were recorded after the addition of increasing amounts of substrate. Chemical shift changes indicated that apart from the active site residues, residues in helix B, helix C, and the basic loop participate in binding of the substrate (Figure 3). The orientation of helix C is established by several hydrophobic contacts with helix D. This interaction enables helix C to correctly position the basic loop toward the nucleic acid substrate. Only then can proper RNA cleavage—and, if necessary, specific cleavage—be guaranteed [78].

6. Protease Activity and Structure

The PR activity of FVs is essential for virus production. When processed Gag in combination with a PR-deficient Pol was provided during virus production, infectious virus particles containing viral DNA were obtained, indicating that PR activity is not absolutely required at cell entry. However, infectivity was reduced to 0.5% to 2% of the wild-type infectivity [23]. Thus, other groups suggest that Gag cleavage is essential for viral infectivity [19,20]. However, PR-mediated Gag processing is absolutely necessary to initiate intraparticle reverse transcription as well as the template switch of reverse transcriptase [23,26]. What is more, Pol processing is essential for genome integration, but not for the RT activity itself [23,72].

Since retroviral PRs have been shown to be only active as dimers and FV PR-RTs are monomeric proteins, the question arises how the activation of PR can be achieved [74,80,115]. The NMR solution structure of the independent SFVmac PR domain (residues 1 to 102) showed that it is a stable monomer and adopts a conformation similar to one subunit of the HIV-1 PR dimer [75,116] (Figure 4). The monomer consists of seven β-strands and a helical turn. The β-strands form a closed barrel-like β-sheet. A β-hairpin is formed by the amino-terminal halves of β4 and β5, which is typical for the so-called flap region of aspartate PRs [75,117]. Similarly to other retroviral PRs, the FV PR domain harbors four characteristic structural features: (a) a hairpin containing the A1 loop, (b) the B loop or the so-called fireman's grip, which includes the conserved amino acid motif DSG (in some PRs DTG) forming the active site in the dimer, (c) an α-helix, and (d) the flap region [75]. Structural analyses of other retroviral PRs revealed that the fireman's grip, the flap, the N-terminal region, and the C-terminal region, which form a four-stranded β-sheet, are involved in dimerization [117], corroborating that the FV PR domain is also able to form dimers.

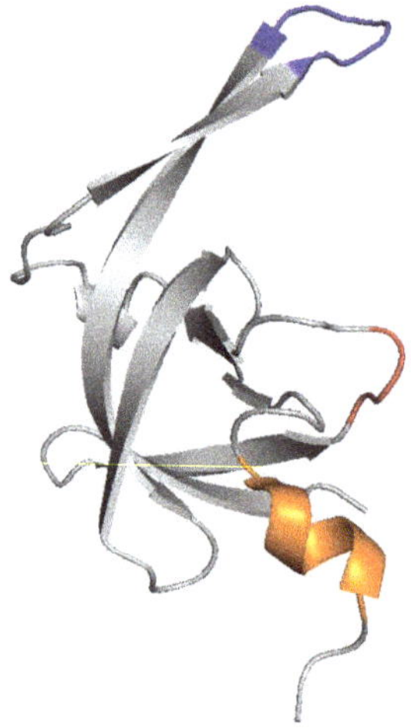

Figure 4. Three-dimensional structure of the SFV from macaques (SFVmac) protease (PR) monomer. The flap region (blue), the a-helix (orange) and the location of the DSG motif (red) forming the active site in the dimer are highlighted (pdb: 2JYS).

Nevertheless, activity of the independent PR domain (1 to 102) as well as of the full-length FV PR-RT could only be achieved using high NaCl concentrations of 2 to 3 M [74,80,118]. The expression of PFV PR as a maltose-binding protein (MBP) or thioredoxin fusion at the N-terminus as well as a C-terminal extension of the PR (residues 1 to 143) appeared to improve the stability of the PR and allowed substrate cleavage, but activity was lost after elimination of the fusion protein [73,118,119]. Based on sequence alignments with HIV-1 PR, single (Q8R, H22L, S25T, T28D) and double (Q8R-T28D, H22L-T28D) mutants of PFV PR were created that harbored amino acid exchanges, making the PR variants more similar to HIV-1 PR. Urea denaturation revealed an increased stability for most mutants, suggesting that the substitutions promote dimer stability [120].

The putative PR dimerization inhibitor cholic acid inhibited the activity HIV-1 and FV PR, whereas darunavir and tipranavir—which are known to prevent HIV-1 PR dimerization—had no effect on FV PR. Determination of the binding site for cholic acid by ^{1}H-^{15}N HSQC experiments using ^{15}N labeled PR indicated that the inhibitor binds in the putative dimerization interface. Paramagnetic relaxation enhancement (PRE), an NMR method that allows the detection of minor conformational species, finally showed that the FV PR domain is able to form transient homodimers. However, in solution, these dimers constitute only a small fraction of less than 5% [80,81].

Obviously, high NaCl concentrations do not represent the situation in a living cell in which the virus replicates. PR activation of HIV-1 is achieved by the formation of transient PR dimers in the Gag–Pol precursor, which leads to N-terminal autoprocessing [121]. Since FVs express Gag and Pol separately, and Pol can only be taken up into the virus particle by binding to the pregenomic viral RNA, it isobvious that FVs developed a different mechanism for PR activation. A PR-activating RNA motif (PARM) was identified in the cis-acting CasII sequence of the RNA, which includes the A and B elements of the purine-rich sequences located at the 3′ end of *pol* (Figure 1) [122].

The addition of PARM RNA to PFV PR-RT initiates substrate cleavage. The corresponding DNA does not lead to PR activation. Truncated PARM RNA or the addition of only the A or B element RNA to the assay also resulted in a loss of PR activation. Gel shift experiments with the PARM RNA and PFV PR-RT showed that the enzyme oligomerizes upon RNA binding [122]. Determination of the PARM RNA secondary structure using selective 2′ hydroxyl acylation analysed by primer extension (SHAPE) revealed that both the A and B elements are located in a stem-loop structure of ca. 15 nucleotides in length. PARM enables the formation of proteolytically active PR-RT dimers (Figure 5). It might also be possible that only the PR domains of two full-length enzyme molecules dimerize upon PARM binding [122]. The data suggest that in the host cell, the PR domain in the Pol precursor is inactive until enough viral RNA is produced. PR activation can only be achieved during packaging upon binding of the RT domain to the PARM of the pregenomic RNA. The IN domain of Pol is not required for PR activation [55]. This order of events creates a regulatory mechanism by which premature Pol or Gag processing can be avoided.

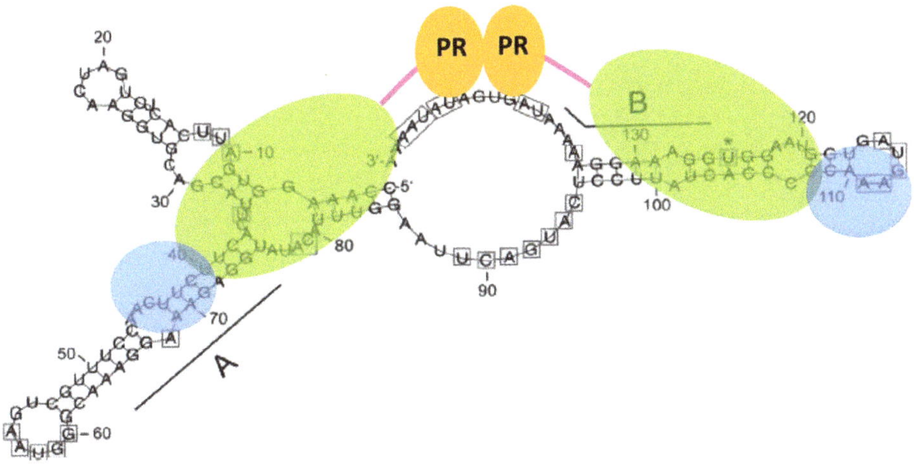

Figure 5. Model of protease (PR) activation upon binding to the PR-activating RNA motif (PARM). Both the A and B elements are required. They are involved in stem structures to which two PR-RT molecules can bind. Upon interaction of the RT domain with the RNA, the PR domains of the two PR-RTs can dimerize. Colors as in Figure 2.

7. Resistance of FV PR-RT against RT Inhibitors

The only known RT inhibitors that impair PFV replication are tenofovir and azido-3′-deoxythymidine (AZT, zidovudine). The addition of 5 μM of AZT to cell cultures are sufficient to prevent virus propagation [45,123,124]. Attempts to generate AZT resistant FV were only successful with SFVmac, but not with SFV from chimpanzee (SFVcpz) or PFV. This is quite astonishing, since the amino acid sequences of the polymerase domains of PFV and SFVmac are 84.5% identical.

Four amino acid substitutions in the RT domain of SFVmac have been identified that together confer high-level resistance to AZT: K211I, I224T, S345T, and E350K (Figure 6). The I224T substitution is probably a polymorphism that does not contribute directly to AZT resistance, but is important for regaining polymerization activity and viral fitness [76,125]. Two different AZT resistance mechanisms have been shown for HIV: HIV-2 is able to discriminate between the natural triphosphate TTP and the phosphorylated inhibitor AZTTP, whereas the major mechanism in HIV-1 is based on the removal of the already incorporated chain-terminating AZTMP in the presence of ATP [126]. In SFVmac, the AZT-resistant RTs can also remove the incorporated AZTMP more readily than the wild-type enzyme in the presence of ATP. The PR-RT harboring the single amino acid exchange S345T is the only single substitution variant exhibiting significant AZTMP excision activity. Excision efficiency doubles when K211I is present together with S345T or E350K [127].

```
                10        20        30        40L       50        60      N
HIV-1   PVKLKPGMDGPKV-KQWPLTEEKIKALVEICTEMEKEGKISKIGPENPYNTPVFAIKKKD
SFVmac  PHNIATGTLAPRPQKQYPINPKAKPSIQIVIDDLLKQGVL--IQQNSTMNTPVYPVPKPD
                    160       170       180       190       200

          R       80        90        100       110       120
HIV-1   STKWRKLVDFRELNKRTQDFW-EVQLGIPHPAGLKKKKSVTVLDVGDAYVSVPLDEDFRK
SFVmac  G-KWRMVLDYREVNKIIPLIAAQNQHSAGILSSIYRGKYKTTLDLTNGFWAHPITPESYW
      210 I       220   T   230       240       250       260

          130       140       150       160       170       180 active site
HIV-1   YTAFTIPSINNETPGIRYQYNVLPQGWKGSPAIFQSSMTKMLEPFKKQNPDIVIYQYMDD
SFVmac  LTAFTWQ-------GKQYCWTRLPQGFLNSPALFTADVVDLL----KEIPN--VQAYVDD
         270               280       290       300             310

          190       200       210  F/Y E/Q          230         240
HIV-1   LYVGSDLEIGQHRTKIEELRQHLLRWGLTTPDKKH---QKEPPFLWMGY--ELHPDKWTV
SFVmac  IYISHD-DPQEHLEQLEKIFSILLNAGYVVSLKKSEIAQREVEFLGFNITKEGRGLTDTF
          320        330       340    T    K       360       370
```

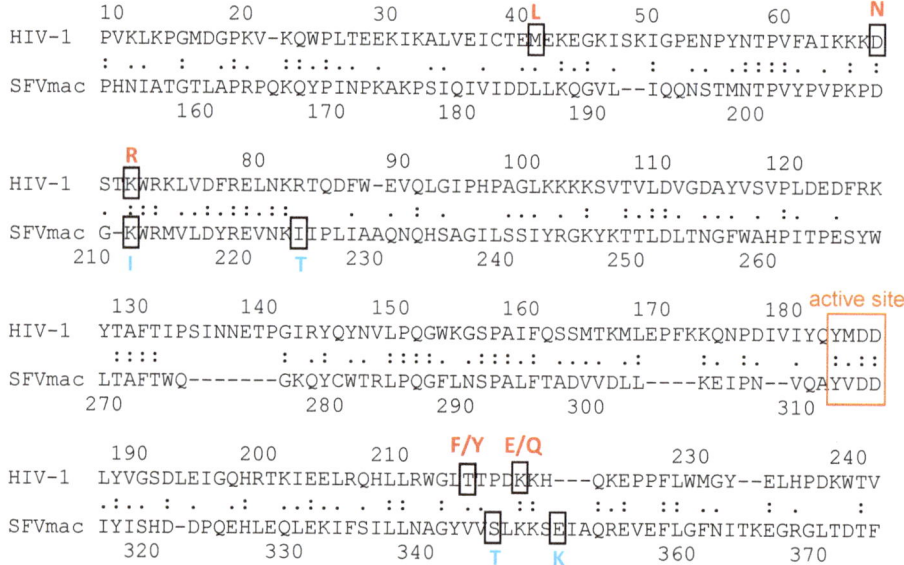

Figure 6. Sequence alignment of the regions of human immunodeficiency virus (HIV)-1 and SFVmac RT, showing the azido-3′deoxythymidine (AZT) resistance amino acid exchanges. The amino acids conferring AZT resistance are shown in red for HIV-1 (M41L, D67N, K70R, T215Y/F, K219E/Q) and blue for SFVmac RT (K211I, I224T, S345T, E350K), respectively. The amino acids of the polymerase active site are highlighted by an orange box. The amino acid identity is 26.2%.

In AZT-resistant HIV-1 RT, the aromatic amino acid exchange T215F/Y allows π–π stacking interactions with the adenine ring of ATP and thus more efficient AZTMP excision [128,129]. In AZT-resistant SFVmac RT, instead of acquiring an aromatic residue, the most important substitution is S345T. NMR ^{1}H-^{15}N HSQC experiments with truncated wild-type and resistant SFVmac RTs harboring the fingers and palm subdomains of the polymerase were recorded in the absence and presence of ATP. Comparison of the spectra revealed that a Trp residue is involved in ATP binding in the S345T variant, which is obscured in the wild-type enzyme, suggesting a direct contact of ATP via π–π stacking interactions similar to HIV-1 RT.

8. Outlook and Persepectives

The life cycle of FVs differs from that of conventional retroviruses in various aspects. Several of the molecular details have been elucidated that make us aware of the differences that have developed during the evolution of FVs. The structure of some FV proteins is already known: PR, RNase H, and IN, as well as parts of the Gag protein [75,78,130–134]. The structure of the full-length FV PR-RT is still missing, but would contribute greatly to our understanding of RTs in general. So far, the only monomeric RT 3D structures known are those of XMRV RT and the closely related MLV RT [70,71]. In addition, the crystal structure of the yeast retrotransposon Ty3 RT has been solved, which is a monomer in solution, but dimerizes upon substrate binding [135]. In order to fully understand the function and mechanistic details of FV proteins and enzymes, more structural and functional information is urgently needed.

Funding: This work was supported by the University of Bayreuth.

Conflicts of Interest: The authors declare no conflict of interest.

References

1. Rethwilm, A.; Lindemann, D. Foamy Viruses. In *Fields Virology*; Knipe, D., Howley, P., Eds.; Lippincott, Williams & Wilkins: Philadelphia, PA, USA, 2013.
2. Vogt, P.K. Historical introduction to the general properties of retroviruses. In *Retroviruses*; Coffin, J.M., Hughes, S.H., Varmus, H.E., Eds.; Cold Spring Harbor Laboratory Press: Cold Spring Harbor, NY, USA, 1997.
3. Achong, B.G.; Mansell, P.W.; Epstein, M.A.; Clifford, P. An unusual virus in cultures from a human nasopharyngeal carcinoma. *J. Natl. Cancer Inst.* **1971**, *46*, 299–307. [PubMed]
4. Herchenröder, O.; Renne, R.; Loncar, D.; Cobb, E.K.; Murthy, K.K.; Schneider, J.; Mergia, A.; Luciw, P.A. Isolation, cloning, and sequencing of simian foamy viruses from chimpanzees (SFVcpz): High homology to human foamy virus (HFV). *Virology* **1994**, *201*, 187–199. [CrossRef] [PubMed]
5. Yu, S.F.; Baldwin, D.N.; Gwynn, S.R.; Yendapalli, S.; Linial, M.L. Human foamy virus replication: A pathway distinct from that of retroviruses and hepadnaviruses. *Science* **1996**, *271*, 1579–1582. [CrossRef] [PubMed]
6. Enssle, J.; Jordan, I.; Mauer, B.; Rethwilm, A. Foamy virus reverse transcriptase is expressed independently from the Gag protein. *Proc. Natl. Acad. Sci. USA* **1996**, *93*, 4137–4141. [CrossRef] [PubMed]
7. Jordan, I.; Enssle, J.; Güttler, E.; Mauer, B.; Rethwilm, A. Expression of human foamy virus reverse transcriptase involves a spliced pol mRNA. *Virology* **1996**, *224*, 314–319. [CrossRef] [PubMed]
8. Löchelt, M.; Yu, S.F.; Linial, M.L.; Flügel, R.M. The human foamy virus internal promoter is required for efficient gene expression and infectivity. *Virology* **1995**, *206*, 601–610. [CrossRef]
9. Campbell, M.; Renshaw-Gegg, L.; Renne, R.; Luciw, P.A. Characterization of the internal promoter of simian foamy viruses. *J. Virol.* **1994**, *68*, 4811–4820. [PubMed]
10. Löchelt, M.; Muranyi, W.; Flügel, R.M. Human foamy virus genome possesses an internal, Bel-1-dependent and functional promoter. *Proc. Natl. Acad. Sci. USA* **1993**, *90*, 7317–7321. [CrossRef] [PubMed]
11. Mergia, A. Simian foamy virus type 1 contains a second promoter located at the 3′ end of the env gene. *Virology* **1994**, *199*, 219–222. [CrossRef]
12. Meiering, C.D.; Rubio, C.; May, C.; Linial, M.L. Cell-type-specific regulation of the two foamy virus promoters. *J. Virol.* **2001**, *75*, 6547–6557. [CrossRef]
13. Alke, A.; Schwantes, A.; Kido, K.; Flötenmeyer, M.; Flügel, R.M.; Löchelt, M. The bet gene of feline foamy virus is required for virus replication. *Virology* **2001**, *287*, 310–320. [CrossRef] [PubMed]
14. Löchelt, M.; Romen, F.; Bastone, P.; Muckenfuss, H.; Kirchner, N.; Kim, Y.-B.; Truyen, U.; Rösler, U.; Battenberg, M.; Saib, A.; et al. The antiretroviral activity of APOBEC3 is inhibited by the foamy virus accessory Bet protein. *Proc. Natl. Acad. Sci. USA* **2005**, *102*, 7982–7987. [CrossRef] [PubMed]

15. Chareza, S.; Slavkovic Lukic, D.; Liu, Y.; Räthe, A.-M.; Münk, C.; Zabogli, E.; Pistello, M.; Löchelt, M. Molecular and functional interactions of cat APOBEC3 and feline foamy and immunodeficiency virus proteins: Different ways to counteract host-encoded restriction. *Virology* **2012**, *424*, 138–146. [CrossRef] [PubMed]
16. Perkovic, M.; Schmidt, S.; Marino, D.; Russell, R.A.; Stauch, B.; Hofmann, H.; Kopietz, F.; Kloke, B.-P.; Zielonka, J.; Ströver, H.; et al. Species-specific inhibition of APOBEC3C by the prototype foamy virus protein bet. *J. Biol. Chem.* **2009**, *284*, 5819–5826. [CrossRef] [PubMed]
17. Jaguva Vasudevan, A.A.; Perkovic, M.; Bulliard, Y.; Cichutek, K.; Trono, D.; Häussinger, D.; Münk, C. Prototype foamy virus Bet impairs the dimerization and cytosolic solubility of human APOBEC3G. *J. Virol.* **2013**, *87*, 9030–9040. [CrossRef] [PubMed]
18. Russell, R.A.; Wiegand, H.L.; Moore, M.D.; Schäfer, A.; McClure, M.O.; Cullen, B.R. Foamy virus Bet proteins function as novel inhibitors of the APOBEC3 family of innate antiretroviral defense factors. *J. Virol.* **2005**, *79*, 8724–8731. [CrossRef]
19. Baldwin, D.N.; Linial, M.L. Proteolytic activity, the carboxy terminus of Gag, and the primer binding site are not required for Pol incorporation into foamy virus particles. *J. Virol.* **1999**, *73*, 6387–6393.
20. Enssle, J.; Fischer, N.; Moebes, A.; Mauer, B.; Smola, U.; Rethwilm, A. Carboxy-terminal cleavage of the human foamy virus Gag precursor molecule is an essential step in the viral life cycle. *J. Virol.* **1997**, *71*, 7312–7317.
21. Lehmann-Che, J.; Giron, M.-L.; Delelis, O.; Löchelt, M.; Bittoun, P.; Tobaly-Tapiero, J.; de Thé, H.; Saïb, A. Protease-dependent uncoating of a complex retrovirus. *J. Virol.* **2005**, *79*, 9244–9253. [CrossRef]
22. Cartellieri, M.; Rudolph, W.; Herchenröder, O.; Lindemann, D.; Rethwilm, A. Determination of the relative amounts of Gag and Pol proteins in foamy virus particles. *Retrovirology* **2005**, *2*, 44. [CrossRef]
23. Hütter, S.; Müllers, E.; Stanke, N.; Reh, J.; Lindemann, D. Prototype foamy virus protease activity is essential for intraparticle reverse transcription initiation but not absolutely required for uncoating upon host cell entry. *J. Virol.* **2013**, *87*, 3163–3176. [CrossRef] [PubMed]
24. Stenbak, C.R.; Linial, M.L. Role of the C terminus of foamy virus Gag in RNA packaging and Pol expression. *J. Virol.* **2004**, *78*, 9423–9430. [CrossRef] [PubMed]
25. Zemba, M.; Wilk, T.; Rutten, T.; Wagner, A.; Flügel, R.M.; Löchelt, M. The carboxy-terminal p3Gag domain of the human foamy virus Gag precursor is required for efficient virus infectivity. *Virology* **1998**, *247*, 7–13. [CrossRef] [PubMed]
26. Spannaus, R.; Schneider, A.; Hartl, M.J.; Wöhrl, B.M.; Bodem, J. Foamy virus Gag p71–p68 cleavage is required for template switch of the reverse transcriptase. *J. Virol.* **2013**, *87*, 7774–7776. [CrossRef] [PubMed]
27. Löchelt, M.; Flügel, R.M. The human foamy virus pol gene is expressed as a Pro-Pol polyprotein and not as a Gag-Pol fusion protein. *J. Virol.* **1996**, *70*, 1033–1040. [PubMed]
28. Bodem, J.; Löchelt, M.; Winkler, I.; Flower, R.P.; Delius, H.; Flügel, R.M. Characterization of the spliced pol transcript of feline foamy virus: The splice acceptor site of the pol transcript is located in gag of foamy viruses. *J. Virol.* **1996**, *70*, 9024–9027. [PubMed]
29. Konvalinka, J.; Löchelt, M.; Zentgraf, H.; Flügel, R.M.; Kräusslich, H.G. Active foamy virus proteinase is essential for virus infectivity but not for formation of a Pol polyprotein. *J. Virol.* **1995**, *69*, 7264–7268. [PubMed]
30. Kögel, D.; Aboud, M.; Flügel, R.M. Molecular biological characterization of the human foamy virus reverse transcriptase and ribonuclease H domains. *Virology* **1995**, *213*, 97–108. [CrossRef]
31. Netzer, K.O.; Schliephake, A.; Maurer, B.; Watanabe, R.; Aguzzi, A.; Rethwilm, A. Identification of pol-related gene products of human foamy virus. *Virology* **1993**, *192*, 336–338. [CrossRef]
32. Goff, S.P. Retroviridae: The retroviruses and their replication. In *Fields Virology*; Knipe, D., Howley, P., Eds.; Lippincott, Williams & Wilkins: Philadelphia, PA, USA, 2007; pp. 1999–2069.
33. Boyer, P.L.; Stenbak, C.R.; Clark, P.K.; Linial, M.L.; Hughes, S.H. Characterization of the polymerase and RNase H activities of human foamy virus reverse transcriptase. *J. Virol.* **2004**, *78*, 6112–6121. [CrossRef]
34. Rinke, C.S.; Boyer, P.L.; Sullivan, M.D.; Hughes, S.H.; Linial, M.L. Mutation of the catalytic domain of the foamy virus reverse transcriptase leads to loss of processivity and infectivity. *J. Virol.* **2002**, *76*, 7560–7570. [CrossRef] [PubMed]
35. Erlwein, O.; Bieniasz, P.D.; McClure, M.O. Sequences in pol are required for transfer of human foamy virus-based vectors. *J. Virol.* **1998**, *72*, 5510–5516. [PubMed]

36. Heinkelein, M.; Dressler, M.; Jármy, G.; Rammling, M.; Imrich, H.; Thurow, J.; Lindemann, D.; Rethwilm, A. Improved primate foamy virus vectors and packaging constructs. *J. Virol.* **2002**, *76*, 3774–3783. [CrossRef] [PubMed]
37. Heinkelein, M.; Leurs, C.; Rammling, M.; Peters, K.; Hanenberg, H.; Rethwilm, A. Pregenomic RNA is required for efficient incorporation of pol polyprotein into foamy virus capsids. *J. Virol.* **2002**, *76*, 10069–10073. [CrossRef] [PubMed]
38. Wu, M.; Chari, S.; Yanchis, T.; Mergia, A. Cis-Acting sequences required for simian foamy virus type 1 vectors. *J. Virol.* **1998**, *72*, 3451–3454. [PubMed]
39. Peters, K.; Wiktorowicz, T.; Heinkelein, M.; Rethwilm, A. RNA and protein requirements for incorporation of the Pol protein into foamy virus particles. *J. Virol.* **2005**, *79*, 7005–7013. [CrossRef] [PubMed]
40. Lee, E.-G.; Linial, M.L. The C terminus of foamy retrovirus Gag contains determinants for encapsidation of Pol protein into virions. *J. Virol.* **2008**, *82*, 10803–10810. [CrossRef] [PubMed]
41. Temin, H.M.; Mizutani, S. RNA-dependent DNA polymerase in virions of Rous sarcoma virus. *Nature* **1970**, *226*, 1211–1213. [CrossRef] [PubMed]
42. Baltimore, D. RNA-dependent DNA polymerase in virions of RNA tumour viruses. *Nature* **1970**, *226*, 1209–1211. [CrossRef]
43. Cain, D.; Erlwein, O.; Grigg, A.; Russell, R.A.; McClure, M.O. Palindromic sequence plays a critical role in human foamy virus dimerization. *J. Virol.* **2001**, *75*, 3731–3739. [CrossRef]
44. Erlwein, O.; Cain, D.; Fischer, N.; Rethwilm, A.; McClure, M.O. Identification of sites that act together to direct dimerization of human foamy virus RNA in vitro. *Virology* **1997**, *229*, 251–258. [CrossRef] [PubMed]
45. Moebes, A.; Enssle, J.; Bieniasz, P.D.; Heinkelein, M.; Lindemann, D.; Bock, M.; McClure, M.O.; Rethwilm, A. Human foamy virus reverse transcription that occurs late in the viral replication cycle. *J. Virol.* **1997**, *71*, 7305–7311. [PubMed]
46. Yu, S.F.; Sullivan, M.D.; Linial, M.L. Evidence that the human foamy virus genome is DNA. *J. Virol.* **1999**, *73*, 1565–1572. [PubMed]
47. Delelis, O.; Saïb, A.; Sonigo, P. Biphasic DNA synthesis in spumaviruses. *J. Virol.* **2003**, *77*, 8141–8146. [CrossRef] [PubMed]
48. Zamborlini, A.; Renault, N.; Saïb, A.; Delelis, O. Early Reverse Transcription Is Essential for Productive Foamy Virus Infection. *PLoS ONE* **2010**, *5*, e11023. [CrossRef]
49. Trono, D. Partial reverse transcripts in virions from human immunodeficiency and murine leukemia viruses. *J. Virol.* **1992**, *66*, 4893–4900. [PubMed]
50. Nassal, M. The arginine-rich domain of the hepatitis B virus core protein is required for pregenome encapsidation and productive viral positive-strand DNA synthesis but not for virus assembly. *J. Virol.* **1992**, *66*, 4107–4116.
51. Hatton, T.; Zhou, S.; Standring, D.N. RNA- and DNA-binding activities in hepatitis B virus capsid protein: A model for their roles in viral replication. *J. Virol.* **1992**, *66*, 5232–5241.
52. Nassal, M.; Schaller, H. Hepatitis B virus replication. *Trends Microbiol.* **1993**, *1*, 221–228. [CrossRef]
53. Beck, J.; Nassal, M. Hepatitis B virus replication. *World J. Gastroenterol. WJG* **2007**, *13*, 48–64. [CrossRef]
54. Lee, E.-G.; Sinicrope, A.; Jackson, D.L.; Yu, S.F.; Linial, M.L. Foamy virus Pol protein expressed as a Gag-Pol fusion retains enzymatic activities, allowing for infectious virus production. *J. Virol.* **2012**, *86*, 5992–6001. [CrossRef] [PubMed]
55. Spannaus, R.; Hartl, M.J.; Wöhrl, B.M.; Rethwilm, A.; Bodem, J. The prototype foamy virus protease is active independently of the integrase domain. *Retrovirology* **2012**, *9*, 41. [CrossRef] [PubMed]
56. Swiersy, A.; Wiek, C.; Reh, J.; Zentgraf, H.; Lindemann, D. Orthoretroviral-like prototype foamy virus Gag-Pol expression is compatible with viral replication. *Retrovirology* **2011**, *8*, 66. [CrossRef] [PubMed]
57. Jackson, D.L.; Lee, E.-G.; Linial, M.L. Expression of prototype foamy virus pol as a Gag-Pol fusion protein does not change the timing of reverse transcription. *J. Virol.* **2013**, *87*, 1252–1254. [CrossRef] [PubMed]
58. Kupiec, J.J.; Tobaly-Tapiero, J.; Canivet, M.; Santillana-Hayat, M.; Flügel, R.M.; Périès, J.; Emanoil-Ravier, R. Evidence for a gapped linear duplex DNA intermediate in the replicative cycle of human and simian spumaviruses. *Nucleic Acids Res.* **1988**, *16*, 9557–9565. [CrossRef] [PubMed]
59. Peters, K.; Barg, N.; Gärtner, K.; Rethwilm, A. Complex effects of foamy virus central purine-rich regions on viral replication. *Virology* **2008**, *373*, 51–60. [CrossRef] [PubMed]

60. Tobaly-Tapiero, J.; Kupiec, J.J.; Santillana-Hayat, M.; Canivet, M.; Peries, J.; Emanoil-Ravier, R. Further characterization of the gapped DNA intermediates of human spumavirus: Evidence for a dual initiation of plus-strand DNA synthesis. *J. Gen. Virol.* **1991**, *72*, 605–608. [CrossRef]
61. Moschall, R.; Denk, S.; Erkelenz, S.; Schenk, C.; Schaal, H.; Bodem, J. A purine-rich element in foamy virus pol regulates env splicing and gag/pol expression. *Retrovirology* **2017**, *14*, 10. [CrossRef]
62. Rausch, J.W.; Le Grice, S.F.J. "Binding, bending and bonding": Polypurine tract-primed initiation of plus-strand DNA synthesis in human immunodeficiency virus. *Int. J. Biochem. Cell Biol.* **2004**, *36*, 1752–1766. [CrossRef]
63. Bieniasz, P.D.; Weiss, R.A.; McClure, M.O. Cell cycle dependence of foamy retrovirus infection. *J. Virol.* **1995**, *69*, 7295–7299.
64. Chen, D.; Song, J.; Sun, Y.; Li, Z.; Wen, D.; Liu, Q.; Liu, W.; He, X. The fourth central polypurine tract guides the synthesis of prototype foamy virus plus-strand DNA. *Virus Genes* **2017**, *53*, 259–265. [CrossRef] [PubMed]
65. Le Grice, S.F.; Grüninger-Leitch, F. Rapid purification of homodimer and heterodimer HIV-1 reverse transcriptase by metal chelate affinity chromatography. *Eur. J. Biochem.* **1990**, *187*, 307–314. [CrossRef] [PubMed]
66. Rodgers, D.W.; Gamblin, S.J.; Harris, B.A.; Ray, S.; Culp, J.S.; Hellmig, B.; Woolf, D.J.; Debouck, C.; Harrison, S.C. The structure of unliganded reverse transcriptase from the human immunodeficiency virus type 1. *Proc. Natl. Acad. Sci. USA* **1995**, *92*, 1222–1226. [CrossRef] [PubMed]
67. Rho, H.M.; Grandgenett, D.P.; Green, M. Sequence relatedness between the subunits of avian myeloblastosis virus reverse transcriptase. *J. Biol. Chem.* **1975**, *250*, 5278–5280. [PubMed]
68. Hizi, A.; Joklik, W.K. RNA-dependent DNA polymerase of avian sarcoma virus B77. I. Isolation and partial characterization of the alpha, beta2, and alphabeta forms of the enzyme. *J. Biol. Chem.* **1977**, *252*, 2281–2289. [PubMed]
69. Werner, S.; Wöhrl, B.M. Asymmetric subunit organization of heterodimeric Rous sarcoma virus reverse transcriptase alphabeta: Localization of the polymerase and RNase H active sites in the alpha subunit. *J. Virol.* **2000**, *74*, 3245–3252. [CrossRef]
70. Das, D.; Georgiadis, M.M. The crystal structure of the monomeric reverse transcriptase from Moloney murine leukemia virus. *Structure* **2004**, *12*, 819–829. [CrossRef] [PubMed]
71. Nowak, E.; Potrzebowski, W.; Konarev, P.V.; Rausch, J.W.; Bona, M.K.; Svergun, D.I.; Bujnicki, J.M.; Le Grice, S.F.J.; Nowotny, M. Structural analysis of monomeric retroviral reverse transcriptase in complex with an RNA/DNA hybrid. *Nucleic Acids Res.* **2013**, *41*, 3874–3887. [CrossRef]
72. Roy, J.; Linial, M.L. Role of the Foamy Virus Pol Cleavage Site in Viral Replication. *J. Virol.* **2007**, *81*, 4956–4962. [CrossRef]
73. Pfrepper, K.-I.; Rackwitz, H.-R.; Schnölzer, M.; Heid, H.; Löchelt, M.; Flügel, R.M. Molecular Characterization of Proteolytic Processing of the Pol Proteins of Human Foamy Virus Reveals Novel Features of the Viral Protease. *J. Virol.* **1998**, *72*, 7648–7652.
74. Hartl, M.J.; Mayr, F.; Rethwilm, A.; Wöhrl, B.M. Biophysical and enzymatic properties of the simian and prototype foamy virus reverse transcriptases. *Retrovirology* **2010**, *7*, 5. [CrossRef] [PubMed]
75. Hartl, M.J.; Wöhrl, B.M.; Rösch, P.; Schweimer, K. The solution structure of the simian foamy virus protease reveals a monomeric protein. *J. Mol. Biol.* **2008**, *381*, 141–149. [CrossRef] [PubMed]
76. Hartl, M.J.; Kretzschmar, B.; Frohn, A.; Nowrouzi, A.; Rethwilm, A.; Wöhrl, B.M. AZT resistance of simian foamy virus reverse transcriptase is based on the excision of AZTMP in the presence of ATP. *Nucleic Acids Res.* **2008**, *36*, 1009–1016. [CrossRef] [PubMed]
77. Leo, B.; Hartl, M.J.; Schweimer, K.; Mayr, F.; Wöhrl, B.M. Insights into the structure and activity of prototype foamy virus RNase H. *Retrovirology* **2012**, *9*, 14. [CrossRef] [PubMed]
78. Leo, B.; Schweimer, K.; Rösch, P.; Hartl, M.J.; Wöhrl, B.M. The solution structure of the prototype foamy virus RNase H domain indicates an important role of the basic loop in substrate binding. *Retrovirology* **2012**, *9*, 73. [CrossRef] [PubMed]
79. Schultz, S.J.; Champoux, J.J. RNase H domain of Moloney murine leukemia virus reverse transcriptase retains activity but requires the polymerase domain for specificity. *J. Virol.* **1996**, *70*, 8630–8638.
80. Hartl, M.J.; Schweimer, K.; Reger, M.H.; Schwarzinger, S.; Bodem, J.; Rösch, P.; Wöhrl, B.M. Formation of transient dimers by a retroviral protease. *Biochem. J.* **2010**, *427*, 197–203. [CrossRef]

81. Hartl, M.J.; Burmann, B.M.; Prasch, S.J.; Schwarzinger, C.; Schweimer, K.; Wöhrl, B.M.; Rösch, P.; Schwarzinger, S. Fast mapping of biomolecular interfaces by Random Spin Labeling (RSL). *J. Biomol. Struct. Dyn.* **2012**, *29*, 793–798. [CrossRef]
82. Schneider, A.; Peter, D.; Schmitt, J.; Leo, B.; Richter, F.; Rösch, P.; Wöhrl, B.M.; Hartl, M.J. Structural requirements for enzymatic activities of foamy virus protease-reverse transcriptase. *Proteins* **2014**, *82*, 375–385. [CrossRef]
83. Steitz, T.A. DNA polymerases: Structural diversity and common mechanisms. *J. Biol. Chem.* **1999**, *274*, 17395–17398. [CrossRef]
84. Singh, K.; Marchand, B.; Kirby, K.A.; Michailidis, E.; Sarafianos, S.G. Structural Aspects of Drug Resistance and Inhibition of HIV-1 Reverse Transcriptase. *Viruses* **2010**, *2*, 606–638. [CrossRef] [PubMed]
85. Gu, Z.; Gao, Q.; Li, X.; Parniak, M.A.; Wainberg, M.A. Novel mutation in the human immunodeficiency virus type 1 reverse transcriptase gene that encodes cross-resistance to 2′,3′-dideoxyinosine and 2′,3′-dideoxycytidine. *J. Virol.* **1992**, *66*, 7128–7135. [PubMed]
86. Murray, S.M.; Picker, L.J.; Axthelm, M.K.; Linial, M.L. Expanded tissue targets for foamy virus replication with simian immunodeficiency virus-induced immunosuppression. *J. Virol.* **2006**, *80*, 663–670. [CrossRef] [PubMed]
87. Martin, J.L.; Wilson, J.E.; Haynes, R.L.; Furman, P.A. Mechanism of resistance of human immunodeficiency virus type 1 to 2′,3′-dideoxyinosine. *Proc. Natl. Acad. Sci. USA* **1993**, *90*, 6135–6139. [CrossRef] [PubMed]
88. Ueno, T.; Shirasaka, T.; Mitsuya, H. Enzymatic characterization of human immunodeficiency virus type 1 reverse transcriptase resistant to multiple 2′,3′-dideoxynucleoside 5′-triphosphates. *J. Biol. Chem.* **1995**, *270*, 23605–23611. [CrossRef] [PubMed]
89. Wilson, J.E.; Aulabaugh, A.; Caligan, B.; McPherson, S.; Wakefield, J.K.; Jablonski, S.; Morrow, C.D.; Reardon, J.E.; Furman, P.A. Human immunodeficiency virus type-1 reverse transcriptase. Contribution of Met-184 to binding of nucleoside 5′-triphosphate. *J. Biol. Chem.* **1996**, *271*, 13656–13662. [CrossRef] [PubMed]
90. Krebs, R.; Immendörfer, U.; Thrall, S.H.; Wöhrl, B.M.; Goody, R.S. Single-step kinetics of HIV-1 reverse transcriptase mutants responsible for virus resistance to nucleoside inhibitors zidovudine and 3-TC. *Biochemistry* **1997**, *36*, 10292–10300. [CrossRef]
91. Wöhrl, B.M.; Krebs, R.; Thrall, S.H.; Le Grice, S.F.; Scheidig, A.J.; Goody, R.S. Kinetic analysis of four HIV-1 reverse transcriptase enzymes mutated in the primer grip region of p66 implications for DNA synthesis and dimerization. *J. Biol. Chem.* **1997**, *272*, 17581–17587. [CrossRef]
92. Santos-Velazquez, J.; Kim, B. Deoxynucleoside triphosphate incorporation mechanism of foamy virus (FV) reverse transcriptase: Implications for cell tropism of FV. *J. Virol.* **2008**, *82*, 8235–8238. [CrossRef]
93. Skasko, M.; Weiss, K.K.; Reynolds, H.M.; Jamburuthugoda, V.; Lee, K.; Kim, B. Mechanistic differences in RNA-dependent DNA polymerization and fidelity between murine leukemia virus and HIV-1 reverse transcriptases. *J. Biol. Chem.* **2005**, *280*, 12190–12200. [CrossRef]
94. Tisdale, M.; Schulze, T.; Larder, B.A.; Moelling, K. Mutations within the RNase H domain of human immunodeficiency virus type 1 reverse transcriptase abolish virus infectivity. *J. Gen. Virol.* **1991**, *72*, 59–66. [CrossRef] [PubMed]
95. Repaske, R.; Hartley, J.W.; Kavlick, M.F.; O'Neill, R.R.; Austin, J.B. Inhibition of RNase H activity and viral replication by single mutations in the 3′ region of Moloney murine leukemia virus reverse transcriptase. *J. Virol.* **1989**, *63*, 1460–1464. [PubMed]
96. Krug, M.S.; Berger, S.L. Ribonuclease H activities associated with viral reverse transcriptases are endonucleases. *Proc. Natl. Acad. Sci. USA* **1989**, *86*, 3539–3543. [CrossRef] [PubMed]
97. DeStefano, J.J.; Buiser, R.G.; Mallaber, L.M.; Bambara, R.A.; Fay, P.J. Human immunodeficiency virus reverse transcriptase displays a partially processive 3′ to 5′ endonuclease activity. *J. Biol. Chem.* **1991**, *266*, 24295–24301. [PubMed]
98. Wöhrl, B.M.; Volkmann, S.; Moelling, K. Mutations of a conserved residue within HIV-1 ribonuclease H affect its exo- and endonuclease activities. *J. Mol. Biol.* **1991**, *220*, 801–818. [CrossRef]
99. Huber, H.E.; Richardson, C.C. Processing of the primer for plus strand DNA synthesis by human immunodeficiency virus 1 reverse transcriptase. *J. Biol. Chem.* **1990**, *265*, 10565–10573. [PubMed]
100. Luo, G.X.; Sharmeen, L.; Taylor, J. Specificities involved in the initiation of retroviral plus-strand DNA. *J. Virol.* **1990**, *64*, 592–597.

101. Wöhrl, B.M.; Moelling, K. Interaction of HIV-1 ribonuclease H with polypurine tract containing RNA-DNA hybrids. *Biochemistry* **1990**, *29*, 10141–10147. [CrossRef]
102. Furfine, E.S.; Reardon, J.E. Human immunodeficiency virus reverse transcriptase ribonuclease H: Specificity of tRNA(Lys3)-primer excision. *Biochemistry* **1991**, *30*, 7041–7046. [CrossRef]
103. Smith, J.S.; Roth, M.J. Specificity of human immunodeficiency virus-1 reverse transcriptase-associated ribonuclease H in removal of the minus-strand primer, tRNA(Lys3). *J. Biol. Chem.* **1992**, *267*, 15071–15079.
104. Yang, W.; Lee, J.Y.; Nowotny, M. Making and breaking nucleic acids: Two-Mg^{2+}-ion catalysis and substrate specificity. *Mol. Cell* **2006**, *22*, 5–13. [CrossRef]
105. Steitz, T.A.; Steitz, J.A. A general two-metal-ion mechanism for catalytic RNA. *Proc. Natl. Acad. Sci. USA* **1993**, *90*, 6498–6502. [CrossRef] [PubMed]
106. Schultz, S.J.; Champoux, J.J. RNase H activity: Structure, specificity, and function in reverse transcription. *Virus Res.* **2008**, *134*, 86–103. [CrossRef] [PubMed]
107. Tanese, N.; Goff, S.P. Domain structure of the Moloney murine leukemia virus reverse transcriptase: Mutational analysis and separate expression of the DNA polymerase and RNase H activities. *Proc. Natl. Acad. Sci. USA* **1988**, *85*, 1777–1781. [CrossRef] [PubMed]
108. Zhan, X.; Crouch, R.J. The isolated RNase H domain of murine leukemia virus reverse transcriptase. Retention of activity with concomitant loss of specificity. *J. Biol. Chem.* **1997**, *272*, 22023–22029. [CrossRef]
109. Kanaya, S.; Katsuda-Nakai, C.; Ikehara, M. Importance of the positive charge cluster in Escherichia coli ribonuclease HI for the effective binding of the substrate. *J. Biol. Chem.* **1991**, *266*, 11621–11627. [PubMed]
110. Telesnitsky, A.; Blain, S.W.; Goff, S.P. Defects in Moloney murine leukemia virus replication caused by a reverse transcriptase mutation modeled on the structure of Escherichia coli RNase H. *J. Virol.* **1992**, *66*, 615–622.
111. Lim, D.; Gregorio, G.G.; Bingman, C.; Martinez-Hackert, E.; Hendrickson, W.A.; Goff, S.P. Crystal structure of the moloney murine leukemia virus RNase H domain. *J. Virol.* **2006**, *80*, 8379–8389. [CrossRef]
112. Zhou, D.; Chung, S.; Miller, M.; Grice, S.F.J.L.; Wlodawer, A. Crystal structures of the reverse transcriptase-associated ribonuclease H domain of xenotropic murine leukemia-virus related virus. *J. Struct. Biol.* **2012**, *177*, 638–645. [CrossRef]
113. Davies, J.F.; Hostomska, Z.; Hostomsky, Z.; Jordan, S.R.; Matthews, D.A. Crystal structure of the ribonuclease H domain of HIV-1 reverse transcriptase. *Science* **1991**, *252*, 88–95. [CrossRef]
114. Corona, A.; Schneider, A.; Schweimer, K.; Rösch, P.; Wöhrl, B.M.; Tramontano, E. Inhibition of foamy virus reverse transcriptase by human immunodeficiency virus type 1 RNase H inhibitors. *Antimicrob. Agents Chemother.* **2014**, *58*, 4086–4093. [CrossRef] [PubMed]
115. Pearl, L.H.; Taylor, W.R. A structural model for the retroviral proteases. *Nature* **1987**, *329*, 351–354. [CrossRef] [PubMed]
116. Hartl, M.J.; Wöhrl, B.M.; Schweimer, K. Sequence-specific ^{1}H, ^{13}C and ^{15}N resonance assignments and secondary structure of a truncated protease from Simian Foamy Virus. *Biomol. NMR Assign.* **2007**, *1*, 175–177. [CrossRef] [PubMed]
117. Wlodawer, A.; Gustchina, A. Structural and biochemical studies of retroviral proteases. *Biochim. Biophys. Acta* **2000**, *1477*, 16–34. [CrossRef]
118. Fenyöfalvi, G.; Bagossi, P.; Copeland, T.D.; Oroszlan, S.; Boross, P.; Tözsér, J. Expression and characterization of human foamy virus proteinase. *FEBS Lett.* **1999**, *462*, 397–401. [CrossRef]
119. Pfrepper, K.I.; Löchelt, M.; Schnölzer, M.; Flügel, R.M. Expression and molecular characterization of an enzymatically active recombinant human spumaretrovirus protease. *Biochem. Biophys. Res. Commun.* **1997**, *237*, 548–553. [CrossRef] [PubMed]
120. Sperka, T.; Boross, P.; Eizert, H.; Tözsér, J.; Bagossi, P. Effect of mutations on the dimer stability and the pH optimum of the human foamy virus protease. *Protein Eng. Des. Sel. PEDS* **2006**, *19*, 369–375. [CrossRef] [PubMed]
121. Tang, C.; Louis, J.M.; Aniana, A.; Suh, J.-Y.; Clore, G.M. Visualizing transient events in amino-terminal autoprocessing of HIV-1 protease. *Nature* **2008**, *455*, 693–696. [CrossRef] [PubMed]
122. Hartl, M.J.; Bodem, J.; Jochheim, F.; Rethwilm, A.; Rösch, P.; Wöhrl, B.M. Regulation of foamy virus protease activity by viral RNA: A novel and unique mechanism among retroviruses. *J. Virol.* **2011**, *85*, 4462–4469. [CrossRef]

123. Rosenblum, L.L.; Patton, G.; Grigg, A.R.; Frater, A.J.; Cain, D.; Erlwein, O.; Hill, C.L.; Clarke, J.R.; McClure, M.O. Differential susceptibility of retroviruses to nucleoside analogues. *Antivir. Chem. Chemother.* **2001**, *12*, 91–97. [CrossRef]
124. Lee, C.C.I.; Ye, F.; Tarantal, A.F. Comparison of growth and differentiation of fetal and adult rhesus monkey mesenchymal stem cells. *Stem Cells Dev.* **2006**, *15*, 209–220. [CrossRef] [PubMed]
125. Kretzschmar, B.; Nowrouzi, A.; Hartl, M.J.; Gärtner, K.; Wiktorowicz, T.; Herchenröder, O.; Kanzler, S.; Rudolph, W.; Mergia, A.; Wöhrl, B.; et al. AZT-resistant foamy virus. *Virology* **2008**, *370*, 151–157. [CrossRef] [PubMed]
126. Boyer, P.L.; Sarafianos, S.G.; Clark, P.K.; Arnold, E.; Hughes, S.H. Why do HIV-1 and HIV-2 use different pathways to develop AZT resistance? *PLoS Pathog.* **2006**, *2*, e10. [CrossRef] [PubMed]
127. Schneider, A.; Schweimer, K.; Rösch, P.; Wöhrl, B.M. AZT resistance alters enzymatic properties and creates an ATP-binding site in SFVmac reverse transcriptase. *Retrovirology* **2015**, *12*, 21. [CrossRef] [PubMed]
128. Tu, X.; Das, K.; Han, Q.; Bauman, J.D.; Clark, A.D.; Hou, X.; Frenkel, Y.V.; Gaffney, B.L.; Jones, R.A.; Boyer, P.L.; et al. Structural basis of HIV-1 resistance to AZT by excision. *Nat. Struct. Mol. Biol.* **2010**, *17*, 1202–1209. [CrossRef] [PubMed]
129. Boyer, P.L.; Sarafianos, S.G.; Arnold, E.; Hughes, S.H. Selective excision of AZTMP by drug-resistant human immunodeficiency virus reverse transcriptase. *J. Virol.* **2001**, *75*, 4832–4842. [CrossRef]
130. Ball, N.J.; Nicastro, G.; Dutta, M.; Pollard, D.J.; Goldstone, D.C.; Sanz-Ramos, M.; Ramos, A.; Müllers, E.; Stirnnagel, K.; Stanke, N.; et al. Structure of a Spumaretrovirus Gag Central Domain Reveals an Ancient Retroviral Capsid. *PLoS Pathog.* **2016**, *12*, e1005981. [CrossRef] [PubMed]
131. Goldstone, D.C.; Flower, T.G.; Ball, N.J.; Sanz-Ramos, M.; Yap, M.W.; Ogrodowicz, R.W.; Stanke, N.; Reh, J.; Lindemann, D.; Stoye, J.P.; et al. A unique spumavirus Gag N-terminal domain with functional properties of orthoretroviral matrix and capsid. *PLoS Pathog.* **2013**, *9*, e1003376. [CrossRef]
132. Valkov, E.; Gupta, S.S.; Hare, S.; Helander, A.; Roversi, P.; McClure, M.; Cherepanov, P. Functional and structural characterization of the integrase from the prototype foamy virus. *Nucleic Acids Res.* **2009**, *37*, 243–255. [CrossRef]
133. Lesbats, P.; Serrao, E.; Maskell, D.P.; Pye, V.E.; O'Reilly, N.; Lindemann, D.; Engelman, A.N.; Cherepanov, P. Structural basis for spumavirus GAG tethering to chromatin. *Proc. Natl. Acad. Sci. USA* **2017**, *114*, 5509–5514. [CrossRef]
134. Hare, S.; Gupta, S.S.; Valkov, E.; Engelman, A.; Cherepanov, P. Retroviral intasome assembly and inhibition of DNA strand transfer. *Nature* **2010**, *464*, 232–236. [CrossRef] [PubMed]
135. Nowak, E.; Miller, J.T.; Bona, M.K.; Studnicka, J.; Szczepanowski, R.H.; Jurkowski, J.; Le Grice, S.F.J.; Nowotny, M. Ty3 reverse transcriptase complexed with an RNA-DNA hybrid shows structural and functional asymmetry. *Nat. Struct. Mol. Biol.* **2014**, *21*, 389–396. [CrossRef] [PubMed]

viruses

MDPI

Review

Structural Insights on Retroviral DNA Integration: Learning from Foamy Viruses

Ga-Eun Lee [1,†], Eric Mauro [2,3], Vincent Parissi [2,3], Cha-Gyun Shin [1] and Paul Lesbats [2,3,*]

1 Department of Systems Biotechnology, Chung-Ang University, Anseong 17546, Korea
2 Fundamental Microbiology and Pathogenicity Laboratory, UMR 5234 CNRS-University of Bordeaux, 33076 Bordeaux, France
3 Viral DNA Integration and Chromatin Dynamics Network (DyNAVir), 33076 Bordeaux, France
* Correspondence: Paul.lesbats@u-bordeaux.fr
† Present address: Department of Veterinary Biosciences, The Ohio State University, Columbus, OH 43210, USA.

Received: 6 August 2019; Accepted: 20 August 2019; Published: 22 August 2019

Abstract: Foamy viruses (FV) are retroviruses belonging to the *Spumaretrovirinae* subfamily. They are non-pathogenic viruses endemic in several mammalian hosts like non-human primates, felines, bovines, and equines. Retroviral DNA integration is a mandatory step and constitutes a prime target for antiretroviral therapy. This activity, conserved among retroviruses and long terminal repeat (LTR) retrotransposons, involves a viral nucleoprotein complex called intasome. In the last decade, a plethora of structural insights on retroviral DNA integration arose from the study of FV. Here, we review the biochemistry and the structural features of the FV integration apparatus and will also discuss the mechanism of action of strand transfer inhibitors.

Keywords: retrovirus; foamy virus; integrase; integration

1. Introduction

The *retroviridae* family is a large group of viruses containing seven genera (alpha, beta, gamma, delta, epsilon lenti, and spuma-virus). The deltaretrovirus and lentivirus genera contain the two major human pathogens, Human T-Lymphotropic Virus (HTLV-1) and Human Immunodeficiency Virus-1 (HIV-1), respectively. One feature that distinguishes retroviruses from the other viruses is the ability to integrate their linear double stranded DNA into host cellular chromatin. This essential activity is catalyzed by the virally encoded integrase (IN) protein and will lead to the covalent insertion of the provirus into the host genome [1]. The mechanism of retroviral integration is also shared by numerous prokaryotic and eukaryotic mobile DNA elements to mobilize genetic information between and within genomes. Moreover, retroviral integrases are closely related to the DD(E/D) polynucleotidyl transferase family of DNA transposases [2]. Although the DNA cutting and strand transfer reactions occur through a similar mechanism between these genetics elements, the structure of DNA to be mobilized differs, i.e., IN cannot act on an already integrated DNA molecule and requires linear DNA to carry out the two essential sequential events, 3′ processing, and strand transfer [3–5]. These processes take place in the context of a nucleoprotein complex called intasome, consisting of the two viral DNA (vDNA) ends and a multimer of IN [6,7]. While the function of retroviral integrases is well described, the molecular mechanisms involved were, for a long time, hampered by the lack of structural information. The propensity of many retroviral integrase to self-associate into high order aggregates in vitro has been a factor limiting structural endeavors. Conversely, FV integrase like prototype foamy virus (PFV) was shown to be very amenable for structural biochemistry and was the source of many breakthroughs on the comprehension on the molecular basis of retroviral integration and strand transfer inhibitors resistance [8–11].

2. Biochemistry of Foamy Virus Integration

Biochemical studies of retroviral integration started with the purification of preintegration complexes (PIC) from infected cells [12,13]. Such complexes can perform vDNA integration into target DNA in vitro. Analysis of the intermediates produced during these integration reactions uncovered the two activities catalyzed by retroviral integrase: 3′ processing and strand transfer (Figure 1) [3,4]. The resulting integration products generate a single strand gap and a two-nucleotide overhang that will be repaired by cellular proteins to complete the integration reaction.

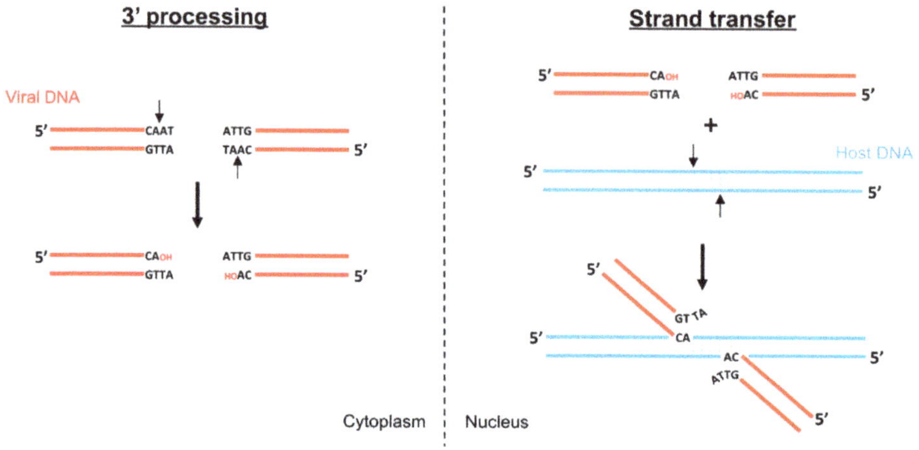

Figure 1. DNA cutting and joining steps catalyzed by retroviral integrases. During 3′ processing (**left**) the integrase removes two (or three) nucleotides from the 3′ ends to expose a conserved terminal CA dinucleotide. The 3′ hydroxyl groups (red OH) will be used in the second step (**right**) to attack the phosphodiester bonds on each target DNA strand.

During 3′ processing, retroviral integrase cleaves two (or, depending on the in vitro conditions, three [14,15]) nucleotides on the 3′ ends of the U3 and U5 vDNA long terminal repeats (LTR). This sequence-specific reaction, a nucleophilic attack by a water molecule, liberates a recessed 3′ hydroxyl group adjacent to an invariant CA dinucleotide [5]. Foamy virus 3′ processing occurs asymmetrically, modifying only the U5 end as the U3 extremity generated after reverse transcription constitutes a bona fide substrate for integration [16,17]. In contrast, the U5 extreme dinucleotides are necessary during the first strand of reverse transcription but have to be cleaved off for integration. During the strand transfer step, the intasome binds host chromosomal DNA, forming the target capture complex (TCC), and utilizes the 3′ hydroxyls as nucleophiles to cut and join simultaneously both 3′vDNA ends to apposing DNA strands with 4–6 bp stagger (4 in the case of FV).

Recombinant retroviral integrases are very efficient at catalyzing 3′ processing and strand transfer reactions in vitro [18–20]. However, the bulk of strand transfer products obtained are generally the result of unpaired products, also called half site integration. Recombinant PFV integrase became a standard model to investigate retroviral integration, as it appeared far more proficient at paired full-site integration. PFV integrase is more soluble in vitro than HIV-1 IN, but the exact biochemical reasons underlying these differences are unclear. Interestingly, comparison of in vitro IN enzymatic reaction conditions among FVs, such as substrate specificity, cofactor usage, and target commitment, showed that the feline foamy virus (FFV) IN has a broader range of substrates and cofactor than other FV INs [21]. FFV IN cleaved PFV U5 LTR substrate, as well as FFV U5 LTR substrate, during in vitro 3′ processing reaction, but not vice versa. The internal six nucleotides in front of terminal CA dinucleotide are identical between the two substrates, indicating that the FFV IN has low substrate specificity compared with PFV IN. Mn^{2+} or Mg^{2+} ions are known as essential cofactors of IN enzyme activities, and in vitro IN activities appear most effectively in the presence of Mn^{2+}. Previous studies have reported that multimerization of HIV-1 IN was promoted by Ca^{2+} as well as Mn^{2+}, although Ca^{2+} could not substitute in strand transfer reaction [22]. Interestingly, Zn^{2+} and Ca^{2+} divalent cations were found to act in FFV 3′ processing in the absence of Mn^{2+} ion, and their inductions of enzymatic reactions were concentration-dependent. Moreover, like FFV IN, PFV integrase was shown to be fairly lax for divalent cations and target DNA commitment. Indeed, while HIV-1 integrase was shown to commit to substrate DNA within 1 min, PFV integrase took more than an hour [23]. Moreover, the same group performed single molecule experiments using PFV intasomes to investigate the mechanics of target DNA capture and catalysis. Using single molecule total internal reflection fluorescence (smTIRF) microscopy, individual PFV intasome were visualized on naked DNA [24]. Theoretical dynamic modelling showed a 1D rotation-coupled translational diffusion of PFV intasome along DNA. 1D diffusion is a phenomenon exploited by many proteins to scan for sequences, lesions, or structures on nucleic acids. Remarkably, this target DNA searching process is very often non-productive as few integration events were recorded, even in the presence of favored PFV integrase sequences. Instead, since PFV intasome prefers supercoiled DNA as the target substrate [8,24], the authors suggested an additional search for DNA conformation rather than sequence alone. However, the question of the search process on the nucleosomal chromatin template remains to be investigated.

3. Domain Organization of Retroviral Integrase

All retroviral IN contain three conserved folded domains that were initially identified using limited proteolysis on HIV-1 IN [25]: the N-terminal domain (NTD), the catalytic core domain (CCD), and the C-terminal domain (CTD). In addition, *spumaretrovirinae* (as well as epsilon and gammaretroviral) integrases harbor a ~40 residues NTD extension domain (NED) (Figure 2A).

The first structural features of individual domains were obtained using nuclear magnetic resonance (NMR) and X-ray crystallography. The structure of HIV-1 and HIV-2 NTD was determined using NMR and shows 3-helical bundles coordinating a single zinc atom via the side chains of a HisHisCysCys (HHCC) motif [26,27] (Figure 2B). The structure confirms the importance of the zinc as an IN cofactor, and also the location of the conserved His and Cys residues involved in the chelation of metal. The CTD structure was also solved in solution by NMR and revealed a high similarity with Src homology 3 (SH3)-like beta barrel and Tudor domains [28,29] (Figure 2D). The NTD and CTD domains play important roles in substrate recognition and assembly of intasome. They are connected to the CCD via flexible linkers whose size varies among retroviral genera. The CCD contains the active site of the enzyme with the invariant D,D-35-E motif. The crystal structure of HIV-1 IN CCD showed a nucleotidyltransferase fold, which is shared with several prokaryotic and eukaryotic transposases, recombinases, and resolvases [30,31]. The structure revealed a dimer of CCD with an extensive interface. The two active sites are facing outward, opposite to each other, and separated by approximately 35 Å. This distance is incompatible with a functional concerted integration of the two viral ends across a major groove of the target DNA that is around 17 Å in a canonical B-form (Figure 2C). Following this observation and the similarity with the mechanistically related transposases [32–34], it appeared clear that an IN multimer must be involved in vDNA concerted integration. Biochemical analysis of IN from various genera failed to establish a relationship between their oligomeric states in solution and the formation of active complexes once bound to their cognate DNA substrates. The breakthrough came from PFV integrase. Monomeric in solution, highly soluble, and exceptionally efficient in catalysis in vitro, this model was the first functional retroviral IN.DNA complex amenable to structural characterization.

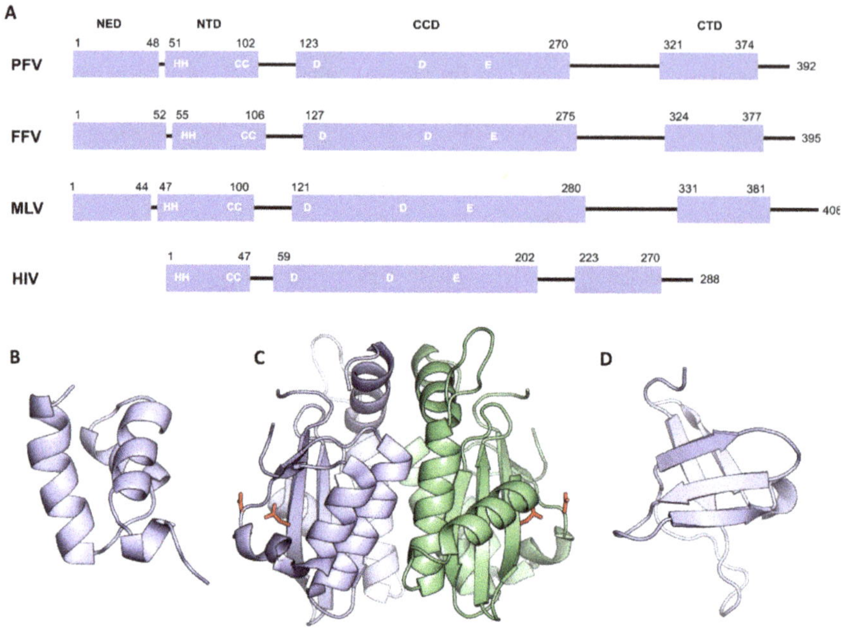

Figure 2. Domain organization of retroviral integrases. (**A**) Schematic of the retroviral IN domain sequences shown as boxes. Isolated domain structures of HIV-1 NTD (**B**), (PDB 1WJC), CCD (**C**), (PDB 1ITG), CTD (**D**), (PDB 1IHV). Chains are shown in cartoon, except active site residues Asp64 and Asp116, which are shown as red sticks (Glu152 residues are disordered and not visible in the structure).

4. Architecture of the PFV Intasome

Determined by X-ray crystallography, the structure of the PFV intasome fundamentally changed the landscape in the field of retroviral integration, as it could both unravel the functional architecture of the integration apparatus and elucidate the mechanism of action of HIV strand transfer inhibitors [9].

The PFV intasome revealed a tetramer of integrases synapsing a pair of vDNA ends. The tetramer consists of a dimer of dimer with two structurally distinct subunits (Figure 3A). The inner subunits mediate all the protein–protein, protein–DNA contacts in an extended conformation and host the active sites to catalyze the 3′ processing and strand transfer reactions. The inner integrases interact via intermolecular NTD–CCD contacts, and by the insertion of a pair of CTDs that rigidly bridge the two halves of the intasome between the CCDs. The outer subunits connect the inner protomers via the canonical CCD–CCD interface. Although the respective positions of the outer NTDs and CTDs are not resolved in the intasome structures published to date, some hints were obtained using SAXS/SANS analysis of PFV intasome [35]. These domains are dispensable for PFV intasome assembly and in vitro activity [36] but they are suspected to provide additional stabilizing interaction with vDNA and/or cellular cofactors. However, the outer CTDs appear to promote aggregation in vitro, as further experiments using intasome lacking the outer domains have shown an increased stability and activity on naked DNA. Solving the structure of the PFV intasome reinforced the hypothesis that the tetrameric architecture was the functional multimer of HIV-1 intasome. Yet, more recently, four additional structures from orthoretroviral intasome; α-retroviral Rous sarcoma virus (RSV) [37], β-retroviral mouse mammary tumor virus (MMTV) [38], lentiviral maedi-visna virus (MVV) [39], and lentiviral HIV-1 [40] were reported, revealing a variety of architectures (see [41] for a more detailed review) (Figure 3B). First, RSV and MMTV intasomes structures solved by X-ray crystallography and Cryo-EM, respectively, revealed an octameric assembly. A core tetramer (called conserved intasome core, CIC [41]) is positioned similarly as in PFV intasome, with the conserved inner catalytic protomers flanked by outer monomer subunits. The position of the synaptic CTDs bridging both halves of the intasome is conserved in the octameric structures, but due to the small size of the CCD–CTD linker, they cannot be supplied by the inner protomer and come from the flanking dimers. Indeed, while in PFV IN the CCD–CTD linker is fifty residues long, in α and β retroviral INs, they are only eight amino acids long. Interestingly, the size of this linker varies among retroviral genera and may predict the requirement for additional oligomers to support CIC assembly [38].

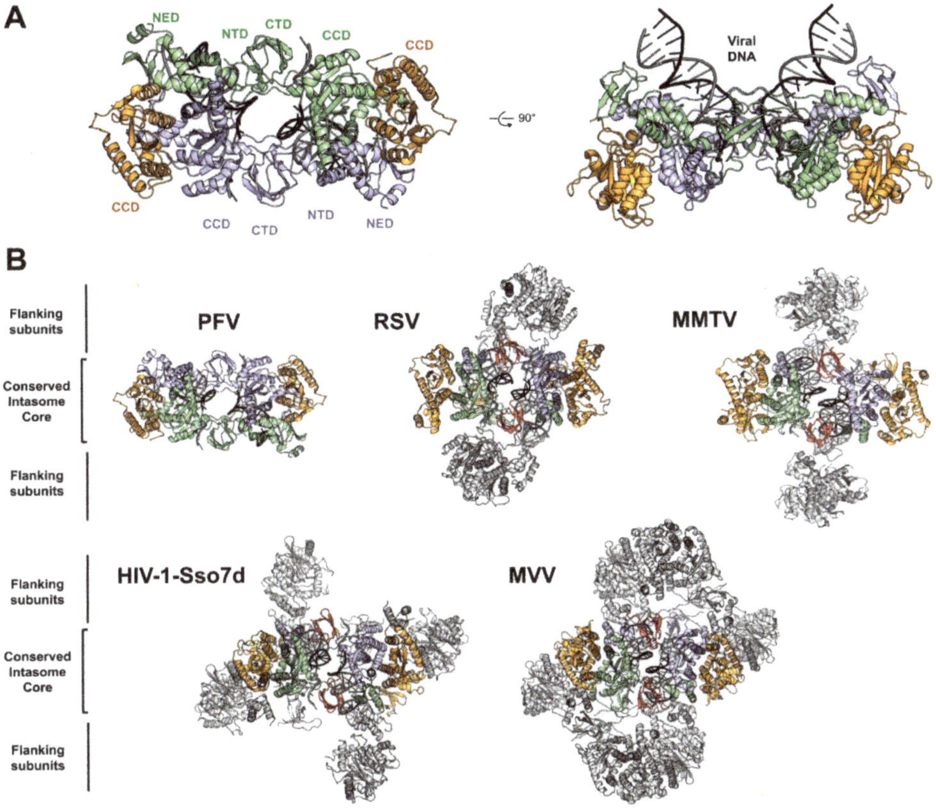

Figure 3. Architecture of PFV and related retroviral intasomes. (**A**) PFV intasome shown in two orthogonal views (PDB 4E7H) with individual domains indicated. Inner IN subunits are colored pale green and light blue, and the outer subunits are in orange. (**B**) Comparison of retroviral intasomes structures (RSV PDB: 5EJK, MMTV PDB: 3JCA, MVV PDB: 5M0Q). Complexes are viewed from below the active site. The conserved intasome core, CIC, is colored as in (A), synaptic CTDs are in red, and flanking subunits are in light grey.

In the case of lentiviral (and δ-retroviral) INs, the size of the CCD–CTD linker is around twenty residues. However, it adopts a compact alpha-helical structure, which is predicted to be incompatible to allow the formation of a minimalist CIC [42].

Fusing HIV-1 IN with the DNA binding domain Sso7d [43] promoted its solubility as well as its in vitro activity [44], allowing the assembly of a complex that could be structurally characterized by Cryo-EM. The structure of the HIV-1-Sso7d intasome revealed a tetramer competent for integration [40]. However, the CCD–CTD linker could not be seen on the electron density map, and assembly of an intasome using HIV-1 IN cofactor lens epithelium-derived growth factor (LEDGF/p75) integrase binding domain (IBD) to stabilize higher-order species revealed a dodecameric structure. In this complex, the core intasome is assembled between two tetramers with a flanking dimer inserting the synaptic CTDs.

The MVV intasome was assembled using wild type integrase proteins and shows a hexadecameric structure (a tetramer of tetramers). Here again, the catalytic core is formed by the CIC. Overall, both intasome architecture are similar and resume the CIC formation. It has been suggested that the extra fusion domain Sso7d in HIV-1 intasome, which cannot be seen in the EM density, may disrupt the dimer–dimer interaction in the flanking HIV-1 IN tetramer, and therefore result in a dodecameric structure, while MVV intasome displays a hexadecamer.

5. Structural Basis for Target DNA Capture

Co-crystallization of the PFV intasome with its target DNA (tDNA) allowed the visualization of both target capture complex (TCC) and strand transfer complex (STC) before and after the reaction, respectively [10,45]. The tDNA binds along the groove created by the two inner subunits, right below the active site (Figure 4A). The intasome does not undergo significant structural rearrangements to accommodate the tDNA, which is severely bent. This deformation is maximal at the center of the integration site, with the widening of the major groove to 26.3 Å. This separation allows the scissile phosphodiester to fit into the active site for in line nucleophilic attack. Because DNA bendability is in large part dictated by the nature of the dinucleotide step, with pyrimidine–purine (YR) being the most flexible and purine-pyrimidine (RY) being the least, it is then not surprising that PFV integration sites are naturally biased towards more flexible pyrimidine–purine dinucleotide at the central position. As expected, due to the low selectivity of tDNA sequence, the majority of contacts between the intasome and tDNA are mediated through the phosphodiester backbone [10], except CCD residue Ala188 and CTD Arg329, that make base-specific contacts. Ala188 makes van der Waals interaction with cytosine at position 6, whereas Arg329 interacts with guanosine 3, guanosine −1, and thymine −2 through hydrogen bonds (Figure 4A, right). Interestingly, these two residues interact with all the consensus bases flanking the flexible central YR dinucleotide. Consequently, PFV IN Ala188 and Arg329 mutants showed in vitro strand transfer defects, as well as new sequence selectivity. The importance of these contacts has been validated for HIV-1 integrase, as mutating Ser119 (the structural equivalent of PFV IN Ala188) showed altered strand transfer and modified sequence selectivity [46–48].

In eukaryotes, host target DNA is compacted within chromatin that strongly distorts DNA around nucleosomes. PFV intasome showed strong integration activity when supplied with purified or recombinant human mononucleosomes [11,49]. Isolation of a stable complex of the PFV intasome and recombinant mononucleosome permitted the characterization by cryo-electron microscopy (Cryo-EM) of the TCC and a nucleosome core particle at 8 Å resolution [11] (Figure 4B). The crystal structures of the intasome and the nucleosome can be unambiguously docked into the electron density map. The intasome harbors the classical tetramer with the two types of subunits. No additional density is seen compared to the previous intasome crystal structures. The intasome sits on nucleosomal DNA above one of the H2A–H2B dimers and makes an extensive nucleosome–intasome interface involving three IN subunits, both turns of the nucleosomal DNA, and one H2A–H2B dimer. The carboxy-terminal helix of H2B is directly poking toward the intasome and is surrounded by a triad of loops from the inner subunits. Integrase residues Pro135, Pro239, and Thr240 wrap the C-terminal helix of H2B (Figure 4B, left) and the double substitution P135E/T240E strongly affected nucleosome binding and nucleosome strand transfer activity. The histone H2A shows density from its N-terminus reaching out to the inner IN CTD, and deletion of the first twelve H2A residues abolished intasome binding and decreased strand transfer activity into nucleosome. Further mutagenesis uncovered a role for the intasome outer domains, specifically the outer CTDs, as its deletion reduced the ability to bind nucleosomes. Additional important contacts between the intasome and the nucleosome involve the canonical CCD–CCD interface and the second gyre of nucleosomal DNA (Figure 4B, right). Residues

Q137, K159, and K168 are located in the vicinity of the contacts with the second gyre of DNA, and their substitution affected nucleosome binding and integration activity in vitro.

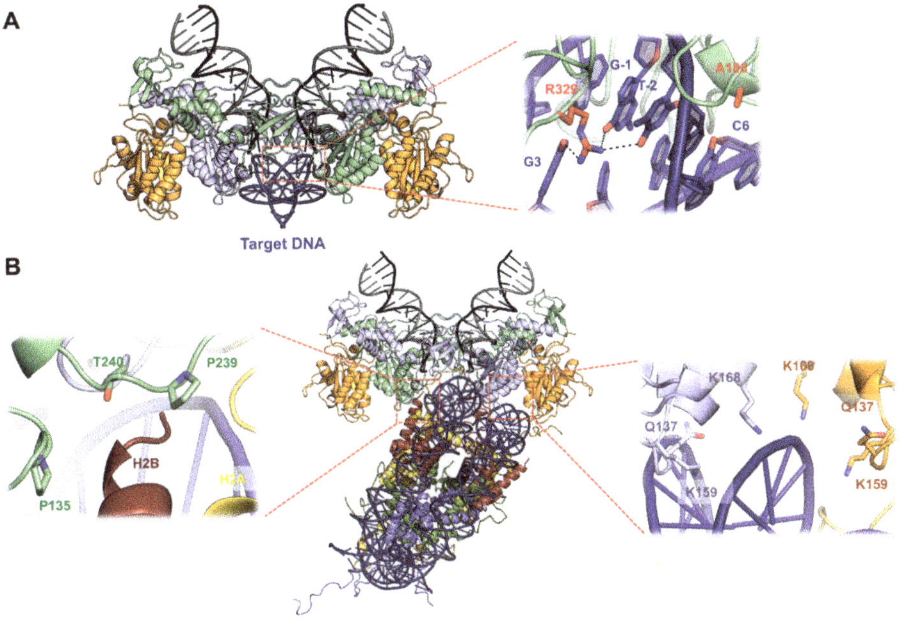

Figure 4. Target DNA capture. (**A**) Crystal structure of the target capture complex TCC (PDB: 3OS1) with sequence specific target DNA interactions shown as a blow up. Arg329 making contacts with guanosine 3, −1, and thymine −2, as well as Ala188 making contact with cytosine 6, are shown as red sticks. (**B**) Structure of the PFV intasome–nucleosome complex displayed as pseudoatomic model by docking PFV intasome (PDB 3L2Q) and nucleosome (PDB 1KX5) structures into the Cryo-EM map (EMDB ID 2992). Histones H2A are colored in yellow, H2B in red, H3 in blue, and H4 in green. IN contacts with H2B (**left**) and with the second gyre of nucleosomal DNA (**right**) are shown as zoomed boxes.

Most striking is the path of DNA captured within the tDNA-binding groove of the intasome. When compared to its structure on a native nucleosome, the captured DNA is kinked and lifted from the surface of the histones, perfectly matching the strong bending seen on the PFV intasome capture complex [11]. The multivalent intasome–nucleosome interactions may aid to reach the energy state required to deform nucleosomal DNA beyond its ground state, and seems to be the only determinant required as, more recently, Yoder and colleagues demonstrated that unwrapping DNA-histones modifications in the vicinity of the intasome integration sites does not impact nucleosome capture [50].

6. Mechanics of PFV Intasome Active Site

Because the IN catalysis requires divalent metal ion cofactor, it has been possible to freeze the PFV enzyme in different ground states before 3′ processing and strand transfer [45] (Figure 5). Both reactive and non-reactive strands of the vDNA are separated via the intrusion of the residues Pro214-Gly218, stacking against the adenine base, leaving three bases unpaired. The scissile dinucleotide phosphodiester backbone makes hydrogen bonds with Tyr212 and Gln186, while the adenine and thymidine bases contacts with the IN are limited to Van der Waals interactions. The binding of the two Mn^{2+} ions in the active site induces a shift of the scissile phosphodiester toward the catalytic triad DDE. The metal ion A is in a near perfect octahedral coordination. It comprises oxygen atoms from

Asp128 and Asp185, the pro-S_P oxygen atom of the scissile phosphodiester and three water molecules, one of them positioned for in-line nucleophilic attack on the scissile CA\AT phosphodiester bond. Both oxygen atoms of Glu221 and one from Asp128 coordinate metal B, as well as one water molecule, a bridging oxygen atom of the scissile phosphodiester and a non-bridging pro-S_P oxygen shared with metal A. This non-ideal environment for metal B may aid scissile phosphodiester bond destabilization during catalysis. Before 3′ processing, the distance between the two metal ions is 3.9 Å, and changes to 3.1 Å after dissociation of the dinucleotide. This metal ions movement has been also described in the RNase H active site and was suggested to allow the nucleophilic water to approach the scissile phosphodiester [51]. In the active site, the metal cofactors move further apart from each other (from 3.1 Å to 3.8 Å) upon target DNA capture. The roles of both metal ions changes between 3′ processing and strand transfer. Metal A and metal B coordination with active site residues stays unchanged, as well as the sharing of the pro-S_P oxygen atom from the target phosphodiester. Accordingly, metal A destabilized the target phosphodiester scissile bond by interacting with the 3′-bridging oxygen atom while metal B activates and positions the 3′OH of the vDNA for nucleophilic attack. After strand transfer catalysis, both metal ions move closer to approximately 3.2 Å.

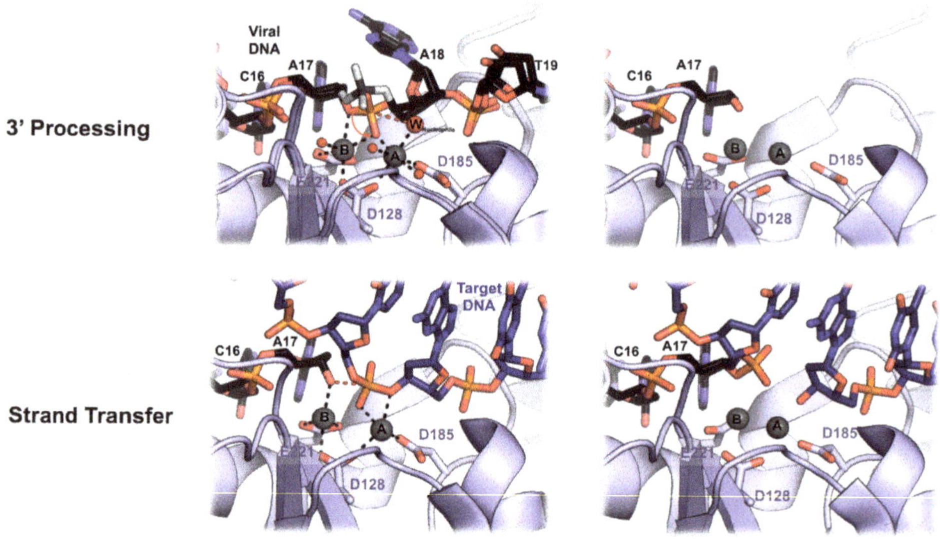

Figure 5. Mechanics of PFV 3′processing and strand transfer. Top panel, a close up of PFV intasome active site during 3′ processing. Superimposition of intasome structures before 3′ processing with and without bound manganese Mn^{2+} (grey spheres A and B) (**left**) and after cleavage (**right**). Relocation of the scissile phosphodiester upon metal binding is shown with a red arrow. The red spheres illustrate the water molecules, and the nucleophile water molecule is shown as a big red sphere. Bottom panel, strand transfer activity upon target DNA binding. The nucleophilic attack is shown with red dashes.

Overlaying the TCC and the STC structure shows that the overall DNA conformations do not change, except the position of the phosphodiester linking the tDNA to vDNA, which is shifted away from the active site. Integrase apply a significant torsional stress to the tDNA, likely providing the displacement force, which is relieved upon cutting of the target phosphodiester bond. This ejection prevents any reversible reaction that would lead to unfruitful viral infection. A soaking experiment with metal cofactor showed an apparent loss of metal B binding affinity after strand transfer, probably due to the ejection of the DNA from the active site. Interestingly, such a tDNA kink within the active site is important for other transpososomes activity like Hermes [34,52], MuA [53], Tn10 [54], and IS231A [55]. This could be an evolutionary conserved feature of DNA transposition apparatus in order to prevent any reversal reaction, while being competent to access tDNA scissile phosphodiester.

7. PFV Intasome and HIV-1 Strand Transfer Inhibitors

Human immunodeficiency virus type 1 (HIV-1) IN has been widely considered as an important target protein for novel anti-acquired immune deficiency syndrome (AIDS) drugs [56]. Based on biochemical assay and biophysical analysis, several classes of retroviral IN inhibitors have been discovered over the last 25 years [57–60]. Hydroxylated natural products and their derivatives were developed, and the most important IN inhibitor family, diketo acids (DKA), emerged [59]. Integrase strand transfer inhibitors (INSTIs) are one of active site inhibitors against HIV-1 integration that act by preventing the strand transfer reaction; however, numerous significant developments and rational designs of INSTIs were reported during recent years. Raltegravir (RAL) was the first INSTIs approved by the United State food and drug administration (FDA) in 2007 [61], providing a new option for highly active antiretroviral therapy (HAART). After that, elvitegravir (EVG) and dolutegravir (DTG) have been approved [62,63] (Figure 6A). RAL, EVG, and DTG belong to the bioisosteres compounds of DKA. DKA derivatives, which contain a 1,3-dicarbonyl aromatic ring, are a class of highly effective HIV-1 INSTIs where the 1,3-dicarbonyl group seizes two Mg2+ ions, preventing the metal ion-mediated retroviral integration [64–66]. More recently, two new molecules, bictegravir (BIC) and cabotegravir (CAB), have been developed [67,68]. Bictegravir was approved by the FDA in early 2018 and is being used as a combination drug. Cabotegravir is currently in phase III development. BIC and CAB are structurally similar to DTG with their tri-cyclic central pharmacophores (Figure 6A), but the latter offers an improved half-life [69].

Despite an increasing drug arsenal, the experimental data related to full-length, wild type HIV-1 intasomes structures are rare. As an alternative, PFV intasome has been adopted for anti-AIDS drug development. A comparison of the CCD structures between HIV-1 and PFV showed that both conserved unique structural features, such as the host cellular factor binding faces and the organization of the active site [8,9,30]. A recent NMR study using the CCD of HIV-1 IN showed that the HIV-1 and PFV IN flexible loops (residues 140–149 in HIV and 209–218 in PFV) are almost similar, and structure prediction of the HIV integrase intasome provided further evidence for the similarities between the active amino acid resides of the PFV and HIV INs [70,71]. Johnson et al. generated a corresponding HIV-1 IN model from the PFV IN crystal structure and they predicted the in vitro anti-INSTI activities using molecular docking and molecular dynamics simulation [72]. Despite the limited sequence similarity and different intasome architecture features (lentiviral: tetramer-of-tetramer, PFV: dimer-of-dimer), PFV IN was highly sensitive to HIV INSTIs [8,73], suggesting that INSTIs target the most conserved regions of IN-DNA complexes. Recently, many studies using PFV IN as a surrogate model in order to investigate HIV-1 INSTIs have been published. Some groups investigated the consistency between in vitro and in vivo resistance profiles for RAL using PFV IN structures mutated at the corresponding to HIV-1 IN active site, Q148, and N155 [74,75]. Hare et al. confirmed the interaction of the pharmacophores of PFV intasome with two metal ions at the IN active site, and they also investigated an interaction between the bound vDNA end and the benzyl group through cocrystal structures of RAL and EVG [9]. Also, they obtained a crystal structure of PFV IN complexed with vDNA and DTG [76] (Figure 6B) (See [1] for more details on the structural basis for INSTIs). Johnson et al. designed a series of INSTIs based on the previous target model through homology modeling and structural superposition method. In their modeling system, the junction between the CCD and CTD adopts a helix-loop-helix motif, which is similar to the corresponding segment of PFV IN [77].

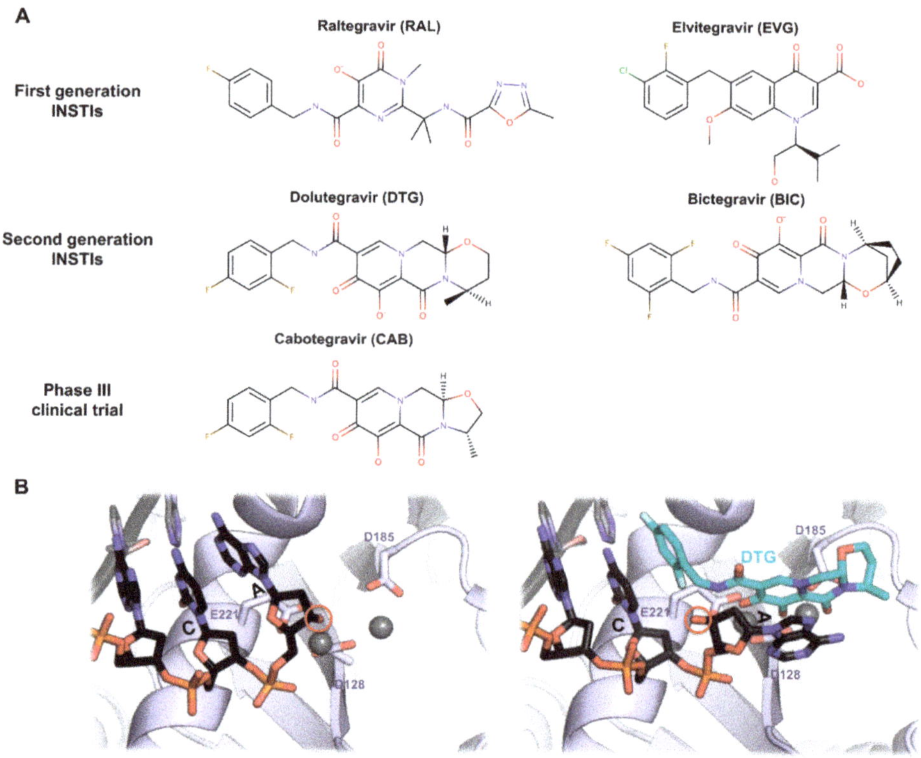

Figure 6. Integrase strand transfer inhibitors. (**A**) Chemical structures of INSTIs. (**B**) Structure of PFV active site with or without DTG. By positioning into the active site, the INSTI engages the metal cofactors and induces a shift of the 3′ reactive hydroxyl (red circle) out of position incompatible for strand transfer.

Hu et al. investigated the inhibitory mechanism of RAL and the recognition of DKA inhibitors with PFV-IN via molecular dynamics and molecular docking methods, and they validated the HIV-1 inhibitor screening platform [73,78]. Du et al. proposed the crystal structure of PFV-IN DNA as a potential HIV-1 INSTI screening platform through a structural biology information survey [79]. They also investigated the molecular recognition system of PFV IN, using six naphthyridine derivatives inhibitors through molecular docking, molecular dynamics simulations, and water-mediated interactions analyses. Besides, there are a lot of studies using PFV intasome to explore the binding mode of compounds for new HIV IN inhibitors. These results have implications for the rational design of HIV-1 IN targeting specific INSTIs with improved affinity and selectivity [80,81].

Some studies have raised doubts on HIV-1 IN inhibitor screening platforms using PFV-IN, indicating that the HIV-1 IN system behaves differently from PFV in terms of folding, recognition, and hydrophobicity of the tDNA binding site, and stability [82]. Although conformational changes and the energy landscape are still unclear, the molecular docking and molecular dynamics study validates the reliability of the platform and reestablishes PFV IN as one of the most credible surrogate model for HIV-1 INSTIs studies and anti-AIDS drug development based on IN structure. Nevertheless, thanks to Cryo-EM advances, future high-resolution structures of primate lentiviral integrases will be of great interest to further improve the structural basis of INSTI mechanisms and development.

8. Conclusions and Perspectives

As an important therapeutic target and molecular tool, retroviral integrase is having a lot of attention from the scientific community. Intensive biochemical studies gave important insights on the functional architecture of the viral enzyme and, little by little, the structural counterpart emerged: from individual domains to active intasomes bound to a nucleosome. The publication in 2010 of the first retroviral intasome structure from PFV was the starting point of a decade-long period of exciting and insightful research on the integration process. The recent revolution in single particle cryo-electron microscopy significantly increased the repertoire of retroviral intasome structures now available that highlight both the conservation and diversity in the architectures. Conservation, because the presence on all retroviral intasome of a PFV-like intasome CIC hosting the catalytic subunits is quite striking, and diversity being on the variety of oligomers needed for the whole assembly. It will be of great interest to expand the catalogue of known intasome structures from the remaining retroviral genera, but also to further investigate new structures derived from wild type primate lentiviral integrases to better understand HIV-1 strand transfer inhibitors.

Many open questions will surely keep the fire of retroviral integration research vivid, notably, what is the precise chronology of intasome assembly during infection. Indeed, HIV-1 virion packages around 250 molecules of integrase, which is far more than needed from the recent structures of lentiviral intasomes. Also, although the structure of the PFV intasome bound to a nucleosome afforded important information on the chromatin capture by retroviral intasomes, the requirement for histones might differs from genus to genus [83,84], highlighting the need for additional structures of intasomes bound to nucleosomes. Additionally, early chromatinisation of retroviral pre-integration complexes has emerged as a feature of two retroviral genera [85,86]. Future studies will be required to determine the functional importance and the conservation among integrative mobile elements and, notably, Foamy viruses.

Funding: This work was supported by a grant from the National Research Foundation of Korea (NRF) funded by the Korean government (NRF-2018R1D1A1A09081872) to Cha-Gyun Shin.

Acknowledgments: We thank Dmitry Lyumkis for providing coordinates of the higher-order HIV-1-IN-Sso7d intasome structure.

Conflicts of Interest: The authors declare no conflict of interest. The funders had no role in the design of the study; in the collection, analyses, or interpretation of data; in the writing of the manuscript, or in the decision to publish the results.

References

1. Lesbats, P.; Engelman, A.N.; Cherepanov, P. Retroviral DNA Integration. *Chem. Rev.* **2016**, *116*, 12730–12757. [CrossRef] [PubMed]
2. Dyda, F.; Chandler, M.; Hickman, A.B. The emerging diversity of transpososome architectures. *Q. Rev. Biophys.* **2012**, *45*, 493–521. [CrossRef] [PubMed]
3. Fujiwara, T.; Mizuuchi, K. Retroviral DNA integration: Structure of an integration intermediate. *Cell* **1988**, *54*, 497–504. [CrossRef]
4. Brown, P.O.; Bowerman, B.; Varmus, H.E.; Bishop, J.M. Retroviral integration: Structure of the initial covalent product and its precursor, and a role for the viral IN protein. *Proc. Natl. Acad. Sci. USA* **1989**, *86*, 2525–2529. [CrossRef] [PubMed]
5. Roth, M.J.; Schwartzberg, P.L.; Goff, S.P. Structure of the termini of DNA intermediates in the integration of retroviral DNA: Dependence on IN function and terminal DNA sequence. *Cell* **1989**, *58*, 47–54. [CrossRef]
6. Bowerman, B.; Brown, P.O.; Bishop, J.M.; Varmus, H.E. A nucleoprotein complex mediates the integration of retroviral DNA. *Genes Dev.* **1989**, *3*, 469–478. [CrossRef] [PubMed]
7. Wei, S.-Q.; Mizuuchi, K.; Craigie, R. A large nucleoprotein assembly at the ends of the viral DNA mediates retroviral DNA integration. *EMBO J.* **1997**, *16*, 7511–7520. [CrossRef]

8. Valkov, E.; Gupta, S.S.; Hare, S.; Helander, A.; Roversi, P.; McClure, M.; Cherepanov, P. Functional and structural characterization of the integrase from the prototype foamy virus. *Nucleic Acids Res.* **2009**, *37*, 243–255. [CrossRef]
9. Hare, S.; Gupta, S.S.; Valkov, E.; Engelman, A.; Cherepanov, P. Retroviral intasome assembly and inhibition of DNA strand transfer. *Nature* **2010**, *464*, 232–236.
10. Maertens, G.N.; Hare, S.; Cherepanov, P. The mechanism of retroviral integration from X-ray structures of its key intermediates. *Nature* **2010**, *468*, 326–329.
11. Maskell, D.P.; Renault, L.; Serrao, E.; Lesbats, P.; Matadeen, R.; Hare, S.; Lindemann, D.; Engelman, A.N.; Costa, A.; Cherepanov, P. Structural basis for retroviral integration into nucleosomes. *Nature* **2015**, *523*, 366–369. [CrossRef]
12. Brown, P.O.; Bowerman, B.; Varmus, H.E.; Bishop, J. Correct integration of retroviral DNA in vitro. *Cell* **1987**, *49*, 347–356. [CrossRef]
13. Farnet, C.M.; Haseltine, W.A. Integration of human immunodeficiency virus type 1 DNA in vitro. *Proc. Natl. Acad. Sci. USA* **1990**, *87*, 4164–4168. [CrossRef] [PubMed]
14. Skinner, L.M.; Sudol, M.; Harper, A.L.; Katzman, M. Nucleophile selection for the endonuclease activities of human, ovine, and avian retroviral integrases. *J. Biol. Chem.* **2001**, *276*, 114–124. [CrossRef] [PubMed]
15. Harper, A.L.; Sudol, M.; Katzman, M. An Amino Acid in the Central Catalytic Domain of Three Retroviral Integrases That Affects Target Site Selection in Nonviral DNA. *J. Virol.* **2003**, *77*, 3838–3845. [CrossRef]
16. Enssle, J.; Mauer, B.; Schweizer, M.; Heinkelein, M.; Neumann-Haefelin, D.; Rethwilm, A.; Panhuysen, M.; Moebes, A. An active foamy virus integrase is required for virus replication. *J. Gen. Virol.* **1999**, *80*, 1445–1452. [CrossRef]
17. Juretzek, T.; Holm, T.; Gärtner, K.; Kanzler, S.; Lindemann, D.; Herchenröder, O.; Picard-Maureau, M.; Rammling, M.; Heinkelein, M.; Rethwilm, A. Foamy Virus Integration. *J. Virol.* **2004**, *78*, 2472–2477. [CrossRef]
18. Fujiwara, T.; Craigie, R. Integration of mini-retroviral DNA: A cell-free reaction for biochemical analysis of retroviral integration. *Proc. Natl. Acad. Sci. USA* **1989**, *86*, 3065–3069. [CrossRef]
19. Katzman, M.; Katz, R.A.; Skalka, A.M.; Leis, J. The avian retroviral integration protein cleaves the terminal sequences of linear viral DNA at the in vivo sites of integration. *J. Virol.* **1989**, *63*, 5319–5327.
20. Vora, A.C.; Fitzgerald, M.L.; Grandgenett, D.P. Removal of 3′-OH-terminal nucleotides from blunt-ended long terminal repeat termini by the avian retrovirus integration protein. *J. Virol.* **1990**, *64*, 5656–5659. [PubMed]
21. Shin, C.-G. Characterization of Biochemical Properties of Feline Foamy Virus Integrase. *J. Microbiol. Biotechnol.* **2010**, *20*, 968–973. [CrossRef]
22. Hazuda, D.J.; Felock, P.J.; Hastings, J.C.; Pramanik, B.; Wolfe, A.L. Differential divalent cation requirements uncouple the assembly and catalytic reactions of human immunodeficiency virus type 1 integrase. *J. Virol.* **1997**, *71*, 7005–7011. [PubMed]
23. Mackler, R.; Lopez, M.; Osterhage, M.; Yoder, K. Prototype foamy virus integrase is promiscuous for target choice. *Biochem. Biophys. Res. Commun.* **2018**, *503*, 1241–1246. [CrossRef] [PubMed]
24. Jones, N.D.; Lopez, M.A., Jr.; Hanne, J.; Peake, M.B.; Lee, J.-B.; Fishel, R.; Yoder, K.E. Retroviral intasomes search for a target DNA by 1D diffusion which rarely results in integration. *Nat. Commun.* **2016**, *7*, 11409. [CrossRef]
25. Engelman, A.; Craigie, R. Identification of conserved amino acid residues critical for human immunodeficiency virus type 1 integrase function in vitro. *J. Virol.* **1992**, *66*, 6361–6369. [PubMed]
26. Cai, M.; Zheng, R.; Caffrey, M.; Craigie, R.; Clore, G.M.; Gronenborn, A.M. Solution structure of the N-terminal zinc binding domain of HIV-1 integrase. *Nat. Genet.* **1997**, *4*, 567–577. [CrossRef]
27. Eijkelenboom, A.P.; Ent, F.M.V.D.; Vos, A.; Doreleijers, J.F.; Hård, K.; Tullius, T.D.; Plasterk, R.H.; Kaptein, R.; Boelens, R. The solution structure of the amino-terminal HHCC domain of HIV-2 integrase: A three-helix bundle stabilized by zinc. *Curr. Biol.* **1997**, *7*, 739–746. [CrossRef]
28. Eijkelenboom, A.P.; Lutzke, R.A.P.; Boelens, R.; Plasterk, R.H.; Kaptein, R.; Hård, K. The DNA-binding domain of HIV-1 integrase has an SH3-like fold. *Nat. Struct. Mol. Biol.* **1995**, *2*, 807–810. [CrossRef]
29. Lodi, P.J.; Ernst, J.A.; Kuszewski, J.; Hickman, A.B.; Engelman, A.; Craigie, R.; Clore, G.M.; Gronenborn, A.M. Solution Structure of the DNA Binding Domain of HIV-1 Integrase. *Biochemistry* **1995**, *34*, 9826–9833. [CrossRef]

30. Dyda, F.; Hickman, A.B.; Jenkins, T.M.; Engelman, A.; Craigie, R.; Davies, D.R. Crystal structure of the catalytic domain of HIV-1 integrase: Similarity to other polynucleotidyl transferases. *Science* **1994**, *266*, 1981–1986. [CrossRef]
31. Nowotny, M. Retroviral integrase superfamily: The structural perspective. *EMBO Rep.* **2009**, *10*, 144–151. [CrossRef]
32. Augé-Gouillou, C.; Brillet, B.; Hamelin, M.-H.; Bigot, Y. Assembly of the mariner Mos1 Synaptic Complex. *Mol. Cell. Biol.* **2005**, *25*, 2861–2870. [CrossRef] [PubMed]
33. Hickman, A.B.; Perez, Z.N.; Zhou, L.Q.; Musingarimi, P.; Ghirlando, R.; Hinshaw, J.E.; Craig, N.L.; Dyda, F. Molecular architecture of a eukaryotic DNA transposase. *Nat. Struct. Mol. Biol.* **2005**, *12*, 715–721. [CrossRef] [PubMed]
34. Hickman, A.B.; Ewis, H.E.; Li, X.; Knapp, J.A.; Laver, T.; Doss, A.-L.; Tolun, G.; Steven, A.C.; Grishaev, A.; Bax, A.; et al. Structural Basis of hAT Transposon End Recognition by Hermes, an Octameric DNA Transposase from Musca domestica. *Cell* **2014**, *158*, 353–367. [CrossRef] [PubMed]
35. Gupta, K.; Curtis, J.E.; Krueger, S.; Hwang, Y.; Cherepanov, P.; Bushman, F.D.; Van Duyne, G.D. Solution Conformations of Prototype Foamy Virus Integrase and its Stable Synaptic Complex with U5 Viral DNA. *Structure* **2012**, *20*, 1918–1928. [CrossRef] [PubMed]
36. Li, M.; Lin, S.; Craigie, R. Outer domains of integrase within retroviral intasomes are dispensible for catalysis of DNA integration. *Protein Sci.* **2016**, *25*, 472–478. [CrossRef]
37. Yin, Z.; Shi, K.; Banerjee, S.; Aihara, H. Crystal structure of the Rous sarcoma virus intasome. Crystal structure of the Rous sarcoma virus intasome. *Nature* **2016**, *530*, 362–366. [CrossRef]
38. Allison Ballandras-Colas, M.B. Cryo-EM reveals a novel octameric integrase structure for β-retroviral intasome function. *Nature* **2016**, *530*, 358–361. [CrossRef]
39. Ballandras-Colas, A.; Maskell, D.P.; Serrao, E.; Locke, J.; Swuec, P.; Jónsson, S.R.; Kotecha, A.; Cook, N.J.; Pye, V.E.; Taylor, I.A.; et al. A supramolecular assembly mediates lentiviral DNA integration. *Science* **2017**, *355*, 93–95. [CrossRef]
40. Passos, D.O.; Li, M.; Yang, R.; Rebensburg, S.V.; Ghirlando, R.; Jeon, Y.; Shkriabai, N.; Kvaratskhelia, M.; Craigie, R.; Lyumkis, D. CryoEM Structures and Atomic Model of the HIV-1 Strand Transfer Complex Intasome. *Science* **2017**, *355*, 89–92. [CrossRef] [PubMed]
41. Engelman, A.N.; Cherepanov, P. Retroviral intasomes arising. *Curr. Opin. Struct. Biol.* **2017**, *47*, 23–29. [CrossRef] [PubMed]
42. Chen, J.C.-H.; Krucinski, J.; Miercke, L.J.W.; Finer-Moore, J.S.; Tang, A.H.; Leavitt, A.D.; Stroud, R.M. Crystal structure of the HIV-1 integrase catalytic core and C-terminal domains: A model for viral DNA binding. *Proc. Natl. Acad. Sci. USA* **2000**, *97*, 8233–8238. [CrossRef] [PubMed]
43. Gao, Y.-G.; Su, S.-Y.; Robinson, H.; Padmanabhan, S.; Lim, L.; McCrary, B.S.; Edmondson, S.P.; Shriver, J.W.; Wang, A.H.-J. The crystal structure of the hyperthermophile chromosomal protein Sso7d bound to DNA. *Nat. Genet.* **1998**, *5*, 782–786. [CrossRef] [PubMed]
44. Li, M.; Jurado, K.A.; Lin, S.; Engelman, A.; Craigie, R. Engineered Hyperactive Integrase for Concerted HIV-1 DNA Integration. *PLoS ONE* **2014**, *9*, e105078. [CrossRef] [PubMed]
45. Hare, S.; Maertens, G.N.; Cherepanov, P. 3′-Processing and strand transfer catalysed by retroviral integrase in crystallo. *EMBO J.* **2012**, *31*, 3020–3028. [CrossRef]
46. Serrao, E.; Krishnan, L.; Shun, M.-C.; Li, X.; Cherepanov, P.; Engelman, A.; Maertens, G.N. Integrase residues that determine nucleotide preferences at sites of HIV-1 integration: Implications for the mechanism of target DNA binding. *Nucleic Acids Res.* **2014**, *42*, 5164–5176. [CrossRef] [PubMed]
47. Serrao, E.; Ballandras-Colas, A.; Cherepanov, P.; Maertens, G.N.; Engelman, A.N. Key determinants of target DNA recognition by retroviral intasomes. *Retrovirology* **2015**, *12*, 1295. [CrossRef] [PubMed]
48. Naughtin, M.; Haftek-Terreau, Z.; Xavier, J.; Meyer, S.; Silvain, M.; Jaszczyszyn, Y.; Levy, N.; Miele, V.; Benleulmi, M.S.; Ruff, M.; et al. DNA Physical Properties and Nucleosome Positions Are Major Determinants of HIV-1 Integrase Selectivity. *PLoS ONE* **2015**, *10*, e0129427. [CrossRef]
49. Benleulmi, M.S.; Matysiak, J.; Henriquez, D.R.; Vaillant, C.; Lesbats, P.; Calmels, C.; Naughtin, M.; Leon, O.; Skalka, A.M.; Ruff, M.; et al. Intasome architecture and chromatin density modulate retroviral integration into nucleosome. *Retrovirology* **2015**, *12*, 469. [CrossRef]

50. Mackler, R.M.; Jones, N.D.; Gardner, A.M.; Lopez, M.A.; Howard, C.J.; Fishel, R.; Yoder, K.E. Nucleosome DNA unwrapping does not affect prototype foamy virus integration efficiency or site selection. *PLoS ONE* **2019**, *14*, e0212764. [CrossRef]
51. Nowotny, M.; Yang, W. Stepwise analyses of metal ions in RNase H catalysis from substrate destabilization to product release. *EMBO J.* **2006**, *25*, 1924–1933. [CrossRef] [PubMed]
52. Gangadharan, S.; Mularoni, L.; Fain-Thornton, J.; Wheelan, S.J.; Craig, N.L. DNA transposon Hermes inserts into DNA in nucleosome-free regions in vivo. *Proc. Natl. Acad. Sci. USA* **2010**, *107*, 21966–21972. [CrossRef] [PubMed]
53. Montano, S.P.; Pigli, Y.Z.; Rice, P.A. The mu transpososome structure sheds light on DDE recombinase evolution. *Nature* **2012**, *491*, 413–417. [CrossRef]
54. Pribil, P.A.; Haniford, D.B. Target DNA Bending is an Important Specificity Determinant in Target Site Selection in Tn10 Transposition. *J. Mol. Biol.* **2003**, *330*, 247–259. [CrossRef]
55. Hallet, B.; Rezsöhazy, R.; Mahilton, J.; Delcour, J. IS231A insertion specificity: Consensus sequence and DNA bending at the target site. *Mol. Microbiol.* **1994**, *14*, 131–139. [CrossRef] [PubMed]
56. Kaur, M.; Rawal, R.K.; Rath, G.; Goyal, A.K. Structure Based Drug Design: Clinically Relevant HIV-1 Integrase Inhibitors. *Curr. Top. Med. Chem.* **2018**, *18*, 2664–2680. [CrossRef] [PubMed]
57. Hazuda, D.J.; Hastings, J.C.; Wolfe, A.L.; Emini, E.A. A novel assay for the DNA strand-transfer reaction of HIV-1 integrase. *Nucleic Acids Res.* **1994**, *22*, 1121–1122. [CrossRef] [PubMed]
58. Hazuda, D.; Felock, P.J.; Hastings, J.C.; Pramanik, B.; Wolfe, A.L. Discovery and analysis of inhibitors of the human immunodeficiency integrase. *Drug Des. Discov.* **1997**, *15*, 17–24. [PubMed]
59. Hazuda, D.J.; Felock, P.; Witmer, M.; Wolfe, A.; Stillmock, K.; Grobler, J.A.; Espeseth, A.; Gabryelski, L.; Schleif, W.; Blau, C.; et al. Inhibitors of Strand Transfer That Prevent Integration and Inhibit HIV-1 Replication in Cells. *Science* **2000**, *287*, 646–650. [CrossRef] [PubMed]
60. Liao, C.; Marchand, C.; Burke, T.R.; Pommier, Y.; Nicklaus, M.C. Authentic HIV-1 integrase inhibitors. *Futur. Med. Chem.* **2010**, *2*, 1107–1122. [CrossRef]
61. Cocohoba, J.; Dong, B.J. Raltegravir: The first HIV integrase inhibitor. *Clin. Ther.* **2008**, *30*, 1747–1765. [CrossRef]
62. Sato, M.; Motomura, T.; Aramaki, H.; Matsuda, T.; Yamashita, M.; Ito, Y.; Kawakami, H.; Matsuzaki, Y.; Watanabe, W.; Yamataka, K.; et al. Novel HIV-1 Integrase Inhibitors Derived from Quinolone Antibiotics. *J. Med. Chem.* **2006**, *49*, 1506–1508. [CrossRef]
63. Johns, B.A.; Kawasuji, T.; Weatherhead, J.G.; Taishi, T.; Temelkoff, D.P.; Yoshida, H.; Akiyama, T.; Taoda, Y.; Murai, H.; Kiyama, R.; et al. Carbamoyl pyridone HIV-1 integrase inhibitors 3. A diastereomeric approach to chiral nonracemic tricyclic ring systems and the discovery of dolutegravir (S/GSK1349572) and (S/GSK1265744). *J. Med. Chem.* **2013**, *56*, 5901–5916. [CrossRef]
64. Barreca, M.L.; Ferro, S.; Rao, A.; De Luca, L.; Zappala', M.; Monforte, A.-M.; Debyser, Z.; Witvrouw, M.; Chimirri, A. Pharmacophore-Based Design of HIV-1 Integrase Strand-Transfer Inhibitors. *J. Med. Chem.* **2005**, *48*, 7084–7088. [CrossRef] [PubMed]
65. Wang, Y.; Rong, J.; Zhang, B.; Hu, L.; Wang, X.; Zeng, C. Design and synthesis of N-methylpyrimidone derivatives as HIV-1 integrase inhibitors. *Bioorg. Med. Chem.* **2015**, *23*, 735–741. [CrossRef]
66. Cuzzucoli Crucitti, G.; Métifiot, M.; Pescatori, L.; Messore, A.; Madia, V.N.; Pupo, G.; Saccoliti, F.; Scipione, L.; Tortorella, S.; Esposito, F.; et al. Structure-activity relationship of pyrrolyl diketo acid derivatives as dual inhibitors of HIV-1 integrase and reverse transcriptase ribonuclease H domain. *J. Med. Chem.* **2015**, *58*, 1915–1928. [CrossRef]
67. Yoshinaga, T.; Kobayashi, M.; Seki, T.; Miki, S.; Wakasa-Morimoto, C.; Suyama-Kagitani, A.; Kawauchi-Miki, S.; Taishi, T.; Kawasuji, T.; Johns, B.A.; et al. Antiviral characteristics of GSK1265744, an HIV integrase inhibitor dosed orally or by long-acting injection. *Antimicrob. Agents Chemother.* **2015**, *59*, 397–406. [CrossRef]
68. Tsiang, M.; Jones, G.S.; Goldsmith, J.; Mulato, A.; Hansen, D.; Kan, E.; Tsai, L.; Bam, R.A.; Stepan, G.; Stray, K.M.; et al. Antiviral Activity of Bictegravir (GS-9883), a Novel Potent HIV-1 Integrase Strand Transfer Inhibitor with an Improved Resistance Profile. *Antimicrob. Agents Chemother.* **2016**, *60*, 7086–7097. [CrossRef] [PubMed]
69. Trezza, C.; Ford, S.L.; Spreen, W.; Pan, R.; Piscitelli, S. Formulation and pharmacology of long-acting cabotegravir. *Curr. Opin. HIV AIDS* **2015**, *10*, 239–245. [CrossRef] [PubMed]

70. Fitzkee, N.C.; Masse, J.E.; Shen, Y.; Davies, D.R.; Bax, A. Solution Conformation and Dynamics of the HIV-1 Integrase Core Domain. *J. Biol. Chem.* **2010**, *285*, 18072–18084. [CrossRef]
71. Krishnan, L.; Li, X.; Naraharisetty, H.L.; Hare, S.; Cherepanov, P.; Engelman, A. Structure-based modeling of the functional HIV-1 intasome and its inhibition. *Proc. Natl. Acad. Sci. USA* **2010**, *107*, 15910–15915. [CrossRef] [PubMed]
72. Johnson, B.C.; Métifiot, M.; Pommier, Y.; Hughes, S.H. Molecular dynamics approaches estimate the binding energy of HIV-1 integrase inhibitors and correlate with in vitro activity. *Antimicrob. Agents Chemother.* **2012**, *56*, 411–419. [CrossRef]
73. Hu, J.-P.; He, H.-Q.; Tang, D.-Y.; Sun, G.-F.; Zhang, Y.-Q.; Fan, J.; Chang, S. Study on the interactions between diketo-acid inhibitors and prototype foamy virus integrase-DNA complex via molecular docking and comparative molecular dynamics simulation methods. *J. Biomol. Struct. Dyn.* **2013**, *31*, 734–747. [CrossRef]
74. Goethals, O.; Van Ginderen, M.; Vos, A.; Cummings, M.D.; Van Der Borght, K.; Van Wesenbeeck, L.; Feyaerts, M.; Verheyen, A.; Smits, V.; Van Loock, M.; et al. Resistance to raltegravir highlights integrase mutations at codon 148 in conferring cross-resistance to a second-generation HIV-1 integrase inhibitor. *Antivir. Res.* **2011**, *91*, 167–176. [CrossRef] [PubMed]
75. Hare, S.; Vos, A.M.; Clayton, R.F.; Thuring, J.W.; Cummings, M.D.; Cherepanov, P. Molecular mechanisms of retroviral integrase inhibition and the evolution of viral resistance. *Proc. Natl. Acad. Sci. USA* **2010**, *107*, 20057–20062. [CrossRef] [PubMed]
76. Hare, S.; Smith, S.J.; Métifiot, M.; Jaxa-Chamiec, A.; Pommier, Y.; Hughes, S.H.; Cherepanov, P. Structural and Functional Analyses of the Second-Generation Integrase Strand Transfer Inhibitor Dolutegravir (S/GSK1349572). *Mol. Pharmacol.* **2011**, *80*, 565–572. [CrossRef]
77. Johnson, B.C.; Metifiot, M.; Ferris, A.; Pommier, Y.; Hughes, S.H. A Homology Model of HIV-1 Integrase and Analysis of Mutations Designed to Test the Model. *J. Mol. Biol.* **2013**, *425*, 2133–2146. [CrossRef]
78. Hu, J.; Liu, M.; Tang, D.; Chang, S. Substrate Recognition and Motion Mode Analyses of PFV Integrase in Complex with Viral DNA via Coarse-Grained Models. *PLoS ONE* **2013**, *8*, e54929. [CrossRef]
79. Du, W.; Zuo, K.; Sun, X.; Liu, W.; Yan, X.; Liang, L.; Wan, H.; Chen, F.; Hu, J. An effective HIV-1 integrase inhibitor screening platform: Rationality validation of drug screening, conformational mobility and molecular recognition analysis for PFV integrase complex with viral DNA. *J. Mol. Graph. Model.* **2017**, *78*, 96–109. [CrossRef]
80. Quashie, P.K.; Han, Y.-S.; Hassounah, S.; Mesplède, T.; Wainberg, M.A. Structural Studies of the HIV-1 Integrase Protein: Compound Screening and Characterization of a DNA-Binding Inhibitor. *PLoS ONE* **2015**, *10*, e0128310. [CrossRef]
81. Reddy, K.K.; Singh, S.K. Combined ligand and structure-based approaches on HIV-1 integrase strand transfer inhibitors. *Chem. Interact.* **2014**, *218*, 71–81. [CrossRef] [PubMed]
82. Dayer, M.R. Comparison of Newly Assembled Full Length HIV-1 Integrase With Prototype Foamy Virus Integrase: Structure-Function Prospective. *Jundishapur J. Microbiol.* **2016**, *9*, e29773. [CrossRef] [PubMed]
83. Benleulmi, M.S.; Matysiak, J.; Robert, X.; Miskey, C.; Mauro, E.; Lapaillerie, D.; Lesbats, P.; Chaignepain, S.; Henriquez, D.R.; Calmels, C.; et al. Modulation of the functional association between the HIV-1 intasome and the nucleosome by histone amino-terminal tails. *Retrovirology* **2017**, *14*, 54. [CrossRef]
84. Mauro, E.; Lesbats, P.; Lapaillerie, D.; Chaignepain, S.; Maillot, B.; Oladosu, O.; Robert, X.; Fiorini, F.; Kieffer, B.; Bouaziz, S.; et al. Human H4 tail stimulates HIV-1 integration through binding to the carboxy-terminal domain of integrase. *Nucleic Acids Res.* **2019**, *47*, 3607–3618. [CrossRef]
85. Wang, G.Z.; Wang, Y.; Goff, S.P. Histones are rapidly loaded onto unintegrated retroviral DNAs soon after nuclear entry. *Cell Host Microbe* **2016**, *20*, 798–809. [CrossRef] [PubMed]
86. Zhu, Y.; Wang, G.Z.; Cingöz, O.; Goff, S.P. NP220 mediates silencing of unintegrated retroviral DNA. *Nature* **2018**, *564*, 278–282. [CrossRef]

viruses

MDPI

Article

The Influence of Envelope C-Terminus Amino Acid Composition on the Ratio of Cell-Free to Cell-Cell Transmission for Bovine Foamy Virus

Suzhen Zhang †, Xiaojuan Liu †, Zhibin Liang, Tiejun Bing, Wentao Qiao and Juan Tan *

Key Laboratory of Molecular Microbiology and Technology, Ministry of Education, College of Life Sciences, Nankai University, Tianjin 300071, China; zhangsuzhen819819@163.com (S.Z.); 1395312330@qq.com (X.L.); liangzhibin@mail.nankai.edu.cn (Z.L.); btj1987@126.com (T.B.); wentaoqiao@nankai.edu.cn (W.Q.)

* Correspondence: juantan@nankai.edu.cn; Tel.: +86-22-2350-4547; Fax: 86-22-2350-0950

† These authors contributed equally to this work.

Received: 12 November 2018; Accepted: 29 January 2019; Published: 31 January 2019

Abstract: Foamy viruses (FVs) have extensive cell tropism in vitro, special replication features, and no clinical pathogenicity in naturally or experimentally infected animals, which distinguish them from orthoretroviruses. Among FVs, bovine foamy virus (BFV) has undetectable or extremely low levels of cell-free transmission in the supernatants of infected cells and mainly spreads by cell-to-cell transmission, which deters its use as a gene transfer vector. Here, using an in vitro virus evolution system, we successfully isolated high-titer cell-free BFV strains from the original cell-to-cell transmissible BFV3026 strain and further constructed an infectious cell-free BFV clone called pBS-BFV-Z1. Following sequence alignment with a cell-associated clone pBS-BFV-B, we identified a number of changes in the genome of pBS-BFV-Z1. Extensive mutagenesis analysis revealed that the C-terminus of envelope protein, especially the K898 residue, controls BFV cell-free transmission by enhancing cell-free virus entry but not the virus release capacity. Taken together, our data show the genetic determinants that regulate cell-to-cell and cell-free transmission of BFV.

Keywords: bovine foamy virus; infectious clone; particle release; cell-free transmission

1. Introduction

Foamy viruses (FVs), also known as spumaviruses, are a group of *Retroviridae* with unique features that differentiate them from orthoretroviruses. FVs infect humans [1,2] and other mammals, including bovines [3], simians [4], felines [5], and equines [6]. However, FV infection does not cause any clinical symptoms in its natural hosts, despite the significant cytopathic effect it causes in fibroblasts or fibroblast-derived cell lines as well as in epithelial cells, such as baby hamster kidney (BHK) cells [7,8].

Viruses have two major transmission strategies: cell-free transmission, involving the release of virus particles into the extracellular space, and cell-to-cell transmission [9–11]. Retroviruses exhibit different degrees of cell-free and cell-to-cell transmission. Unlike most other retroviruses, such as the human immunodeficiency virus (HIV) [12–16], murine leukemia virus (MLV), feline foamy virus (FFV), prototype foamy virus (PFV), and simian foamy virus (SFV), which transmit through both cell-to-cell and cell-free pathways, bovine foamy virus (BFV) infection is tightly cell-associated [17,18].

In contrast to other retroviruses, the envelope (Env) protein of PFV plays an important function in the budding and release of PFV particles [19]. In particular, the leader peptide (LP) in the N-terminal region of PFV Env is essential for virus budding. In LP, the three lysine residues (K14, K15, and K18) undergo ubiquitination, which regulates PFV release [20].

The Env protein determines FV's wide host range [1–6]. The cellular receptor of FVs has not been determined; however, it was reported that heparin sulfate might act as an attachment factor facilitating PFV and SFV entry [21,22]. Different from orthoretroviruses, the assembly and budding of FV particles require direct and specific interaction between the N-terminus of Gag and the Env leader protein Elp [23,24]. FV Gag, lacking the myristoylation membrane targeting signal, cannot produce cell-free Gag-only virus-like particles [18,24,25]. Instead, co-expression of FV Gag and Env leads to the generation of Env-dependent sub-viral particles (SVPs), which sets FVs apart from orthoretroviruses [23,24,26–28].

Bao and colleagues selected high-titer (HT) cell-free BFV-Riems isolates using the in vitro evolution procedure [18]. Yet, they did not generate infectious viral DNA clones and did not explore the molecular mechanisms that have enabled BFV cell-free transmission. Using the BFV strain BFV3026, which we isolated in 1996, we generated an infectious clone called pBS-BFV-B [29]. BFV-B is deficient in cell-free transmission, which does not allow for the development of a BFV vector. We have now screened for BFV variants with enhanced cell-free transmission in BICL cells (derived from BHK-21 cells) by serial virus passaging and successfully created a BFV infectious clone—called pBS-BFV-Z1—with cell-free transmission ability. Through sequence alignment and mutagenesis, we determined the C-terminal region of Env as one determinant for BFV cell-free transmission, and thus uncovered the molecular mechanism by which BFV spreads via cell-free transmission.

2. Materials and Methods

2.1. Cell Lines and Viruses

BHK-21, Cf2Th, HEK293T, BFVL (BHK21-derived indicator cells containing a *luciferase* gene under the control of the BFV LTR) [30], and BICL (BHK21-derived indicator cells containing an enhanced green fluorescent protein under the control of the BFV LTR) cells [31,32] were maintained in Dulbecco's modified Eagle's medium (Thermo Fisher, Waltham, MA, USA) containing 10% fetal bovine serum (GE Healthcare, Cincinnati, OH, USA) and 1% penicillin-streptomycin (Thermo Fisher, Waltham, MA, USA) at 37 °C in a 5% CO_2 atmosphere. BFV3026 was stored in our lab and cultured with Cf2Th and BICL cells. No mycoplasma and viruses contamination were detected in any cells we used.

2.2. Plasmids and Transfection

BFV3026 full-length genomic DNA clone pBS-BFV-B was generated by amplifying viral DNA extracted from BFV3026-infected Cf2Th cells. The BFV infectious clone pBS-BFV-Z1 was constructed using the same methods of pBS-BFV-B as previously reported [29]. Chimeric BFV clones between clone B and Z1 were generated by shared different restriction sites. Mutations were generated using site-direct PCR mutagenesis (Toyobo, Osaka, Japan), and all mutations were verified by DNA sequencing (Genewiz, Beijing, China). The plasmids expressing Env and Gag were constructed by inserting the coding sequences of BFV Env and Gag into the indicated vectors, including pCMV-3HA and pCE-puro-3Flag. HEK293T and BHK-21 cells were transfected using polyethylenimine (PEI) (Polysciences, Warrington, PA, USA) according to the manufacturer's protocol [33]. BHK-21 cells (2×10^5) were seeded in six-well plates. Twenty-four hours later, 2 µg empty vector pBS, pBS-BFV-B, pBS-BFV-Z1, or chimeric infectious clones were transfected into BHK-21 cells. Eight µL PEI (1 mg/mL) was added at DNA:PEI (µg:µg) ratios of 1:4 and incubated for 10 min at room temperature. Cells were harvested 48 h after transfection. Cf2Th cells were transfected using Lipofectamine 2000 (Thermo Fisher, Waltham, MA, USA).

2.3. Titration of Cell-Free BFV3026

BFV3026 was isolated from lymphocytes of peripheral blood of cattle by our lab in 1996 and cultured with Cf2Th cells. The parental cell-free BFV3026 virus was obtained by freezing-thawing highly infected Cf2Th cells. The later serial passage screening was carried in BICL cell lines. BFV was adapted to cell-free transmission in BICL cells by serial passaging using cell-free culture supernatants as previously reported [18]. In the case of viral infection, BICL cells expressed GFP and green signals were visible under a fluorescent microscope.

BFV cell-free titers were determined by infecting BICL indicator cells with gradient diluted BFV-containing supernatants. BICL cells were seeded (2×10^4 cells/well) in 48-well plates. Twenty-four hours later, BFV-containing supernatants were serially diluted 1:5 (triplicate for each dilution) and added to BICL cells. Six days post-infection, BFV titers were determined by fluorescence microscopy for GFP signals in BICL cells. If at least two of the three wells were positive for GFP, that dilution was considered positive for infection.

2.4. *Cell-Free Infection*

BHK-21 cells were transfected with indicated infectious clones for 2, 4, and 6 days. Then, cell culture supernatants were collected and filtered with a 0.45 μm membrane. BFVL cells in 12-well plates (2.5×10^5 cells/well) were then infected with equal volumes of these filtered supernatants for 48 h and subjected to luciferase assay. The infectivity of the cell-free virus was determined by luciferase activity.

2.5. *Cell Co-Culture Assay*

BHK-21 cells were transfected with indicated infectious clones for 2, 4, and 6 days. Then, the 5% of cells were harvested and co-cultured with 1.5×10^5 BFVL cells in 12-well plates. Forty-eight hours post co-culture, luciferase activity was measured to quantitate virus titer.

2.6. *Luciferase Reporter Assay*

Forty-eight hours after infection or co-culture, the BFVL cells were harvested in lysis buffer. Then, luciferase assays were performed using the luciferase reporter assay system (Promega, Madison, WI, USA). In addition to normalizing the luciferase activities, we also detected the GAPDH expression of cell lysates by western blotting. All of the results from the luciferase reporter assay were the averages of three independent experiments.

2.7. *Hirt DNA Extraction*

BICL cells infected with cell-free BFV p43 (passage 43) were harvested, washed with 1.5 mL 1× PBS, and lysed with 250 μL buffer K (20 mM HEPES, 140 mM KCl, 5 mM $MgCl_2$, 1 mM Dithiothreitol) and 7.5 μL 0.5% Triton X-100 for 10 min at room temperature. Following centrifugation (10 min at 1500× *g*), the pellet was dissolved in 400 μL TE and 90 μL 5 M NaCl at 4 °C overnight. The supernatant post centrifugation was extracted with phenol chloroform: isoamylalcohol (24:1), then precipitated for DNA in ethanol with 0.3 M NaAc at −20 °C for 1 h. The purified DNA was then washed with 70% ethanol, dissolved in 20 μL TE, and stored at −20 °C.

2.8. *Enrichment of Wt and Sub-Viral BFV Particles*

Six milliliters of cell culture supernatants containing BFV particles or SVPs (including Env-only and Gag-Env SVPs) were filtered through 0.45 μm membranes and layered on a 1 mL cushion of 20% sucrose in PBS (*w*/*v*). After ultracentrifugation (Optima LE-80K, Beckman Coulter) at 4 °C for 1.5 h at 210,053× *g*, the non-visible pellet was re-suspended in 30 μL loading buffer containing 2% SDS and subjected to western blotting.

2.9. *Co-Immunoprecipitation*

HEK293T cells transfected with pCMV-3HA-Gag and pCMV-3HA-Env were lysed in lysis buffer (50 mM Tris, pH 7.4; 150 mM NaCl; 2 mM EDTA; 3% Glycerol; 1% NP-40; complete, EDTA-free protease inhibitor cocktail tablets). The cell lysates were sonicated and centrifuged at 13,000× *g* for 10 min at 4 °C. Following centrifugation, supernatants were incubated with mouse anti-Gag antibody for 2 h at 4 °C and rotated with Protein A-agarose (Merck Millipore, Darmstadt, Germany) for 3 h or overnight at 4 °C. After six washes with lysis buffer, the immunoprecipitated materials were boiled in 40 μL of 2× SDS loading buffer and subjected to western blotting using rabbit anti-HA antibody.

2.10. *Immunofluorescent Assay*

BHK-21 cells seeded in 12-well plates containing coverslips were infected with infectious clones. After 48 h, BHK-21 cells were fixed with 500 μL of 4% formaldehyde in PBS for 10 min on a shaker. Cell membranes were permeabilized with 500 μL of penetration solution (0.1% Triton X-100 in 4% formaldehyde) for 10 min. Then, cells were blocked in 500 μL of blocking solution (50% serum, 6% non-fat milk power, 15% BSA, 5% NaN_3, 20% Triton in PBS) for 2 h at room temperature or 4 °C overnight. Cells were then incubated in diluted primary antibody for 2 h at room temperature. The coverslips were washed in the 12-well plates with PBST and incubated in diluted fluorochrome-conjugated secondary antibody for 40 min in the dark. After 5 washes, cells were incubated in 500 μL of DAPI for 10 min in the dark. The coverslips were mounted onto glass slides and allowed to air dry for 1 h. For long-term storage, slides were stored flat at 4 °C protected from light.

2.11. *Western Blotting*

Proteins were separated by SDS-PAGE (polyacrylamide gel electrophoresis). Then, the separated proteins were transferred onto a polyvinylidene difluoride (PVDF) membrane (GE Healthcare, Cincinnati, OH, USA) by electroblotting for 1 h at 100 V in 4 °C. Following incubation in PBS containing 5% nonfat milk for 45 min at room temperature, the PVDF membranes were subsequently incubated with primary antibody for 90 min. Then, the membranes were incubated with secondary antibodies—goat anti-mouse or goat anti-rabbit IgG conjugated to horseradish peroxidase, for an additional 45 min. Protein bands were detected by chemiluminescence (Merck Millipore, Darmstadt, Germany).

2.12. *Statistical Analysis*

Data were expressed as the mean ± SD of the results of three independent experiments in which each assay was performed in triplicate. Data were compared using the unpaired two-tailed t test. A p value of <0.05 was considered significant (* $p < 0.05$, ** $p < 0.01$, *** $p < 0.001$, **** $p < 0.0001$).

3. Results

3.1. *Construction of a Cell-Free BFV Infectious Clone pBS-BFV-Z1*

To isolate a high-titer cell-free BFV stain, we performed in vitro evolution experiments in BICL cells, which express GFP upon BFV infection. The original virus strain used for selection was Cf2Th-associated BFV3026, which was isolated in China. After 53 passages, the cell-free infectivity of BFV reached a plateau of 10^5 IU/mL (Figure 1A). The full-length viral genomic DNA was amplified from the hirt DNA extracted from BICL cells infected with cell-free BFV (passage 43) and then inserted into the pBluescript SK-(pBS) vector. The constructed infectious viral DNA clone was named pBS-BFV-Z1.

We next characterized the pBS-BFV-Z1 clone for its ability to produce infectious cell-free particles by harvesting viruses in the supernatants of BHK-21 cells that were transfected with BFV infectious clones. As shown in Figure 1B, the BFV particle release was observed in Z1-transfected cells but not in cells transfected with the cell-associated clone, pBS-BFV-B. At the same time, we also analyzed the intracellular Gag expression levels and observed that Gag expression in BFV-B was less than BFV-Z1 (Figure 1B). Furthermore, we observed that the replication capacity of the Z1 clone was 40 times greater than that of the B clone, as measured by co-culture assay (Figure 1C). Notably, the cell-free Z1 virus particles were infectious (Figure 1C) and spread in a long-term infection (Figure 1D). Together, these data demonstrate that the pBS-BFV-Z1 clone is highly infectious and produces infectious cell-free virus particles.

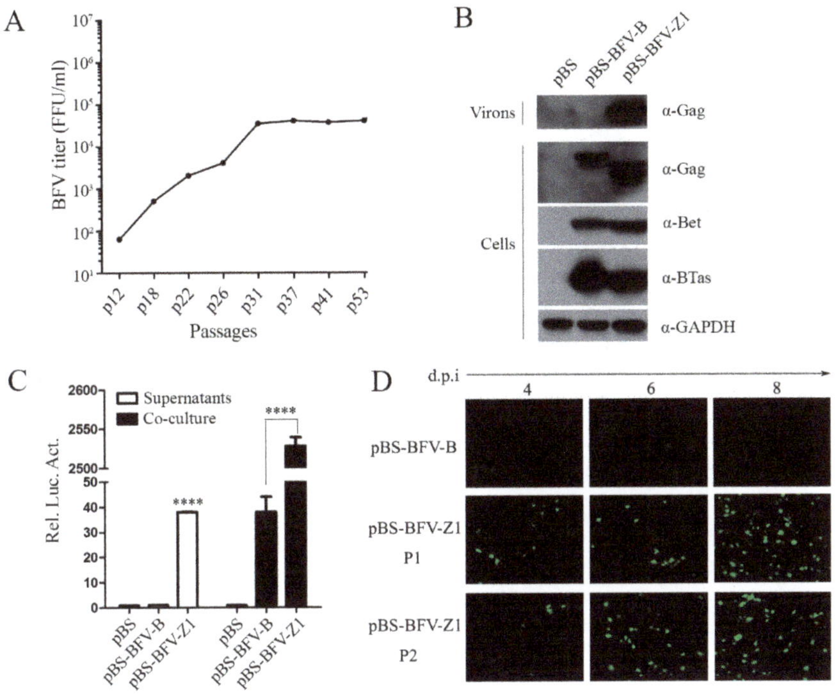

Figure 1. The cell-free and cell-to-cell transmission activity of BFV-Z1. (**A**) Screen of the high-titer cell-free bovine foamy virus (BFV) strain in BICL cells with cleared supernatants. Around 53 passages, BFV cell-free titers were determined by gradient dilution. BICL cells were seeded in 48-well plates (2×10^4 cells/well), then BFV-containing supernatants were serially diluted 1:5 in the plate (triplication for each dilution). Four to six days post-infection, the cell-free BFV titers were calculate and analyzed, as determined by fluorescence microscopy for GFP signals in BICL cells. (**B–C**) BHK-21 (baby hamster kidney) cells (2×10^5) were seeded in 6-well plates. After 24 h, 2 µg empty vector pBS, pBS-BFV-B, or pBS-BFV-Z1 were transfected into BHK-21 cells. Four days later, 5% cells co-cultured with 1.5×10^5 BFVL cells and part of supernatants infected 2.5×10^5 BFVL cells, respectively, for cell-to-cell and cell-free transmission activity using a luciferase activity assay after 48 h, and the results were the averages of three independent experiments and data were analyzed using GraphPad Prism software (compared with BFV-B, * $p < 0.05$, ** $p < 0.01$, *** $p < 0.001$, **** $p < 0.0001$). The remainder of the supernatants and cells transfected for 2 days were harvested for western blot with the indicated antibodies (B). (**D**) Part of the supernatants were collected to infect fresh BICL cells (marked P1) prior to ultracentrifugation, and the expression of GFP was observed. If more than 80% BICL cells were positive for green fluorescence, then the supernatants were collected and cleared to infect fresh BICL cells (marked P2).

3.2. The C Terminus of Env Determines the Ability of BFV to Generate Infectious Cell-Free Particles

To identify which regions in the sequence of pBS-BFV-Z1 changed and enabled the production of infectious cell-free virus particles, we aligned the sequences of the two BFV clones, B and Z1. Changes were identified at multiple nucleotide positions (Tables S1 and S2). We then swapped the sequences between the B and Z1 clones and generated six chimeric BFV clones (*Eco*R I within *pol* gene, and *Nde* I within *env*) (Figure 2A). As shown in Figure 2, clone S1S2 and clone Z1 produced similar levels of intracellular Gag (Figure 2B) as well as comparable cell-to-cell transmission activity (Figure 2D). Unfortunately, none of these chimeric clones produced infectious cell-free BFV particles (Figure 2C). Notably, the expression of Gag in BFV-B could be detected for two days (Figure 1B) but not for four days that was passaged one time with a low ratio of transfected cells (Figure 2B). One possibility is that the activity of clone B is much weaker than clone Z1 (Figure 1C).

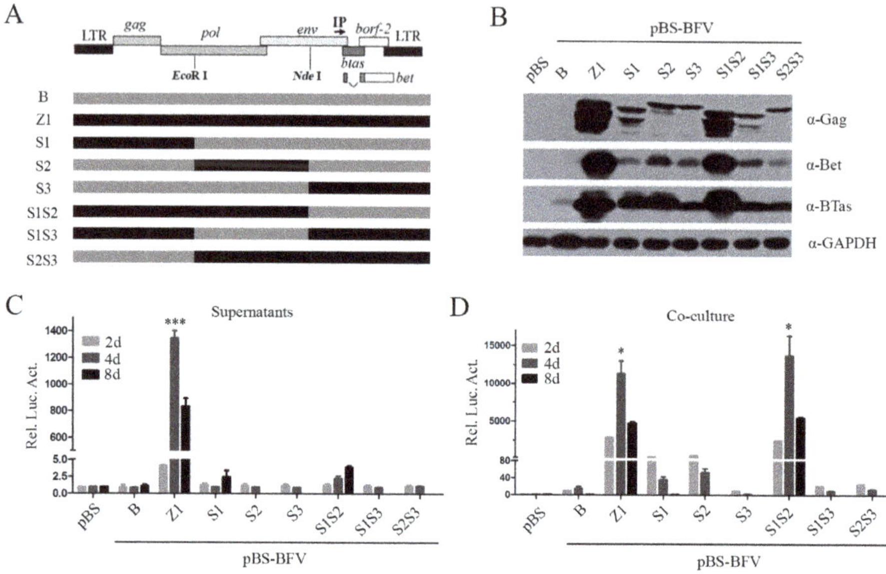

Figure 2. Activities of chimeric BFV infectious clones between pBS-BFV-B and pBS-BFV-Z1. (**A**) The structure model of BFV proviral genome is shown on the top, followed with a schematic overview of the chimeric virus between BFV-B and BFV-Z1. The gray box represents the BFV3026 proviral genomic DNA of pBS-BFV-B, and the black box represents pBS-BFV-Z1. The full-length viral DNA was divided into three segments based on the single restriction enzyme sites of *Eco*R I and *Nde* I, and the new chimeric clones were generated by exchanging the fragments between pBS-BFV-B and pBS-BFV-Z1 plasmids. (**B–D**) BHK-21 (2×10^5) cells were transfected with 2 μg empty vector pBS, pBS-BFV-B, pBS-BFV-Z1, or chimeric infectious clones as indicated for 2, 4, or 8 days. Cells transfected for 4 days were subjected to western blotting with indicated antibodies (**B**). The activity of cell-free and cell-to-cell transmission was measured by a luciferase activity assay at the indicated times (**C**,**D**), and the data were the averages of three independent experiments. Compared with BFV-B, * $p < 0.05$, ** $p < 0.01$, *** $p < 0.001$, **** $p < 0.0001$.

Previous studies have shown that Env protein is essential for PFV release and entry [26,34,35]. Clone S1S2 contains a chimeric *env* gene, including the N terminus of EnvZ1 and the C terminus of EnvB, but lacks cell-free transmission ability. To test the role of Env in the ability of the Z1 clone to produce infectious cell-free virus particles, we engineered another two chimeric clones, Z1(1–9554) and Z1(EnvcB). Clone Z1(1–9554) contained an entire *env* gene from clone Z1, whereas clone Z1(EnvcB) had the clone Z1 sequence except for the C-terminal region of Env, which was derived from clone B (Figure 3A). The intracellular Gag expression from Z1(1–9554) and Z1(EnvcB) was similar to that from clones Z1 and S1S2 (Figure 3B). Excitingly, the Z1(1-9554) clone produced high levels of infectious cell-free virus particles, although still two to three-fold lower than the parental clone Z (Figure 3C). In contrast, the cell-to-cell transmission of Z1(EnvcB) was two-fold more efficient than that of clone Z1, as measured by co-culture assay (Figure 3D). However, compared with clone Z1, chimera Z1(EnvcB) was unable to transmit by cell-free particles, which suggests that replacement of the C-terminal

Env with that from clone B abrogated the cell-free infectivity of clone Z1 (Figure 3C). Furthermore, Z1(1–9554) exhibited cell-free transmission activity, although to a lesser degree than Z1 (Figure 3C). Overall, these results indicate that the C-terminus of Env is crucial for BFV cell-free infectivity.

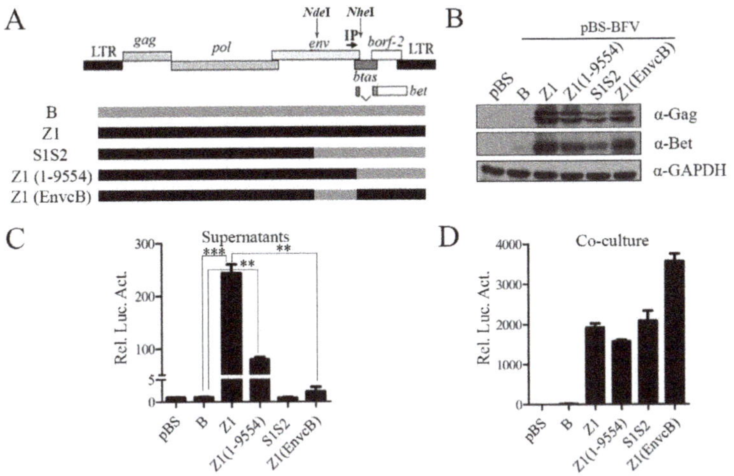

Figure 3. The C terminus of Env determines the ability of BFV to generate infectious cell-free particles. (**A**) We constructed clone BFV-Z1(1-9554) by the single restriction enzyme sites of *Nhe* I, which cuts downstream of Env in the BFV proviral genome, and clone BFV-Z1(EnvcB) was constructed by *Nde* I and *Nhe* I. The gray box represents the BFV3026 proviral genomic DNA of pBS-BFV-B, and the black box represents pBS-BFV-Z1. (**B–D**) BHK-21 cells (2×10^5) were transfected with 2 μg empty vector pBS, pBS-BFV-B, pBS-BFV-Z1, pBS-BFV-Z1(1-9554), pBS-BFV-S1S2, or pBS-BFV-Z1(EnvcB) for 4 days, and cells were subjected to western blotting with indicated antibodies (**B**). The cell-free and cell-to-cell transmission activity was measured with the indicated assays (**C**,**D**), and the data were the averages of three independent experiments.

To identify the specific sites that affect the cell-free transmission ability of clone Z1, we compared the amino acid sequence of the C-terminal region of Env between clone Z1 and clone B and found differences at five sites: H816Y, P823S, E898K, R976K, and L978S (Figure 4A), which are all located in the C-terminus of transmembrane (TM) protein gp48 (aa 572–990). Using chimera S1S2 that bears the C-terminal region of the clone B Env, we mutated the amino acids at the above five positions to the counterparts in clone Z1. Our results showed that two single point mutations—H816Y and E898K, especially E898K—rendered clone S1S2 to produce infectious cell-free virus particles. Furthermore, the cell-free infectivity of clone S1S2-898/976/978, which had the amino acids at position 898, 976, and 978 of Z1 Env, was similar to that of Z1(1–9554) (Figure 4B). We also mutated the above five positions in clone Z1 Env to the respective amino residues in clone B Env. The K898E mutation markedly impaired the cell-free infectivity of Z1, and mutations Y816H and K898E together abrogated the cell-free infectivity of Z1 (Figure 4D). These results indicate that amino acid K898 together with Y816 in the Env protein are major determinants of BFV cell-free transmission.

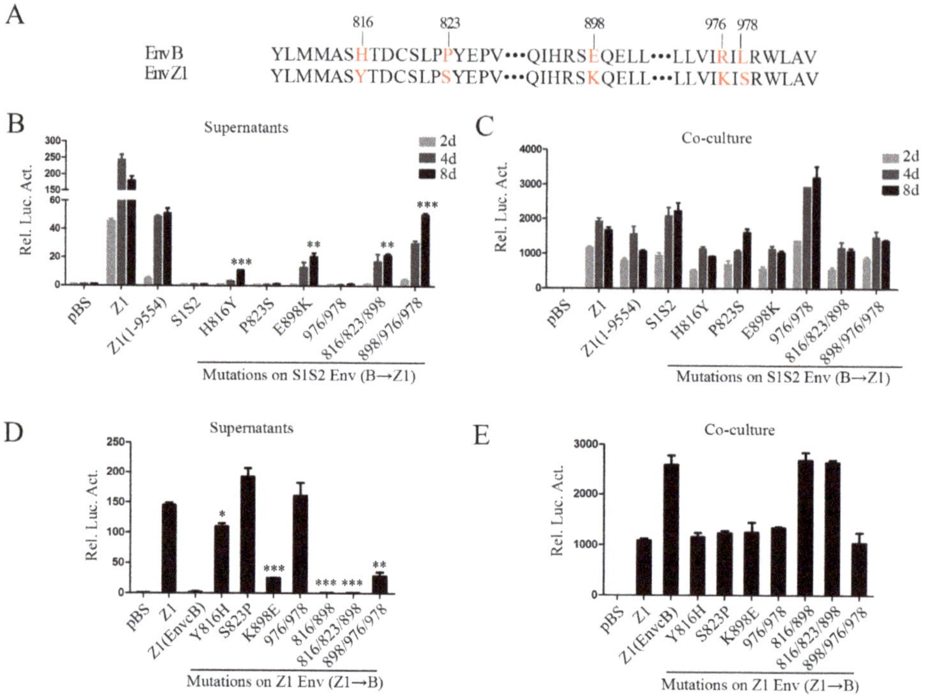

Figure 4. K898 in the *env* gene of BFV-Z1 is crucial for BFV cell-free transmission. (**A**) Amino acid site mutations, marked in red, in the C terminus of Env by sequence alignment analyses are shown. (**B**,**C**) Construction of infectious clones with point mutations on the basis of pBS-BFV-S1S2 from B to Z1 and their transfection to BHK-21 cells. The transmission activity was analyzed by measuring luciferase activity, and the data were the averages of three independent experiments. Compared with BFV-S1S2, * $p < 0.05$, ** $p < 0.01$, *** $p < 0.001$, **** $p < 0.0001$. (**D**,**E**) Construction of clones with point mutations based on pBS-BFV-Z1 from Z1 to B. Then, these were transfected into BHK-21 cells and the transmission activity was analyzed. Compared with BFV-Z1, * $p < 0.05$, ** $p < 0.01$, *** $p < 0.001$, **** $p < 0.0001$. "•" stands for omission.

3.3. The 14-AA Deletion in Gag Gene Increases BFV Cell-Free Transmission Activity

Gag plays an indispensable role in the assembly and release of PFV particles. We found that Gag of the Z1 clone is 14 aa shorter than Gag of the B clone (Figure 5A). We tested whether this 14-aa deletion had an effect on BFV cell-free transmission by constructing two chimeric clones, Z1(Gag60) and Z1(1-9554; Gag60), which had the 14 aa inserted back in clones Z1 and Z1(1-9554). BICL cells were transfected with the above BFV clones and observed similar levels of Gag expression from all viral DNA clones (Figure 5B). However, the cell-free infectivity of Z1(Gag60) was four- to five-fold lower than that of Z1 (Figure 5C), although the cell-to-cell transmission activities of these two clones were comparable (Figure 5D). We further observed that Gag-B, Gag-Z1, and Gag60 were similarly distributed in the cytoplasm, suggesting that this 14-aa sequence does not affect the cellular localization of Gag (Figure 5E).

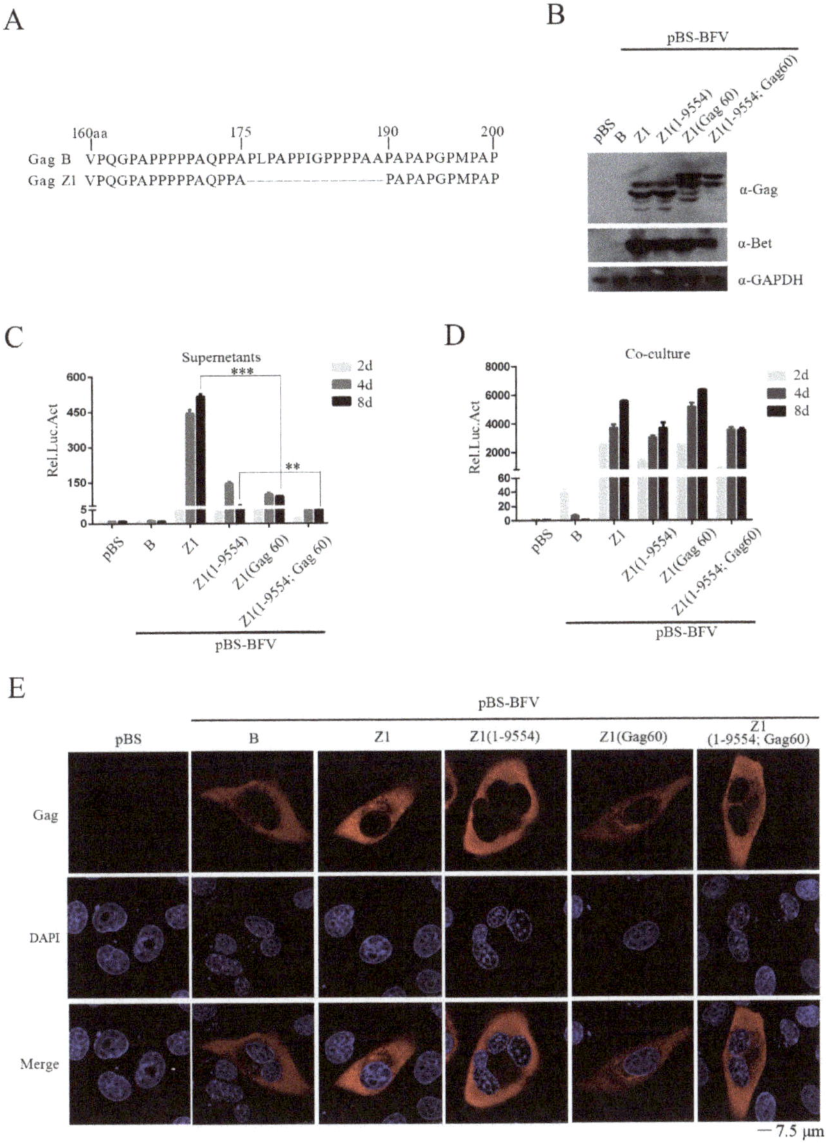

Figure 5. The 14 aa deletion in *gag* gene increases BFV cell-free transmission activity. (**A**) Partial results—sequence alignment of amino acids in Gag-B and Gag-Z1 is shown in the top left corner. Starting with the 176th amino acid, 14 consecutive amino acids are missing in Gag-Z1. (**B**) BHK-21 cells were transfected with empty vector pBS, pBS-BFV-B, pBS-BFV-Z1, pBS-BFV-Z1(1-9554), pBS-BFV-Z1(Gag60), or pBS-BFV-Z1(1-9554; Gag60), and partial lysates of cells after 4 d of transfection were tested by western blotting analysis. (**C**,**D**) The cell-free and cell-to-cell transmission activity was detected separately at the indicated transfection time, and the data were the averages of three independent experiments. (**E**) BHK-21 cells were transfected with indicated infectious clones, then subjected to immunofluorescent assays. Confocal microscopy was adopted for observation and image capture. "-" stands for missing.

Unlike orthoretroviruses, the release of FV virions requires both Gag and Env proteins [36]. FV can form Gag-Env SVPs or Env-only SVPs [26,34,37]. We therefore examined the ability of Env-B and Env-Z1 to mediate SVPs release. Different *env* and *gag* genes were cloned into the pCMV-3HA or the pCE-puro-3Flag vector. Gag plasmids alone or together with different Env plasmids were transfected into HEK293T cells. Two days post-transfection, virus particles in the culture supernatants were harvested through ultracentrifugation and analyzed by western blotting. As shown in Figure 6A, SVPs were detected when Gag was expressed together with Env but not when Gag was expressed alone. Similar levels of SVPs were produced by Env and Gag from both clone B and clone Z1. However, Env-Z1, but not Env-B, was completely processed in virus particles.

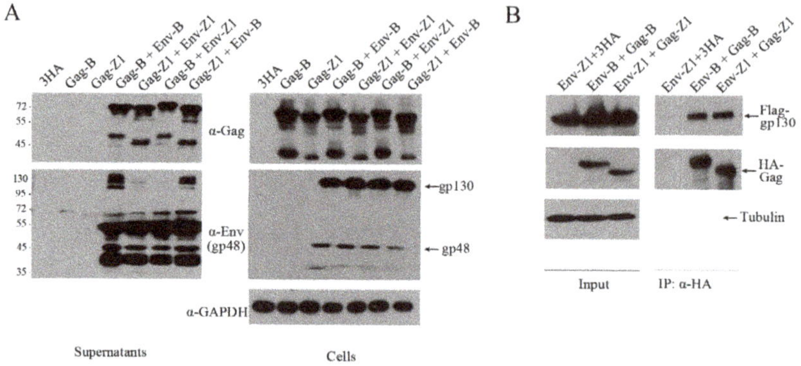

Figure 6. The interaction between Gag and Env. (**A**) HEK293T (4×10^6) cells were transfected with different eukaryotic expression plasmids, 3HA-Gag and 3HA-Env, for 2 days. Cells and supernatants were harvested separately, and the cell culture supernatants were cleared by ultracentrifugation following filtration with a 0.45 μm membrane. Levels of Gag and Env in cells and supernatants were measured by western blotting. (**B**) Immunoprecipitation (with anti-HA) and immunoblot (with anti-HA and anti-Flag) of HEK293T (4×10^6) cells co-transfected with the same source of eukaryotic expression plasmids encoding 3HA-Gag and 3Flag-Env.

Next, co-immunoprecipitation (Co-IP) assays were performed to measure the interaction between Env and Gag. 3Flag-Env and 3HA-Gag were co-transfected into HEK293T cells followed by IP with anti-HA antibody. The results of western blots showed similar levels of interaction between Env and Gag of both the B and Z1 clones (Figure 6B). Taken together, the 14-amino acid sequence that is missing in the Z1 Gag contributes to the increased cell-free transmission of clone Z1, but this activity is not a result of greater ability of assembling SVPs nor interacting with Env.

3.4. *The C-Terminal Region of Env Modulates the Entry of Cell-Free BFV Particles But Does Not Affect Virus Release*

We showed that chimeric clone Z1(EnvcB), which contains the C-terminus of Env-B, is defective in cell-free transmission (Figure 3C). To further understand the underlying causes, we examined the ability of EnvcB in mediating the assembly and release of Gag-Env particles. The results showed similar levels of SVPs that were produced with either EnvcB, Env-Z1 or Env-B together with Gag (Figure 7A). In addition, all three Env proteins formed Env-only SVPs (Figure 7A), which is consistent with the previous reports [26,34,37]. We also observed that there were more uncleaved gp130 in Env-B-containing SVPs that were produced with Gag-Env and Env alone compared to Env-Z1 SVPs and EnvcB SVPs, which suggests that this C-terminal region of Env affects Env protein processing.

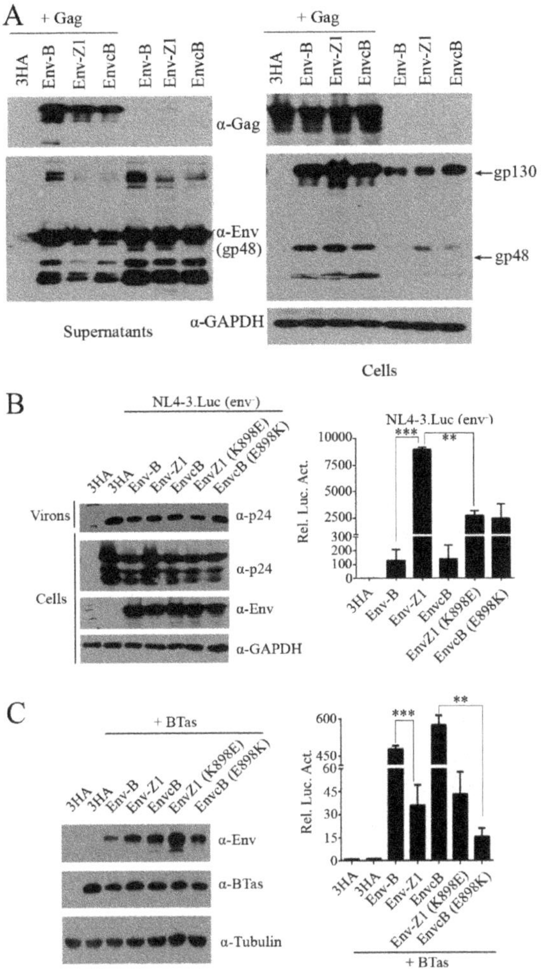

Figure 7. The C-terminal region of Env modulates the entry of cell-free BFV particles but does not affect virus release. (**A**) Immunoblot analysis of Gag and Env in HEK293T cells co-transfected with the indicated plasmids for 48 h and viral particles in supernatants. (**B**) Immunoblot analysis of HEK293T cells transfected with different HA-Env and NL4-3.luc (env⁻). Luciferase reporter assays to analyze the infectivity of viral particles in supernatant, and the data were the averages of three independent experiments. (**C**) Immunoblot analysis of HEK293T cells transfected for 48 h with plasmids encoding different Env and BTas, and luciferase reporter assays to analyze the membrane fusion ability mediated by different Env. The data were the averages of three independent experiments.

To determine whether the defective processing of BFV Env diminishes Env entry function, we used BFV Env proteins to pseudotype HIV-1(env-) viruses and measured virus infectivity. BFV Env proteins were co-expressed with HIV-1 DNA clone NL4-3.Luc.env-, which harbors a luciferase reporter gene and does not express HIV-1 Env. The culture supernatants containing BFV Env-pseudotyped HIV-1 particles were used to infect Cf2Th cells. Luciferase expression in Cf2Th cells reflects virus entry mediated by BFV Env proteins. The results showed that both Env-B and EnvcB were able to mediate HIV-1 entry, but the efficiency was 85-fold lower than Env-Z1. Furthermore, the K898E mutation reduced the entry efficiency of Env-Z1, which is in agreement with the increased entry of EnvcB harboring the E898K mutation (Figure 7B). We also tested the efficiency of these Env proteins in mediating cell-cell fusion. HEK293T cells were co-transfected with BTas DNA and different Env DNA and then co-cultured with the BFVL indicator cells. Env-mediated fusion of 293T and BFVL cells allows BTas to activate the expression luciferase reporter gene in BFVL cells. These results showed that EnvcB and EnvB led to much higher cell fusion than EnvZ1 (Figure 7C). The E898K mutation impaired the ability of EnvcB to mediate cell fusion (Figure 7C). Together, these data suggest that the C-terminal region of Env affects Env processing and therefore has a key role in the function of Env to mediate virus-cell or cell-cell fusion.

4. Discussion

In this study, we generated high-titer cell-free BFV variants by serial virus passaging in vitro and further constructed a cell-free infectious clone, pBS-BFV-Z1. We also identified the viral genes and key amino acids that regulate BFV cell-free transmission. In particular, we found that the C-terminal region of Env, especially the K898 residue, is essential for BFV cell-free transmission activity.

It is known that BFV is highly cell-associated and spreads mainly through cell-to-cell transmission [17,18]. Although FFV, SFV, and PFV can transmit by both cell-to-cell and cell-free pathways, the sequence similarity between BFV and other FVs (FFV, SFV, and PFV) is low, and it is thus difficult to identify the viral genetic determinants through sequence alignment. We thus performed in vitro evolution to generate high-titer cell-free BFV variants. There are two factors that influence cell-free transmission, the number and the infectivity of the released virions [9,10]. Using the two distinct isolates, BFV-B and BFV-Z1, we detected Env-dependent production of BFV Gag-Env SVPs and demonstrated that Env-B was as efficient as Env-Z1 and EnvcB in mediating SVPs release (Figure 7A). However, Env-B was not completely processed in virus particles when compared with Env-Z1. It is reported that all known FV Env proteins contain a conserved optimal cleavage site RX(K/R)R between the SU and TM subunits and processing of SU/TM does not affect the egress of viral particles but is essential for the infectivity of the released virus particles [26,38,39]. Indeed, Env-Z1 was 85-fold more efficient than EnvcB and EnvB in mediating cell-free virus entry (Figure 7B). Our study demonstrates that the C-terminal sequence of Env regulates BFV cell-free entry efficiency rather than virion release capacity.

BFV Env is essential for virus budding, release, entry, and membrane fusion [18,19]. Compared with BFV-B, there are a few mutations in BFV-Z1 Env (eight changes among 990 residues), including three mutations in the N-terminus and five in the C-terminus. Previous reports state that the ubiquitination of three lysine sites in the N-terminal cytoplasmic tail region of PFV Env protein increases virus infectivity and decreases the production of SVPs [20]. In our study, the four N-terminal mutations (D42N, V55I, and P134H) did not change cell-free virus infectivity (Figure 3C). In contrast, the C-terminal mutations H816Y, P823S, E898K, R976K, and L978S, especially the E898K mutation, enhance cell-free transmission (Figure 4B,D). It is well-known that lysine (K) can undergo methylation, acetylation, succinylation, ubiquitination, and other modifications, which play an important role in regulating the protein activity and structure adjustment. Interestingly, we found that the equivalent position of the 898 residue in four currently described BFV isolates from the United States (GenBank accession number NC001831.1) [40], China (accession number AY134750.1) [41], Poland (accession number JX307861) [42,43], and Germany (accession number JX307862) [43], which spread only through cell-to-cell, is not a lysine (K). Nevertheless, the equivalent position is occupied by a lysine in other high titer cell-free strains, such as SFV and PFV. These suggest that the K898 in Env has an important role in FV cell-free transmission. The underlying mechanism warrants further study.

The Gag protein of BFV-Z1 lost a 14-amino acid sequence compared to BFV-B. This 14-residue deletion led to a smaller Gag-Z1, as shown by the results of western blotting (Figure 5B). Interestingly, Gag-Z1 enhanced cell-free infectivity by four- to five-fold (Figure 5C). Similar deletions have also been reported in other high titer cell-free BFV strains, although there is differing in the number of missing amino acids and their locations (Professor Martin Löchelt's unpublished data). It is known that the

Gag-Env interaction is very important for the budding and release of BFV virions. Yet, in our study, the interaction of Gag and Env in BFV-B and BFV-Z1 was almost the same, which suggests that the contribution of Gag-Z1 to enhanced cell-free transmission is not through promoting interaction with Env. The other changes of the BFV-Z1 genome contributed little to BFV cell-free transmission.

In summary, we demonstrated that the C-terminus of Env, especially the K898 residue, is critical for BFV cell-free transmission. This function of Env C-terminal sequence results from promoting BFV cell-free entry efficiency rather than viral particle release capacity. Our study thus suggests the possibility of generating high-titer BFV vectors through engineering viral Env—in particular, the C-terminal sequence.

Supplementary Materials: The following are available online at http://www.mdpi.com/1999-4915/11/2/130/s1, Table S1: The mutation amino acid (aa) sites in coding region of Cell-free BFV; Table S2: The mutation sites in noncoding region of Cell-free BFV.

Author Contributions: Conceptualization, S.Z., X.L., J.T.; Methodology, S.Z., X.L.; Formal Analysis, S.Z., X.L., J.T.; Resources, Z.L., T.B.; Writing-Original Draft Preparation, S.Z., X.L., Z.L.; Writing-Review & Editing, W.Q., J.T.; Supervision, W.Q., J.T.; Project Administration, W.Q., J.T.; Funding Acquisition, J.T.

Funding: This work was supported by grants from the National Natural Science Foundation of China (31670151).

Acknowledgments: We thank Martin Löchelt (German Cancer Research Center) for his generous sharing of screening basis for high-titer cell-free BFV strain. We also thank Chen Liang (McGill University, Canada) for the critical reading of the manuscript.

Conflicts of Interest: The authors declare no conflict of interest.

References

1. Achong, B.G.; Mansell, P.W.; Epstein, M.A.; Clifford, P. An unusual virus in cultures from a human nasopharyngeal carcinoma. *J. Natl. Cancer Inst.* **1971**, *46*, 299–307. [PubMed]
2. Switzer, W.M.; Bhullar, V.; Shanmugam, V.; Cong, M.E.; Parekh, B.; Lerche, N.W.; Yee, J.L.; Ely, J.J.; Boneva, R.; Chapman, L.E.; et al. Frequent simian foamy virus infection in persons occupationally exposed to nonhuman primates. *J. Virol.* **2004**, *78*, 2780–2789. [CrossRef] [PubMed]
3. Johnson, R.H.; Oginnusi, A.A.; Ladds, P.W. Isolations and serology of bovine spumavirus. *Aust. Vet. J.* **1983**, *60*, 147. [CrossRef] [PubMed]
4. Broussard, S.R.; Comuzzie, A.G.; Leighton, K.L.; Leland, M.M.; Whitehead, E.M.; Allan, J.S. Characterization of new simian foamy viruses from african nonhuman primates. *Virology* **1997**, *237*, 349–359. [CrossRef] [PubMed]
5. Mochizuki, M.; Akuzawa, M.; Nagatomo, H. Serological survey of the iriomote cat (felis iriomotensis) in Japan. *J. Wildl. Dis.* **1990**, *26*, 236–245. [CrossRef]
6. Tobaly-Tapiero, J.; Bittoun, P.; Neves, M.; Guillemin, M.C.; Lecellier, C.H.; Puvion-Dutilleul, F.; Gicquel, B.; Zientara, S.; Giron, M.L.; de The, H.; et al. Isolation and characterization of an equine foamy virus. *J. Virol.* **2000**, *74*, 4064–4073. [CrossRef]
7. Linial, M. Why aren't foamy viruses pathogenic? *Trends Microbiol.* **2000**, *8*, 284–289. [CrossRef]
8. Rethwilm, A. Molecular biology of foamy viruses. *Med. Microbiol. Immunol.* **2010**, *199*, 197–207. [CrossRef]
9. Zhong, P.; Agosto, L.M.; Munro, J.B.; Mothes, W. Cell-to-cell transmission of viruses. *Curr. Opin. Virol.* **2013**, *3*, 44–50. [CrossRef]
10. Johnson, D.C.; Huber, M.T. Directed egress of animal viruses promotes cell-to-cell spread. *J. Virol.* **2002**, *76*, 1–8. [CrossRef]
11. Sattentau, Q. Avoiding the void: Cell-to-cell spread of human viruses. *Nat. Rev. Microbiol.* **2008**, *6*, 815–826. [CrossRef] [PubMed]
12. Jolly, C.; Mitar, I.; Sattentau, Q.J. Requirement for an intact t-cell actin and tubulin cytoskeleton for efficient assembly and spread of human immunodeficiency virus type 1. *J. Virol* **2007**, *81*, 5547–5560. [CrossRef] [PubMed]
13. Agosto, L.M.; Uchil, P.D.; Mothes, W. Hiv cell-to-cell transmission: Effects on pathogenesis and antiretroviral therapy. *Trends Microbiol.* **2015**, *23*, 289–295. [CrossRef] [PubMed]

14. Mazurov, D.; Ilinskaya, A.; Heidecker, G.; Lloyd, P.; Derse, D. Quantitative comparison of htlv-1 and hiv-1 cell-to-cell infection with new replication dependent vectors. *PLoS Pathog.* **2010**, *6*, e1000788. [CrossRef] [PubMed]
15. Martin, N.; Sattentau, Q. Cell-to-cell HIV-1 spread and its implications for immune evasion. *Curr. Opin. HIV AIDS* **2009**, *4*, 143–149. [CrossRef] [PubMed]
16. Talbert-Slagle, K.; Atkins, K.E.; Yan, K.K.; Khurana, E.; Gerstein, M.; Bradley, E.H.; Berg, D.; Galvani, A.P.; Townsend, J.P. Cellular superspreaders: An epidemiological perspective on hiv infection inside the body. *PLoS Pathog.* **2014**, *10*, e1004092. [CrossRef] [PubMed]
17. Liebermann, H.; Riebe, R. Isolation of bovine syncytial virus in east germany. *Arch. Exp. Veterinarmed.* **1981**, *35*, 917–919. [PubMed]
18. Bao, Q.; Hipp, M.; Hugo, A.; Lei, J.; Liu, Y.; Kehl, T.; Hechler, T.; Lochelt, M. In vitro evolution of bovine foamy virus variants with enhanced cell-free virus titers and transmission. *Viruses* **2015**, *7*, 5855–5874. [CrossRef] [PubMed]
19. Lindemann, D.; Pietschmann, T.; Picard-Maureau, M.; Berg, A.; Heinkelein, M.; Thurow, J.; Knaus, P.; Zentgraf, H.; Rethwilm, A. A particle-associated glycoprotein signal peptide essential for virus maturation and infectivity. *J. Virol.* **2001**, *75*, 5762–5771. [CrossRef] [PubMed]
20. Stanke, N.; Stange, A.; Luftenegger, D.; Zentgraf, H.; Lindemann, D. Ubiquitination of the prototype foamy virus envelope glycoprotein leader peptide regulates subviral particle release. *J. Virol.* **2005**, *79*, 15074–15083. [CrossRef] [PubMed]
21. Plochmann, K.; Horn, A.; Gschmack, E.; Armbruster, N.; Krieg, J.; Wiktorowicz, T.; Weber, C.; Stirnnagel, K.; Lindemann, D.; Rethwilm, A.; et al. Heparan sulfate is an attachment factor for foamy virus entry. *J. Virol.* **2012**, *86*, 10028–10035. [CrossRef] [PubMed]
22. Nasimuzzaman, M.; Persons, D.A. Cell membrane-associated heparan sulfate is a receptor for prototype foamy virus in human, monkey, and rodent cells. *Mol. Ther.* **2012**, *20*, 1158–1166. [CrossRef] [PubMed]
23. Wilk, T.; Geiselhart, V.; Frech, M.; Fuller, S.D.; Flugel, R.M.; Lochelt, M. Specific interaction of a novel foamy virus env leader protein with the n-terminal gag domain. *J. Virol.* **2001**, *75*, 7995–8007. [CrossRef] [PubMed]
24. Pietschmann, T.; Heinkelein, M.; Heldmann, M.; Zentgraf, H.; Rethwilm, A.; Lindemann, D. Foamy virus capsids require the cognate envelope protein for particle export. *J. Virol.* **1999**, *73*, 2613–2621. [PubMed]
25. Liu, Y.; Kim, Y.B.; Lochelt, M. N-terminally myristoylated feline foamy virus gag allows env-independent budding of sub-viral particles. *Viruses* **2011**, *3*, 2223–2237. [CrossRef]
26. Hutter, S.; Zurnic, I.; Lindemann, D. Foamy virus budding and release. *Viruses* **2013**, *5*, 1075–1098. [CrossRef] [PubMed]
27. Fischer, N.; Heinkelein, M.; Lindemann, D.; Enssle, J.; Baum, C.; Werder, E.; Zentgraf, H.; Muller, J.G.; Rethwilm, A. Foamy virus particle formation. *J. Virol.* **1998**, *72*, 1610–1615.
28. Geiselhart, V.; Schwantes, A.; Bastone, P.; Frech, M.; Lochelt, M. Features of the env leader protein and the N-terminal gag domain of feline foamy virus important for virus morphogenesis. *Virology* **2003**, *310*, 235–244. [CrossRef]
29. Bing, T.; Yu, H.; Li, Y.; Sun, L.; Tan, J.; Geng, Y.; Qiao, W. Characterization of a full-length infectious clone of bovine foamy virus 3026. *Virol. Sin.* **2014**, *29*, 94–102. [CrossRef]
30. Guo, H.Y.; Liang, Z.B.; Li, Y.; Tan, J.; Chen, Q.M.; Qiao, W.T. A new indicator cell line established to monitor bovine foamy virus infection. *Virol. Sin.* **2011**, *26*, 315–323. [CrossRef]
31. Ma, Z.; Hao, P.; Yao, X.; Liu, C.; Tan, J.; Liu, L.; Yang, R.; Geng, Y.; Chen, Q.; Qiao, W. Establishment of an indicator cell line to quantify bovine foamy virus infection. *J. Basic Microbiol.* **2008**, *48*, 278–283. [CrossRef] [PubMed]
32. Ma, Z.; Qiao, W.T.; Xuan, C.H.; Xie, J.H.; Chen, Q.M.; Geng, Y.Q. Detection and analysis of bovine foamy virus infection by an indicator cell line. *Acta Pharmacol. Sin.* **2007**, *28*, 994–1000. [CrossRef] [PubMed]
33. Durocher, Y.; Perret, S.; Kamen, A. High-level and high-throughput recombinant protein production by transient transfection of suspension-growing human 293-ebna1 cells. *Nucleic Acids Res.* **2002**, *30*, E9. [CrossRef] [PubMed]
34. Shaw, K.L.; Lindemann, D.; Mulligan, M.J.; Goepfert, P.A. Foamy virus envelope glycoprotein is sufficient for particle budding and release. *J. Virol.* **2003**, *77*, 2338–2348. [CrossRef]
35. Picard-Maureau, M.; Jarmy, G.; Berg, A.; Rethwilm, A.; Lindemann, D. Foamy virus envelope glycoprotein-mediated entry involves a ph-dependent fusion process. *J. Virol.* **2003**, *77*, 4722–4730. [CrossRef]

36. Cartellieri, M.; Herchenroder, O.; Rudolph, W.; Heinkelein, M.; Lindemann, D.; Zentgraf, H.; Rethwilm, A. N-terminal gag domain required for foamy virus particle assembly and export. *J. Virol.* **2005**, *79*, 12464–12476. [CrossRef]
37. Swiersy, A.; Wiek, C.; Zentgraf, H.; Lindemann, D. Characterization and manipulation of foamy virus membrane interactions. *Cell Microbiol.* **2013**, *15*, 227–236. [CrossRef]
38. Bansal, A.; Shaw, K.L.; Edwards, B.H.; Goepfert, P.A.; Mulligan, M.J. Characterization of the R572T point mutant of a putative cleavage site in human foamy virus Env. *J. Virol.* **2000**, *74*, 2949–2954. [CrossRef]
39. Sun, Y.; Wen, D.D.; Liu, Q.M.; Yi, X.F.; Wang, T.T.; Wei, L.L.; Li, Z.; Liu, W.H.; He, X.H. Comparative analysis of the envelope glycoproteins of foamy viruses. *Acta Virol.* **2012**, *56*, 283–291. [CrossRef]
40. Holzschu, D.L.; Delaney, M.A.; Renshaw, R.W.; Casey, J.W. The nucleotide sequence and spliced pol mrna levels of the nonprimate spumavirus bovine foamy virus. *J. Virol.* **1998**, *72*, 2177–2182.
41. Yu, H.; Li, T.; Qiao, W.; Chen, Q.; Geng, Y. Guanine tetrad and palindromic sequence play critical roles in the rna dimerization of bovine foamy virus. *Arch. Virol.* **2007**, *152*, 2159–2167. [CrossRef] [PubMed]
42. Materniak, M.; Bicka, L.; Kuzmak, J. Isolation and partial characterization of bovine foamy virus from polish cattle. *Pol. J. Vet. Sci.* **2006**, *9*, 207–211. [PubMed]
43. Hechler, T.; Materniak, M.; Kehl, T.; Kuzmak, J.; Lochelt, M. Complete genome sequences of two novel european clade bovine foamy viruses from germany and poland. *J. Virol.* **2012**, *86*, 10905–10906. [CrossRef] [PubMed]

viruses

MDPI

Review

In-Vivo Gene Therapy with Foamy Virus Vectors

Yogendra Singh Rajawat [1], Olivier Humbert [1] and Hans-Peter Kiem [1,2,3,*]

[1] Stem Cell and Gene Therapy Program, Fred Hutchinson Cancer Research Center, Seattle, WA 98109, USA; ohumbert@fredhutch.org (O.H.); yrajawat@fredhutch.org (Y.S.R.)
[2] Departments of Medicine, University of Washington School of Medicine, Seattle, WA 98195, USA
[3] Departments of Pathology, University of Washington School of Medicine, Seattle, WA 98195, USA
* Correspondence: hkiem@fredhutch.org; Tel.: +1-206-667-4425

Received: 29 September 2019; Accepted: 20 November 2019; Published: 23 November 2019

Abstract: Foamy viruses (FVs) are nonpathogenic retroviruses that infect various animals including bovines, felines, nonhuman primates (NHPs), and can be transmitted to humans through zoonotic infection. Due to their non-pathogenic nature, broad tissue tropism and relatively safe integration profile, FVs have been engineered as novel vectors (foamy virus vector, FVV) for stable gene transfer into different cells and tissues. FVVs have emerged as an alternative platform to contemporary viral vectors (e.g., adeno associated and lentiviral vectors) for experimental and therapeutic gene therapy of a variety of monogenetic diseases. Some of the important features of FVVs include the ability to efficiently transduce hematopoietic stem and progenitor cells (HSPCs) from humans, NHPs, canines and rodents. We have successfully used FVV for proof of concept studies to demonstrate safety and efficacy following in-vivo delivery in large animal models. In this review, we will comprehensively discuss FVV based in-vivo gene therapy approaches established in the X-linked severe combined immunodeficiency (SCID-X1) canine model.

Keywords: gene therapy; in-vivo gene therapy; hematopoietic stem and progenitor cells; foamy virus vector; pre-clinical canine model; SCID-X1

1. Introduction

Therapies based on gene transfer to hematopoietic stem and progenitor cells (HSPCs) have achieved tremendous curative outcomes over the past decade and due to revolutionary success in some of these gene therapy clinical trials, these outcomes will redefine the clinical management of patients [1–3]. Pioneering gene therapy trials have shown that the genetic engineering of HSPCs can be a potentially superior alternative to allogeneic transplantation in the treatment of hematological monogenetic disorders including primary immunodeficiencies [4–6]. Transfer of therapeutic genes into long-term repopulating HSPCs can potentially cure blood disorders such as hemoglobinopathies and primary immunodeficiencies. Specifically, with regards to X-linked severe combined immunodeficiency (SCID-X1), recent data showed that this approach could be curative in animal models [7,8] together with very promising clinical results using gene therapy in SCID-X1 patients [1,9]. Despite these advances, gene therapy continues to face a number of challenges which, if not resolved, could be detrimental to the clinical translation of these approaches [4]. These challenges range from the translation of research findings to clinical practice, covering issues with regards to the need for a conditioning regimen, vector-related genotoxicity, specific vector design, and the requirement of sophisticated manufacturing facilities, all of which present various obstacles towards efficacious and practically feasible gene therapy. Manipulation of HSPCs ex-vivo in clinical trials have several drawbacks including a cumbersome and expensive process of extracting and purifying HSPCs from the patient and returning the genetically modified cells to the patient, which also causes a delay in treatment. Further, relative refractoriness of human hematopoietic stem cells to clinically available vector systems remains a significant obstacle for most applications. To circumvent the current challenges and achieve practical HSPCs gene therapy, much work has focused on the development of newer delivery vehicles (viral vector based, or non-viral vector based using nanoparticles), alternative conditioning regimens (non-genotoxic), or simpler methods to target HSPCs in-situ by in vivo administration of the therapeutic transgene which bypasses the need for ex-vivo manipulation of these cells.

Priority should be given to the development of new viral vectors that overcome the known obstacles to stem cell transduction, such as the ability to transduce nondividing cells and utilization of virus that target receptors specific to primitive repopulating cells. With keeping in mind application and clinical translatability, various vectors such as γ-retroviral vector (γ-RVV, [9]), lentiviral (LVV, [1,10–12]), adenoviral [13–16] and adeno-associated viral [17,18] vectors have been designed to target refined cell populations with varying clinical and preclinical success. Although, significant progress has been made in the design of viral vectors, there are several limitations that still need considerable attention, particularly in the large-scale production of viral vectors under good manufacturing practice (GMP), which constitutes a major bottleneck. In recent times, AAV vectors have achieved clinical success; however, pre-existing immunity, relatively low transduction efficacy to non-dividing cells and relatively low transgene/cDNA (~4.4 kb) delivery capacity restricted their use [19,20]. Adenoviral vectors offer several advantages, including large cloning capacity and transduction of a number of tissues based on serotype, but their use has been restricted mainly due to their potent induction of acute immune response that could be fatal [21,22]. γ-RVV and LVV have shown very encouraging clinical outcomes specifically in monogenetic disorders of hematopoietic origin. However, the most commonly used envelope (VSV-G) to pseudotype clinical γ-RVV and LVV vectors targets HSPCs inefficiently and these vectors have significant batch to batch variability in large scale manufacturing and in their subsequent transduction of target cells [23,24]. Further, VSV-G pseudotyped lentiviral vectors are immunogenic, which leads to the elimination of corrected HSPCs in-vivo due to potent humoral and cellular immune responses, resulting in lower engraftment in patients [25,26]. To circumvent limitations of the currently available viral vector platform, there is an unmet need to either improve the current viral vector platform or to identify novel viral vectors applicable to HSPCs gene therapy.

More than two decades ago, a new vector system based on foamy viruses from the spumavirus family was described that can be used for gene transfer into murine hematopoietic stem cells (HSCs) [27,28]. Foamy viruses are non-pathogenic retroviruses with a wide tissue tropism that are commonly found in mammalian species. David Russell and his group developed replication-defective foamy virus vectors (FVVs) and demonstrated that these vector particles efficiently transfer a marker gene into repopulating mouse HSCs and into human CD34+ cells ex-vivo [29,30]. Since then, our laboratory has optimized parameters for efficient transduction of human and canine CD34+ HSPCs by FVVs [31–33]. In the last decade, our group has demonstrated efficacy of FVV in correction of monogenetic diseases of hematopoietic origin in large animal models (non-human primates and canine) and has established the safety of FVV in-vivo [7,8,34,35]. In these pre-clinical studies, FVV-mediated transgene delivery maintained high and persistent levels of marker-gene expression possibly due to improved transduction of quiescent cells and to the novel envelope/receptor system used for stem cell entry [7,8]. In the following sections, we will discuss advantages of FVV for therapeutic gene therapy applications and will specifically focus on our studies using in-vivo FVV delivery for the treatment of canine model of SCID-X1 since general characteristics and different aspects of FV biology have already been discussed elsewhere in this special issue.

2. Limitations of Ex-Vivo Gene Therapy

Hematopoietic stem and progenitor cells ex-vivo gene therapy utilizing viral vectors have been used in multiple clinical trials to circumvent the complications associated with allogeneic bone marrow transplantation. Despite the undeniable therapeutic benefits offered by HSPCs gene therapy treatment for various monogenetic disorders such as hemoglobinopathies [36,37], primary immunodeficiencies [1,9,38,39] and inborn metabolic disorders [40,41], this approach poses several limitations which include requirement of cytotoxic conditioning regimen to promote engraftment of donor cells, lifelong administration of immunoglobulins in cases of immunodeficiencies, safety concerns due to vector genotoxicity (insertional mutagenesis), invasive procedure to procure HSPCs, and requirement of costly GMP facility for production of the cell product. Further, ex-vivo transduction protocols used in SCID-X1 clinical trials using SIN lentiviral vectors [1,42] required manipulation of HSCs by culture in multiple cytokines for approximately 3–4 days that may compromise HSCs pluripotency due to entry into pathways of differentiation and limit their engraftment potential and long-term repopulating capacity. Similar findings were reported in SCID-X1 dogs transplanted with bone marrow CD34+ cells from normal healthy donors [43]. Therefore, innovation is needed for long-term efficacy of ex-vivo gene therapies [44]. Alternatively, to circumvent these problems, an attractive approach is to transduce HSCs in-vivo within their natural environment by direct intravenous injection (in-vivo gene therapy). For comprehensive information of ex-vivo studies using FVV in HSPCs, we refer the reader to the excellent review by Vassilopoulos et al., in the same edition. In the current review, we will focus on FVV as an in-vivo gene therapy platform established in the canine model of SCID-X1. We will also discuss progress made in vector design and regimen used to mobilize HSCs out of the bone marrow.

3. Viral and Non-Viral Vectors Platforms for In-Vivo Gene Therapy

In lieu of various shortcomings of ex-vivo gene therapy, an alternative strategy that overcomes current limitations and still utilizes the benefits of gene therapy would provide a great advancement toward clinical translation. We propose that a possible answer lies in the use of in-vivo gene therapy. In-vivo gene transfer strategies administer the therapeutic vector either directly to the target organ or via the vascular system into blood vessels feeding that organ. In-vivo gene transfer offers several advantages over ex-vivo strategies including ease of administration, no need for HSPCs collection, manipulation and culture outside the body and thus no requirement for costly cell processing GMP facilities, and increased safety due to absence of myeloablative conditioning and transplantation procedures. Finally, this novel platform is portable and easy to disseminate worldwide particularly in under-developed countries with a large patient population needing treatment.

Multiple approaches and various delivery vehicles have been utilized for in-vivo transfer of therapeutic genes. These platforms include the use of non-viral [45] and viral vectors (integrating and non-integrating) [46] based approaches. Non-viral gene delivery systems have gained considerable attention as a promising alternative to viral delivery to treat various diseases [47,48]. However, despite extensive research, little is known about the parameters that underline the safe and effective in-vivo use of the nanoparticle-based delivery. So far, nanoparticles have shown promise in targeting and delivering cargo to various tumors very effectively. This success has been attributed to enhanced permeability and retention (the EPR effect) that can permit passive accumulation into tumor interstitial tissue. However, sub-optimal delivery is achieved with most nanoparticles because of heterogeneity of vascular permeability, which limits nanoparticle penetration. With regards to in- vivo gene therapy using nanoparticles, we cannot rely on passive accumulation and need to target tissue specific delivery of therapeutic cargo. Moreover, slow drug release limits bioavailability, which also restricts the use of nanoparticles for delivery of therapeutic cDNA. Overall, the modest efficacy, limited stability of nanoparticle conjugated to delivery cargo and lack of specificity of non-viral delivery are the central issues that need to be addressed. Thus, although nanoparticle-based approaches remain an attractive potential choice for in-vivo gene therapy, many questions still need to be answered for their effective clinical translation.

In early attempts with in-vivo gene therapy with viral vectors, VSV-G pseudotyped lentiviral vectors were used for direct intravenous injections in female rat brains using a stereotactic approach and showed effective transduction in multiple cell types including terminally differentiated neurons [49]. These early studies showed that LVVs can successfully be administered intravenously, transgene expression could be sustained for several months without detectable pathology, and they provided proof of concept which eventually led to multiple follow-up studies with various vector systems. Intravenous administration of early adenoviral vector platforms in ornithine transcarbamylase deficiency (OTCD) clinical trials [50] resulted in fatal systemic inflammatory response syndrome in one patient [22]. Further, the use of first generation γ-RVVs (non-SIN γ-RVV) derived from Moloney murine leukemia virus (MMLV) with duplicated viral enhancer sequences within the long terminal repeats (LTRs) led to leukemogenesis in early SCID-X1 clinical trials [51–53]. These early setbacks paved the path for the design of novel and safe viral vectors. In the past two decades, not only have there been inventions of a variety of safer viral vector such as "gutless adenoviral vectors" [54–56] and self-inactivating (SIN) γ-RVVs [9,57] and LVVs [12,58], but these vectors have also become the backbone of ex-vivo gene therapy clinical trials [24,59–61].

With regards to use of integrating viral vectors (γ-RVVs and LVV's) in-vivo, intravenous administration of the retroviral replicating vector, Toca 511, recently demonstrated efficacy in orthotopic immune-competent mouse glioma model [62]. Further, a phase 1/2 study of a non-primate lentiviral vector based upon the equine infectious anemia virus (EIAV) expressing three genes involved in dopamine metabolism demonstrated safety of local lentiviral gene delivery into the central nervous system with evidence of clinical benefit [63]. In-vivo gene delivery using a lentiviral vector has also been applied clinically to the eye [64] and demonstrated that EIAV vectors provide a safe platform with robust and sustained transgene expression for ocular gene therapy. Cantore et al. reported the efficacy and safety of liver-directed in-vivo gene therapy in large and small animal models using lentiviral vectors. These vectors targeting the expression of a canine factor IX transgene in hepatocytes were well tolerated and provided a stable long-term production of coagulation factor IX in dogs with hemophilia B [65]. Even though these studies represent evidence of tremendous improvement in γ-RVV's and LVV's design for use as in-vivo gene delivery vehicles, major hurdles such as safety and host immune response against the vector and envelope used for pseudotyping restricts their use in clinical applications. Therefore, various strategies have been proposed to improve existing platforms to be utilized for in-vivo gene delivery [66–68].

Existing viral vectors have shown varying degrees of therapeutic efficacy in ex-vivo gene therapy clinical trials; nonetheless, little progress has been made for in-vivo clinical use with the exception of AAV vectors. In recent times, AAV vector-based in-vivo gene therapy has seen tremendous success for monogenetic disorders, which is evident with the recent approval of alipogene tiparvovec (Glybera, EMA, Amsterdam, Netherlands; year 2012) for the treatment of a rare inherited disorder, lipoprotein lipase deficiency, voretigene neparvovec (Luxturna, USFDA, Silver spring, Maryland, USA; year 2017) for the treatment of Leber's congenital amaurosis and for the treatment of pediatric spinal muscular atrophy (SMA) with bi-allelic mutations in the survival motor neuron 1 (SMN1), geneonasemnogene abeparvovec-xioi (Zolgensma, USFDA, year 2019). Although AAV based approaches have seen clinical success, these vectors have several drawbacks including limited scope with regard to target tissues and cell types that do not divide rapidly. AAV is largely maintained episomally, with very limited vector getting integrated in genome that will limit long-term efficacy. Although AAV vectors have little or no acute toxicity, there are reports of development of hepatocellular carcinoma in the mice model [69], ocular toxicity in mice [70], and the use of AAV vectors resulted into severe toxicity in non-human primates and pigs [71]. Altogether, current viral vector-based approaches for in-vivo gene therapy need to be further improved by leveraging recent discoveries in viral biology, progress in vector design and transduction, or exploring the use of novel viral vectors. In the following section, we discuss our promising data using in-vivo administration of FVV's for the treatment of SCID-X1 in the dogs.

4. In-Vivo Gene Therapy for Canine SCID-X1 with FVVs

FVs are unique retroviruses which belong to Spumaretrovirus and are nonpathogenic to their natural host [72]. FVs are prevalent in many mammals including nonhuman primates but they are not endemic in human populations [73]. Cell membrane associated heparan sulfate is a receptor for the prototype foamy virus in many species including humans [74]. As heparan sulfate is expressed in a variety of cell types, FVs are able to infect many tissues. Prototype FVVs were developed owing to several unique properties including lack of pathogenicity [75], broad tropism (can transduce many therapeutic targets), large transgene capacity, unique replication strategy which provides the ability to persist in quiescent cells, safer integration profile [31,76,77] and resistance to serum complement inhibition [27,78] which is a determining factor for in-vivo gene therapy. FVVs system have evolved from early replication competent vectors to third generation non replicating viral vectors which are efficient gene delivery vehicles that have shown great promise for gene therapy in various preclinical animal models including our SCID-X1 dogs [79].

The SCID-X1 dog model provides a fantastic opportunity to delineate various therapeutic strategies that are very much translatable to human SCID-X1 patients. Our collaborators, Felsburg and colleagues, have established a SCID-X1 dog model in basset hounds breed in which immunodeficiency is caused by a naturally occurring genetic mutation in the common gamma chain (γC) [80,81]. The mutation is a four base pair frameshift deletion in the signal peptide region that results in a pre-mature termination codon in exon1 [82]. Unlike genetically engineered γC deficient mice, canine SCID-X1 has a clinical and immunologic phenotype representative of human SCID-X1, thus making it an ideal pre-clinical model to improve gene therapy strategies for human SCID-X1.

In our very first study, we evaluated the efficacy of FVV gene therapy in treating SCID-X1 [7]. Five neonatal SCID-X1 dogs were treated by in-vivo administration of the FVV, containing Green Fluorescent Protein (GFP) and the coding sequence for the human common gamma chain (γC) linked by a 2A element, and expressed under control of the elongation factor 1 promoter (EF1α) (EF1α-EGFP-2A-γC). All five animals were intravenously injected with 4.0–8.4 $\times$ 10^8 infectious unit of FVV (age at injection varied from one day old to 13 days old). The injection of FVV was well tolerated by all five pups with no adverse effect. γC+ lymphocytes were detected in peripheral blood within 14 days post-treatment and, by 84 days, γC+ cells comprised 30%–58% of the total lymphocytes. Four out of five dogs showed a parallel trend for GFP+ lymphocytes. While promising, these results were limited by the relatively slow rate of lymphocyte reconstitution in these animals. The dogs surviving long-term eventually recovered normal lymphocyte counts at 112 days post-treatment (R2202 and 2203, Figure 1 inset, blue lines, Figure 1 includes selected results of two dogs from first study [7]). GFP+ (i.e., gene corrected) lymphocytes eventually accounted for 73% to 91% of circulating lymphocytes and expression of γC was sufficient for the development of CD3+ T cells, comprising 7% to 43% of total lymphocytes in peripheral blood by six weeks after administration of FVV. As expected, the majority of CD3+ cells expressed GFP that originated from the gene therapy vector and stained positive for CD4 and CD8. Most of the CD3+ cells also stained positively for CD45RA, a marker for naïve T cells, indicating recent thymic emigration.

We further assessed the T-cell receptor (TCR) diversity in each treated animal by spectratyping that analyzes genetic rearrangement of the 17 families of TCR Vβ segments. The longest surviving dog, R2202, initially expressed polyclonal TCR at early timepoints but eventually lost TCR diversity by 322 days post-treatment. These results demonstrated that delivery of the γC gene via FVV in-vivo in SCID-X1 dogs enabled thymocyte development and maturation as demonstrated by robust TCR rearrangement. Normal T cells counts as well as functionality of the γC-dependent signaling pathway were also restored, as demonstrated by tyrosine phosphorylation of the downstream STAT5 effector via activation of the γC pathway by IL-2 stimulation in peripheral blood mononuclear cells (PBMCs). Moreover, these γC+ lymphocytes were able to proliferate and re-enter into the cell cycle upon mitogen (phytohemagglutinin, PHA) stimulation as assessed by BrdU incorporation. Overall, FVV injection restored T-cell-mediated immunity with normal number and functionality of T cells generated. Specific antibody responses and immunoglobulin class switching was also evaluated in treated animals after immunization with the T cell-dependent neoantigen bacteriophage, ΦX174. This neoantigen is routinely being used in human patients with SCID-X1 to evaluate success of treatment with bone marrow transplantation or gene therapy. We found that treated animals showed a primary and secondary antibody response that is very similar to that seen in healthy human and canine subjects, indicating that our treatment restored both the B and T cell cytokine signaling required for class switching and memory responses to this neoantigen.

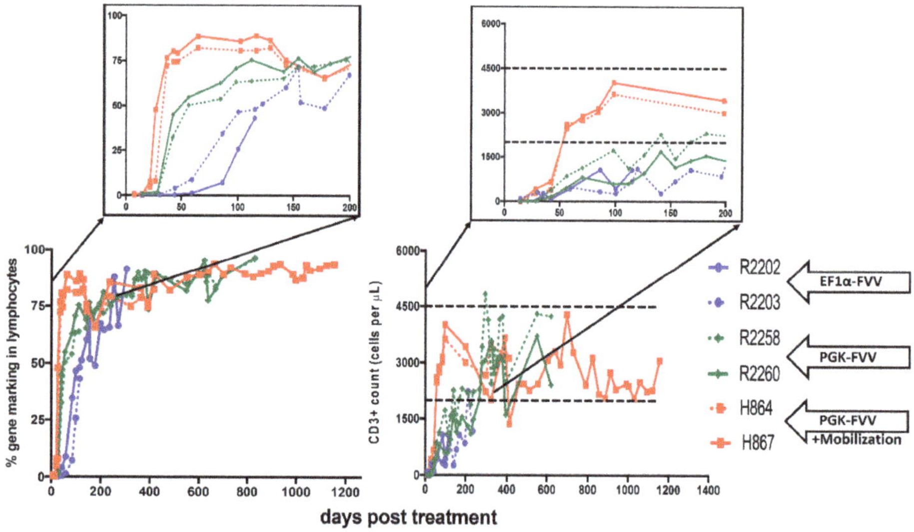

Figure 1. Immune reconstitution in foamy virus vector (FVV) treated X-linked severe combined immunodeficiency (SCID-X1) dogs: Bottom left graph shows % gene corrected lymphocytes in peripheral blood of various animals. Top left inset highlights the early kinetics of gene marking in treated animals (blue vs. green vs. red lines). The mobilized dog H867 had a stable level of gene marking almost 1260 days post treatment. Bottom right graph represents absolute number of CD3+ T lymphocytes in peripheral blood of treated dogs. Top right inset emphasizes the days required to attain normal numbers of absolute T lymphocytes (blue vs. green vs. red lines; dashed black lines shows counts in healthy dogs). H867 maintained normal levels of CD3+ T cell counts for over three years. Data in this figure was reproduced from previous studies [7,8] and contains extended data on H864 and H867. R2202 and R2203 were part of the cohort of five dogs from our first study [7] and R2258, R2260, H864 and H867 were part of our second study [8], additional details are included in the text. EF1α-FVV: elongation factor 1 α promoter (EF1α-GFP-2A-γC) carrying foamy virus vector (FVV); PGK-FVV: human phosphoglycerokinase (PGK-mCherry-γC) promoter carrying FVV.

To assess the safety and potential genotoxicity of FVV, retroviral integration site (RIS) analysis was performed longitudinally on peripheral blood of treated animals. Based on the identification of only 20 unique RISs across all samples, we concluded that all dogs displayed a polyclonal hematopoietic contribution in gene-modified cells over time. To determine if our in-vivo FVV treatment resulted in significant off-target activity (intended target cell population was bone marrow or blood derived HSCs or HSPCs), we assessed the biodistribution of the DNA provirus from various tissues by RIS. The majority of the identified integrants originated from the perfused blood into the tissues except for one event detected in the gut. We also found two integration events in the ovaries of R2202 but no integration was observed in the testis of R2203. Taken together, intravenous FVV gene therapy resulted in a very low frequency of off-target transduction events and are thus not likely to be passed on in the germline. Although clonal diversity and TCR repertoire were relatively low in these animals, these results provided proof of concept that FVV can safely be used in a pre-clinical model for in-vivo gene therapy. In conclusion, this first study demonstrated feasibility and safety of FVV in-vivo gene therapy in SCID-X1 dogs. Further, this study proved that in-vivo gene therapy using FVVs could achieve immune reconstitution in a clinically relevant large animal model of SCID-X1.

5. Optimization of FVV In-Vivo Gene Delivery

Our preliminary study using FVV, EF1α-EGFP-2A-γC was equally efficacious (in terms of T lymphocyte reconstitution) to earlier studies using in-vivo γ-retroviral vectors (γ-RVV) to treat canine SCID-X1 [83] or to ex-vivo γ-RVV clinical trial results reported in human patients [9]. However, this study demonstrated limited gene marking in the B and myeloid cell lineages as was reported in γ-RVV studies. In particular, treated animals still developed opportunistic infections (Table 1) and produced low immunoglobulin (Ig)G levels, and marking levels in granulocytes and monocytes were very low (0.6%), indicating that more efficient transduction of multipotent HSCs is required to achieve long-term phenotypic correction.

Table 1. Description of SCID-X1 dogs treated by intravenous injection of FVV in various in-vivo gene therapy studies [7,8]. Two out of five dogs from the EF1α-EGFP-2A-γC study [7] were selected for inclusion in the table.

ID	Age at Injection (Days Old.)	Foamy Viral Vector	Dose of Vector (Infectious Units)	Mobilization	Survival of Dogs (Days Post Treatment)	Health Status or Infectious Complications
H867	16	PGK.mCherry.2A.γC	4.0×10^8	G-CSF/AMD3100	1260	Healthy and Alive
H864	16	PGK.mCherry.2A.γC	4.0×10^8	G-CSF/AMD3100	~486	*Bordetella bronchiseptica*
R2258	18	EF1α.EGFP.2A.γC PGK.mCherry.2A.γC	4.0×10^8 4.0×10^8	NO	~820	Papillomavirus
R2260	18	EF1α.mCherry.2A.γC PGK.EGFP.2A.γC	4.0×10^8 4.0×10^8	NO	~820	Papillomavirus
R2202	1	EF1α-EGFP-2A-γC	4.2×10^8	NO	~334	Coccidiosis; Canine Distemper virus
R2203	1	EF1α-EGFP-2A-γC	4.2×10^8	NO	~120	Canine Parainfluenza virus

The suboptimal immune reconstitution observed in the preliminary dog study prompted us to evaluate several strategies to further optimize our FVV in-vivo gene delivery protocol. The kinetics of immune reconstitution may be enhanced by modifying FVVs design, for example, by using a stronger promoter in place of the short form of the human EF1α promoter to drive expression of γC. In addition, targeting HSCs more efficiently may increase gene marking in other cell lineages that do not have a selective advantage like T lymphocytes. This could, in principle, be achieved by using mobilizing agents to increase the number of circulating HSCs in peripheral blood at the time of vector administration.

In our next study using FVV for in-vivo gene therapy [8], we hypothesized that utilizing an alternative promoter to EF1α promoter could result in more robust γC expression in cells of hematologic origin. For this purpose, we redesigned our FVV with a human phosphoglycerokinase (hPGK) promoter to drive expression of the codon optimized human γC cDNA. Performance of each vector was compared side by side in a competitive repopulation assay by intravenous injection of equal doses of the FVVs, EF1α-EGFP -γC and PGK-mCherry -γC, in two newborn SCID-X1 animals. Competitive injection of EF1α-EGFP-γC and PGK-mCherry-γC in the same SCID-X1 dog bestowed an ideal opportunity to study the efficacy of each promoter under similar physiological conditions in the same animal. The absolute number of circulating lymphocytes steadily increased in both treated dogs during the first six months post-treatment, plateaued around 6–8 months, and remained within the normal range during the course of 2.5 years post-treatment (dogs R2258 and R2260, Figure 1, Green Lines). Strikingly, the majority of gene marking (70% to 90%) in peripheral blood came from the PGK-mCherry-γC vector in both animals, whereas marking from the EF1α-EGFP-γC vector comprised only a small fraction (5% to 10%). Interestingly, the early kinetics of gene marking in peripheral blood lymphocytes in these two animals was substantially improved as compared with animals treated with the EF1α-EGFP-γC vector from our previous study (R2202 and R2203, Figure 1). The fraction of gene-corrected peripheral lymphocytes reached 40% in both R2258 and R2260 at six weeks post-injection, as compared with 5% for the EF1α-EGFP-γC alone treated animal, demonstrating superior therapeutic performance of the PGK-mCherry-γC vector as compared to EF1α-EGFP-γC. Nevertheless, this new vector did not result in improved targeting of the most primitive HSCs as showcased by limited gene marking in non-T cell lineages (B and myeloid cells).

In an attempt to target HSCs more effectively, we chose to treat a new animal cohort with a mobilization agent to increase the frequency of HSCs in peripheral blood at the time of FVV administration. Stem cell mobilization is defined as a process in which certain drugs are used to cause the trafficking of stem cells from the bone marrow into the blood and is commonly used to collect and store stem cells that may be used later as for bone marrow replacement therapy during a stem cell transplant. Granulocyte colony-stimulating factor (G-CSF) mobilized HSPCs from peripheral blood is the most widely used source of HSPCs for clinical transplantation [84]. As an alternative, plerixafor (AMD3100) was shown to not only efficiently mobilize the HSPCs in various species including humans [85,86], but also augment the mobilization and yield of CD34+ HSPCs when used in combination with G-CSF for clinical transplantation [87,88]. Furthermore, plerixafor was found to be very effective at mobilizing CD34+ HSPCs in dogs (3–10 fold increase in circulating CD34+ HSPCs count) [89]. Therefore, we hypothesized that mobilization prior to injection of FVV may enhance HSPCs transduction efficiency in-vivo. In the next cohort of animals, we treated two SCID-X1 dogs with both plerixafor (4 mg/kg, subcutaneously, single dose) and G-CSF (5 μg/kg, subcutaneously, twice a day for five days), which resulted in a 6.4–7.2-fold increase in circulating CD34+ cells [8]. Plerixafor treatment significantly increased the kinetics of lymphocyte expansion and gene marking as compared to non-mobilized PGK-mCherry-γC-treated animals. The fraction of gene-corrected lymphocytes in peripheral blood of mobilized animals reached 80% at six weeks post-treatment, whereas it took >20 weeks in non-mobilized animals to reach similar levels (green lines vs. red lines comparison in Figure 1). Accordingly, the time required to reach normal lymphocyte counts was markedly reduced in the mobilized animals (red lines, Figure 1). The two non-mobilized FV vector-treated animals (R2258 and R2260) initially showed normal frequency (90%) of CD3+CD45RA+ T cells in peripheral blood, but their frequency subsequently declined to 50% at one-year post-treatment. In comparison, levels of CD3+CD45RA+ cells have remained stable for both mobilized dogs, up to 18 months in H864 and for over 36 months post-treatment in H867, which continues to be monitored.

Thymic output was assessed by analysis of T cell receptor excision circles (TRECs) originating from TCR genes rearrangement that occurs during T-lymphocyte maturation. In the non-mobilized animals, TRECs were initially 10-fold lower in treated dogs (1000–1200 TREC/million peripheral blood mononuclear cells, PBMCs), as compared with a normal littermate control (12,000–14,000 TREC/million PBMCs), and then gradually declined over time. In contrast, TRECs in the mobilized animals reached normal levels as early as three months post-treatment and remained similar to the littermate control for up to three years post-treatment. In summary, we found that mobilization before FVV injection of SCID-X1 canines improved kinetic of T-lymphocyte reconstitution and increased thymic output to levels comparable to those in a healthy control.

The majority of expanded CD3+ lymphocytes were mature and expressed the coreceptor CD4 or CD8, with a small fraction of cells being CD4/CD8 double positive or double negative. Both mobilized animals H864 and H867 showed normal CD4:CD8 cell ratios, averaging two. The majority of circulating T lymphocytes in non-mobilized (R2258/R2260) and mobilized (H864/H867) also stained positive for TCR α/β starting at two months post-treatment, consistent with observations from healthy canines and humans. When assessing TCR diversity in each treated animal by TCR β spectratyping, we found that the two animals mobilized with G-CSF/AMD3100 showed robust spectratype profiles comparable to that of an aged-matched normal littermate, characterized by Gaussian distribution of fragments sized across 17 families of TCR vector β segments, and stable for up to three years post-treatment.

Similar to what we described in our previous study, we also verified functionality of the γC-dependent signaling pathways in all FVV-treated animals as well as effective stimulation in response to T-cell mitogen phytohemagglutinin. Primary and secondary antibody responses, and immunoglobulin class switching after immunization with the T cell–dependent neoantigen bacteriophage ΦX174 was also documented in these animals. In addition, polyclonal IgM, IgG, and IgA concentrations were measured from serum of mobilized dogs at multiple timepoints post-treatment and showed IgG (1850–3152 mg/dL) and IgM levels (250–382 mg/dL) in the treated SCID animals that were comparable to a healthy littermate control (IgG: 670–1650 mg/dL: IgM: 100–400 mg/dL), indicating partial restoration of B-lymphocyte function. Although, antibody levels were within normal range for the mobilized FVV treated dogs (H864 and H867), the gene marking levels in B lymphocytes were low throughout the study. In fact, despite substantially improving T-lymphocyte reconstitution, HSPC mobilization did not increase gene marking in myeloid cells (0–1.5%) or B lymphocytes (0–4%) in mobilized dogs, which is consistent with the levels of gene marking in myeloid and B lymphocytes in non-mobilized dogs. Thus, FVV in-vivo gene therapy can result in low levels of correction of HSCs or myeloid progenitors in addition to circulating common lymphoid or T cell progenitors that experience a selective growth advantage after gene correction.

To assess the safety and potential genotoxicity of FVVs, tissues from non-mobilized animals (R2258 and R2260) were collected and analyzed by RIS for biodistribution assessment of the foamy provirus. The vast majority of RISs (90%) detected in tissues were also found in peripheral blood at the same time point, suggesting that they originated from contaminating blood cells present in perfused tissues. Interestingly, ovaries and testes showed the smallest number of integration events (37 and 56, respectively, as compared with 766 and 469 in blood), and none of the RISs found exclusively in the gonadal tissues appeared at notable frequencies except for one integration site in the ovaries (chromosome 38; 34,522; 4.28%). No unique RIS at a noteworthy frequency was detected in semen from mobilized male H867. Taken together, these results suggested that off-target transduction events by in-vivo FVV treatment are rare and thus unlikely to be passed on in the germline, a finding also supported by the study of progeny issued from FVV-treated male R2260. RIS analysis from peripheral white blood cell DNA showed a marked increase in integration events in mobilized dogs H864 and H867 as compared with non-mobilized dogs R2258 and R2260, despite the use of an equal dose of FVV PGK-γC, consistent with the greater therapeutic activity of this vector. No clonal dominance was observed in any animal, but some persisting clones contributing to 0.1% of total gene marking were found in the non-mobilized animals, albeit with no indication of expansion. Taken together, our studies indicated that the use of G-CSF/AMD3100 mobilization before intravenous FVV delivery increases both the kinetics of lymphocyte recovery and diversity of immune reconstitution in SCID-X1 canines.

Altogether, we have so far treated nine dogs (five with EF1α-EGFP-2A-γC; two with both EF1α-EGFP-2A-γC and PGK-mCherry-2A-γC and two dogs with PGK-mCherry-2A-γC and G-CSF/AMD3100 mobilization) [5,6] and all treated dogs demonstrated efficacy and safety of FVV in-vivo gene therapy in canine model. Out of nine treated SCID-X1 dogs, five lived more than a year and three lived for over 2.5 years. Most importantly, the kinetics of lymphocyte reconstitution in our study using PGK-mCherry-2A-γC and G-CSF/AMD3100 mobilization is comparable that of SCID-X1 patients treated using ex-vivo gene therapy [9]. The long-term treated dogs demonstrated that correction of cellular and humoral immune compartment is sustained for over three years. Even though we have seen therapeutic correction of SCID phenotype in the dogs, particularly in T cell immune reconstitution, there is still room for improvement in myeloid and B cell gene marking. This could be achieved by treatment with more effective HSC mobilization regimen, by directly targeting primitive HSCs in their niche through intra-osseous delivery [90] of the viral vector, or with the use of a selection strategy for gene-modified HSCs [34,91]. Our findings from FVV-treated dogs are directly translatable to human SCID-X1 patients and validate FVVs as an effective vehicle for in-vivo delivery of the therapeutic transgene to correct SCID-X1 and potentially for other hematologic disorder.

6. Summary and Future Perspective

Ex-vivo HSPCs gene therapy clinical trials using non-SIN γ-RVV, SIN γ-RVV and LVV for SCID-X1 patients have demonstrated tremendous clinical success and will change the current practice of patient care. However, these therapies still require, in most cases, high doses of conditioning with chemotherapy, and thus patients are myelosuppressed for prolonged periods requiring hospitalization.

In addition, conditioning can lead to genotoxicity and secondary malignancies. All ex-vivo approaches require invasive procedures to procure HSPCs and appropriate facilities, with very high cost. Due to these limitations, it will be challenging to apply current ex-vivo gene therapy strategies using integrating viral vectors on a broad scale. Therefore, there is an unfulfilled and ongoing quest for a safer and affordable treatment option for SCID-X1 patients. In-vivo gene therapy offers several advantages and could be a potential alternative to mitigate some of the challenges seen with ex-vivo HSPCs gene therapy. In terms of in-vivo gene therapy, γ-RVV and LVV have been used pre-clinically for disease models (as discussed briefly in this review) other than SCID-X1, with varying degree of therapeutic efficacy. However, challenges such as safety and immunogenicity remain a major hurdle for clinical translation of these vectors involving in-vivo delivery.

In-vivo gene therapy with FVVs has provided encouraging long term safety and efficacy results in the pre-clinical SCID-X1 dog model. These findings demonstrate comparable efficacy in terms of immune reconstitution and T cell functionality to human SCID-X1 clinical trials with the use of γ-RVV and LVV in ex-vivo gene therapy. Interestingly, in our SCID-X1 model, we have seen production of immunoglobulins that show normal B cell function with no prior conditioning, whereas, in human clinical trials normal function of B cells and production of immunoglobulin's (IgG and IgA) was attributed to use of conditioning regimen. Therefore, FVV's could provide an alternative platform for in-vivo gene therapy to mitigate some of the challenges possessed by γ-RVV and LVV. Our current pre-clinical FVV in-vivo gene therapy offers a path forward as an effective, safe, and accessible platform that may provide prompt treatment of newborn SCID-X1 patients without the complications associated with conditioning or manipulation of HSPCs. Moreover, this treatment scheme could be applied in other hematological disorders with monogenetic mutations, particularly in those disorders where manipulation of HSPCs ex-vivo is near impossible and where transfer of the therapeutic gene in few stem cells could be curative such as Fanconi anemia.

The excellent therapeutic benefits reported in patients and regulatory approval of viral vector-based gene therapy products such as Glybera, Luxturna, and Zolzensma are providing enough impetus to continue the exploration of novel in-vivo gene transfer approaches. However, the choices of viral vector for in-vivo gene therapy will depend on specific disease, target tissue in hand, size of transgene delivered, and packaging capacity of vector. Specific challenges that need to overcome for in-vivo gene transfer strategies include the induction of immunity by the viral vector, access of the gene therapy vector to the targeted cells/organ, efficient targeting of the vector to the cell and translocation of the genetic material to the nucleus, and any toxicity induced by expression of virus and/or transgene. Further, ideal in-vivo gene therapy that should be affordable as Glybera (now withdrawn from market), Luxturna, and Zolzensma are very expensive and could be a concern for widespread usage and commercial interest. Among the integrating viral vectors, FVV provides a suitable platform due to several advantages offered as compared to γ-RVV and LVV as discussed in this study. With our recent pre-clinical data in the canine model of SCID-X1, FVV have so far successfully shown clear long-term safety and therapeutic efficacy. This portable in-vivo gene delivery platform circumvents some of the challenges imposed by some clinically used viral vectors. Importantly, with the advent of novel gene-editing approaches, FVV, in its engineered integration-deficient form, provides an attractive option for the in-vivo delivery of editing reagents (Cas9, gRNA and donor template) due to its large packaging capacity. Altogether, FVV could be an answer to some of the challenges faced today in clinical translation via the in-vivo delivery of gene therapeutics.

Author Contributions: Conceptualization—H.-P.K. and Y.S.R.; writing—original draft preparation, Y.S.R.; writing—review and editing, Y.S.R., O.H., H.-P.K.; supervision, H.-P.K.; funding acquisition, H.-P.K.

Funding: This research was funded by National Institutes of Health, National Institute of Allergy and Infectious Diseases grant P01: AI097100, National Heart, Lung, and Blood Institute grant P01: HL122173 and Fred Hutchinson Cancer Research Center support grant P30: CA15704.

Acknowledgments: We thank Helen Crawford for her assistance with manuscript and figure preparation.

Conflicts of Interest: The authors declare no conflicts of interest.

References

1. Mamcarz, E.; Zhou, S.; Lockey, T.; Abdelsamed, H.; Cross, S.J.; Kang, G.; Ma, Z.; Condori, J.; Dowdy, J.; Triplett, B.; et al. Lentiviral gene therapy combined with low-dose busulfan in infants with SCID-X1. *N. Engl. J. Med.* **2019**, *380*, 1525–1534. [CrossRef]
2. Anguela, X.M.; High, K.A. Entering the modern era of gene therapy. *Annu. Rev. Med.* **2019**, *70*, 273–288. [CrossRef]
3. Naldini, L. Genetic engineering of hematopoiesis: Current stage of clinical translation and future perspectives. *EMBO Mol. Med.* **2019**, *11*, e9958. [CrossRef]
4. Cavazzana, M.; Bushman, F.D.; Miccio, A.; Andre-Schmutz, I.; Six, E. Gene therapy targeting haematopoietic stem cells for inherited diseases: Progress and challenges. *Nat. Rev. Drug Discov.* **2019**, *18*, 447–462. [CrossRef]
5. Coquerelle, S.; Ghardallou, M.; Rais, S.; Taupin, P.; Touzot, F.; Boquet, L.; Blanche, S.; Benaouadi, S.; Brice, T.; Tuchmann-Durand, C.; et al. Innovative curative treatment of beta thalassemia: Cost-efficacy analysis of gene therapy versus allogenic hematopoietic stem-cell transplantation. *Hum. Gene Ther.* **2019**, *30*, 753–761. [CrossRef]
6. Touzot, F.; Moshous, D.; Creidy, R.; Neven, B.; Frange, P.; Cros, G.; Caccavelli, L.; Blondeau, J.; Magnani, A.; Luby, J.M.; et al. Faster T-cell development following gene therapy compared with haploidentical HSCT in the treatment of SCID-X1. *Blood* **2015**, *125*, 3563–3569. [CrossRef]
7. Burtner, C.R.; Beard, B.C.; Kennedy, D.R.; Wohlfahrt, M.E.; Adair, J.E.; Trobridge, G.D.; Scharenberg, A.M.; Torgerson, T.R.; Rawlings, D.J.; Felsburg, P.J.; et al. Intravenous injection of a foamy virus vector to correct canine SCID-X1. *Blood* **2014**, *123*, 3578–3584. [CrossRef]
8. Humbert, O.; Chan, F.; Rajawat, Y.S.; Torgerson, T.R.; Burtner, C.R.; Hubbard, N.W.; Humphrys, D.; Norgaard, Z.K.; O'Donnell, P.; Adair, J.E.; et al. Rapid immune reconstitution of SCID-X1 canines after G-CSF/AMD3100 mobilization and in vivo gene therapy. *Blood Adv.* **2018**, *2*, 987–999. [CrossRef]
9. Hacein-Bey-Abina, S.; Pai, S.Y.; Gaspar, H.B.; Armant, M.; Berry, C.C.; Blanche, S.; Bleesing, J.; Blondeau, J.; Buckland, K.F.; Caccavelli, L.; et al. A modified gamma-retrovirus vector for X-linked severe combined immunodeficiency. *N. Engl. J. Med.* **2014**, *371*, 1407–1417. [CrossRef]
10. Cronin, J.; Zhang, X.Y.; Reiser, J. Altering the tropism of lentiviral vectors through pseudotypin. *Curr. Gene Ther.* **2005**, *5*, 387–398. [CrossRef]
11. Kafri, T.; Blomer, U.; Peterson, D.A.; Gage, F.H.; Verma, I.M. Sustained expression of genes delivered directly into liver and muscle by lentiviral vectors. *Nat. Genet.* **1997**, *17*, 314–317. [CrossRef]
12. Zufferey, R.; Dull, T.; Mandel, R.J.; Bukovsky, A.; Quiroz, D.; Naldini, L.; Trono, D. Self-inactivating lentivirus vector for safe and efficient in vivo gene delivery. *J. Virol.* **1998**, *72*, 9873–9880.
13. Richter, M.; Saydaminova, K.; Yumul, R.; Krishnan, R.; Liu, J.; Nagy, E.E.; Singh, M.; Izsvak, Z.; Cattaneo, R.; Uckert, W.; et al. In vivo transduction of primitive mobilized hematopoietic stem cells after intravenous injection of integrating adenovirus vectors. *Blood* **2016**, *128*, 2206–2217. [CrossRef]
14. Schmid, M.; Ernst, P.; Honegger, A.; Suomalainen, M.; Zimmermann, M.; Braun, L.; Stauffer, S.; Thom, C.; Dreier, B.; Eibauer, M.; et al. Adenoviral vector with shield and adapter increases tumor specificity and escapes liver and immune control. *Nat. Commun.* **2018**, *9*, 450. [CrossRef]
15. Wold, W.S.; Toth, K. Adenovirus vectors for gene therapy, vaccination and cancer gene therapy. *Curr. Gene Ther.* **2013**, *13*, 421–433. [CrossRef]
16. Wang, H.; Georgakopoulou, A.; Psatha, N.; Li, C.; Capsali, C.; Samal, H.B.; Anagnostopoulos, A.; Ehrhardt, A.; Izsvak, Z.; Papayannopoulou, T.; et al. In vivo hematopoietic stem cell gene therapy ameliorates murine thalassemia intermedia. *J. Clin. Investig.* **2019**, *129*, 598–615. [CrossRef]
17. Zhong, L.; Zhao, W.; Wu, J.; Maina, N.; Han, Z.; Srivastava, A. Adeno-associated virus-mediated gene transfer in hematopoietic stem/ progenitor cells as a therapeutic tool (Review). *Curr. Gene Ther.* **2006**, *6*, 683–698. [CrossRef]
18. Srivastava, A. In vivo tissue-tropism of adeno-associated viral vectors. *Curr. Opin. Virol.* **2016**, *21*, 75–80. [CrossRef]
19. Colella, P.; Ronzitti, G.; Mingozzi, F. Emerging issues in AAV-mediated in vivo gene therapy. *Mol. Ther. Methods Clin. Dev.* **2018**, *8*, 87–104. [CrossRef]

20. Manno, C.S.; Pierce, G.F.; Arruda, V.R.; Glader, B.; Ragni, M.; Rasko, J.J.; Ozelo, M.C.; Hoots, K.; Blatt, P.; Konkle, B.; et al. Successful transduction of liver in hemophilia by AAV-Factor IX and limitations imposed by the host immune response. *Nat. Med.* **2006**, *12*, 342–347. [CrossRef]
21. Marshall, E. Gene therapy death prompts review of adenovirus vector. *Science* **1999**, *286*, 2244–2245. [CrossRef]
22. Raper, S.E.; Chirmule, N.; Lee, F.S.; Wivel, N.A.; Bagg, A.; Gao, G.P.; Wilson, J.M.; Batshaw, M.L. Fatal systemic inflammatory response syndrome in a ornithine transcarbamylase deficient patient following adenoviral gene transfer. *Mol. Genet. Metab.* **2003**, *80*, 148–158. [CrossRef]
23. Van der Loo, J.C.; Wright, J.F. Progress and challenges in viral vector manufacturing. *Hum. Mol. Genet.* **2016**, *25*, R42–R52. [CrossRef]
24. Milone, M.C.; O'Doherty, U. Clinical use of lentiviral vectors. *Leukemia* **2018**, *32*, 1529–1541. [CrossRef]
25. Follenzi, A.; Santambrogio, L.; Annoni, A. Immune responses to lentiviral vectors. *Curr. Gene Ther.* **2007**, *7*, 306–315. [CrossRef]
26. Annoni, A.; Gregori, S.; Naldini, L.; Cantore, A. Modulation of immune responses in lentiviral vector-mediated gene transfer. *Cell. Immunol.* **2019**, *342*, 103802. [CrossRef]
27. Russell, D.W.; Miller, A.D. Foamy virus vectors. *J. Virol.* **1996**, *70*, 217–222.
28. Vassilopoulos, G.; Trobridge, G.; Josephson, N.C.; Russell, D.W. Gene transfer into murine hematopoietic stem cells with helper-free foamy virus vectors. *Blood* **2001**, *98*, 604–609. [CrossRef]
29. Trobridge, G.D.; Russell, D.W. Helper-free foamy virus vectors. *Hum. Gene Ther.* **1998**, *9*, 2517–2525. [CrossRef]
30. Hirata, R.K.; Miller, A.D.; Andrews, R.G.; Russell, D.W. Transduction of hematopoietic cells by foamy virus vectors. *Blood* **1996**, *88*, 3654–3661. [CrossRef]
31. Trobridge, G.D.; Miller, D.G.; Jacobs, M.A.; Allen, J.M.; Kiem, H.P.; Kaul, R.; Russell, D.W. Foamy virus vector integration sites in normal human cells. *Proc. Natl. Acad. Sci. USA* **2006**, *103*, 1498–1503. [CrossRef]
32. Kiem, H.P.; Allen, J.; Trobridge, G.; Olson, E.; Keyser, K.; Peterson, L.; Russell, D.W. Foamy virus-mediated gene transfer to canine repopulating cells. *Blood* **2007**, *109*, 65–70. [CrossRef]
33. Trobridge, G.D.; Allen, J.M.; Peterson, L.; Ironside, C.G.; Russell, D.W.; Kiem, H.P. Foamy and lentiviral vectors transduce canine long-term repopulating cells at similar efficiency. *Hum. Gene Ther.* **2009**, *20*, 519–523. [CrossRef]
34. Trobridge, G.D.; Beard, B.C.; Wu, R.A.; Ironside, C.; Malik, P.; Kiem, H.P. Stem cell selection in vivo using foamy vectors cures canine pyruvate kinase deficiency. *PLoS ONE* **2012**, *7*, e45173. [CrossRef]
35. Trobridge, G.D.; Horn, P.A.; Beard, B.C.; Kiem, H.P. Large animal models for foamy virus vector gene therapy. *Viruses* **2012**, *4*, 3572–3588. [CrossRef]
36. Thompson, A.A.; Walters, M.C.; Kwiatkowski, J.; Rasko, J.E.J.; Ribeil, J.A.; Hongeng, S.; Magrin, E.; Schiller, G.J.; Payen, E.; Semeraro, M.; et al. Gene therapy in patients with transfusion-dependent beta-thalassemia. *N. Engl. J. Med.* **2018**, *378*, 1479–1493. [CrossRef]
37. Ribeil, J.A.; Hacein-Bey-Abina, S.; Payen, E.; Magnani, A.; Semeraro, M.; Magrin, E.; Caccavelli, L.; Neven, B.; Bourget, P.; El Nemer, W.; et al. Gene therapy in a patient with sickle cell disease. *N. Engl. J. Med.* **2017**, *376*, 848–855. [CrossRef]
38. Hacein-Bey-Abina, S.; Hauer, J.; Lim, A.; Picard, C.; Wang, G.P.; Berry, C.C.; Martinache, C.; Rieux-Laucat, F.; Latour, S.; Belohradsky, B.H.; et al. Efficacy of gene therapy for X-linked severe combined immunodeficiency. *N. Engl. J. Med.* **2010**, *363*, 355–364. [CrossRef]
39. Aiuti, A.; Biasco, L.; Scaramuzza, S.; Ferrua, F.; Cicalese, M.P.; Baricordi, C.; Dionisio, F.; Calabria, A.; Giannelli, S.; Castiello, M.C.; et al. Lentiviral hematopoietic stem cell gene therapy in patients with Wiskott-Aldrich syndrome. *Science* **2013**, *341*, 1233151. [CrossRef]
40. Biffi, A.; Montini, E.; Lorioli, L.; Cesani, M.; Fumagalli, F.; Plati, T.; Baldoli, C.; Martino, S.; Calabria, A.; Canale, S.; et al. Lentiviral hematopoietic stem cell gene therapy benefits metachromatic leukodystrophy. *Science* **2013**, *341*, 1233158. [CrossRef]
41. Sessa, M.; Lorioli, L.; Fumagalli, F.; Acquati, S.; Redaelli, D.; Baldoli, C.; Canale, S.; Lopez, I.D.; Morena, F.; Calabria, A.; et al. Lentiviral haemopoietic stem-cell gene therapy in early-onset metachromatic leukodystrophy: An ad-hoc analysis of a non-randomised, open-label, phase 1/2 trial. *Lancet* **2016**, *388*, 476–487. [CrossRef]

42. De Ravin, S.S.; Wu, X.; Moir, S.; Anaya-O'Brien, S.; Kwatemaa, N.; Littel, P.; Theobald, N.; Choi, U.; Su, L.; Marquesen, M.; et al. Lentiviral hematopoietic stem cell gene therapy for X-linked severe combined immunodeficiency. *Sci. Transl. Med.* **2016**, *8*, 335ra57. [CrossRef] [PubMed]
43. Kennedy, D.R.; McLellan, K.; Moore, P.F.; Henthorn, P.S.; Felsburg, P.J. Effect of ex vivo culture of CD34+ bone marrow cells on immune reconstitution of XSCID dogs following allogeneic bone marrow transplantation. *Biol. Blood Marrow Transplant.* **2009**, *15*, 662–670. [CrossRef] [PubMed]
44. Cavazzana, M. Innovations needed for effective implementation of ex vivo gene therapies. *Front. Med.* **2017**, *4*, 29. [CrossRef]
45. Yin, H.; Kanasty, R.L.; Eltoukhy, A.A.; Vegas, A.J.; Dorkin, J.R.; Anderson, D.G. Non-viral vectors for gene-based therapy. *Nat. Rev. Genet.* **2014**, *15*, 541–555. [CrossRef]
46. Lundstrom, K. Viral vectors in gene therapy. *Diseases* **2018**, *6*, 42. [CrossRef]
47. Adams, D.; Gonzalez-Duarte, A.; O'Riordan, W.D.; Yang, C.C.; Ueda, M.; Kristen, A.V.; Tournev, I.; Schmidt, H.H.; Coelho, T.; Berk, J.L.; et al. Patisiran, an RNAi therapeutic, for hereditary transthyretin amyloidosis. *N. Engl. J. Med.* **2018**, *379*, 11–21. [CrossRef]
48. Pardi, N.; Secreto, A.J.; Shan, X.; Debonera, F.; Glover, J.; Yi, Y.; Muramatsu, H.; Ni, H.; Mui, B.L.; Tam, Y.K.; et al. Administration of nucleoside-modified mRNA encoding broadly neutralizing antibody protects humanized mice from HIV-1 challenge. *Nat. Commun.* **2017**, *8*, 14630. [CrossRef]
49. Naldini, L.; Blömer, U.; Gallay, P.; Ory, D.; Mulligan, R.; Gage, F.H.; Verma, I.M.; Trono, D. In vivo gene delivery and stable transduction of nondividing cells by a lentiviral vector. *Science* **1996**, *272*, 263–267. [CrossRef]
50. Raper, S.E.; Yudkoff, M.; Chirmule, N.; Gao, G.P.; Nunes, F.; Haskal, Z.J.; Furth, E.E.; Propert, K.J.; Robinson, M.B.; Magosin, S.; et al. A pilot study of in vivo liver-directed gene transfer with an adenoviral vector in partial ornithine transcarbamylase deficiency. *Hum. Gene Ther.* **2002**, *13*, 163–175. [CrossRef]
51. Hacein-Bey-Abina, S.; von Kalle, C.; Schmidt, M.; Le Deist, F.; Wulffraat, N.; McIntyre, E.; Radford, I.; Villeval, J.L.; Fraser, C.C.; Cavazzana-Calvo, M.; et al. A serious adverse event after successful gene therapy for X-linked severe combined immunodeficiency. *N. Eng. J. Med.* **2003**, *348*, 255–256. [CrossRef]
52. Hacein-Bey-Abina, S.; von Kalle, C.; Schmidt, M.; McCormack, M.P.; Wulffraat, N.; Leboulch, P.; Lim, A.; Osborne, C.S.; Pawliuk, R.; Morillon, E.; et al. LMO2-associated clonal T cell proliferation in two patients after gene therapy for SCID-X1. *Science* **2003**, *302*, 415–419. [CrossRef]
53. Hacein-Bey-Abina, S.; Garrigue, A.; Wang, G.P.; Soulier, J.; Lim, A.; Morillon, E.; Clappier, E.; Caccavelli, L.; Delabesse, E.; Beldjord, K.; et al. Insertional oncogenesis in 4 patients after retrovirus-mediated gene therapy of SCID-X1. *J. Clin. Investig.* **2008**, *118*, 3132–3142. [CrossRef] [PubMed]
54. Alba, R.; Bosch, A.; Chillon, M. Gutless adenovirus: Last-generation adenovirus for gene therapy. *Gene Ther.* **2005**, *12* (Suppl. S1), S18–S27. [CrossRef]
55. Li, C.; Psatha, N.; Wang, H.; Singh, M.; Samal, H.B.; Zhang, W.; Ehrhardt, A.; Izsvak, Z.; Papayannopoulou, T.; Lieber, A. Integrating HDAd5/35++ vectors as a new platform for HSC gene therapy of hemoglobinopathies. *Mol. Ther. Methods Clin. Dev.* **2018**, *9*, 142–152. [CrossRef] [PubMed]
56. Lee, C.S.; Bishop, E.S.; Zhang, R.; Yu, X.; Farina, E.M.; Yan, S.; Zhao, C.; Zheng, Z.; Shu, Y.; Wu, X.; et al. Adenovirus-mediated gene delivery: Potential applications for gene and cell-based therapies in the new era of personalized medicine. *Genes Dis.* **2017**, *4*, 43–63. [CrossRef] [PubMed]
57. Thornhill, S.I.; Schambach, A.; Howe, S.J.; Ulaganathan, M.; Grassman, E.; Williams, D.; Schiedlmeier, B.; Sebire, N.J.; Gaspar, H.B.; Kinnon, C.; et al. Self-inactivating gammaretroviral vectors for gene therapy of X-linked severe combined immunodeficiency. *Mol. Ther.* **2008**, *16*, 590–598. [CrossRef]
58. Miyoshi, H.; Blomer, U.; Takahashi, M.; Gage, F.H.; Verma, I.M. Development of a self-inactivating lentivirus vector. *J. Virol.* **1998**, *72*, 8150–8157.
59. Rio, P.; Navarro, S.; Wang, W.; Sanchez-Dominguez, R.; Pujol, R.M.; Segovia, J.C.; Bogliolo, M.; Merino, E.; Wu, N.; Salgado, R.; et al. Successful engraftment of gene-corrected hematopoietic stem cells in non-conditioned patients with Fanconi anemia. *Nat. Med.* **2019**, *25*, 1396–1401. [CrossRef]
60. High, K.A.; Roncarolo, M.G. Gene Therapy. *N. Engl. J. Med.* **2019**, *381*, 455–464. [CrossRef]
61. Kotterman, M.A.; Chalberg, T.W.; Schaffer, D.V. Viral vectors for gene therapy: Translational and clinical outlook. *Annu. Rev. Biomed. Eng.* **2015**, *17*, 63–89. [CrossRef] [PubMed]

62. Huang, T.T.; Parab, S.; Burnett, R.; Diago, O.; Ostertag, D.; Hofman, F.M.; Espinoza, F.L.; Martin, B.; Ibanez, C.E.; Kasahara, N.; et al. Intravenous administration of retroviral replicating vector, Toca 511, demonstrates therapeutic efficacy in orthotopic immune-competent mouse glioma model. *Hum. Gene Ther.* **2015**, *26*, 82–93. [CrossRef] [PubMed]
63. Palfi, S.; Gurruchaga, J.M.; Ralph, G.S.; Lepetit, H.; Lavisse, S.; Buttery, P.C.; Watts, C.; Miskin, J.; Kelleher, M.; Deeley, S.; et al. Long-term safety and tolerability of ProSavin, a lentiviral vector-based gene therapy for Parkinson's disease: A dose escalation, open-label, phase 1/2 trial. *Lancet* **2014**, *383*, 1138–1146. [CrossRef]
64. Campochiaro, P.A.; Lauer, A.K.; Sohn, E.H.; Mir, T.A.; Naylor, S.; Anderton, M.C.; Kelleher, M.; Harrop, R.; Ellis, S.; Mitrophanous, K.A. Lentiviral vector gene transfer of endostatin/angiostatin for macular degeneration (GEM) study. *Hum. Gene Ther.* **2017**, *28*, 99–111. [CrossRef]
65. Cantore, A.; Ranzani, M.; Bartholomae, C.C.; Volpin, M.; Valle, P.D.; Sanvito, F.; Sergi, L.S.; Gallina, P.; Benedicenti, F.; Bellinger, D.; et al. Liver-directed lentiviral gene therapy in a dog model of hemophilia B. *Sci. Transl. Med.* **2015**, *7*, 277ra28. [CrossRef]
66. Milani, M.; Annoni, A.; Bartolaccini, S.; Biffi, M.; Russo, F.; Di Tomaso, T.; Raimondi, A.; Lengler, J.; Holmes, M.C.; Scheiflinger, F.; et al. Genome editing for scalable production of alloantigen-free lentiviral vectors for in vivo gene therapy. *EMBO Mol. Med.* **2017**, *9*, 1558–1573. [CrossRef]
67. Bernadin, O.; Amirache, F.; Girard-Gagnepain, A.; Moirangthem, R.D.; Levy, C.; Ma, K.; Costa, C.; Negre, D.; Reimann, C.; Fenard, D.; et al. Baboon envelope LVs efficiently transduced human adult, fetal, and progenitor T cells and corrected SCID-X1 T-cell deficiency. *Blood Adv.* **2019**, *3*, 461–475. [CrossRef]
68. Munis, A.M.; Mattiuzzo, G.; Bentley, E.M.; Collins, M.K.; Eyles, J.E.; Takeuchi, Y. Use of heterologous vesiculovirus G proteins circumvents the humoral anti-envelope immunity in lentivector-based in vivo gene delivery. *Mol. Ther. Nucleic Acids* **2019**, *17*, 126–137. [CrossRef]
69. Donsante, A.; Miller, D.G.; Li, Y.; Vogler, C.; Brunt, E.M.; Russell, D.W.; Sands, M.S. AAV vector integration sites in mouse hepatocellular carcinoma. *Science* **2007**, *317*, 477. [CrossRef]
70. Xiong, W.; Wu, D.M.; Xue, Y.; Wang, S.K.; Chung, M.J.; Ji, X.; Rana, P.; Zhao, S.R.; Mai, S.; Cepko, C.L. AAV cis-regulatory sequences are correlated with ocular toxicity. *Proc. Natl. Acad. Sci. USA* **2019**, *116*, 5785–5794. [CrossRef]
71. Hinderer, C.; Katz, N.; Buza, E.L.; Dyer, C.; Goode, T.; Bell, P.; Richman, L.K.; Wilson, J.M. Severe toxicity in nonhuman primates and piglets following high-dose intravenous administration of an adeno-associated virus vector expressing human SMN. *Hum. Gene Ther.* **2018**, *29*, 285–298. [CrossRef] [PubMed]
72. Lindemann, D.; Rethwilm, A. Foamy virus biology and its application for vector development. *Viruses* **2011**, *3*, 561–585. [CrossRef] [PubMed]
73. Meiering, C.D.; Linial, M.L. Historical perspective of foamy virus epidemiology and infection. *Clin. Microbiol. Rev.* **2001**, *14*, 165–176. [CrossRef] [PubMed]
74. Nasimuzzaman, M.; Persons, D.A. Cell membrane-associated heparan sulfate is a receptor for prototype foamy virus in human, monkey, and rodent cells. *Mol. Ther.* **2012**, *20*, 1158–1166. [CrossRef] [PubMed]
75. Linial, M. Why aren't foamy viruses pathogenic? *Trends Microbiol.* **2000**, *8*, 284–289. [CrossRef]
76. Everson, E.M.; Olzsko, M.E.; Leap, D.J.; Hocum, J.D.; Trobridge, G.D. A comparison of foamy and lentiviral vector genotoxicity in SCID-repopulating cells shows foamy vectors are less prone to clonal dominance. *Mol. Ther. Methods Clin. Dev.* **2016**, *3*, 16048. [CrossRef]
77. Beard, B.C.; Keyser, K.A.; Trobridge, G.D.; Peterson, L.J.; Miller, D.G.; Jacobs, M.; Kaul, R.; Kiem, H.P. Unique integration profiles in a canine model of long-term repopulating cells transduced with gammaretrovirus, lentivirus, and foamy virus. *Hum. Gene Ther.* **2007**, *18*, 423–434. [CrossRef]
78. Takeuchi, Y.; Liong, S.H.; Bieniasz, P.D.; Jager, U.; Porter, C.D.; Friedman, T.; McClure, M.O.; Weiss, R.A. Sensitization of rhabdo-, lenti-, and spumaviruses to human serum by galactosyl(alpha1-3)galactosylation. *J. Virol.* **1997**, *71*, 6174–6178.
79. Trobridge, G.D. Foamy virus vectors for gene transfer (Review). *Expert Opin. Biol. Ther.* **2009**, *9*, 1427–1436. [CrossRef]
80. Jezyk, P.F.; Felsburg, P.J.; Haskins, M.E.; Patterson, D.F. X-linked severe combined immunodeficiency in the dog. *Clin. Immunol. Immunopathol.* **1989**, *52*, 173–189. [CrossRef]

81. Felsburg, P.J.; Somberg, R.L.; Hartnett, B.J.; Henthorn, P.S.; Carding, S.R. Canine X-linked severe combined immunodeficiency. A model for investigating the requirement for the common gamma chain (gamma c) in human lymphocyte development and function (Review). *Immunol. Res.* **1998**, *17*, 63–73. [CrossRef] [PubMed]
82. Henthorn, P.S.; Somberg, R.L.; Fimiani, V.M.; Puck, J.M.; Patterson, D.F.; Felsburg, P.J. IL-2R gamma gene microdeletion demonstrates that canine X-linked severe combined immunodeficiency is a homologue of the human disease. *Genomics* **1994**, *23*, 69–74. [CrossRef] [PubMed]
83. Ting-De Ravin, S.S.; Kennedy, D.R.; Naumann, N.; Kennedy, J.S.; Choi, U.; Hartnett, B.J.; Linton, G.F.; Whiting-Theobald, N.L.; Moore, P.F.; Vernau, W.; et al. Correction of canine X-linked severe combined immunodeficiency by in vivo retroviral gene therapy. *Blood* **2006**, *107*, 3091–3097. [CrossRef] [PubMed]
84. Hopman, R.K.; DiPersio, J.F. Advances in stem cell mobilization. *Blood Rev.* **2014**, *28*, 31–40. [CrossRef] [PubMed]
85. Liles, W.C.; Broxmeyer, H.E.; Rodger, E.; Wood, B.; Hubel, K.; Cooper, S.; Hangoc, G.; Bridger, G.J.; Henson, G.W.; Calandra, G.; et al. Mobilization of hematopoietic progenitor cells in healthy volunteers by AMD3100, a CXCR4 antagonist. *Blood* **2003**, *102*, 2728–2730. [CrossRef]
86. Broxmeyer, H.E.; Orschell, C.M.; Clapp, D.W.; Hangoc, G.; Cooper, S.; Plett, P.A.; Liles, W.C.; Li, X.; Graham-Evans, B.; Campbell, T.B.; et al. Rapid mobilization of murine and human hematopoietic stem and progenitor cells with AMD3100, a CXCR4 antagonist. *J. Exp. Med.* **2005**, *201*, 1307–1318. [CrossRef]
87. DiPersio, J.F.; Stadtmauer, E.A.; Nademanee, A.; Micallef, I.N.; Stiff, P.J.; Kaufman, J.L.; Maziarz, R.T.; Hosing, C.; Fruehauf, S.; Horwitz, M.; et al. Plerixafor and G-CSF versus placebo and G-CSF to mobilize hematopoietic stem cells for autologous stem cell transplantation in patients with multiple myeloma. *Blood* **2009**, *113*, 5720–5726. [CrossRef]
88. Flomenberg, N.; Devine, S.M.; DiPersio, J.F.; Liesveld, J.L.; McCarty, J.M.; Rowley, S.D.; Vesole, D.H.; Badel, K.; Calandra, G. The use of AMD3100 plus G-CSF for autologous hematopoietic progenitor cell mobilization is superior to G-CSF alone. *Blood* **2005**, *106*, 1867–1874. [CrossRef]
89. Burroughs, L.; Mielcarek, M.; Little, M.T.; Bridger, G.; MacFarland, R.; Fricker, S.; LaBrecque, J.; Sandmaier, B.M.; Storb, R. Durable engraftment of AMD3100-mobilized autologous and allogeneic peripheral blood mononuclear cells in a canine transplantation model. *Blood* **2005**, *106*, 4002–4008. [CrossRef]
90. Wang, X.; Shin, S.C.; Chiang, A.F.; Khan, I.; Pan, D.; Rawlings, D.J.; Miao, C.H. Intraosseous delivery of lentiviral vectors targeting factor VIII expression in platelets corrects murine hemophilia A. *Mol. Ther.* **2015**, *23*, 617–626. [CrossRef]
91. Wang, H.; Richter, M.; Psatha, N.; Li, C.; Kim, J.; Liu, J.; Ehrhardt, A.; Nilsson, S.K.; Cao, B.; Palmer, D.; et al. A combined in vivo HSC transduction/selection approach results in efficient and stable gene expression in peripheral blood cells in mice. *Mol. Ther. Methods Clin. Dev.* **2018**, *8*, 52–64. [CrossRef] [PubMed]

viruses

MDPI

Review

FV Vectors as Alternative Gene Vehicles for Gene Transfer in HSCs

Emmanouil Simantirakis [1], Ioannis Tsironis [1] and George Vassilopoulos [1,2,*]

1 Gene Therapy Lab, Biomedical Research Foundation of the Academy of Athens, Division of Genetics and Gene Therapy, Basic Research II, 11527 Athens, Greece; esimantirakis@bioacademy.gr (E.S.); tsironis@upatras.gr (I.T.)
2 Division of Hematology, University of Thessaly Medical School, 41500 Larissa, Greece
* Correspondence: gvasilop@bioacademy.gr

Received: 8 January 2020; Accepted: 15 March 2020; Published: 19 March 2020

Abstract: Hematopoietic Stem Cells (HSCs) are a unique population of cells, capable of reconstituting the blood system of an organism through orchestrated self-renewal and differentiation. They play a pivotal role in stem cell therapies, both autologous and allogeneic. In the field of gene and cell therapy, HSCs, genetically modified or otherwise, are used to alleviate or correct a genetic defect. In this concise review, we discuss the use of SFVpsc_huHSRV.13, formerly known as Prototype Foamy Viral (PFV or FV) vectors, as vehicles for gene delivery in HSCs. We present the properties of the FV vectors that make them ideal for HSC delivery vehicles, we review their record in HSC gene marking studies and their potential as therapeutic vectors for monogenic disorders in preclinical animal models. FVs are a safe and efficient tool for delivering genes in HSCs compared to other retroviral gene delivery systems. Novel technological advancements in their production and purification in closed systems, have allowed their production under cGMP compliant conditions. It may only be a matter of time before they find their way into the clinic.

Keywords: foamy virus; gene therapy; HSC; gene marking; FV gene transfer to HSCs; gene therapy alternatives

1. Introduction

Hematopoietic Stem Cells (HSCs) are rare cells residing in the Bone Marrow (BM) that can support blood cell production for the lifetime of an individual. This is achieved through HSCs potential to differentiate and self-renew [1]. The self-renewal process is the central dogma in stem cell biology and is a character that is lost when HSCs are extensively manipulated ex vivo; this observation argues for the substantial contribution of the BM milieu in supporting HSCs. Practically, both HSC nature and BM nurture, in a coordinated interplay, allow HSCs to express their unique characters [2]. What has been elusive is the HSC per se; HSC cannot be identified by morphology but only by surface markers and functional assays.

In humans, HSCs are considered as CD34+ cells residing in the mononuclear cell population of the BM. Not all HSCs are CD34+ but a significant fraction of CD34+ cells are HSCs; this circular argument can be rephrased to convey that CD34+ cells are enriched in HSC and CD34 marking is used to assay whether a certain cell population has enough HSC to serve as a donor for a transplantation experiment [3]. The latter is the sole surrogate marker to assay whether a population of cells has the potential to support hematopoiesis in a myeloablated host. In addition, Stem Cell Transplantation (SCT), is the ultimate marker to support the potential of a viral vector to correct a genetic defect in a HSC; the marked or corrected cells of the donor will be present in the blood cells of the recipient host and will provide phenotypic correction for a lifetime.

Allogeneic SCT (ASCT) has been used since around the '70s for the treatment of acute leukemias. ASCT for genetic defects such as thalassemia was introduced in the 90s and achieved high cure rates for those who had a suitable donor [4]. In contrast, transplantation with autologous gene-corrected HSCs entered the therapeutic armamentarium around the year 2000 and was only recently endorsed as a therapeutic option by the FDA [5]. Gene correction for HSC requires the permanent integration of the vector in the host-HSC genome; if episomal, the vector is destined to dilute out at some point in the subsequent cell divisions since episomes do not faithfully follow the cell's DNA mitotic cycles [6]. Retroviruses are viruses with potential of permanent integration, which is a prerequisite for viral gene expression and a productive life cycle.

There are two subfamilies of Retroviruses: the first is the *Orthoretrovirinae* that includes the Genera *Lentivirus* and *Gammaretrovirus* (GV), and the second is *Spumaretrovirinae* that includes the genera *Simiispumavirus* and *Felispumavirus* [7]. The human foamy virus isolates are actually chimpanzee foamy viruses. There are three to date: human isolate HSRV clone 13 SFVpsc_huHSRV.13, human isolate BAD327 SFVptr_huBAD327, and human isolate AG15 SFVptr_huAG15 [7]. For simplicity and familiarity reasons, in this article, wherever we refer to SFVpsc_huHSRV.13 we shall use the name PFV, HSRV, or FV vectors. The first vectors to be developed for gene transfer purposes were those with the gamma-retroviral backbones and were used for genetic correction of immunodeficiency syndromes after extended preclinical validations [8,9]. However, along with the successes, novel problems emerged; The not-so-random insertion of the retroviruses close to oncogenes, resulted in the development of leukemias [10]. The development of high throughput technologies allowed the mapping of Retroviral Integration Sites (RIS) and shed light on the gammaretroviral vector potential to cause leukemias, in relation to their preference for specific genomic sites. Gammaretroviral vectors as well as Lentiviral vectors demonstrate a preference for the integration of their retroviral cDNA into transcriptionally active sites in the host genome [11]. In addition, the Gammaretroviral vectors showed an increased preference for landing near oncogenes, a potentially dangerous condition [12]. Further data showed that different genera of retroviruses have distinct preferences for genomic integrations: Gammaretroviral vectors and Foamy Viral vectors prefer to integrate in proximity to transcription start sites and regulatory elements like CpG islands, while Lentiviral vectors tend to integrate within coding sequences [13–15]. Beyond safety, a problem that retroviruses had in relation to the need for long-term expression in the context of HSCs, was the frequent observed silencing of the transferred transgene. Although silencing was related to the methylation of the retroviral DNA [16,17], a problem that could be solved with the use of insulator elements [18] or partially reversed with hypomethylating agents [19], the quest for a more efficient gene transfer vehicle did not seize.

In a chronological order, the two other kinds of retroviruses that were tested for their HSC gene transfer potential were the Lenti- and the Foamy- or Spuma- derived vectors. In a seminal paper on Lenti-vectors, the authors reported long-term gene marking in CD34+ cells transplanted in NOD/SCID mice [20]. Reports on the potential of Spuma- (or Foamy Virus, FV) derived vectors to transduce efficiently both murine and human HSCs and to express the transferred gene in a long-term manner, came soon after [21]. Although, currently, Lenti has gained tremendous popularity as a gene transfer tool and has obtained commercial approval for human use, FV-derived vectors are a safe and efficient alternative for gene transfer into HSCs [22,23]. Beyond HSC gene transfer, FV vectors of feline origin have been developed as gene transfer vehicles and have been tested so far in cell lines [24]; an interesting application of these vectors is their use as vehicles for the transfer of genes that induce immune responses to feline viruses [25]. In this review, we will present all the relative data that confirm the potential of FV-derived vectors as a non-inferior vehicle for HSC gene transfer and therapy. The main features of each retroviral gene delivery system are summarized in Table 1.

Table 1. Features of Retroviral gene delivery systems.

Vector System	Lenti-	Gammaretro-	Foamy-
Transgene Capacity (kb)	9 [26]	10 [27]	At least 9 [28]
Self-Inactivating (SIN) design	+ [29]	+ [30]	+ [31]
Generation	3rd	3rd	3rd
Presence of insulators in design	+	+	+
Pseudotyping	+	+	-
Cell cycle requirement			
cGMP complience	+	+	possible
Preferred integration sites in host genome	Active transcriptional units [11]	Transcriptional start sites and CpG islands [11,32]	Constitutively lamina associated regions (cLAD) and less often CpGs [15]

2. Features of FV Vectors for HSC Gene Delivery

A number of features are essential for any vector to be suitable for HSC gene transfer. Target cell tropism is the principal condition, and FV vectors have shown that they can transduce a number of cell lines and murine hematopoietic progenitors and stem cells early on during the vector development history [21,33,34]. The broad spectrum of permissive cells for FV transduction, suggested that an abundant molecule on the cell surface was facilitating FV attachment and/or entry. This molecule was later identified as heparan sulfate [35,36]. The expression of heparan sulfate in a wide variety of cells and its use by FVs as a non-specific receptor could explain the wide cell tropism that this vector demonstrates.

Another key principal for any gene transfer vehicle is its ability to deliver its cargo into non-dividing cells such as the HSCs. This principle was assessed through experiments that tested FV vector transgene expression in vivo after transplantation of transduced HSCs. Given that reporter gene expression can be traced in transplant recipients, it can be inferred that true, non-dividing HSCs were transduced by FV vectors [21,37]. However, gene transfer in HSCs occurs after the 5FU treatment of the HSC donor animals and the ex vivo manipulation of cells under strong cytokine stimulation; in such conditions, HSCs are practically forced to divide. Thus, conclusions on FV gene transfer into non-dividing cells from such experiments could not be confidently reached. It was later shown in a different cellular system that although FV DNA lacks nuclear localization signals, the FV DNA can survive long enough in the cytoplasm in anticipation of a subsequent cell division that will result in nuclear membrane break down [38,39]. Under such conditions, FV DNA can enter the nucleus and establish a productive infection or transduction. However, it should be clarified that FVs are complex retroviruses. Their replication demands an RNA intermediate from which viral cDNA synthesis occurs by the activity of viral reverse transcriptase. Furthermore, in in vitro systems, it has been observed that the reverse transcription of viral RNA is completed before virus budding [13].

Following cellular entry and nuclear penetration, gene transfer vehicles must also have long-term expression in daughter cells. This is a prerequisite for therapeutic procedures whose results are expected to span the lifetime of an individual. Vector gene silencing occurs through DNA methylation/histone acetylation and has been a central problem in gene transfer with retroviral vectors [16,17]. This does not seem to be a problem with FV vectors, since (i) transgene silencing has not been reported in any of the in vivo studies published so far and (ii) it has been shown that FV Long Terminal Repeats (LTRs) have the potential to insulate the vector genome when integrated in the host cell DNA [31,40]. The FV insulation can be seen as a double-edged sword; it protects the transgene from external effects but also protects the genomic environment from the effects of the FV vectors. This prompts the issue of activation of neighboring oncogenes at the integration site. Compared to LVs and GVs in in vitro immortalization assays, FV vectors had the lowest rate of read-through transcripts. When the LMO2 site was targeted for insertion, LMO2 mRNA increments were 280x for GV, 200x for LV, and 45x for FV vectors, normalized for genomic integration site, indicating insulator properties of the LTR. This low read-through transcription of an integrated FV vector occurs due to a 36 bp long CTCF binding motif inside its LTR. CTCF is the major chromatin insulator protein in vertebrates and binds the CCCTC sequence via various combinations of 11 zinc fingers [41].

After cell tropism and long-term expression is the issue of safety. From data on zookeepers that are chronic FV carriers, we have reassuring evidence that wtFV, causes no harm to its hosts [42,43]. However, beyond the wtFV non-pathogenic characteristics, foamy viral vectors possess a number of features making them attractive for use in gene therapy. Current FV designs consist of a split four plasmid system: the transfer vector and three accessory or helper packaging plasmids [44,45]. The packaging plasmids encode the Gag, Pol, and Env proteins; the Tas (or Bel1) and Bet proteins required for the infection and replication of the wtFV are dispensable for vector production and can be omitted. Furthermore, the vectors have a self-inactivating (SIN) design; deletion of the 3′LTR U3 region in the transfer plasmid is copied in in the 5′LTR sequence during packaging, rendering the deleted FVs safe for gene therapy applications. Bet deletion also renders the host cell susceptible to superinfection (multiple rounds of infection), a desirable feature for difficult to transduce cell targets [15,31,46]. PFV vectors were developed independently in the States and in Europe by Russel's [44] and Rethwilm's [47] groups, respectively. Here, we shall elaborate on the vectors developed by the Russel group. The FV vectors originated from the wtFV strain SFVpsc_huHSRV.13 [48]. The wt provirus map is presented in Figure 1. The viral cDNA contains three overlapping open reading frames (ORFs). The viral cDNA also encodes the genes *gag*, *pol*, and *env*. The latter three are typical of all retroviruses. The aforementioned overlapping ORF encodes the genes *bel1/tas*, *bel2*, and *bel3*. Tas is a transactivator protein that binds into the internal promoter present in *env* and 5′LTR promoters and enhances the transcription of the wt integrated FV viral genome. Additionally, Bet results from the translation of spliced *bel1* and *bel2* ORF mRNA. Bel1-3 and Bet are not required for viral replication in vitro. Thus, they are omitted from vector designs. The current vectors comprise of four plasmids. A transfer vector with deleted viral LTRs. Some important cis-acting elements exist between the 5′LTR and *gag*, a part of the 5′ *gag* (CAS I) sequence, a part of the 3′ *pol* (CAS II) sequence, and a part of the 5′ *env* sequence. The 3′ LTR bears a deletion in the U3 region. Additionally, the 5′ LTR is fused with the CMV promoter to render the vector Tas independent. In order to avoid the generation of the replication competent virus in the packaging cell lines, the Gag, Pol, and Env are expressed by separate plasmids. The coding sequences bear minimal overlap [21,28,44,49].

In the recent years, more light has been shed on the integration site profile of FVs on the host cell genome. On studies performed on human HSCs transduced with FV vectors, the vectors seemed to prefer integrating upstream of transcription start sites specifically within CpG islands, with only 4.4% of the integration sites to be 50kb proximal to proto-oncogenes [13,31,41]. Although Integration Sites (IS) proximity to the genes remains largely random, the preference that the FV vectors display makes them relatively safer than GV and LV vectors, as they prefer constitutively lamina associated regions (cLAD) and less often CpGs [15] to integrate.

An issue of interest in gene therapy applications is the transgene payload that a vector can carry. Transgene payload is of paramount importance because regulated gene expression requires non-coding sequences of significant length. As a rule of thumb, one should not exceed the length of the wt genome or a significant drop in titer is inevitable. Foamy viruses have the largest genome among retroviruses and as a result, FV vectors have enough space to accommodate a little over 9 kb of exogenous DNA [44].

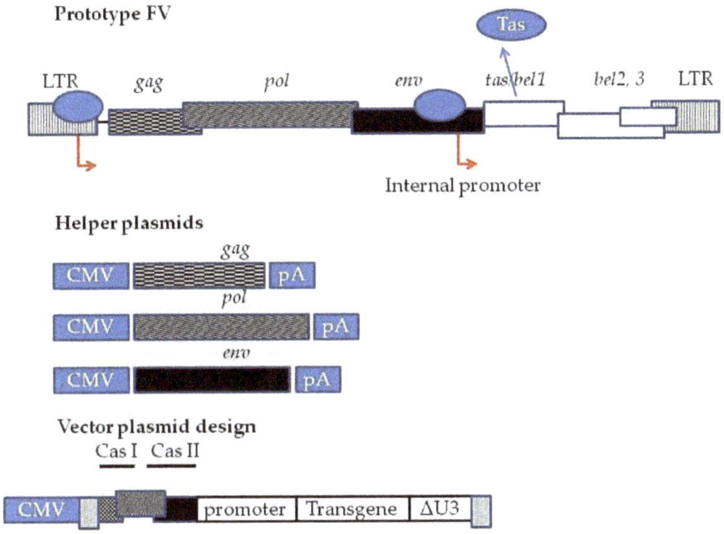

Figure 1. Third generation Foamy Virus (FV) vector system. At the top wtPFV provirus genome is depicted. The LTR contains the entire U3 region of the Human Foamy Virus (HFV.). Red arrows indicated the promoters driving the expression of FV genes, as well as the internal promoter present inside the *env* sequence driving the expression of *tas*. *tas* is expressed at basal levels when the provirus integrates into host cell genome. Upon translation, Tas binds to the LTR and internal promoter and enhances the transcription of *gag*, *pol*, and *env*. Additionally, Tas enhances the transcription of *bel1*, *bel2*, and *bel3*. *bel1* and *bel2* transcripts splice into a single mRNA whose translation generates Bet. In third -generation systems, the FV genome is split into a four-plasmid system comprised of three helper plasmids encoding *gag*, *pol*, and *env* under the control of a CMV promoter and a pA (polyadenylation signal) to allow the packaging cell lines to express the proteins at high levels. Transfer vector is comprised of deleted LTRs. Viral RNA expression is driven by a CMV promoter and an important cis-acting element sequence between the 5′LTR and *gag*, a part of the 5′ *gag* (CAS I) sequence, a part of the 3′ *pol* (CAS II) sequence and a part of the 5′ *env* sequence. These sequences are necessary for efficient virion assembly. The CMV 5′LTR fusion renders the viral vector production in packaging cell lines (HEK293T) Tas independent. Moreover, there is a deletion of the U3 region of LTR. Following integration into the transduced cell genome, the Tas dependent LTR promoter is regenerated. This fact renders the vector SIN and shuts the expression driven by 5′ LTR off. Transgene expression is driven by internal promoters.

Finally, and aiming at practical applications, comes the issue of titers and storage. FV vectors can be concentrated by ultracentrifugation [44,45]. The codon optimization and expression design optimization of packaging and transfer vector plasmid sequences have allowed for the generation of high titer FV vector supernatants. These modifications rendered FV vectors as efficient as lentiviral vectors producing 10×10^7 TU/mL of crude supernatant [44]. Finally, FV supernatants can be concentrated and purified in closed systems using affinity chromatography with POROS-Heparin columns, followed by Tangential Flow Filtration and ultracentrifugation [50] or size exclusion chromatography using CaptoCore columns followed by sepharose-heparin affinity chromatography and ultracentrifugation [51]. Both purification approaches are performed in closed systems compliant with cGMP and yield significantly pure preparations. Lastly, in regard to storage, although not reported in the literature per se, we have developed a freezing medium that allows repeated freeze/thaw cycles with 80–90% yields in vector titer.

3. Gene Marking Studies in Small Animals

Replication incompetent FV vectors were shown to transduce nearly every cell line including hematopoietic cell lines [33,34]. As the next leap forward, FV vectors were tested for their gene marking potential with murine HSCs after transplantation into lethally irradiated hosts [21]. The data showed that FV vectors could transduce murine HSC with a marking efficiency of about 50% and after transplantation there was sustained expression of the transgene for over 6 months. Similarly, when human HSCs (CD34+) cells were transduced and transplanted in ablated NOD/SCID animals, high levels of gene marking were observed across all lineages, indicating the transduction of a true human HSC [37]. In a direct head-to-head comparison between GV, LV and FV vectors with identical constructs, FV vectors performed as efficiently as the LV vectors, indicating FV vectors' potential for clinical applications [52].

Another notable mention is that in close to 500 animals that we have transplanted, we never encountered an adverse outcome such as leukemia or lymphomaThese early observations on murine and human HSCs were the first indications that FV derived vectors were a relatively safe vector system that did not cause any harm in the HSC genomes and could thus be further tested in preclinical animal models as a therapeutic gene transfer vehicle.

4. Therapeutic Gene Transfer in Murine Preclinical Models

The testing ground for any gene therapy vector has traditionally been the genetic correction of β-thalassemia. Two such FV vectors have been developed and tested side-by-side. The expression cassette had the complete human β-globin gene under the control of the short native β-globin gene promoter with either an α-globin HS40 sequence, or a mini-LCR with the core sequences of the HS2 and HS3 regulatory elements from the β-globin LCR. Both vector viral stocks were used to transduce erythroleukemia lines, murine Lin- HSCs from normal and thalassemic mice and human CD34+ cells from β-thalassemia patients. The vectors had comparable efficiency in all settings, although the HS40 was marginally superior and more stable in vivo. In the thalassemic mouse model Hbbth3/+, the transplantation of FV-transduced HSCs with the HS40 vector resulted in 43% of peripheral blood expressing human β globin at 6 months post transplantation. This level of expression is adequate to establish a thalassemia carrier phenotype and a therapeutic effect [53].

Another monogenic recessive disorder amenable to treatment with gene therapy is chronic granulomatous disease (CGD) [54]; the X-linked form of the disease results from mutations in the CYBB gene that encodes the gp91phox, the larger subunit of the oxidase flavocytochrome b558. Patients with CGD lack production of microbicidal superoxide, resulting in recurrent infections and early deaths in childhood. An FV vector carrying the *gp91phox* gene under the control of a PGK or a MSCV-LTR promoter was tested for its ability to restore superoxide levels in transplanted animals. With an average of 41.5% chimerism, the transplanted animals displayed phagoburst activity that reached 40% of the wt animals, clearly indicating a robust therapeutic effect in the preclinical model [55,56]. Overall, superoxide production reached 70% of normal with low vector copy numbers per cell (<2), a finding that argues for copy number dependent expression and minimal cytotoxic effects. These levels of superoxide production are similar to what has been reported for lenti-based vectors [57].

FV vectors have also been used for the genetic correction of the Wiskott-Aldrich syndrome (WAS) mouse model [58]. WAS is an X-linked disorder characterized by eczema, immunodeficiency, and micro-thrombocytopenia resulting in bleeding tendency [59]. Uchiyama et al., used a WAS cDNA under the control of two different promoters (an endogenous and an A2UOCE-derived 631 bp fragment) and demonstrated the correction of the WAS phenotypic disorders. T-cell receptor-mediated responses, B-cell migration, platelet adhesion, and podosome formation in dendritic cells (DCs) were restored at levels that can translate into a therapeutic effect. In addition, they showed improvement in gene transfer rates with repeated transduction cycles and confirmed earlier integration site analyses. The IS distribution showed FV vectors landing within transcriptional units at a frequency of 22%–44%, versus 46%–72% for a similar WAS protein-expressing Lenti vector and a low tendency for integration near oncogenes (<5%). As the authors state, the combination of complete phenotypic restoration with low copy numbers (<2) and a relatively safe IS profile, make the WAS protein-expressing FV vectors attractive for clinical applications.

One of the first attempts of gene therapy in humans targeted the SCID-X1 disorder with retroviral vectors. The attempt was considered a success [8] but it was also an alarm on the side effects that should be addressed before the wide application of gene therapy [10]. The disease was targeted with an FV vector to test whether FVs could be an alternative vector system and to test whether the integration sites in T cells were relatively "safer" when FVs were used to transfer the γc gene [60]. In the ED40515 (γc-) T cell line, the FV vector integration sites were located in close proximity to the transcriptional start sites in 13% of integration events relative to 25% with the retroviral vectors. In addition, in the 100 IS analyzed, there were none located within oncogenes, as opposed to three, present in the retrovirally-transduced cells. Finally, animals transplanted with FV-corrected HSC cells, recovered their T and B cell counts and their serum levels of IgM, IgG, and IgA.

A relative problem with HSC gene transfer applications, specifically where in vivo selective advantage of transduced cells does not apply, has been the low gene transfer rates. A potential solution to this problem could be the use of pharmacologic agents that could selectively eliminate non-transduced cells. In an attempt to test whether resting HSC can be transduced and selected in vivo, investigators used the MGMT(P140K) DNA repair protein in an FV backbone. Transplanted mice were treated at 4 weeks post Bone Marrow Transplantation (BMT), with sub-myeloablative conditioning with O6-BG (O-6-Benzylguanine) and BCNU(bis-chloroethylnitrosourea) at different doses and analyzed 6 months later, the mock-transduced animals had undetectable levels of MGMT expression as compared to 55% of positive animals in the FV transduced group [61]. These results confirm the potential of FV vectors to transduce relatively resting HSC cells at low Multiplicity Of Infection (MOIs) and to selectively enhance their presence in the peripheral blood with pharmacologic manipulations. This approach was also used in the design of FV vectors that could block HIV replication. A cassette, that carried three anti-HIV targets in the form of short hairpins (*tat/rev* at site I and site II and to human CCR5), was able to confer 4 log reductions in HIV replication assays [49]. FV vectors are particularly useful for anti-HIV gene therapy, since using Lenti-based vectors for RNAi delivery could be problematic since the anti-HIV sequences can jeopardize the vector packaging process [62]. Beyond therapeutic gene transfer targeting single gene disorders, FV vectors designed to deliver shRNA through PolIII promoters after HSC transfer and transplantation provided a significant long-term downregulation of target genes [63].

Overall, the potential of FV vectors to correct the genetic defect in monogenic disorders amenable to HSC gene addition has been well established in various disease settings. In addition, FV vectors perform as good as their LV counterpart and have not been linked to any adverse effects.

5. Large Animal Preclinical Models

Large animal models offer the potential to simulate conditions that are much closer to the clinical setting as compared to the murine preclinical models. FV vectors have been used to treat two such conditions, the leukocyte adhesion deficiency (LAD) and the pyruvate kinase deficiency (PKD).

LAD is a stem cells disorder that affects white blood cell migration in response to chemotactic signals and as a result, affects immune responses. Patients suffer from bacterial and fungal infections that most commonly occur on the skin and mucous membranes. The defects affect the leukocyte integrin ITGB2 gene (CD18) that prevents the expression of the CD11/CD18 adhesion complex on the cell surface [64]. The canine form of the disease (CLAD) recapitulates the severe deficiency phenotype of LAD-1 in children [65].

Canine HSCs were transduced with an FV vector expressing normal CD18 cDNA and were transplanted to affected dogs [66]. After a year, the dogs had their WBC counts restored to normal and survived without antibiotics, both signs of a functional cure of their disease. The observed long-term (24 months) lymphocyte marking rates of 5–10% are compatible with normal life expectancy. This result was achieved with a single overnight exposure to the vector and a nonmyeloablative conditioning regimen. Furthermore, the copy number per cell was low and in the order of 0.83-1.25 provirus copies per diploid cell.

In the canine setting, FV vectors have also been used to treat a Basenji pyruvate kinase deficient dog model. Pyruvate kinase deficiency causes severe hemolytic anemia, which is potentially lethal [67]. Since PKD does not provide survival advantage to the successfully transduced cells, the vector was enhanced by co-expressing the mutant MGMTP140K that provides resistance to O6-benzylguanine and BCNU, potent inhibitors of the wt MGMTP protein that is expressed in all normal tissues. At 100 days post HSC transplantation with transduced cells, the gene marking rates were 3.5% for granulocytes and 0.4% for lymphocytes. After three rounds of treatment with O6BG and BCNU, gene marking raised to 33% in granulocytes and 5.5% in lymphocytes [68]. This also translated to the correction of the phenotypic disorder, as evidenced by the normalization of LDH (an indicator of hemolysis) and the achievement of transfusion independence.

Finally, it has to be mentioned that FV vectors are resistant to lysis by human serum, a property that has sparked interest for direct in vivo delivery of the vectors, avoiding all ex vivo manipulations of HSCs. This has been tried with the X-SCID canine model [69]. A total of five newborn SCID-X1 dogs received i.v. infusions of FV vector preparations with doses ranging from 4.0-8.4 x10^8 particles. The functional outcomes showed marginal immune reconstitution. The dogs did not survive past one year and succumbed to infections. In regard to off target viral integrations, two such sites were recorded: one in the gut, another (potential) at the virus infusion site and none in the germ cells. An improved protocol was later implemented from the same group that included stem cell mobilization with G-CSF/AMD3100 prior to FV vector delivery and the substitution of the EF1a promoter with that of the *pgk* gene in the FV vector [59]. The data argue for the faster recovery of T cell numbers and a broad TcR repertoire, and are clinically relevant when considering the overall survival that climbed to 2.5 years as compared to 330 days in the previous study. On the issue of safety, a major concern when a vector with broad cell tropism is tested, two conclusions emerged from this study: (i) the vast majority of integration sites were shared between tissues and blood indicating blood contamination and (ii) the gonads had the smallest number of integration events (37 and 56 for ovaries and testes, respectively, as compared to 766 and 469 in blood) with none of them being unique except for one integration site in the ovaries that may have been derived from non-germ cells.

6. Conclusions

Foamy virus vectors have been extensively tested in marking and in gene therapy studies with small and big preclinical animal models. The gene therapy trials featured in this review are summarized in Table 2. Their non-pathogenic nature is an attractive feature for clinical applications. This is further supported by all the positive outcomes that the gene therapy community has communicated from two decades of testing.It is therefore strange that these vectors have not found their way into the clinic. It seems from the relative literature that most manufacturing issues have been overcome and what is missing is the interest of pharmaceutical companies to develop it as a product. In the meantime, the gene therapy world has been dominated by LV vectors that are offered as pharmaceutical products often at extraordinary prices [70]. FVs with the relative ease of production, concentration, and purification could become a poor man's Ferrari for nations and insurance systems that cannot afford million-dollar price tags for a relatively simple and one-off treatment.

Table 2. Gene therapy trials with FV-derived vectors.

Disease	Animal Model	FV Vector Systems	Promoter	Transgene	Target Cells	Method of Application	Outcome	Reference
β-thalassemia	β-Thal3 mice	3rd 3rd	Hu-α-globin HS40-short hu-β-globin Hu-β-globin HS2-HS3 LCR-short hu-β-globin	hu-β-globin	Lin- BM HSCs	Ex vivo	Conversion to thalassemia carrier phenotype	[53]
Chronic Granulomatus Disease (CGD)	B6.129S-Cybb^{tm1Din}/J mice	3rd 3rd	PGK MSCV-LTR	c-o hu-gp91phox c-o hu-gp91phox IRES.EGFP	Lin-BM HSCs	Ex vivo	Complete phenotypic restoration	[55]
Wiskott-Aldrich Syndrome (WAS)	WAS KO mice	3rd 3rd	Native promoter UCO631	hu-was	Lin- BM HSCs	Ex vivo	Complete phenotypic restoration	[58]
SCID-X1	NOD/SCID γc KO mice	3rd	UCO631	Human γc gene (IL2RG)	Lin- BM HSCs	Ex vivo	Reconstitution of T and B cells. No NK correction	[60]
SCID-X1	SCID-X1 dogs	3rd	EF1a (intronless)	GFP.T2A.hIL2RG	i.v. infusion	In vivo	Partial lymphocyte reconstitution	[69]
					i.v. infusion in HSC mobilized animals		Lymphocyte reconstitution. Successful treatment	[59]
SCID-X1	SCID-X1 dogs	3rd	PGK	GFP.T2A.hIL2RG	i.v. infusion in mobilized HSC	In vivo	Lymphocyte reconstitution. Phenotypic correction	
Leukocyte adhesion deficiency	CLAD dogs	3rd	MSCV	hu-CD18	BM derived CD34+ cells	Ex vivo	Phenotypic correction	[66]
Pyruvate Kinase deficiency	Basenji Dog PKD	3rd	PGK	SFFVMGMT.T2AEGFP.PGK.cPK	Mobilized CD34+ HSCs	Ex vivo	Phenotypic correction	[67]

Author Contributions: G.V. set the conceptual frame for the manuscript; E.S. authored the manuscript; I.T. was instrumental in assigning the references. All authors have read and agreed to the published version of the manuscript.

Funding: There are no financial resources to be declared.

Acknowledgments: The authors would like to thank Christian Yanes for English text editing.

Conflicts of Interest: The authors declare no conflict of interest.

References

1. Seita, J.; Weissman, I.L. Hematopoietic stem cell: Self-renewal versus differentiation. *Wiley Interdiscip. Rev. Syst. Biol. Med.* **2010**, *2*, 640–653. [CrossRef] [PubMed]
2. Lucas, D. The Bone Marrow Microenvironment for Hematopoietic Stem Cells. *Adv. Exp. Med. Biol.* **2017**, *1041*, 5–18. [PubMed]
3. Heimfeld, S. Bone marrow transplantation: How important is CD34 cell dose in HLA-identical stem cell transplantation? *Leukemia* **2003**, *17*, 856–858. [CrossRef] [PubMed]
4. Lucarelli, G.; Isgro, A.; Sodani, P.; Gaziev, J. Hematopoietic stem cell transplantation in thalassemia and sickle cell anemia. *Cold Spring Harb. Perspect. Med.* **2012**, *2*, a011825. [CrossRef] [PubMed]
5. Dunbar, C.E.; High, K.A.; Joung, J.K.; Kohn, D.B.; Ozawa, K.; Sadelain, M. Gene therapy comes of age. *Science* **2018**, *359*, eaan4672. [CrossRef]
6. Papapetrou, E.P.; Ziros, P.G.; Micheva, I.D.; Zoumbos, N.C.; Athanassiadou, A. Gene transfer into human hematopoietic progenitor cells with an episomal vector carrying an S/MAR element. *Gene Ther.* **2006**, *13*, 40–51. [CrossRef]
7. Khan, A.S.; Bodem, J.; Buseyne, F.; Gessain, A.; Johnson, W.; Kuhn, J.H.; Kuzmak, J.; Lindemann, D.; Linial, M.L.; Lochelt, M.; et al. Corrigendum to "Spumaretroviruses: Updated taxonomy and nomenclature" [Virology 516 (2018) 158-164]. *Virology* **2019**, 528. [CrossRef]
8. Cavazzana-Calvo, M.; Hacein-Bey, S.; de Saint Basile, G.; Gross, F.; Yvon, E.; Nusbaum, P.; Selz, F.; Hue, C.; Certain, S.; Casanova, J.L.; et al. Gene therapy of human severe combined immunodeficiency (SCID)-X1 disease. *Science* **2000**, *288*, 669–672. [CrossRef]
9. Aiuti, A.; Cattaneo, F.; Galimberti, S.; Benninghoff, U.; Cassani, B.; Callegaro, L.; Scaramuzza, S.; Andolfi, G.; Mirolo, M.; Brigida, I.; et al. Gene therapy for immunodeficiency due to adenosine deaminase deficiency. *N. Engl. J. Med.* **2009**, *360*, 447–458. [CrossRef]
10. Hacein-Bey-Abina, S.; Garrigue, A.; Wang, G.P.; Soulier, J.; Lim, A.; Morillon, E.; Clappier, E.; Caccavelli, L.; Delabesse, E.; Beldjord, K.; et al. Insertional oncogenesis in 4 patients after retrovirus-mediated gene therapy of SCID-X1. *J. Clin. Investig.* **2008**, *118*, 3132–3142. [CrossRef]
11. Lesbats, P.; Engelman, A.N.; Cherepanov, P. Retroviral DNA Integration. *Chem. Rev.* **2016**, *116*, 12730–12757. [CrossRef] [PubMed]
12. Cattoglio, C.; Facchini, G.; Sartori, D.; Antonelli, A.; Miccio, A.; Cassani, B.; Schmidt, M.; von Kalle, C.; Howe, S.; Thrasher, A.J.; et al. Hot spots of retroviral integration in human CD34+ hematopoietic cells. *Blood* **2007**, *110*, 1770–1778. [CrossRef]
13. Trobridge, G.D.; Miller, D.G.; Jacobs, M.A.; Allen, J.M.; Kiem, H.P.; Kaul, R.; Russell, D.W. Foamy virus vector integration sites in normal human cells. *Proc. Natl. Acad. Sci. USA* **2006**, *103*, 1498–1503. [CrossRef] [PubMed]
14. Nowrouzi, A.; Dittrich, M.; Klanke, C.; Heinkelein, M.; Rammling, M.; Dandekar, T.; von Kalle, C.; Rethwilm, A. Genome-wide mapping of foamy virus vector integrations into a human cell line. *J. Gen. Virol.* **2006**, *87 Pt 5*, 1339–1347. [CrossRef]
15. Lesbats, P.; Serrao, E.; Maskell, D.P.; Pye, V.E.; O'Reilly, N.; Lindemann, D.; Engelman, A.N.; Cherepanov, P. Structural basis for spumavirus GAG tethering to chromatin. *Proc. Natl. Acad. Sci. USA* **2017**, *114*, 5509–5514. [CrossRef] [PubMed]
16. Challita, P.M.; Kohn, D.B. Lack of expression from a retroviral vector after transduction of murine hematopoietic stem cells is associated with methylation in vivo. *Proc. Natl. Acad. Sci. USA* **1994**, *91*, 2567–2571. [CrossRef] [PubMed]
17. Ellis, J. Silencing and variegation of gammaretrovirus and lentivirus vectors. *Hum. Gene Ther.* **2005**, *16*, 1241–1246. [CrossRef] [PubMed]

18. Li, C.L.; Emery, D.W. The cHS4 chromatin insulator reduces gammaretroviral vector silencing by epigenetic modifications of integrated provirus. *Gene Ther.* **2008**, *15*, 49–53. [CrossRef] [PubMed]
19. McInerney, J.M.; Nawrocki, J.R.; Lowrey, C.H. Long-term silencing of retroviral vectors is resistant to reversal by trichostatin A and 5-azacytidine. *Gene Ther.* **2000**, *7*, 653–663. [CrossRef] [PubMed]
20. Miyoshi, H.; Smith, K.A.; Mosier, D.E.; Verma, I.M.; Torbett, B.E. Transduction of human CD34+ cells that mediate long-term engraftment of NOD/SCID mice by HIV vectors. *Science* **1999**, *283*, 682–686. [CrossRef]
21. Vassilopoulos, G.; Trobridge, G.; Josephson, N.C.; Russell, D.W. Gene transfer into murine hematopoietic stem cells with helper-free foamy virus vectors. *Blood* **2001**, *98*, 604–609. [CrossRef] [PubMed]
22. Lindemann, D.; Rethwilm, A. Foamy virus biology and its application for vector development. *Viruses* **2011**, *3*, 561–585. [CrossRef] [PubMed]
23. Vassilopoulos, G.; Rethwilm, A. The usefulness of a perfect parasite. *Gene Ther.* **2008**, *15*, 1299–1301. [CrossRef] [PubMed]
24. Liu, W.; Lei, J.; Liu, Y.; Lukic, D.S.; Rathe, A.M.; Bao, Q.; Kehl, T.; Bleiholder, A.; Hechler, T.; Lochelt, M. Feline foamy virus-based vectors: Advantages of an authentic animal model. *Viruses* **2013**, *5*, 1702–1718. [CrossRef] [PubMed]
25. Ledesma-Feliciano, C.; Hagen, S.; Troyer, R.; Zheng, X.; Musselman, E.; Slavkovic Lukic, D.; Franke, A.M.; Maeda, D.; Zielonka, J.; Munk, C.; et al. Replacement of feline foamy virus bet by feline immunodeficiency virus vif yields replicative virus with novel vaccine candidate potential. *Retrovirology* **2018**, *15*, 38. [CrossRef] [PubMed]
26. Lamsfus-Calle, A.; Daniel-Moreno, A.; Urena-Bailen, G.; Raju, J.; Antony, J.S.; Handgretinger, R.; Mezger, M. Hematopoietic stem cell gene therapy: The optimal use of lentivirus and gene editing approaches. *Blood Rev.* **2019**, 100641. [CrossRef] [PubMed]
27. Maetzig, T.; Galla, M.; Baum, C.; Schambach, A. Gammaretroviral vectors: Biology, technology and application. *Viruses* **2011**, *3*, 677–713. [CrossRef]
28. Trobridge, G.D. Foamy virus vectors for gene transfer. *Expert Opin. Biol. Ther.* **2009**, *9*, 1427–1436. [CrossRef]
29. Miyoshi, H.; Blomer, U.; Takahashi, M.; Gage, F.H.; Verma, I.M. Development of a self-inactivating lentivirus vector. *J. Virol.* **1998**, *72*, 8150–8157. [CrossRef]
30. Thornhill, S.I.; Schambach, A.; Howe, S.J.; Ulaganathan, M.; Grassman, E.; Williams, D.; Schiedlmeier, B.; Sebire, N.J.; Gaspar, H.B.; Kinnon, C.; et al. Self-inactivating gammaretroviral vectors for gene therapy of X-linked severe combined immunodeficiency. *Mol. Ther.* **2008**, *16*, 590–598. [CrossRef]
31. Goodman, M.A.; Arumugam, P.; Pillis, D.M.; Loberg, A.; Nasimuzzaman, M.; Lynn, D.; van der Loo, J.C.M.; Dexheimer, P.J.; Keddache, M.; Bauer, T.R., Jr.; et al. Foamy Virus Vector Carries a Strong Insulator in Its Long Terminal Repeat Which Reduces Its Genotoxic Potential. *J. Virol.* **2018**, *92*, e01639-17. [CrossRef] [PubMed]
32. Roth, S.L.; Malani, N.; Bushman, F.D. Gammaretroviral integration into nucleosomal target DNA in vivo. *J. Virol.* **2011**, *85*, 7393–7401. [CrossRef] [PubMed]
33. Russell, D.W.; Miller, A.D. Foamy virus vectors. *J. Virol.* **1996**, *70*, 217–222. [CrossRef]
34. Hirata, R.K.; Miller, A.D.; Andrews, R.G.; Russell, D.W. Transduction of hematopoietic cells by foamy virus vectors. *Blood* **1996**, *88*, 3654–3661. [CrossRef] [PubMed]
35. Plochmann, K.; Horn, A.; Gschmack, E.; Armbruster, N.; Krieg, J.; Wiktorowicz, T.; Weber, C.; Stirnnagel, K.; Lindemann, D.; Rethwilm, A.; et al. Heparan sulfate is an attachment factor for foamy virus entry. *J. Virol.* **2012**, *86*, 10028–10035. [CrossRef] [PubMed]
36. Nasimuzzaman, M.; Persons, D.A. Cell Membrane-associated heparan sulfate is a receptor for prototype foamy virus in human, monkey, and rodent cells. *Mol. Ther.* **2012**, *20*, 1158–1166. [CrossRef] [PubMed]
37. Josephson, N.C.; Vassilopoulos, G.; Trobridge, G.D.; Priestley, G.V.; Wood, B.L.; Papayannopoulou, T.; Russell, D.W. Transduction of human NOD/SCID-repopulating cells with both lymphoid and myeloid potential by foamy virus vectors. *Proc. Natl. Acad. Sci. USA* **2002**, *99*, 8295–8300. [CrossRef]
38. Trobridge, G.; Russell, D.W. Cell cycle requirements for transduction by foamy virus vectors compared to those of oncovirus and lentivirus vectors. *J. Virol.* **2004**, *78*, 2327–2335. [CrossRef]
39. Lehmann-Che, J.; Renault, N.; Giron, M.L.; Roingeard, P.; Clave, E.; Tobaly-Tapiero, J.; Bittoun, P.; Toubert, A.; de The, H.; Saib, A. Centrosomal latency of incoming foamy viruses in resting cells. *PLoS Pathog.* **2007**, *3*, e74. [CrossRef]
40. Hendrie, P.C.; Huo, Y.; Stolitenko, R.B.; Russell, D.W. A rapid and quantitative assay for measuring neighboring gene activation by vector proviruses. *Mol. Ther.* **2008**, *16*, 534–540. [CrossRef]

41. Ong, C.T.; Corces, V.G. CTCF: An architectural protein bridging genome topology and function. *Nat. Rev. Genet.* **2014**, *15*, 234–246. [CrossRef]
42. Heneine, W.; Switzer, W.M.; Sandstrom, P.; Brown, J.; Vedapuri, S.; Schable, C.A.; Khan, A.S.; Lerche, N.W.; Schweizer, M.; Neumann-Haefelin, D.; et al. Identification of a human population infected with simian foamy viruses. *Nat. Med.* **1998**, *4*, 403–407. [CrossRef] [PubMed]
43. Switzer, W.M.; Bhullar, V.; Shanmugam, V.; Cong, M.E.; Parekh, B.; Lerche, N.W.; Yee, J.L.; Ely, J.J.; Boneva, R.; Chapman, L.E.; et al. Frequent simian foamy virus infection in persons occupationally exposed to nonhuman primates. *J. Virol.* **2004**, *78*, 2780–2789. [CrossRef] [PubMed]
44. Trobridge, G.; Josephson, N.; Vassilopoulos, G.; Mac, J.; Russell, D.W. Improved foamy virus vectors with minimal viral sequences. *Mol. Ther.* **2002**, *6*, 321–328. [CrossRef]
45. Nasimuzzaman, M.; Kim, Y.S.; Wang, Y.D.; Persons, D.A. High-titer foamy virus vector transduction and integration sites of human CD34+ cell-derived SCID-repopulating cells. *Mol. Ther. Methods Clin. Dev.* **2014**, *1*, 14020. [CrossRef]
46. Bock, M.; Heinkelein, M.; Lindemann, D.; Rethwilm, A. Cells expressing the human foamy virus (HFV) accessory Bet protein are resistant to productive HFV superinfection. *Virology* **1998**, *250*, 194–204. [CrossRef]
47. Heinkelein, M.; Dressler, M.; Jarmy, G.; Rammling, M.; Imrich, H.; Thurow, J.; Lindemann, D.; Rethwilm, A. Improved primate foamy virus vectors and packaging constructs. *J. Virol.* **2002**, *76*, 3774–3783. [CrossRef]
48. Lochelt, M.; Zentgraf, H.; Flugel, R.M. Construction of an infectious DNA clone of the full-length human spumaretrovirus genome and mutagenesis of the bel 1 gene. *Virology* **1991**, *184*, 43–54. [CrossRef]
49. Kiem, H.P.; Wu, R.A.; Sun, G.; von Laer, D.; Rossi, J.J.; Trobridge, G.D. Foamy combinatorial anti-HIV vectors with MGMTP140K potently inhibit HIV-1 and SHIV replication and mediate selection in vivo. *Gene Ther.* **2010**, *17*, 37–49. [CrossRef]
50. Nasimuzzaman, M.; Lynn, D.; Ernst, R.; Beuerlein, M.; Smith, R.H.; Shrestha, A.; Cross, S.; Link, K.; Lutzko, C.; Nordling, D.; et al. Production and purification of high-titer foamy virus vector for the treatment of leukocyte adhesion deficiency. *Mol. Ther. Methods Clin. Dev.* **2016**, *3*, 16004. [CrossRef]
51. Spannaus, R.; Miller, C.; Lindemann, D.; Bodem, J. Purification of foamy viral particles. *Virology* **2017**, *506*, 28–33. [CrossRef]
52. Leurs, C.; Jansen, M.; Pollok, K.E.; Heinkelein, M.; Schmidt, M.; Wissler, M.; Lindemann, D.; Von Kalle, C.; Rethwilm, A.; Williams, D.A.; et al. Comparison of three retroviral vector systems for transduction of nonobese diabetic/severe combined immunodeficiency mice repopulating human CD34+ cord blood cells. *Hum. Gene Ther.* **2003**, *14*, 509–519. [CrossRef]
53. Morianos, I.; Siapati, E.K.; Pongas, G.; Vassilopoulos, G. Comparative analysis of FV vectors with human alpha- or beta-globin gene regulatory elements for the correction of beta-thalassemia. *Gene Ther.* **2012**, *19*, 303–311. [CrossRef]
54. Kang, E.M.; Malech, H.L. Gene therapy for chronic granulomatous disease. *Methods Enzymol.* **2012**, *507*, 125–154.
55. Chatziandreou, I.; Siapati, E.K.; Vassilopoulos, G. Genetic correction of X-linked chronic granulomatous disease with novel foamy virus vectors. *Exp. Hematol.* **2011**, *39*, 643–652. [CrossRef]
56. Marciano, B.E.; Zerbe, C.S.; Falcone, E.L.; Ding, L.; DeRavin, S.S.; Daub, J.; Kreuzburg, S.; Yockey, L.; Hunsberger, S.; Foruraghi, L.; et al. X-linked carriers of chronic granulomatous disease: Illness, lyonization, and stability. *J. Allergy Clin. Immunol.* **2018**, *141*, 365–371. [CrossRef]
57. Chiriaco, M.; Farinelli, G.; Capo, V.; Zonari, E.; Scaramuzza, S.; Di Matteo, G.; Sergi, L.S.; Migliavacca, M.; Hernandez, R.J.; Bombelli, F.; et al. Dual-regulated lentiviral vector for gene therapy of X-linked chronic granulomatosis. *Mol. Ther.* **2014**, *22*, 1472–1483. [CrossRef]
58. Uchiyama, T.; Adriani, M.; Jagadeesh, G.J.; Paine, A.; Candotti, F. Foamy virus vector-mediated gene correction of a mouse model of Wiskott-Aldrich syndrome. *Mol. Ther.* **2012**, *20*, 1270–1279. [CrossRef]
59. Humbert, O.; Chan, F.; Rajawat, Y.S.; Torgerson, T.R.; Burtner, C.R.; Hubbard, N.W.; Humphrys, D.; Norgaard, Z.K.; O'Donnell, P.; Adair, J.E.; et al. Rapid immune reconstitution of SCID-X1 canines after G-CSF/AMD3100 mobilization and in vivo gene therapy. *Blood Adv.* **2018**, *2*, 987–999. [CrossRef]
60. Horino, S.; Uchiyama, T.; So, T.; Nagashima, H.; Sun, S.L.; Sato, M.; Asao, A.; Haji, Y.; Sasahara, Y.; Candotti, F.; et al. Gene therapy model of X-linked severe combined immunodeficiency using a modified foamy virus vector. *PLoS ONE* **2013**, *8*, e71594. [CrossRef]

61. Cai, S.; Ernstberger, A.; Wang, H.; Bailey, B.J.; Hartwell, J.R.; Sinn, A.L.; Eckermann, O.; Linka, Y.; Goebel, W.S.; Hanenberg, H.; et al. In vivo selection of hematopoietic stem cells transduced at a low multiplicity-of-infection with a foamy viral MGMT (P140K) vector. *Exp. Hematol.* **2008**, *36*, 283–292. [CrossRef] [PubMed]
62. Olszko, M.E.; Trobridge, G.D. Foamy virus vectors for HIV gene therapy. *Viruses* **2013**, *5*, 2585–2600. [CrossRef] [PubMed]
63. Papadaki, M.; Siapati, E.K.; Vassilopoulos, G. A foamy virus vector system for stable and efficient RNAi expression in mammalian cells. *Hum. Gene Ther.* **2011**, *22*, 1293–1303. [CrossRef]
64. Leukocyte Adhesion Deficiency Type 1. Available online: https://ghr.nlm.nih.gov/condition/leukocyte-adhesion-deficiency-type-1 (accessed on 3 March 2020).
65. Kijas, J.M.; Bauer, T.R., Jr.; Gafvert, S.; Marklund, S.; Trowald-Wigh, G.; Johannisson, A.; Hedhammar, A.; Binns, M.; Juneja, R.K.; Hickstein, D.D.; et al. A missense mutation in the beta-2 integrin gene (ITGB2) causes canine leukocyte adhesion deficiency. *Genomics* **1999**, *61*, 101–107. [CrossRef]
66. Bauer, T.R., Jr.; Allen, J.M.; Hai, M.; Tuschong, L.M.; Khan, I.F.; Olson, E.M.; Adler, R.L.; Burkholder, T.H.; Gu, Y.C.; Russell, D.W.; et al. Successful treatment of canine leukocyte adhesion deficiency by foamy virus vectors. *Nat. Med.* **2008**, *14*, 93–97. [CrossRef]
67. Takegawa, S.; Fujii, H.; Miwa, S. Change of pyruvate kinase isozymes from M2- to L-type during development of the red cell. *Br. J. Haematol.* **1983**, *54*, 467–474. [CrossRef]
68. Trobridge, G.D.; Beard, B.C.; Wu, R.A.; Ironside, C.; Malik, P.; Kiem, H.P. Stem cell selection in vivo using foamy vectors cures canine pyruvate kinase deficiency. *PLoS ONE* **2012**, *7*, e45173. [CrossRef]
69. Burtner, C.R.; Beard, B.C.; Kennedy, D.R.; Wohlfahrt, M.E.; Adair, J.E.; Trobridge, G.D.; Scharenberg, A.M.; Torgerson, T.R.; Rawlings, D.J.; Felsburg, P.J.; et al. Intravenous injection of a foamy virus vector to correct canine SCID-X1. *Blood* **2014**, *123*, 3578–3584. [CrossRef]
70. Macaulay, R. How CAR-T Cell and Gene Therapies Are Redefining the Traditional Pharmaceutical Pricing and Reimbursement Model. Available online: https://www.parexel.com/news-events-resources/blog/how-car-t-cell-and-gene-therapies-are-redefining-traditional-pharmaceutical-pricing-and-reimbursement-model (accessed on 16 March 2020).

MDPI
St. Alban-Anlage 66
4052 Basel
Switzerland
Tel. +41 61 683 77 34
Fax +41 61 302 89 18
www.mdpi.com

Viruses Editorial Office
E-mail: viruses@mdpi.com
www.mdpi.com/journal/viruses

www.ingramcontent.com/pod-product-compliance
Lightning Source LLC
LaVergne TN
LVHW070228100526
838202LV00015B/2104